Quick Reference Guide to Medicine and Surgery

CRASH COURSE

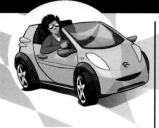

SERIES EDITOR:

Dan Horton-Szar
BSc(Hons) MBBS(Hons) MRCGP
Northgate Medical Practice
Canterbury
Kent, UK

FACULTY ADVISORS:

John Rees
MD, FRCP, FKC
Professor of Medical Education
King's College London School
   of Medicine
London, UK

Adrian Wagg
MBBS FRCP (Lond) FRCP (Edin) FHEA
Professor of Healthy Ageing
University of Alberta, Canada

Quick Reference Guide to Medicine and Surgery

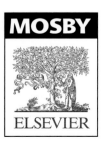

MOSBY

ELSEVIER

Leonora Weil
MBBS, MA (Cantab), MSc, DFPH,
Public Health Registrar
London, UK

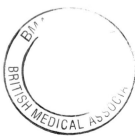

Edinburgh London NewYork   Oxford Philadelphia StLouis Sydney Toronto 2014

MOSBY
ELSEVIER

Commissioning Editor: Jeremy Bowes
Development Editor: Fiona Conn
Project Manager: Andrew Riley
Designer: Stewart Larking
Icon Illustrations: Geo Parkin
Illustration Manager: Jennifer Rose
Illustrator: Antbits Ltd.

First edition 2014

ISBN: 978-0-7234-3553-2

British Library Cataloguing in Publication Data
A catalogue record for this book is available from the British Library

Library of Congress Cataloging in Publication Data
A catalog record for this book is available from the Library of Congress

Notices
Knowledge and best practice in this field are constantly changing. As new research and experience broaden our understanding, changes in research methods, professional practices, or medical treatment may become necessary.

Practitioners and researchers must always rely on their own experience and knowledge in evaluating and using any information, methods, compounds, or experiments described herein. In using such information or methods they should be mindful of their own safety and the safety of others, including parties for whom they have a professional responsibility.

With respect to any drug or pharmaceutical products identified, readers are advised to check the most current information provided (i) on procedures featured or (ii) by the manufacturer of each product to be administered, to verify the recommended dose or formula, the method and duration of administration, and contraindications. It is the responsibility of practitioners, relying on their own experience and knowledge of their patients, to make diagnoses, to determine dosages and the best treatment for each individual patient, and to take all appropriate safety precautions.

To the fullest extent of the law, neither the Publisher nor the authors, contributors, or editors, assume any liability for any injury and/or damage to persons or property as a matter of products liability, negligence or otherwise, or from any use or operation of any methods, products, instructions, or ideas contained in the material herein.

ELSEVIER your source for books, journals and multimedia in the health sciences
www.elsevierhealth.com

  Working together to grow libraries in developing countries

www.elsevier.com • www.bookaid.org

The Publisher's policy is to use **paper manufactured from sustainable forests**

Printed in China

Contents

Series editor foreword

We are delighted to present this brand new addition to the Crash Course series. The Quick Reference Guide is different: designed as a companion book to the other titles, it collates the key learning points from the medical curriculum and presents them in one compact volume. It's perfect for keeping in your bag to make the most of those quick opportunities for revision while travelling, or on the wards.

The Crash Course series first published in 1997 and now, 17 years on, we are still going strong. Medicine never stands still, and the work of keeping this series relevant for today's students is an ongoing process. The latest books in the series, including this brand new title, build on the success of the previous titles and incorporate new and revised material, to keep the series up to date with current guidelines for best practice, and recent developments in medical research and pharmacology.

For this new title, we hold fast to the principles upon which we first developed the series. Crash Course will always bring you the information you need to revise in compact, manageable volumes that integrate basic medical science and clinical practice. The books still maintain the balance between clarity and conciseness, and provide sufficient depth for those aiming at distinction. The authors are medical students and junior doctors who have recent experience of the exams you are now facing, and the accuracy of the material is checked by a team of faculty advisors from across the UK.

Dr Dan Horton-Szar

Series Editor

Author preface

The main purpose of the book is to provide a clear, core text for medical students that includes everything that you need to understand and pass the final medical and surgical examinations. It can be used at each stage of your early medical career: from learning about a new disease, as a quick reference on the wards, for the MBBS examinations and even in your first years as a junior doctor.

Each chapter is co-written by experts, specialists in their field to ensure that the information is up to date and clearly presented. The chapters are prefaced with an 'overview section' that includes the key information that you should recall for each system so that you do not need to keep referring back to other books and includes key investigations applicable for each specialty. We have also included a chapter on the acutely unwell patient to prepare you to deal with emergency situations with confidence.

Within the chapters, each disease is presented in a consistent format to help you find what you need quickly and easily; each includes:

- A clear outline to ensure that you really understand what the disease is about and to help you remember the key points.
- Key pathology and physiology to aid understanding and provide the background knowledge needed for examinations.
- A section that includes associations and 'the typical patient' (a format that repeatedly comes up in examinations).
- Key symptoms, signs, tests, prognoses and complications deliberately not exhaustive and focused on the most commonly occurring for easy recall.
- Management, consistently divided into conservative, medical and surgical categories and clearly presented so that they are as useful for junior doctors as for those learning the theory for each disease. This section includes the main guidelines and what to do in an emergency situation so that everything can be found in one location.
- Mnemonics, memory aids and figures to help with revision.

This book was written with the medical student constantly in mind. We hope you find this book useful and we wish you the best of luck for your future medical career.

Leonora Weil
Adrian Wagg
John Rees

Acknowledgements

There are many people to thank for all their hard work, patience and support in pulling this book together. Firstly a big thank you to all the expert faculty contributors who co-wrote each chapter; Jonathan Behar, Anita Jayadev, Nasser Khan, Daniel Abeles, Rimona Weil, Laurie Sharman, Sarah Barsam, Anisur Rahman, Philip Gothard, Nicolas Alexander and Gideon Lipman. Each of you brought a high level of specialist knowledge and originality to each chapter and ensured that what was written was not only accurate but clear and understandable. Thank you for your patience and enthusiasm in rewriting, rechecking and reediting at various stages of this project. Thanks also to Dr John Hurst and Dr Malin Roesner for their early work on the respiratory and endocrinology chapters respectively. A big thank you to everyone at Elsevier for all their help and encouragement in taking this book from vision to print: Jeremy Bowes, Alison Taylor, Fiona Conn, Dan Horton Szar and Laurence Hunter. I am so grateful for all your time, patience and support. I am particularly grateful to Andrew Riley for bringing this project together at the final crucial stages. Thanks also to Martin and Ruth Dunitz for persuading me to take my ideas further and showing me how and to Dr Anna Remington (as talented in design as in the lab) for drafting early mock-ups that got the project started. Thanks to Dr Hannah Handstater, Dr Deborah Ragol-Levy and Lisa Stock for their very helpful comments, additions and improvements to the early drafts of this book and to Robin Landy for his technical expertise.

Finally, there are three people without whom this book would not have been possible. A special thanks to both Adrian Wagg and John Rees for their roles as Faculty Advisors in overseeing the project as a whole, providing creative input, co-writing sections and ensuring accuracy, relevance to the curriculum and a high standard of the text. I am particularly grateful to Adrian for your belief in this project from the very beginning and encouragement at every stage. Most of all, many thanks to Gideon Lipman for not just co-writing many chapters, but particularly for editing, rewriting, formatting, correcting and standardising the book as a whole throughout this process.

Thank you all

L.W.

PICTURE CREDITS

We are grateful to the following individuals and organizations for permission to reproduce the figures and tables listed below:

Chapter 1

Fig.1.1 http://www.resus.org.uk/
Fig 1.2 Adamas-Rappaport, W, Brannan, S: Crash Course Surgery Mosby 2005

Chapter 2

Figs 2.1, 2.6, 2.7 and 2.12 Lim EKS et al Medicine and surgery Churchill Livingstone 2007
Figs 2.2, 2.3 and 2.18 Colledge N et al (eds) Davidson's Principles and Practice of Medicine 20th edition Churchill Livingstone 2006
Figs 2.4, 2.5, 2.6 and 2.10 Russ R Crash Course Cardiovascular system Mosby 2006
Fig 2.9 **http://www.resus.org.uk/**
Fig 2.10 Witham, M et al Crash Course: Foundation Doctor's Guide to Medicine and Surgery 2nd edition Mosby 2008
Fig 2.11 Hampton J: ECG made easy 7th edition Churchill Livingstone 2008
Figs 2.13, 2.15, 2.19, 2.22 Baliga R: CC internal medicine Mosby 2006
Fig 2.14 Ferri F: Practical guide to the care of the medical patient 7th edition Mosby 2007
Fig.2.16 **http://www.resus.org.uk/**
Fig 2.24 Baliga R: CC Cardiology 978-0323035644 Mosby 2005
Figs 2.25, 2.26, 2.27, 2.28, 2.29 Fishback J CC pathology Mosby 2005
Fig 2.30 Pang D: Crash Course Paediatrics Mosby 2nd edition
Fig 2.31 NICE clinical guideline 127: Hypertension. Clinical management of primary hypertension in adults © NICE 2011 (http://guidance.nice.org.uk/CG127/QuickRefGuide/pdf/English)

Chapter 3

Fig 3.1 Myers A Crash Course Respiratory system Mosby 2005
Fig 3.2A Swash M, Glynn M: Hutchison's clinical methods 22nd edition Saunders 2007
Fig 3.2B Kumar P, Clark M: Kumar and Clark's Clinical Medicine 6th edition Saunders 2005
Fig 3.3 Ter Meulen D Crash Course Imaging Mosby 2008
Figs 3.4, 3.5, 3.8, 3.12 Corne J et al: Chest Xray made easy 3rd edition Churchill Livingstone 2010
Fig 3.9 Colledge N et al (eds) Davidson's Principles and Practice of Medicine 2nd edition Churchill Livingstone 2006
Fig 3.10 CXR showing a left pleural effusion (arrowed). Dalton H et al: Final MB 4th edition Churchill Livingstone 2005
Figs 3.11, 3.13 Herring W: Learning radiology: recognising the basics 2nd edition Saunders 2011
Fig 3.14 Pretorius and Solomon: Radiology secrets Mosby 2005 2/e
Fig 3.15 Corne J, Pointon, K: 100 Chest Xray problems Churchill Livingstone 2006

Chapter 4

Fig 4.1 Begg J Abdominal Xray made easy Churchill Livingstone 2006
Fig 4.2 McNally P: GI/Liver secrets 3rd edition Mosby 2005
Fig 4.3 Andreoli T et al: Cecil Essentials of medicine 7th edition Saunders 2007

Chapter 5

Fig 5.1 Colledge N et al (eds) Davidson's Principles and Practice of Medicine 20th edition Churchill Livingstone 2006
Fig 5.2 Fishback J Crash Course Pathology Mosby 2005

Figs 5.4, 5.6 Thuluvath P Crash Course Gastroenterology Mosby 2006
Figs 5.5, 5.7. Kumar P, Clark M Kumar and Clark's Clinical Medicine 6th edition Saunders 2005
Fig 5.8 From http://www.mhra.gov.uk/Safetyinformation/DrugSafetyUpdate/CON185624
Fig 5.10 Seidel E Crash Course Gastrointestinal system Mosby 2005
Fig 5.11 Ter Meulen D Crash Course Imaging Mosby 2008

Chapter 6

Fig 6.1 Fitzgerald MJT et al: Clinical neuroanatomy and neuroscience 5th edition Saunders 2006
Fig 6.2 Fishback J Crash Course Pathology Mosby 2005
Fig 6.3, 6.4, 6.5, 6.6, 6.9 Liporace J Crash Course neurology Mosby 2006
Fig 6.7, 6.8 Parker R, Sharma A CC General Medicine 3rd edition Mosby 2008
Fig 6.10 Kumar P, Clark M Kumar and Clark's Clinical Medicine 6th edition Saunders 2005
Fig 6.11 Swash M, Glynn M: Hutchison's clinical methods 22nd edition Saunders 2007
Fig 6.12 Gordon P Crash Course History and examination Mosby 2005

Chapter 7

Fig 7.1 Meszaros J CC Endocrine and reproductive system Mosby 2005
Fig 7.2 Lim EKS et al Medicine and surgery Churchill Livingstone 2007
Fig 7.3 Begg J: Abdominal X ray made easy Churchill Livingstone 2006
Fig 7.4 Brenner B: Brenner and Rector's the kidney 8th edition Saunders 2008
Fig 7.5 Adamas-Rappaport, W, Brannan, S: Crash Course Surgery Mosby 2005

Chapter 8

Fig 8.1 Novak J Crash Course Immunology Mosby 2006
Fig 8.2A, 8.5, 8.7 Ferri F Practical guide to the care of the medical patient 7th edition Mosby 2007
Fig 8.2B Forbes C, Jackson Colour Atlas and Text of Clinical Medicine 3rd edition Mosby 2003
Fig 8.2C, E Kumar P, Clark M Kumar and Clark's Clinical Medicine 6th edition Saunders 2005
Fig 8.2D Colledge N et al (eds) Davidson's Principles and Practice of Medicine 20th edition
   Churchill Livingstone 2006

Chapter 9

Fig 9.1 Meszaros J CC Endocrine and reproductive system Mosby 2005
Fig 9.2, 9.5 Baliga R: CC internal medicine Mosby 2006
Fig 9.3 Stevenson F: Crash Course Renal and Urinary Systems Mosby 2005
Fig 9.6, 9.9 Lim EKS et al Medicine and surgery Churchill Livingstone 2007
Fig 9.7 Neville, B et al Oral and Maxillofacial Pathology 3rd edn Saunders 2009
Fig 9.8 Witham M, Al-Khairalla M: 100 plus diseases for the MRCP Part 2 Churchill Livingstone 2001
Fig 9.10, 9.11 Hall T PACES for the MRCP Churchill Livingstone 2008

Chapter 10

Fig 10.1, 10.3, 10.10 Walji A: Crash Course musculoskeletal system Mosby 2006
Fig 10.4, 10.7.10.9 Ter Meulen D Crash Course Imaging Mosby 2008
Fig 10.5A, 10.11 Colledge N et al (eds) Davidson's Principles and Practice of Medicine 20th edition
   Churchill Livingstone 2006
Fig 10.5B Baliga R: CC internal medicine Mosby 2006
Fig 10.6 Ballinger A: Essentials of Kumar and Clark's clinical medicine 5th edition Saunders 2012
Fig 10.8 Noble J Textbook of primary care medicine 3rd edition Mosby 2001

Chapter 11

Fig 11.1 Kumar P, Clark M: Kumar and Clark's Clinical Medicine 6th edition Saunders 2005

Chapter 13

Fig 13.1 Hall, T PACES for the MRCP: with 250 Clinical Cases, 2e Churchill Livingstone 2008

Fig 13.2 Ferri, F: Ferri's clinical advisor 2009 Mosby 2008

Fig 13.3, 13.17 Ter Meulen D Crash Course Imaging Mosby 2008

Fig 13.4, 13.5, 13.6, 13.7, 13.8, 13.9, 13.20 Adamas-Rappaport, W, Brannan, S: Crash Course Surgery Mosby 2005

Fig 13.10, 13.11 Siedel H et al: Mosby's Guide to Physical Examination 6th edition Mosby 2006

Fig 13.12, 13.18 Fishback J Crash Course Pathology Mosby 2005

Fig 13.13, 13.16 Herring W: Learning radiology Saunders 2011

Fig 13.14, 13.22 Lim EKS et al Medicine and surgery Churchill Livingstone

Fig 13.15 Begg J Abdominal X ray made easy Churchill Livingstone 2006

Fig 13.19 Thuluvath P Crash Course Gastroenterology Mosby 2006

Fig 13.23 Russ R Crash Course Cardiovascular system Mosby 2006

Fig 13.25 Gordon P Crash Course History and examination Mosby 2005

Fig 13.26, 13.28 Colledge N et al (eds) Davidson's Principles and Practice of Medicine 20th edition Churchill Livingstone 2006

Fig 13.27 Ferri F: Practical guide to the care of the medical patient 7th edition Mosby 2007

Fig 13.29 Walji A: Crash Course musculoskeletal system Mosby 2006

Chapter 14

Fig 14.1 Liporace J: Crsh Course Neurology Mosby 2006

Chapter 15

Fig 15.1 Baliga R: Crash Course Cardiology Mosby 2005

Fig 15.2 Seidel E Crash Course Gastrointestinal system Mosby 2005

Fig 15.3 Patel, H: Crash Course Respiratory System 3rd edition Mosby 2008

Fig 15.4 Baliga R: Crash Course Internal Medicine Mosby 2006

Fig 15.5 Bhangu A Flesh and bones surgery Mosby 2007

Fig 15.6 Granger N Crash Course Anatomy Mosby 2006

Fig 15.7 Liporace J: Crash Course neurology Mosby 2006

Dedication

For Mum, Dad, Gideon, Carmelle and Gavriel for your encouragement, patience, love and enthusiasm at every new adventure and challenge.

This book is in memory of Marc Weinberg, a special brother-in-law for whom education always came first. He would have loved this book.

L.W.

(These vary. Please check with your local laboratory)

Haematology	
Haemoglobin	
Male	13.5–17.7 g/dL
Female	11.5–15.5 g/dL
Mean corpuscular haemoglobin (MCH)	27–32 pg
Mean corpuscular haemoglobin concentration (MCHC)	32–36 g/dL
Mean corpuscular volume (MCV)	80–96 fL
Packed cell volume (PCV) or haematocrit	
Male	0.40–0.54 L/L
Female	0.37–0.47 L/L
White blood count (WBC)	$4–11 \times 10^9$/L
Basophil granulocytes	$<0.01–0.1 \times 10^9$/L
Eosinophil granulocytes	$0.04–0.4 \times 10^9$/L
Lymphocytes	$1.5–4.0 \times 10^9$/L
Monocytes	$0.2–0.8 \times 10^9$/L
Neutrophil granulocytes	$2.0–7.5 \times 10^9$/L
Platelet count	$150–400 \times 10^9$/L
Serum B_{12}	160–925 ng/L (150–675 pmol/L)
Serum folate	4–18 mcg/L (5–63 nmol/L)
Red cell folate	160–640 mcg/L
Red cell mass	
Male	25–35 mL/kg
Female	20–30 mL/kg
Reticulocyte count	0.5–2.5% of red cells ($50–100 \times 10^9$/L)
Erythrocyte sedimentation rate (ESR)	<20 mm in 1 hour
Coagulation	
Bleeding time (Ivy method)	3–10 min
Activated partial thromboplastin time (APTT)	26–37 s
Prothrombin time	12–16 s
International Normalized Ratio (INR)	1.0–1.3
D-dimer	<500 ng/mL

BIOCHEMISTRY

(Serum/plasma in alphabetical order)	
Alanine aminotransferase (ALT)	<40 U/L
Albumin	35–50 g/L
Alkaline phosphatase	39–117 U/L
Amylase	25–125 U/L
Angiotensin-converting enzyme	10–70 U/L
α_1-Antitrypsin	2–4 g/L
Aspartate aminotransferase (AST)	12–40 U/L
Bicarbonate	22–30 mmol/L
Bilirubin	<17 µmol/L (0.3–1.5 mg/dL)
Brain natriuretic peptide (BNP) threshold	100 pg/mL
Caeruloplasmin	1.5–2.9 µmol/L
Calcium	2.20–2.67 mmol/L (8.5–10.5 mg/dL)
Chloride	98–106 mmol/L
Complement	
C3	0.75–1.65 g/L
C4	0.20–0.60 g/L
C-reactive protein	<5 mg/L
Creatinine	79–118 µmol/L (0.6–1.5 mg/dL)
Creatine kinase (CPK)	
Female	20–170 U/L
Male	30–200 U/L
Ferritin	
Female	15–200 µg/L
Post-menopausal	4–230 µg/L
Male	30–300 µg/L
α-Fetoprotein	<10 kU/L
Glucose (fasting)	4.5–5.6 mmol/L (70–110 mg/dL)
γ-Glutamyl transpeptidase (γ-GT)	
Male	11–58 U/L
Female	7–32 U/L
Glycosylated (glycated) haemoglobin (HbA$_{1c}$)	3.7–5.1 %
Immunoglobulins (11 years and over)	
IgA	0.8–4 g/L
IgG	5.5–16.5 g/L
IgM	0.4–2.0 g/L
Iron	13–32 µmol/L (50–150 µg/dL)
Iron binding capacity (total) (TIBC)	42–80 µmol/L (250–410 µg/dL)

Lactate dehydrogenase	240–480 U/L
Magnesium	0.7–1.1 mmol/L
Osmolaity	275–295 mOsm/kg
Phosphate	0.8–1.5 mmol/L
Potassium	3.5–5.0 mmol/L
Prostate-specific antigen (PSA)	up to 4.0 µg/L
Protein (total)	62–77 g/L
Sodium	135–146 mmol/L
Urate	0.18–0.42 mmol/L (3.0–7.0 mg/dL)
Urea	2.5–6.7 mmol/L (8–25 mg/dL)
Vitamin D (seasonal variation)	
25-hydroxy	37–200 nmol/L (0.15–0.80 ng/L)
1,25-dihydroxy	60–108 pmol/L (0.24–0.45 pg/L)
Lipids and lipoproteins	
Cholesterol	3.5–6.5 mmol/L (ideal <5.2 mmol/L)
Lipids (total)	4.0-10.0 g/L
Lipoproteins	
VLDL	0.128–0.645 mmol/L
LDL	1.55-4.4 mmol/L
HDL (male)	0.70–2.1 mmol/L
HDL (female)	0.50–1.70 mmol/L
Phospholipid	2.9–5.2 mmol/L
Triglycerides	
Male	0.70–2.1 mmol/L
Female	0.50–1.70 mmol/L
Thyroid-stimulating hormone	0.3–3.5 mU/L
Blood gases (arterial)	
$Paco_2$	4.8–6.1 kPa (36–46 mmHg)
Pao_2	10–13.3 kPa (75–100 mmHg)
[H+]	35–45 nmol/L
pH	7.35–7.45
Bicarbonate	22–26 mmol/L
Urine values	
5-hydroxyindole acetic acid (5HIAA)	<47 µmol daily; amounts lower in females than males
Protein (quantitative)	<0.15 g per 24 hours
Sodium	60–180 mmol per 24 hours
Serum values	
eGFR	
Male	90–140 mL/min
Female	80–125 mL/min

Normal values

Clinical observations	
Temperature, normal	36.2–37.5 °C
Heart rate, normal	60–100 bpm
Blood pressure	120/80 mmHg average; systolic blood pressure is high if >140 mmHg, low if <100 mmHg
Oxygen saturation, normal	>94% on air (except in COPD)
Respiratory rate, normal	12–15 breaths/min

ABG	arterial blood gas		**EBV**	Epstein–Barr virus
ACE	angiotensin-converting enzyme		**ECG**	electrocardiography
ACTH	adrenocorticotrophic hormone		**Echo**	echocardiography
ADH	antidiuretic hormone (vasopressin)		**EEG**	electroencephalography
AF	atrial fibrillation		**ELISA**	enzyme-linked immunosorbent assay
AIDS	acquired immunodeficiency syndrome		**EMG**	electromyography (electrical activity produced by skeletal muscle)
ALF	acute liver failure			
ALL	acute lymphoblastic leukaemia		**ENT**	ears nose and throat
ALP	alkaline phosphatase		**ERCP**	endoscopic retrograde cholangiopancreatography
ALT	alanine aminotransferase			
AMA	anti-mitochondrial antibodies		**ESR**	erythrocyte sedimentation rate (measure of inflammation)
AML	acute myeloid leukaemia			
ANA	anti-nuclear antibodies		**FBC**	full blood count
ANCA	antineutrophil cytoplasmic antibodies: c-ANCA, cytoplasmic (commonly against proteinase 3); p-ANCA, perinuclear (commonly against myeloperoxidase)		**FEV1**	forced expiratory volume in 1 second
			FSH	follicle-stimulating hormone
			FVC	forced vital capacity
			GFR	glomerular filtration rate
APTT	activated partial thromboplastin time		**GGT**	gamma-glutamyl transpeptidase
ARDS	acute respiratory distress syndrome		**GH**	growth hormone
ASD	atrial septal defect		**GHRH**	growth hormone-releasing hormone/factor
AST	asparatate aminotransferase		**GI**	gastrointestinal
AV	atrioventicular		**GnRH**	gonadotrophin-releasing hormone
AXR	abdominal radiography		**GORD**	gastro-oesophageal reflux disease
BCG	Bacille–Calmette–Guerin (vaccination)		**GPI, GPII**	glycoproteins I and II
BMI	body mass index		**HAV**	hepatitis A virus
BP	blood pressure		**Hb**	haemoglobin (HbF, fetal Hb; HbA, normal adult variant)
bpm	beats per minute			
CHD	congenital heart disease		**HBV**	hepatitis B virus
CJD	Creutzfeldt–Jakob disease		**HCC**	hepatocellular carcinoma
CLL	chronic lymphocytic leukaemia		**HCV**	hepatitis C virus
CML	chronic myeloid leukaemia		**HDL**	high density lipoprotein
CMV	cytomegalovirus		**HDU**	high-dependency unit
CNS	central nervous system		**HDV**	hepatitis D virus
COPD	chronic obstructive airway disease		**HEV**	hepatitis E virus
CPAP	continuous positive airway pressure		**HIV**	human immunodeficiency virus
CRF	chronic renal failure		**HLA**	human leucocyte antigen
CRH	corticotrophin-releasing hormone/factor		**HSV**	herpes simplex virus
CRP	C-reactive protein (an inflammatory marker)		**IBD**	inflammatory bowel disease
CSF	cerebrospinal fluid		**ICP**	intracranial pressure
CT	computed tomography		**IDL**	intermediate density lipoprotein
CTPA	computed tomography pulmonary angiography		**IDU**	intravenous or injection drug use/user
			Ig	immunoglobulin
CXR	chest radiography		**IHD**	ischaemic heart disease
DEXA	dual energy X-ray absorptiometry		**IL**	interleukin
DIC	disseminated intravascular coagulation		**IM**	intramuscular
DMARD	disease-modifying anti-rheumatic drug		**INR**	international normalized ratio
dsDNA	double-stranded DNA		**ITP**	idiopathic thrombocytopenic purpura
DVT	deep vein thrombosis		**ITU**	intensive care unit

IV	intravenous	PR	per rectum
IVU	intravenous urogram	PT	prothrombin time
JVP	jugular venous pressure	PTH	parathyroid hormone (parathormone)
KUB	kidneys, ureter, bladder radiography	RA	right atrium
LA	left atrium	RBC	red blood cells
LDL	low density lipoprotein	RIF	right iliac fossa
LFT	liver function tests	RV	right ventricle
LH	luteinizing hormone	SC	subcutaneous
LMN	lower motor neuron	SIADH	syndrome of inappropriate ADH secretion
LMWH	low-molecular-weight heparin	SLE	systemic lupus erythromatosus
LV	left ventricle	SOB	shortness of breath
MCV	mean cell volume	T_3	triiodothyronine
MEN	multiple endocrine neoplasia	T_4	thyroxine
MI	myocardial infarction	TB	tuberculosis
MRCP	magnetic resonance cholangiopancreatography	TFT	thyroid function test
		TIA	transient ischaemic attack
MRI	magnetic resonance imaging	TIPS	transjugular intrahepatic portosystemic shunt
MRSA	methicillin-resistant *Staphylococcus aureus*		
MS	multiple sclerosis	TNF	tumour necrosis factor
NASH	non-alcoholic steatohepatitis/fatty liver disease	TRH	thyrotropin-releasing hormone
		TSH	thyroid-stimulating hormone
NHL	non-Hodgkin lymphoma	TTE	transthoracic echocardiography
NSAID	non-steroidal anti-inflammatory drug	U&Es	urea and electrolytes
NYHA	New York Heart Association	UMN	upper motor neuron
OGD	oesophagogastroduodenoscopy	US	ultrasound
PCR	polymerase chain reaction	UTI	urinary tract infection
PDA	patent ductus arteriosus	VLDL	very low density lipoprotein
PEFR	peak expiratory flow rate	VSD	ventricular septal defect
PET	positron emission tomography	VTE	venous thromboembolism
PFA-100	platelet function analyser 100	WBC	white blood cell count

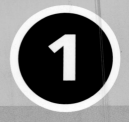

Patients who are acutely unwell in the emergency setting need to be dealt with quickly and effectively.

Throughout this book, this will be referred to as the ABC approach.

Patient has collapsed or is acutely unwell

Perform DR ABC DE

DR: danger and response

Danger: ensure the area is safe to approach

Response: squeeze, shake and shout; if there is no response, call for help.

ABC

Proceed to the primary survey ABC (Table 1.1).

D: Disability

Assess responsiveness according to the AVPU scale:

- Alert
- Voice: responds to voice
- Pain: responds to pain
- Unresponsive.
- Or use the Glasgow Coma Scale (GCS; Table 1.2). The scale assesses eye, verbal and motor responses; the lowest possible total score is 3 (deep coma or death), while the highest is 15 (fully awake person).

E: Examine and everything else:

- Expose top to toes work down systematically, look for rashes, active bleeding, fractures
- Check patient's notes, past history
- Do routine investigations
- Treat any pain
- Eyes: examine the eyes and their reaction to light:
  - bilateral pinpoint pupils: pontine lesions, opiate drugs, Argyll–Robertson pupil (syphilis)
  - bilateral dilated pupils: brainstem death, drugs: atropine, adrenaline, tricyclic antidepressants
  - unilateral dilated pupils: third nerve palsy, extra-dural haematoma, Holmes—Adie pupil
  - unilateral constricted pupil: Horner's syndrome (with ptosis).

DEFG: Don't ever forget glucose

Check blood glucose as hypo/hyperglycaemia is a reversible cause of collapse

Criteria to call the outreach team from the intensive care unit

- Respiratory rate: <8 or >25 breaths/min
- Pulse < 50 or >125 bpm
- Systolic BP: <90 or >200 mmHg
- Oliguria: <0.5 mL/kg per hour
- Sudden fall in GCS >2 points.

The patient in respiratory or circulatory arrest

If the acutely unwell patient goes into respiratory or circulatory arrest, call for help and begin basic life support:

Basic life support: ABC approach

Danger: Check it is safe to approach

Response: Gently shake the patient and ask 'Are you alright?'. If there is no response shout for help

Airway: look for anything that may be obstructing the mouth, then perform the head tilt-chin lift manoeuvre or jaw thrust if spinal injury is suspected.

Breathing: listen for breath sounds, feel for their breath on your cheek and look for movements of the chest at the same time to a total of 10 seconds

Circulation: feel for carotid pulse at the same time to a total of 10 seconds:

- if there are no signs of life, call the emergency switchboard to call the resuscitation team
- start 30 chest compressions at 100 beats/min to a depth of one third of the sternum
- then deliver 2 rescue breaths; in hospital use a bag-valve mask
- continue CPR at a ratio of 30 compressions:2 breaths until a defibrillator arrives.

If there is no pulse present, or a defibrillator arrives, proceed to advanced life support.

Table 1.1   Primary ABC survey

	A: airway	B: breathing	C: circulation
Look	*Is airway clear?*	Depth and symmetry of chest movements Use of accessory muscles Cyanosis Nasal flaring	Pallor Peripheral cyanosis JVP Oedema: sacral, ankle
Feel	Breathing on your cheek	Tracheal deviation Percussion of chest	Clamminess Peripheral pulses
Listen	Upper respiratory sounds: gurgle, stridor (inspiratory), wheeze (expiratory/inspiratory)	Breath sounds: equal, bronchial, additional sounds?	Heart sounds
Measure	O_2 saturations: normally >94% on air (may be lower if pre-existing pathology)	Respiratory rate (Normally 12–15 breaths/min) Arterial blood gas (ABG, see p. 73) Chest radiography (CXR)	Capillary refill (normally <2 s) Heart rate (normally 60–100 bpm) Urine output (>0.5 ml/kg per hour) Blood pressure (BP) Temperature ECG
Treat	*Obstruction* Fluid/vomit with Yankuer sucker Solid with McGill forceps *Position of the patient* Immobilise the cervical spine if a spinal injury is suspected Head tilt, chin lift (or jaw thrust if spinal injury is suspected) *Airway adjuncts* Oropharyngeal airway Nasopharyngeal airway Advanced airway intervention: laryngeal mask airway, endotracheal tube	*Patient not breathing*: put out an arrest call and start with basic life support *Patient breathing*: O_2 at 10–15 L/min with a non-rebreathing Hudson mask and reservoir bag (caution in those with CO_2 retention to maintain O_2 saturation at 88–92%) *Ventilatory support* Bag-valve mask Continuous positive airway pressure (CPAP) Bilevel positive airway pressure (BIPAP)	*No palpable pulse* Put out an arrest call and start basic life support *With a pulse* Insert 2 wide-bore cannulae in antecubital fossa Obtain blood sample for: full blood count (FBC), urea and electrolytes (U&Es), liver function tests (LFTs), C-reactive protein (CRP), glucose, clotting, cultures, group and save IV fluid if in shock Active bleeding: colloid or blood as soon as possible

Table 1.2   Glasgow Coma Scale

Test	Score					
	1	2	3	4	5	6
Eyes	Eyes remain closed	Eyes open to painful stimuli	Eyes open to command or voice	Spontaneous eye opening	–	–
Verbal	No speech	Incomprehensible sounds	Inappropriate speech	Confused, disoriented	Oriented, converses normally	–
Motor	No response	Extensor response to painful stimuli	Abnormal flexion to painful stimuli	Withdraws from painful stimuli	Localizes painful stimuli	Obeys commands

Advanced life support (figure 1.1)

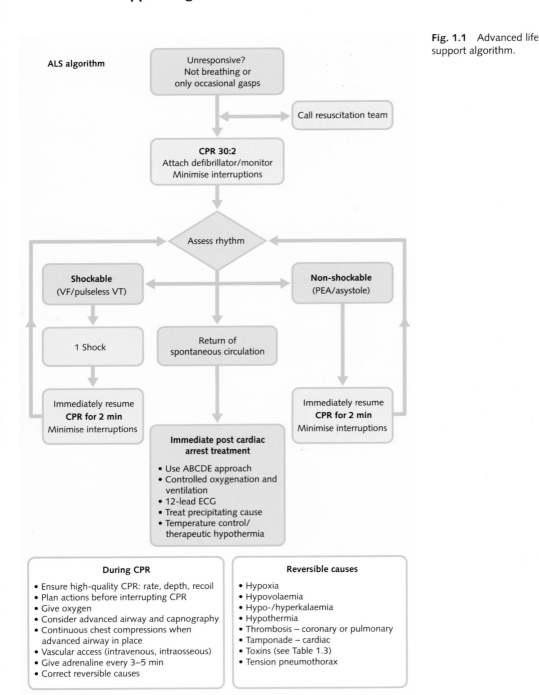

Fig. 1.1 Advanced life support algorithm.

ALS algorithm

Unresponsive?
Not breathing or
only occasional gasps

Call resuscitation team

CPR 30:2
Attach defibrillator/monitor
Minimise interruptions

Assess rhythm

Shockable
(VF/pulseless VT)

Non-shockable
(PEA/asystole)

1 Shock

Return of
spontaneous circulation

Immediately resume
CPR for 2 min
Minimise interruptions

Immediately resume
CPR for 2 min
Minimise interruptions

**Immediate post cardiac
arrest treatment**

- Use ABCDE approach
- Controlled oxygenation and
  ventilation
- 12-lead ECG
- Treat precipitating cause
- Temperature control/
  therapeutic hypothermia

During CPR	**Reversible causes**
• Ensure high-quality CPR: rate, depth, recoil • Plan actions before interrupting CPR • Give oxygen • Consider advanced airway and capnography • Continuous chest compressions when advanced airway in place • Vascular access (intravenous, intraosseous) • Give adrenaline every 3–5 min • Correct reversible causes	• Hypoxia • Hypovolaemia • Hypo-/hyperkalaemia • Hypothermia • Thrombosis – coronary or pulmonary • Tamponade – cardiac • Toxins (see Table 1.3) • Tension pneumothorax

If there are signs of life following advanced life support, reassess the respiratory rate, BP and heart rate followed by ABCDEFG:

A: arterial blood gases (ABGs)
B: bloods and BP repeated

C: CXR
D: disposal: transfer patient to appropriate department
E: ECG
F: inform family of patient status
G: gratitude: thank the resuscitation team.

Table 1.3 Lists toxins and their antidotes.

Table 1.3 Toxins and their antidotes

Toxin	Effect	Antidote
Benzodiazepines	Respiratory depression, coma	Flumazenil (benzodiazepine antagonist)
Beta-blockers	Bradycardia, cardiac failure, coma	Atropine: side effect bradycardia Glucagon IV for severe overdose
Carbon monoxide (faulty heaters)	Headache, nausea, confusion, pulse oximetry rarely useful (can be artificially high)	O_2; consider hyperbaric O_2 therapy (O_2 at higher than atmospheric pressure may quicken dissociation of carbon monoxide from carboxyhaemoglobin and cytochrome oxidase)
Cyanide (often due to smoke inhalation)	Collapse, neurological symptoms of progressive hypoxia, cherry red skin colour	100% O_2 Can consider hydoxycobalamin (binds cyanide so that it can be excreted in the urine)
Digoxin	Nausea and vomiting, diarrhoea, arrhythmias, delirium, xanthopsia (yellow vision)	Digibind: digoxin specific antibody fragments (prevents digoxin binding to target cells)
Heparin (anticoagulant)	Haemorrhage	IV protamine sulphate (binds heparin). Less effective for LMWH
Iron	Haemorrhage, nausea and vomiting, abdominal pain, coma	Desferioxamine (an iron chelating agent)
Opiates (e.g. heroin, morphine)	Respiratory depression, pinpoint pupils, bradycardia, coma	Naloxone (short acting)
Organophosphate insecticides(sarin)	**SLUDGE**: **s**alivation, **l**acrimation, **u**rination, **d**iarrhoea, **g**astrointestinal upset, **e**mesis	Atropine (muscarinic acetylcholine receptor antagonist)
Warfarin	Haemorrhage	Oral or IV vitamin K depending on INR and if active haemorrhage (warfarin acts by inhibiting enzyme recycling oxidised vitamin K). Consider also recombinant factor VIIa or prothrombin complex concentrate

Consult toxbase (www.toxbase.org) for advice on any poisons or overdose or call the National Poisons Centre (08448920111)
For alcohol and paracetamol overdose, see Ch. 5.
For aspirin overdose, see p. 10.

SHOCK

SHOCK: GENERAL FEATURES

Outline

- Inadequate delivery of O_2 and other vital substances to respiring cells from an abnormality in the circulatory system
- Due to a failure in the pumping action of the heart or a problem within the peripheral circulation
- **A medical emergency**.

Pathogenesis/aetiology

Classification

- Based on the cause of the inadequate delivery
- Hypovolaemic
- Cardiogenic
- Obstructive (obstruction to outflow or restricted cardiac filling)

- Septic
- Anaphylactic

Each type of shock can be considered generally (as outlined here) and with the additional specific features, investigations and treatments as below.

Symptoms and signs

- ABC approach

Measure:

- Prolonged capillary refill (>2 s)
- Tachycardia
- BP: systolic <90 mmHg or diastolic <60 mmHg.

Investigations

Blood tests

- FBC
- U&Es
- Glucose
- LFTs

- Cross match
- Clotting
- ABG.

Infection screen

- Blood and urine cultures.

Imaging

- CXR
- Computed tomography (CT)

- US.

Other tests

- Dependent on suspected cause, e.g. echocardiography (echo).

Treatment

- ABC approach

Airway, breathing:
- May include oxygenation and ventilation

Circulation:
- IV access with fluids to restore BP: fast crystalloid infusion (care with cardiogenic shock)
- Inotropes if persistent hypotension

- Raise foot of bed

Then:
- Treat underlying cause
- Treat complications
- Hourly observations including urine output (may need a catheter).

HYPOVOLAEMIC SHOCK

Outline

- Insufficient circulating fluid due to internal or external loss.

Pathogenesis/aetiology

Causes

- Haemorrhage
- Fluid loss, e.g. vomiting, diarrhoea, burns.

Symptoms and signs

As for shock and:
- Blue, cold skin
- Sweating
- JVP not visible

- Cool peripheries
- Dry
- Confusion
- Restlessness.

Investigations

- Look for fluid loss including haemorrhage and third space losses (movement of fluid into interstitial tissues).

Treatment

- Fluids: crystalloid or colloid
- If haemorrhagic cause consider transfusing blood products.

CARDIOGENIC SHOCK

Outline

- Heart is unable to maintain the circulation
- There is evidence of heart failure

- Raised JVP
- Basal crackles (evidence of pulmonary oedema).

Pathogenesis/aetiology

Causes

- Cardiac failure
- Pulmonary embolus
- Tension pneumothorax

- Cardiac tamponade
- Arrhythmias
- Myocardial infarct.

Symptoms and signs

- Evidence of pulmonary oedema
- Increased respiratory effort
- Bibasal crackles
- Tachypnoea

- Clammy
- JVP raised
- Cool peripheries.

Investigations

Blood tests

As for shock in general and:
- Serum troponin

- Creatine kinase.

Other tests

- ECG
- CXR
- Echocardiogram: to exclude cardiac tamponade, valve lesions and to quantify cardiac function

- Swan-Ganz catheter: to calculate pulmonary wedge pressures, a measure of intravascular filling.

Treatment

- Calculate pulmonary wedge pressure:
  - if <15 mmHg continue giving IV fluids until adequately filled. Swan-Ganz catheter required.
  - when >15 mmHg give inotropes

- Correct arrhythmias
- Treat underlying cause
- Refer to Intensive Care Unit (ICU) for inotropic support
- Diamorphine for pain.

SEPTIC SHOCK

Outline

- Sepsis causing hypotension and perfusion abnormalities
- Vasodilatation and a reduction in peripheral vascular resistance result in hypotension

See also chapter 11 for 'the septic patient'.

Pathogenesis/aetiology

Causes

- Infection.

Symptoms and signs

- Respiratory crackles: if due to respiratory sepsis
- Sweating
- Warm peripheries

- Pyrexia
- Oliguria
- Confusion.

Investigations

Blood tests

- Clotting and platelet abnormalities can occur

- ABG: arterial hypoxaemia, metabolic acidosis.

Infection screen

- Cultures: blood, urine, sputum

- Lumbar puncture: CSF analysis and culture.

Imaging

- CXR.

Treatment

- IV fluids
- Inotropes if necessary

- Urgent antibiotic therapy: refer to local guidelines
- Consider referral to ICU.

ANAPHYLACTIC SHOCK

Outline

- Shock caused by exposure to a specific allergen that precipitates a type 1 IgE hypersensitivity reaction

- Release of histamine results in capillary leak and oedema causing vasodilation and a reduction in peripheral vascular resistance.

Pathogenesis/aetiology

Causes

- Common precipitants: peanuts, shellfish, drugs (most commonly penicillins).

Symptoms and signs

- Stridor: if upper airway obstruction
- Increased respiratory effort
- Wheeze
- Cyanosis

- Tachycardia
- Skin: rash, erythema, urticaria, itch
- Face: angioedema, oedema.

Investigations

Blood tests

As for shock in general and:
- Tryptase (an enzyme raised within one hour of anaphylaxis, useful for diagnosis).

Other tests

- Allergy testing: for investigation of precipitant.

Treatment

- O₂ 100%
- Remove precipitant
- Alert anaesthetist if necessary
- Adrenaline 0.5 mg IM, repeated after 5 min if needed
- Chlorphenamine 10 mg IV over 1–2 min

- Hydrocortisone 200 mg IV
- IV fluids
- If wheeze persists: nebulised salbutamol

Patients at risk may carry an Epipen with adrenaline and Medilert bracelet.

BURNS

Outline

- Tissue damage from a variety of causes including chemical, electrical, radiation and thermal.

- Thermal: dry (fire) or wet (scald): danger of inhalation injury and carbon monoxide poisoning with smoke inhalation.

Pathogenesis/aetiology

Pathogenesis

- Danger of infection and hypovolaemia due to increased capillary permeability

Thickness of burn:

Superficial:
- Painful due to vasodilation and release of kinins
- ~2 weeks to heal

Partial:
- Swelling and blisters
- ~3–4 weeks to heal, most do not scar

Full thickness:
- Nerve endings are damaged, and sensation is lost
- Skin is dry and pale, skin will scar.

Who

- Burns from hot water: common in infants

Symptoms and signs

- Severe pain
- Blistering
- Erythema.

Assess area of burn:

- Rule of nines used to estimate the percentage of skin burned (Fig. 1.2)

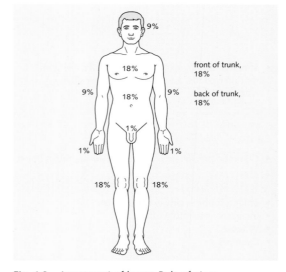

Fig. 1.2   Assessment of burns: Rule of nines.

Investigations

Blood tests

- ABG

- Carboxyhaemoglobin.

Treatment

- Transfer to a burns unit if appropriate (check local guidelines, will depend on extent of burns)

ABC approach:

- Airway: hot gases can lead to airway obstruction, involve anaesthetist early
- Circulation: fluid requirement if extensive burns
- Analgesia

- Cover the burns with cling film if transferring: burns become painful when exposed to air

- Dress the burns:
  - *superficial burns*: sulphadiazine cream, dressings
  - *full thickness burns*: surgical debridement and skin grafts
- Prevent 2° infection: may need antibiotics.

Prognosis and complications

Prognosis

- Dependent on area and thickness of burns and pre-existing morbidity

- High mortality if >50% burns.

Complications

- Infection
- Scarring

- Care if burn is circumferential around the limbs as may constrict and act like a tourniquet.

HYPOTHERMIA

Outline

- Core body temperature <35 °C
- Mild 32–35 °C

- Moderate 28–32 °C
- Severe <28 °C.

Pathogenesis/aetiology

Causes

- ↓ heat production:
  - Hypothyroidism
  - Hypopituitarism
  - Hypoadrenalism
- ↑ heat loss:
  - Immersion in water
  - Exposure

- Impaired thermoregulation:
  - Hypothalamic failure, e.g. trauma, stroke, tumours
  - Autonomic neuropathy, e.g. diabetes, Parkinson's disease
  - Toxic: alcohol overdose
  - Drugs: hypnotics, benzodiazepines.

Who

Increased risk:

- Elderly
- Alcoholic excess

- Dementia
- Socioeconomically deprived.

Symptoms and signs

- Shivering
- Mental confusion
- Dehydration
- Respiration slow and shallow

- Muscle stiffness
- Drowsiness
- Coma
- Death.

Investigations

- Core temperature (rectal).

Blood tests

- U&Es
- Plasma glucose

- Amylase
- Thyroid function.

ECG

- Bradycardia
- J waves

- Cardiac arrhythmias including ventricular fibrillation.

Treatment

- Ventilate if necessary
- Warm slowly (0.5–2 °C/h)
- Cardiac monitor to indentify and then treat arrhythmias
- Correction of metabolic abnormalities
- Broad spectrum antibiotics
- Monitor every 30 min

Sudden hypothermia:
- Mediastinal warm lavage
- Haemodialysis
- Cardiopulmonary bypass.

Prognosis and complications

Prognosis

- Age and temperature dependent, worse in the elderly

- Moderate and severe hypothermia mortality ∼40% (despite hospital treatment).

Complications

- Arrhythmias
- Acute renal failure

- Sepsis.

SALICYLATE OVERDOSE

Outline

- Aspirin overdose
- >150 mg/kg

- Severe toxicity >500 mg/kg
- Fatal overdose >700 mg/kg.

Pathogenesis/aetiology

Pathogenesis

- Aspirin directly stimulates the respiratory centre leading to hyperventilation and an early respiratory alkalosis
- Aspirin also uncouples oxidative phosphorylation, ↓ ATP production which is compensated for by ↑ glycolysis

which leads to accumulation of lactic acid and therefore a later metabolic acidosis
- Aspirin decreases platelet function directly.

Who

- Risk factors for death in severe poisoning:
  - Extremities of age
  - CNS features
  - Metabolic acidosis

- Pyrexia
- Late presentation
- Pulmonary oedema.

Symptoms and signs

Early features:
- Hyperventilation
- Tinnitus
- Nausea and vomiting
- Sweating
- Dehydration
- Lethargy
- Tremor
- Vertigo

Later features:
- Seizures
- Pulmonary or cerebral oedema
- Renal failure
- Coma and death

Metabolic features:
- Hypoglycaemia
- Hypokalaemia.

Investigations

Blood tests

- FBC
- U&Es
- LFTs: repeat 12 hourly
- Glucose
- INR

- ABG: respiratory alkalosis then metabolic acidosis
- Plasma drug levels: may need to repeat due to continuing absorption.

Urine

- Aspirin levels

- pH.

Treatment

- O_2
- Correct dehydration: IV fluids
- Correct acidosis: bicarbonate 8.4%
- Correct hypokalaemia

- Control hyperthermia
- Correct clotting: vitamin K
- Monitor

Overdose <1 h previously:

- Activated charcoal

- Gastric lavage

Level dependent treatment:

- If levels >500 mg/L consider alkalinisation of urine

- Levels >700 mg/L refer for haemodialysis.

Prognosis and complications

Prognosis

- 1% mortality with severe toxicity.

Complications

- Renal failure with chronic use.

ALCOHOL OVERDOSE

Outline

- Recommendations for maximal weekly intake: 21 units for males, 14 for females

Chronic abuse:

Affects multiple systems:
- Liver: alcoholic hepatitis, chronic liver disease and cirrhosis (see also alcoholic liver disease p. 175)
- GI: gastritis, oesophagitis, pancreatitis
- CNS: Wernickes's encephalopathy, Korsakoff' syndrome (see Neurology Chapter 6), cerebellar dysfunction

- Cardiovascular: restrictive cardiomyopathy, arrhythmias
- Endocrine: gynaecomastia, testicular atrophy
- Social complications.

Pathogenesis/aetiology

- Alcoholic: a compulsive need for alcohol that interferes with work of social life
- Alcohol dependence: physical dependence or addiction when the individual takes the drug to experience its psychic effects or to avoid the symptoms of withdrawal
- Alcohol tolerance: increased quantity is required to produce the original effect.

Who

- 1% of population is alcohol dependent: 20–30% of them develop alcoholic liver disease
- 20% of hospital admissions in males related to alcohol consumption
- ♀ < ♂
- Commonest cause of chronic liver disease in Western world.

Symptoms and signs

Acute intoxication:

- Impaired coordination and judgement
- Loss of inhibition
- Hypoglycaemia
- Hypothermia
- Euphoria
- Slurred speech
- Lability
- Nausea and vomiting
- Memory lapse
- Respiratory failure
- Coma and death

Chronic abuse:

- Signs dependent on system/s or organ involved

Acute withdrawal:

- 10–72 h after drinking
- Hallucinations
- Tremor
- Fits
- Confusion
- Delirium tremens: intense hallucinations.

Investigations

CAGE questionnaire:

- Quick assessment of alcoholic dependency, if yes to any question take detailed history:
- Do they want to cut down
- Do they get annoyed when criticised about drinking
- Do they feel guilty about drinking
- Have they used alcohol as an eye opener.

Blood tests

- FBC: macrocytosis (↑ MCV), leucocytosis, thrombocytopenia, anaemia
- LFTs: ↑ GGT, ↑ AST, ↑ ALT, ↑ ALP, ↑ bilirubin, ↓ albumin
- U&Es: ↓ urea (unless recent GI bleed)
- Blood alcohol level.

Treatment

Support:
- Circulatory support and fluid
- Thiamine IV to prevent Wernicke's encephalopathy and then glucose (always thiamine first)
- Alcohol cessation: alcohol cessation services including group therapy such as alcoholics anonymous
- Good nutrition
- Antibiotics if septic

Withdrawal symptoms:
- Chlodiazepoxide for 3 days with a gradually reducing dose

To reduce relapse:
- Acamprosate: for anxiety and insomnia
- Disulfiram: leads to unpleasant side effects by increasing acetaldehyde levels when taken with alcohol

Hepatic encephalopathy or severe disease:
- See hepatology chapter.

Prognosis and complications

Prognosis

- Chronic abusers have a 2–3 times ↑ risk of dying compared with non-drinkers.

Complications

- Cirrhosis: 10–20% of heavy drinkers
- Depends on organs affected.

Faculty Contributor: Jonathan Behar

BP = cardiac output × peripheral vascular resistance
Cardiac output = heart rate × stroke volume.

Blood supply to the heart

The blood supply to the heart is from three main coronary arteries:

- Left anterior descending artery
- Left circumflex artery
- Right coronary artery.

Occlusion of each vessel affects a certain region and is associated with specific ECG changes, as illustrated in Table 2.1.

Electrical conductivity

- Conduction of electricity starts is initiated with depolarisation of pacemaker cells within the sino-atrial node (SAN) of the right atrium.
- Electrical activity spreads from the sinoatrial node towards the atrioventricular (AV) node where conduction is held up before electricity spreads down, the bundle of His in the septum, where it divides into left and right bundle branches to supply the respective ventricles
- Sinoatrial node depolarisation frequency is influenced by autonomic nerves; parasympathetic vagal nerves (inhibit) and sympathetic nerves (stimulate).

Important causes of sudden cardiac death in the young adult

- Cardiomyopathy, e.g. hypertrophic obstructive cardiomyopathy
- Arrhythmogenic right ventricular cardiomyopathy:
  - primary electrophysiological abnormality
  - Brugada syndrome
  - long QT syndrome
- Acute chest trauma, e.g. road traffic accident
- Aortic dissection
- Congenital heart disease (CHD).

Bradycardias

Bradycardia is defined as a heart rate <60 bpm.

Symptoms and signs

- Often asymptomatic
- Can cause reduced cardiac output and therefore patients have hypotension, presyncope and syncope.
- JVP: cannon waves in complete heart block.

Common causes

- Coronary artery disease (ischaemia/infarction)
- Degenerative calcific aortic stenosis (valve near AV node)
- Idiopathic conduction system fibrosis (elderly)
- Electrolyte disturbance (hyperkalaemia)
- Hypoxia
- Digoxin toxicity (direct nodal blocker)
- Anti-arrhythmic drugs, e.g. beta-blockers, calcium antagonist, digoxin
- Radiotherapy
- Hypothermia
- Physiological, e.g. athletes.

Uncommon causes

- Collagen vascular diseases, e.g. rheumatoid arthritis, lupus, systemic sclerosis
- Myocarditis (viral, bacterial, protozoal, e.g. Chagas' disease)
- Neuromuscular disease, e.g. myotonic dystrophy
- Sarcoidosis
- CHD, e.g. Ebstein's abnormality, atrial septal defect (ASD)
- Cardiomyopathy, e.g. haemochromotosis.

Classification and origin

Figure 2.1 shows the conduction of electricity through the heart.

Sinus bradycardia

Sinoatrial node discharge <60 bpm.
Causes:

- can be physiologically normal, e.g. sleep, athletes, children
- drugs: beta-blockers, amiodarone, calcium antagonists, lithium
- metabolic: hypothermia, hypothyroid, hyperkalaemia
- raised vagal tone: nausea and vomiting, vasovagal attack, carotid sinus hypersensitivity.

Table 2.1 Vessel occlusion and ECG changes

Coronary artery	Associated region of myocardium perfused	ECG changes when artery is occluded
Left anterior	Anterior or septal	Q waves, ST elevation V1–4
Circumflex	Lateral	Q waves, ST elevation V4–6, I, aVL
Right	Inferior	Q waves, ST elevation II, III, aVF
Right or circumflex	Posterior (often coexistent with inferior or lateral MI)	Prominent R wave in V1 and V2, with ST depression V1–V3

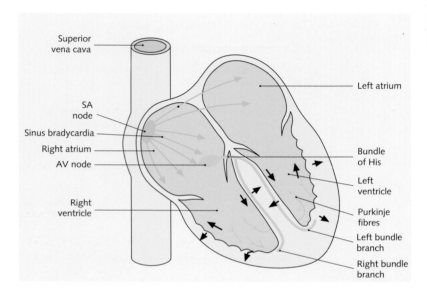

Fig. 2.1 Conduction of electricity through the heart and origin of bradycardias.

Sick sinus syndrome (tachy-brady syndrome)

A disease of the sinoatrial node (SAN) where patients experience tachycardias and bradycardias due to sinus node dysfunction.

Causes:

- common in elderly patients (often have fibrosis of conductive tissue, sometimes secondary to ischaemia/infarction).

AV node block: first-degree heart block

Prolonged delay at the AV node causing slowed conduction time between the atria and ventricles (Fig. 2.2):

- ECG: prolonged PR interval >200 ms.

AV node block: second-degree heart block

Intermittent failure of conduction at the AV node. Two types:

- Mobitz I (Wenckebach):
  - benign
  - common in children and athletes.

- ECG (Fig. 2.3): progressive lengthening of PR interval until a lone P wave is not followed by a QRS (arrowed)
- Mobitz II:
  - more sinister, at risk of complete block
  - ECG (Fig. 2.4): fixed PR interval with some P waves that are not followed by a QRS complex. Description determined by number of P waves *per* QRS complex (this can vary), e.g. 2:1, 3:1.

AV node block: third-degree (complete block)

Complete failure of conduction at the AV node:

- Atrial and ventricular depolarisations occur independently from each other
- As conduction fails, escape rhythms from just below the AVN (~50 bpm) or ventricular myocardium (~30 bpm) take over pacemaker function
- ECG: no relationship between P waves and QRS complexes (Fig. 2.5). Conduction with ventricular escape rhythms travels through adjacent coupled myocardium rather than the usual circuit (His–Purkinje) and therefore is represented by broad QRS complexes.

Fig. 2.2   First-degree AVN block.

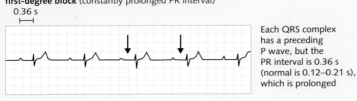

first-degree block (constantly prolonged PR interval)

0.36 s

Each QRS complex has a preceding P wave, but the PR interval is 0.36 s (normal is 0.12–0.21 s), which is prolonged

Fig. 2.3   ECG showing second-degree block.

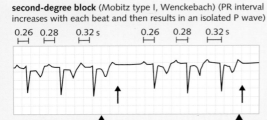

second-degree block (Mobitz type I, Wenckebach) (PR interval increases with each beat and then results in an isolated P wave)

0.26   0.28   0.32 s   0.26   0.28   0.32 s

The PR interval progressively increases and then there is one isolated P wave without a following QRS complex; the PR interval then goes back to normal and starts to increase again

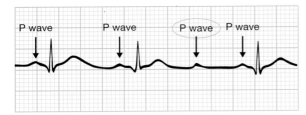

P wave   P wave   P wave   P wave

Fig. 2.4   ECG showing second-degree block 2:1.

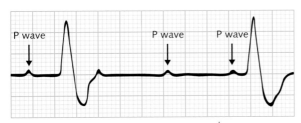

P wave   P wave   P wave

Fig. 2.5   ECG illustrating third-degree block.

Bundle branch block

Delay in conduction along the His–Purkinje system and bundle fibres. There is one right bundle and two left bundles (split into anterior and posterior fascicles). The ECG pattern will help determine which of the bundles is blocked.

- ECG: wide QRS complex (WILLIAM MORROW: helps to remember ECG appearance).

Causes:

- ischaemic heart disease (IHD)
- hypertension

- valvular disease
- conduction tissue fibrosis
- myocarditis/endocarditis
- any cardiomyopathy, e.g. hypertrophic obstructive cardiomyopathy
- cor pulmonale, right ventricle hypertrophy, pulmonary hypertension (usually right bundle branch block)
- secundum artrial septal defect (right bundle branch block), primum atrial septal defect (left bundle branch block)
  - bifascicular block: two of three fascicles of the bundle of His are blocked
  - ECG will usually show: right bundle branch block, left axis deviation
  - trifascicular block: all three fascicles of the bundle of His are blocked (right bundle branch block with both left anterior fascicular block and left posterior fascicular block)
  - ECG: usually the same as bifascicular block but with the addition of a prolonged PR interval.

Emergency management of bradycardias

- Follow adult bradycardia algorithm (Fig. 2.6)
- Remember to stop precipitants, e.g. beta-blockers, and correct/treat any reversible causes such as hypothermia, electrolyte disturbance, acute ischaemia hypothermia, electrolyte disturbance

Tachycardias

Tachycardias are defined as a heart rate >100 bpm.

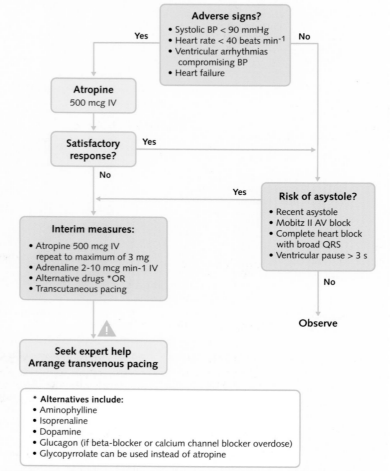

Adult bradycardia algorithm
(includes rates inappropriately slow for haemodynamic state)

Fig. 2.6 Adult bradycardia algorithm.

If appropriate, give oxygen, cannulate a vein, and record a 12-lead ECG

Adverse signs?
- Systolic BP < 90 mmHg
- Heart rate < 40 beats min⁻¹
- Ventricular arrhythmias compromising BP
- Heart failure

Yes — No

Atropine
500 mcg IV

Satisfactory response? — Yes

No

Yes — **Risk of asystole?**
- Recent asystole
- Mobitz II AV block
- Complete heart block with broad QRS
- Ventricular pause > 3 s

No

Interim measures:
- Atropine 500 mcg IV repeat to maximum of 3 mg
- Adrenaline 2-10 mcg min-1 IV
- Alternative drugs *OR
- Transcutaneous pacing

Observe

⚠ **Seek expert help**
Arrange transvenous pacing

* **Alternatives include:**
- Aminophylline
- Isoprenaline
- Dopamine
- Glucagon (if beta-blocker or calcium channel blocker overdose)
- Glycopyrrolate can be used instead of atropine

Contact your local cardiology service to decide upon temporary vs. permanent pacing options.

Symptoms and signs

- Syncope/presyncope
- Chest pain
- Shortness of breath (SOB)
- Heart failure.

Classification and origin

Table 2.2 shows the ECG classification of ventricular and supraventricular tachycardias.

Supraventricular tachycardias

Electrical focus of depolarisation originates from myocytes above the division of the bundle of His.

- ECG: usually demonstrates a narrow complex tachycardia on ECG (QRS <120 ms) because conduction follows the conventional electrical pathways in the heart. If however, conduction follows an aberrant pathway, supraventricular tachycardias may cause broad QRS complex tachycardia (e.g. atrial fibrillation with bundle branch block or with pre-excitation).

Ventricular tachycardia (VT)

Tachyarrhythmia originates in the ventricles:

- ECG: broad QRS complex tachycardias.

Sinus tachycardia

- ECG: Each P wave is followed by QRS with a rate >100 bpm.

Table 2.2 ECG classification of ventricular and supraventricular tachycardias

Classification by ECG	Supraventricular tachycardias	Ventricular tachycardias
Regular	Atrial • Sinus tachycardia • Atrial flutter • Atrial fibrillation (AF) • Atrial tachycardia (focal/multi focal) AV • AV re-entry tachycardia, e.g. Wolff–Parkinson–White • AV node re-entry tachycardia	Ventricular
Irregular	Atrial fibrillation (AF): AF with bundle branch block or pre excitation Multifocal atrial tachycardia	Ventricular fibrillation: Polymorphic VT, e.g. torsade de pointes

Causes:

- physiological: emotion, stress, exercise, pain
- stimulants: caffeine, cocaine, salbutamol
- pathology: sepsis, thyrotoxicosis, hypovolaemia
- treatment is to treat or remove the underlying cause.

Atrial flutter

Regular atrial discharges at a rate of 300 bpm, usually around a counter clockwise circuit in the floor of the right atrium (cavo-tricuspid isthmus).

- The AV node has a maximum speed of electrical activity it will allow through, and therefore, classically conducts only half (i.e. 2:1) of the electrical signals and results in a ventricular response of 150 bpm. If the AV node conducts 1 in 3 (3:1), the ventricular response is 100 bpm
- ECG: P waves resemble a 'saw tooth' (arrowed) in typical cavo-tricuspid isthmus dependent atrial flutter (Fig. 2.7).

Atrial fibrillation

Fibrillating atrial myocytes at a rate of ~600 bpm:

- ECG (Fig. 2.8): no P waves, fibrillating baseline (sometimes difficult to see), an irregularly irregular ventricular response (may be slow or fast). If bundle

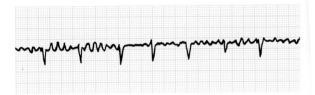

Fig. 2.8 ECG showing atrial fibrillation.

branch block exists, one will often see an irregular broader complex ventricular response. If complete AVN block exists, ventricular response may still be regular (due to complete atrioventricular dissociation).

See p. 30 for more on atrial fibrillation (AF).

AV re-entry tachycardia, e.g. Wolff–Parkinson–White

A congenital accessory pathway (bundle of Kent) whereby electrical conduction can spread to the His–Purkinje system, bypassing the AVN:

- If atrial arrhythmias exist, there is risk of rapid conduction to the ventricles without the slowing effect of the AVN.
- ECG (Fig. 2.9): short PR interval followed by slurred upstroke in QRS (delta wave, arrowed) in resting ECG of Wolff–Parkinson–White syndrome.

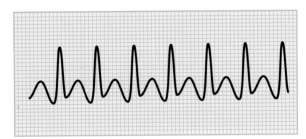

Fig. 2.7 ECG showing atrial flutter.

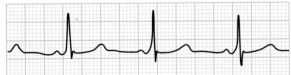

Fig. 2.9 ECG of Wolff–Parkinson–White syndrome.

Treatment:

- antiarrhythmics
- implantable cardiac defibrillators
- surgery: curative radiofrequency ablation, performed percutaneously, ~90% success rate.

Monomorphic ventricular tachycardias

- Regular broad complex tachycardia, often QRS >160 ms
- If persistent often results in cardiac arrest
- ECG morphology (Fig. 2.10): wide regular waveforms.

Treatment:

- DC shock (synchronised)
- amiodarone or other anti-arrhythmics
- if recurrent, consider implantable cardiac defibrillators to prevent sudden death.

Torsade de pointes (polymorphic ventricular tachycardias)

- Uncommon
- A consequence of a long QT interval (Fig. 2.11).

Causes of long QT:

- congenital conditions
- drugs: sotalol, chlorpromazine and many others.

Treatment:

- IV magnesium sulphate
- may precipitate VF.

Ventricular fibrillation

Ineffective ventricular contraction causing a cessation of cardiac output:

- ECG morphology (Fig. 2.12): random waveform with no pattern.

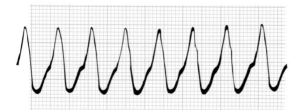

Fig. 2.10 ECG showing characteristic VT.

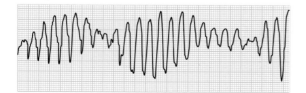

Fig. 2.11 ECG showing torsade de pointes.

Treatment:

- DC shock and advanced life support protocol.

Emergency management of tachycardias

- Follow adult tachycardia algorithm (Fig. 2.13)
- Once acute rhythm control is achieved consider starting a maintenance anti-arrhythmic agent. This is often a beta-blocker, calcium channel antagonist or amiodarone.

Investigations

Blood tests: serum cardiac enzymes

- Levels of cardiac enzymes in the blood increase with myocardial damage (Table 2.3), e.g. during a myocardial infarction (MI)
- Troponin I or T is the most widely used cardiac biomarker and is highly specific. More modern assays have increasing sensitivity as well. For patients with ischaemic sounding chest pain, a blood test is performed at baseline (on admission) and then 6–12 hours after the onset of pain.

ECG

A graphical representation of the electrical activity of the heart (Fig. 2.14). Used to assess abnormal cardiac rhythms, myocardial ischaemia or infarction and the likely location of arterial blockage.

Normal ECG (parameters):

PR: 120–200 ms (3–5 small squares)
QRS: <120 ms (3 small squares)
QT: <440 ms (11 small squares).

Exercise tolerance test

An ECG is taken during exercise on a treadmill and used to demonstrate or unmask cardiac ischaemia.

Echocardiogram

Ultrasound of the heart which assesses ventricular function, valvular function, severity of stenoses or valve incompetence and chamber size (Fig. 2.15).

Two main echo modalities used in practice:

- Transthoracic (TTE): images obtained non invasively with the probe on the anterior chest wall.
- Transoesophageal (TOE): images obtained invasively with the probe inserted into the oesophagus (similar to endoscopy). The picture resolution is greater and this modality is usually reserved for cases where more structural detail is required, for example, possible endocarditis or valvular disease.

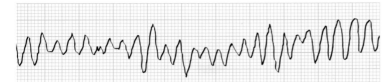

Fig. 2.12 ECG of ventricular fibrillation.

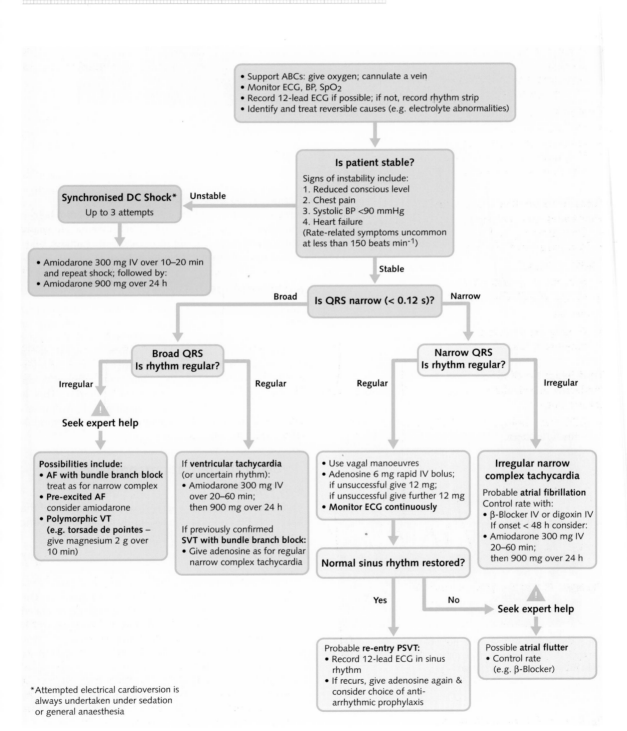

- Support ABCs: give oxygen; cannulate a vein
- Monitor ECG, BP, SpO₂
- Record 12-lead ECG if possible; if not, record rhythm strip
- Identify and treat reversible causes (e.g. electrolyte abnormalities)

Is patient stable?

Signs of instability include:
1. Reduced conscious level
2. Chest pain
3. Systolic BP <90 mmHg
4. Heart failure
(Rate-related symptoms uncommon at less than 150 beats min⁻¹)

Unstable

Synchronised DC Shock*
Up to 3 attempts

- Amiodarone 300 mg IV over 10–20 min and repeat shock; followed by:
- Amiodarone 900 mg over 24 h

Stable

Broad ← **Is QRS narrow (< 0.12 s)?** → **Narrow**

Broad QRS
Is rhythm regular?

Irregular

Seek expert help

Possibilities include:
- **AF with bundle branch block** treat as for narrow complex
- **Pre-excited AF** consider amiodarone
- **Polymorphic VT** (e.g. torsade de pointes – give magnesium 2 g over 10 min)

Regular

If **ventricular tachycardia** (or uncertain rhythm):
- Amiodarone 300 mg IV over 20–60 min; then 900 mg over 24 h

If previously confirmed
SVT with bundle branch block:
- Give adenosine as for regular narrow complex tachycardia

Narrow QRS
Is rhythm regular?

Regular

- Use vagal manoeuvres
- Adenosine 6 mg rapid IV bolus; if unsuccessful give 12 mg; if unsuccessful give further 12 mg
- **Monitor ECG continuously**

Normal sinus rhythm restored?

Yes

Probable **re-entry PSVT:**
- Record 12-lead ECG in sinus rhythm
- If recurs, give adenosine again & consider choice of anti-arrhythmic prophylaxis

No

Seek expert help

Irregular

Irregular narrow complex tachycardia

Probable **atrial fibrillation**
Control rate with:
- β-Blocker IV or digoxin IV
If onset < 48 h consider:
- Amiodarone 300 mg IV 20–60 min; then 900 mg over 24 h

Possible **atrial flutter**
- Control rate (e.g. β-Blocker)

*Attempted electrical cardioversion is always undertaken under sedation or general anaesthesia

Fig. 2.13 Adult tachycardia algorithm.

Table 2.3 Cardiac enzyme release with myocardial damage

Cardiac enzyme	Time to peak (h)	Time in the blood (h)
Troponins	12	168
Creatine kinase MB	24	48
Aspartate aminotransferase (AST)	30	60
Lactate dehydrogenase (LDH)	72	240

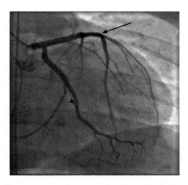

Fig. 2.16 Coronary angiogram showing the left coronary artery which splits into the left anterior descending (arrow) and left circumflex artery (arrowhead) upon injection of contrast dye.

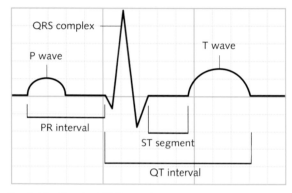

Fig. 2.14 Standard ECG complex.

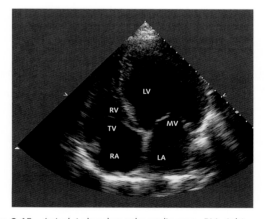

Fig. 2.15 Apical 4 chamber echocardiogram. RV, right ventricle; LV, left ventricle; MV, mitral valve; LA, left atrium; RA, right atrium; TV, tricuspid valve.

Stress echocardiogram

Cardiac function is observed on echocardiogram before and after the heart is stressed, either pharmacologically with intravenous dobutamine or on an exercise bike. This is to demonstrate cardiac ischaemia.

Myocardial perfusion scan

Another imaging modality performed by the nuclear medicine department. A radioisotope (thallium or technetium) is injected intravenously and the heart scanned at rest and during pharmacological stress usually with dobutamine or adenosine. Areas of myocardium which are ischaemic will have reduced tracer uptake during stress, as compared with rest. This is therefore another functional imaging test to demonstrate cardiac ischaemia. Some centres use this modality more than others.

Cardiac catheterisation/coronary angiography

An invasive procedure whereby the blood vessels of the heart can be visualised for diagnostic and therapeutic purposes:

- This is the gold standard for assessment of coronary artery disease.
- Catheters are passed to the aortic root retrogradely via an arterial puncture (femoral or radial arteries). The coronary ostia in the aortic root are then cannulated by manipulation of the catheters and contrast dye is injected to demonstrate the coronary anatomy. Any obstructive lesions can be visualised and any further treatment planned.

Cardiac CT (computed tomography)

A useful screening modality to visualise the coronary arteries non invasively by injecting intravenous contrast and scanning the chest in a CT scanner. An estimate of coronary artery obstruction can be made as well as the calcium content, which correlates with atheroma burden. However, if this test estimates >50% obstruction in one or more of the coronary arteries, invasive coronary angiography is advised.

Cardiac MRI

A recent addition to the non invasive tools used to image the heart. This provides exquisite resolution images of the cardiac structure and function. Stress/perfusion sequences using a pharmacological stress (intravenous adenosine) can demonstrate regions of the myocardium which become ischaemic. High resolution images are an invaluable tool for investigation of the cardiomyopathies.

HEART FAILURE

- Clinical syndrome where the heart is unable to maintain sufficient cardiac output to meet the demands of the body.

- Caused by failure of either the right side of the heart, or left side, or both.

Types

Left ventricular failure
Due to either:
- Low output, where the heart cannot pump sufficiently (i.e. ejection fraction (EF) <40%, on echo).

- OR high output, where body demand for perfusion or oxygenation is increased.

Right ventricular failure
From increased right ventricle (RV) pressure.

Congestive heart failure
Both sides of the heart fail.

Severity: New York Heart Association (NYHA) classification

I: no symptoms on physical activity
II: symptoms on moderate effort (climbing flights of stairs)
III: symptoms with mild effort (walking 100 m on flat ground)

IV: symptoms at rest.

Acute vs. chronic heart failure

In acute failure, there is no time for acclimatisation and so acute pulmonary oedema ensues, with a poor prognosis (e.g. post MI).

Pathogenesis/aetiology

Pathogenesis

Acute failure of the heart leads to back pressure in the venous system and congestion in the form of pulmonary and peripheral oedema.

This leads to poor renal perfusion which activates the renin–angiotensin system and the sympathetic nervous system,

causing vasoconstriction, fluid retention and further myocardial stretch. The heart can compensate through increased inotropy but eventually failure with left ventricle (LV) dilatation occurs

This is illustrated in Figure 2.17.

Causes

Left ventricular failure
- Low output
  - IHD
  - hypertension
  - valvular heart disease
  - dilated cardiomyopathy.
- High output
  - anaemia
  - pregnancy
  - Paget's (elderly men)
  - arteriovenous malformations
  - beriberi (wet and dry).

Right ventricular failure
- 2° to left ventricular failure
- Pulmonary hypertension (from chronic hypoxia, cor pulmonale)
- Pulmonary embolism
- Constrictive pericarditis.

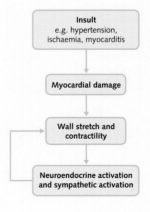

Fig. 2.17 Heart failure.

Pathogenesis/aetiology

Precipitants

Often patients with heart failure are admitted to hospital because of sudden deterioration, precipitants include:
- infection
- reduced diuretic therapy
- therapy related (e.g. negatively inotropic medications)
- NSAIDs, causing fluid accumulation
- new arrhythmias (e.g. fast AF)
- further disease (e.g. new MI).

Who

Epidemiology

- 10% of those over 65 years
- 1 million people in the UK.

A typical patient

A 65-year-old man complains to his GP that he becomes breathless even when walking to the local shops. He has a history of heart disease and high BP. He adds that he sleeps with three pillows at night.

Clinical features

Symptoms

- SOB
- ↓ Exercise tolerance
- Orthopnoea: breathlessness on lying flat (ask how many pillows are used at night)
- Paroxysmal nocturnal dyspnoea: breathlessness waking the patient at night
- Nocturia
- Ankle swelling
- Wheeze: 'cardiac asthma'
- Cough with pink frothy sputum
- Fatigue
- ↓ appetite, often with weight loss (accelerated catabolism in heart failure)
- Abdominal pain and nausea
- Abdominal swelling
- Depression (very common).

Signs

- Tachycardia
- Tachypnoea
- Pulsus alternans (altering large and small volume pulse)
- Peripheral cyanosis
- Inferolaterally displaced apex
- Third heart sound (S3)
- Basal crepitations
- Dependent oedema (sacrum and feet).
- Specific signs indicating right ventricular failure:
  - ↑ JVP
  - RV heave
  - pan-systolic murmur of tricuspid regurgitation (TR)
  - tender pulsatile hepatomegaly (TR)
- Pitting oedema.

Investigations

Suspicion of heart failure:
- ECG: evidence of left ventricular failure or IHD
- N-terminal B type natruretic peptide:
  - released from ventricles in response to dilation/stretch
  - >20 pmol/L is abnormal.

If either ECG or B type natruretic peptide is abnormal: request echo for diagnosis.

Imaging

Echo:
- Gold standard for diagnosis:
  - measures ejection fraction, indicating left and RV function
  - may demonstrate cause

CXR:
- Look for features of heart failure (LV). Features given by ABCDE (Fig. 2.18):
  - **A**lveolar oedema
  - Kerley **B** lines
  - **C**ardiomegaly
  - **D**ilated prominent upper lobe vessels
  - pleural **E**ffusion.

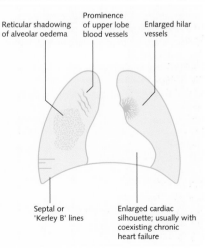

Reticular shadowing of alveolar oedema | Prominence of upper lobe blood vessels | Enlarged hilar vessels

Septal or 'Kerley B' lines | Enlarged cardiac silhouette; usually with coexisting chronic heart failure

Fig. 2.18 Schematic illustrating the five key features of heart failure.

Investigations

Blood tests

- U&E, LFTs, bone and clotting profile
- TFTs
- Fasting glucose and lipids.

Urine

Dipstick.

(See also pulmonary oedema p. 121.)

Treatment

Acute presentation

Medical emergency (pulmonary oedema results):
- ABC (see Chapter 1), including O_2
- Sit patient up
- Cardiac monitor with ECG.
- Bloods: FBC, U&E, LFT, clotting, ABG (evidence of hypoxia, acidosis)
- CXR.
Systolic BP >100 mmHg:
- Diuretics: IV furosemide

- Glyceryl trinitrate infusion
- Opiates IV: for anxiety associated with SOB and for venodilation to reduce preload.
Systolic BP <100 mmHg:
- Consider CPAP ventilation to cause venodilation and reduce preload without reducing BP
- If the patient is unwell, acidotic and not responding to treatment, consult ITU.

Chronic management

- Identify and treat the cause
- Improve quality of life
- Patient education:
  - pneumococcal vaccine
  - fluid intake

- ↑ exercise
- ↓ alcohol, smoking, salt.
- Specialist heart failure nurse input (often managed in the community).

Medication

- Diuretics: first-line therapy, for symptom relief, reducing fluid retention and preload; no effect in reducing mortality (side effect: ↓ potassium, ↓ sodium, ↓ BP, incontinence, renal impairment, gout)
  - loop diuretic: furosemide
  - thiazide diuretic: bendroflumethiazide
  - potassium-sparing diuretics: spironolactone; aldosterone antagonist; **of prognostic benefit** (side effects: gynaecomastia, ↑ potassium)
- Angiotensin-converting enzyme (ACE) inhibitors: inhibit aldosterone production thereby reducing water retention, vasodilating so reduce preload
  - all patients should be treated with an ACE inhibitor, e.g. enalapril, ramipril
  - side effects: renal impairment, hypotension, ↑ potassium, rash, **cough** (in 10%; switch to angiotensin II receptor antagonist, e.g. losartan)
  - prognostic and symptomatic benefit
- Beta-blockers: cardioselective drugs (e.g. bisoprolol, carvedilol, metoprolol); block sympathetic system and should be avoided in the acute setting (precipitate decompensation)

  - side effects: hypotension
  - prognostic and symptomatic benefit.
- Other drugs:
  - vasodilators: to reduce preload
  - nitrates: reduce preload; little outcome on mortality but good for **symptom control** (e.g. isosorbide mononitrate (particularly in angina), hydralazine (second line))
  - positive inotropes: increase contraction force
  - digoxin: good for rate control in those with AF (less clear for those in sinus rhythm); reduces hospitalisation from exacerbations but no decrease in mortality
  - anticoagulation: for AF, LV thrombus, etc.
Device therapy for heart failure:
- Implantable cardiac defibrillators: deliver DC shock to dangerous arrhythmias; indications are ischaemia-related heart failure with EF <35% and QRS of <120 ms
- Cardiac resynchronisation therapy: biventricular pacemakers enable synchronous contraction of the ventricles.

Surgical interventions

- Coronary artery bypass graft/valve surgery

- Transplantation: for end-stage.

Prognosis and complications

Prognosis

40% die within 1 year.
Heart failure is a progressive disease with a poor prognosis.
Palliative care plays an important role with these patients
(particularly when back in the community).

Poor prognostic indicators:
- Low serum sodium
- High NYHA score
- Raised B type natruretic peptide or its precursor.

Complications

NSAIDs and calcium channel blockers are contraindicated in these patients as they can precipitate decompensation:
NSAIDs via fluid retention and calcium channel blockers via LV function

ISCHAEMIC HEART DISEASE

GENERAL FEATURES

Outline

- Ischaemia results from insufficient O_2 delivery to organs or tissues usually as a result of reduced blood flow
- Atherosclerosis (plaques obstruct blood flow in vessels) is the hallmark of this disease.

Pathogenesis/aetiology

Pathogenesis of atherosclerosis

Progression is in stages:
1. Fatty streaks develop in arteries (young adults)
2. Endothelial dysfunction
3. Atheromatous plaques develop containing lipids, macrophages, smooth muscle cells and fibroblasts
4. Plaques can be flow limiting, causing symptoms of angina

5. Unstable plaques can rupture to create thrombi, which may obstruct vessels.

In the heart these events are broadly termed acute coronary syndromes.

Who

IHD
- Commonest cause of death in the developed world
- Results in >100,000 deaths per year in the UK

- >40 000 premature deaths (<75 years of age) per year in the UK.

Clinical features

Atherosclerosis causes:
- IHD
- peripheral vascular disease
- cerebrovascular disease (strokes, TIAs)

- multi-infarct (vascular) dementia
- renal artery stenosis
- aortic aneurysmal disease.

Investigations

Depends on presentation.

Treatment

Depends on cause and symptom severity

Cardiac drugs

- Aspirin: inhibits platelet function by inhibiting thromboxane A_2
- Clopidogrel: inhibits platelet function by inhibiting ADP-induced platelet aggregation
- Prasugrel and Ticagrelor also inhibit platelet function through similar pathways
- Statins: hydroxymethylglutaryl (HMG)-CoA reductase inhibitors (e.g. simvastatin, atorvastatin); inhibit cholesterol formation

- Beta-blockers (e.g. atenolol), −ve inotrope, chronotrope. These are first line in suspected IHD as they are prognostic in IHD:
  - caution advised in asthma
  - side effects: bradycardia. heart block, hypotension, fatigue, impotence
- Calcium channel blockers (e.g. amlodipine, diltiazem) block membrane calcium channels in myocardium and vessel wall:

Treatment

- side effects: peripheral oedema, headache, flushing, postural hypotension
- Nitrates: (isosorbide mononitrate/dinitrate) tablets, glyceryl trinitrate spray facilitate smooth muscle cell relaxation in vessel walls:
  - tolerance can develop if used constantly
  - side effects: caution in asthmatics and severe aortic stenosis, flushing, headache
- GpIIb/IIIa inhibitors (e.g. abciximab, tirofiban) block the adherence of fibrinogen to platelet receptors and inhibit platelet aggregation. These are powerful antiplatelet medications reserved for use in ACS and in those undergoing angiography.
  - side effects: bleeding, ↓ platelets.

Prognosis and complications

Prognosis

Depends on cause.

ANGINA PECTORIS

Outline

Chest pain from myocardial ischaemia:
- Usually results from atherosclerosis
- Other causes include prolonged hypotension and anaemia
- Angina is not a disease but a clinical presentation of IHD.

Classification

- Stable:
  - relieved by rest and/or glyceryl trinitrate
  - pain often occurs at a constant level of exertion
- Unstable:
  - severe and persistent, not relieved by rest
- may be new or a sudden worsening of existing stable angina
- results from rupture of unstable plaque and partial or complete obstruction to blood flow

Canadian Cardiovascular Society angina classification

Angina occurs:
I: on strenuous or prolonged physical activity
II: on vigorous physical activity (slight limitation)

III: on performing everyday living activities (moderate limitation)
IV: at rest (severe limitation).

Pathogenesis/aetiology

Causes

- Atherosclerosis
- Anaemia
- Aortic stenosis
- Tachyarrythmias
- Hypertrophic obstructive cardiomyopathy
- Coronary artery spasm (e.g. with cocaine)
- Arteritis: inflammatory
- Pulmonary hypertension
- Prolonged hypotension.

Who

Cardiovascular risks

- Modifiable:
  - smoking
  - hypertension
  - hyperlipidaemia
  - diabetes
  - obesity
  - sedentary lifestyle
  - metabolic syndrome
  - psychological stress
  - excess alcohol.
- Non-modifiable:
  - ↑ age
  - males
  - postmenopause
  - **family history**
  - Asian race.

Emerging risk factors
- Homocysteinuria
- Inflammation
- Oxidative stress
- Chronic kidney disease.

Clinical features

Features:
- Crushing or squeezing retrosternal chest pain
- Often diffuse and deep: patient is unable to pin-point location

- The patient often clutches the left-centre of the chest with a clenched right fist (Levine's sign)
- Pain may radiate to the left arm, jaw and occasionally to the back (consider aortic dissection causing infarction)
- Average duration: <10 min.

Precipitating factors

Physical exertion or stress, with immediate relief on resting or administration of nitrates (highly predictive of angina pectoris).

Investigations

Acute setting

ECG
Demonstrates ST depression

Non-acute setting

Exercise tolerance test
- Monitor for ST depression, reproducible chest pain, failure of heart rate or BP to rise, ventricular arrhythmias and inability to complete the test.

Stress echo
- Visual assessment before, during and after 'work' induced pharmacologically.

Myocardial perfusion scan (MPS)
- Identifies healthy and dead myocardial tissue and demonstrates whether there is *reversible* ischaemia.

Coronary angiography
- Demonstrates condition of coronary arteries and guides potential revascularisation.

NB: Both MPS and stress echo are useful in patients who cannot physically perform exercise (e.g. with osteoarthritis or claudication from peripheral vascular disease).

Treatment

Stable angina

- Acute: nitrate (sublingual glyceryl trinitrate)

Medication
- Beta-blockers (e.g. atenolol) excellent anti-anginal drugs; first line in suspected IHD
- Calcium channel blockers (e.g. amlodipine, diltiazem) used if beta-blockers are contraindicated, not tolerated or if maximal beta blockade is insufficient
- Nitrates: isosorbide mononitrate/dinitrate tablets and glyceryl trinitrate spray; often used as an adjunct to a beta-blocker or calcium channel blocker for breakthrough angina.

Elective reperfusion strategies
- Percutaneous coronary intervention:
  - same procedure as a coronary angiogram but coronary lesions are dilated and stented to improve coronary blood flow
  - two types of stent used: bare metal or drug eluting
  - patients with IHD tend to take aspirin for life; if stents inserted clopidogrel also added for at least 12 months (drug eluting) or 1 month (bare metal).

- Chronic: optimise ischaemic risk factors/up titrate anti anginal medications.

- Potassium channel activator: nicorandil is a vasodilator
- Others
  - ivabradine: −ve inotrope acting on the sino-atrial node to reduce heart rate; useful in those intolerant of beta-blockers
  - ranolazine: useful adjunct in chronic angina for those already on a beta-blocker, calcium channel blocker and nitrate.

- Coronary artery bypass grafting:
  - use of veins (e.g. long saphenous vein) or arteries (e.g. left internal mammary artery) to bypass blocked arteries
  - preferred option for young, diabetic patients with triple vessel disease.

Unstable angina

See acute coronary syndromes, below.

Prognosis

- 10-year-MI risk ~20%
- Annual death rate: 1.6–3.2%.

MYOCARDIAL INFARCTION

Outline

Necrosis (cell death) following myocardial ischaemia – a medical emergency.

WHO definition of MI

Two of the following:
- good clinical history: including chest pain lasting >15 min
- dynamic ECG changes: ST elevation or depression, Q waves, T wave inversion

- rise in biochemical markers of myocardial necrosis: troponin T or I.

Acute coronary syndromes

Encompasses those with persistent chest pain and autonomic symptoms and who you suspect are having an MI:
- STEMI (ST elevation MI):
  - ECG criteria of ST elevation >2 mm in two congruent chest leads (V1–V6), or >1 mm in limb leads or new left bundle branch block
  - usually troponin positive

- Non-STEMI:
  - troponin positive
  - usually without ECG STEMI criteria but may have ischaemic changes
- Unstable angina:
  - usually minimal ECG changes
  - troponin − ve
  - high risk of having an MI within 30 days.

Pathogenesis/aetiology

Causes

- Rupture of atherosclerotic plaque
- As above for stable angina

- Acute aortic dissection: retrograde dissection into the aortic arch obliterating the ostium of the coronary artery coming from the coronary sinuses.

Who

45% of MIs occur in patients <65 years

♀ < ♂.

A typical patient

A 50-year-old man presents by ambulance to A&E with severe chest pain that has gone on for some time. He describes it as central and crushing and radiating to his jaw. He is sweating profusely and is very anxious. ECG shows convex ST elevation in several leads.

Clinical features

Symptoms

Chest pain:
- acute central/left-sided chest pain
- radiates to left arm/neck/jaw
- crushing, dull, tight or squeezing pain

- sudden onset
- usually occurs at rest
- often lasts for >15 min.

Associated symptoms

Often 2° to an autonomic nervous system response or pump failure:
- nausea and vomiting
- sweatiness
- dyspnoea
- palpitations

- syncope/presyncope
- pale/grey complexion
- feeling of impending doom
- elderly patients and those with diabetes may have no symptoms.

Signs

Often very few specific clinical signs but autonomic activation will often cause:
- tachycardia: unless heart block present resulting in a bradycardia

- features of heart failure.

Investigations

Blood tests

↑ Cardiac enzymes:
- ↑troponin 12 h after onset of chest pain

- other enzymes measured including creatine kinase MB (see Table 2.2. p. 14).

ECG

The ECG leads affected indicate the region of the infarct (Fig. 2.19):
- changes in minutes:
  - ST elevation: can stay elevated for days but usually comes down with treatment
  - hyperacute T waves (similar to hyperkalaemia tenting)

- changes in hours–days:
  - pathological Q waves
  - ST segment returns to baseline
  - T wave inversion: may be immediate or delayed, often persists until resolution of ST segment.

Imaging:

CXR:
- Widened mediastinum in aortic dissection: anti-platelets are contraindicated
- Evidence of heart failure
- Look for other causes of chest pain.

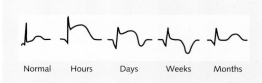

Normal   Hours   Days   Weeks   Months

Fig. 2.19 Progressive changes seen on ECG following a myocardial infarction.

Treatment

Acute coronary syndrome

- MONA: morphine, O₂, nitrate, aspirin
- Treat in a monitored bay: cardiac monitor with resuscitation facilities

- ABC approach: airway, breathing (high-flow O_2), circulation.

Anti-platelet therapy
- Aspirin 300 mg
- 2nd anti platelet agent (Clopidogrel 300 mg, Prasugrel 60 mg or Ticagrelor 180 mg)

- Those on dual antiplatelet therapy are at higher risk of bleeding so also give gastric protection if >65, prior GI bleeding or peptic ulceration, e.g. lansoprazole.

Anti-thrombotic therapy
Low-molecular-weight heparin (LMWH) e.g. Clexane 1 mg/kg sc or Fondaparinux 2.5 mg sc.

Analgesia
- IV morphine/diamorphine with IV antiemetic (metoclopramide)

- glyceryl trinitrate infusion: titrate until pain resolves while maintaining systolic BP >100 mmHg.

Reperfusion strategy
- If good clinical history: emergency reperfusion with 1° percutaneous coronary intervention or angioplasty. Ideally within 12 h of onset of chest pain. Often involves ambulance transfer to a tertiary centre (see angina). Some hospitals still

  attempt reperfusion with IV thrombolysis (streptokinase/tissue plasminogen activator)
- If percutaneous coronary intervention is imminent, add an extra 300 mg clopidogrel (total of 600 mg) and an infusion of a GpIIb/IIIa inhibitor, e.g. abciximab.

Treatment

Further medications to reduce mortality

- Beta-blocker: can start immediately and titrate up. Reduces likelihood of myocardial rupture and incidence of fatal arrhythmias. Caution with inferior MI or those in heart block
- ACE inhibitors: start within 24 h of MI and titrate up. Monitor renal function
- Statins: can be started immediately for plaque stabilising effect.

Newer antiplatelet therapies

Prasugrel, ticagrelor: recently licensed.

Post MI care (>24 h)

- Titrate up beta-blocker and ACE inhibitor.
- Continue LMWH for 3–5 days but usually stopped after angiogram.
- Echo to assess LV function and regional wall motion abnormalities
- Cardiac rehabilitation
- Optimise risk factors (see above):
  - no sex for 4 weeks
- no driving for 4 weeks after an MI or coronary artery bypass graft (reduced to 1 week if patient had percutaneous coronary intervention and good LV function on echocardiogram)
- Cardiology follow-up
- Aspirin lifelong and 2nd antiplatelet for 12 months if drug-eluting stent inserted, 1 month if bare metal stent.

Prognosis and complications

Prognosis

Mortality with STEMI:
- At 30 days:
  - 13% with medical therapy
  - 7% with thrombolysis
  - 3–5% with percutaneous coronary intervention
- At 6 years:
  - 20% have a recurrent MI
  - 20% have heart failure

Complications

- Further pain associated with:
  - coronary occlusion
  - post-infarct angina
- Arrhythmias (e.g. AV node block, particularly with right coronary artery lesions, ectopic beats)
- Ruptured or damaged structures:
  - acute mitral regurgitation
  - ventricular septal defect (VSD)
  - myocardial free wall rupture
  - LV aneurysm: at 4–6 weeks, persistent ST elevation
- Pump failure/dysfunction:
  - hypotension
  - heart failure
  - cardiogenic shock
- Post-necrosis inflammation:
  - pericarditis
  - Dressler syndrome: an autoimmune phenomena of pericarditis usually many weeks after MI; often responsive to steroids
- Venous thromboembolism (VTE): if prolonged immobilisation.

ARRHYTHMIAS

(see pp. 15 and 17 for tachycardias and bradycardias)

ATRIAL FIBRILLATION

Outline

All the cardiac atrial myocytes discharge electrical energy at the same time creating disorganised ineffectual contraction, known as fibrillation:
- The myocytes discharge at 300–400 bpm but the AV node (the cardiac fail-safe mechanism) only conducts up to 150–180 bpm to the ventricles.
- Rapid heart rate and an inefficient pumping mechanism leads to a poor cardiac output, reducing cardiac output by up to 30%
- A fibrillating atrium also causes 'relative' stasis of blood within the left atrial appendage and is a risk factor for thrombus formation, which can embolise causing a stroke.

Outline

Classification

- Paroxysmal: self terminates within 7 days
- Persistent: lasts >7 days

- Permanent: does not terminate with cardioversion or will revert within 24 h of successful cardioversion.

Pathogenesis/aetiology

Causes

Any condition resulting in increased atrial pressure or volume:
- Common causes:
  - IHD
  - hypertension
  - valve disease (particularly mitral)
  - hypertrophic obstructive cardiomyopathy
  - LV dysfunction
  - post-cardiac surgery (30% cases)
  - pericarditis
- Common medical causes:
  - alcohol excess

- metabolic disturbance (e.g. hypoxia, acidotic)
- infection (e.g. pneumonia)
- drugs (e.g. cocaine)
- hyperthyroidism
- cor pulmonale from chronic obstructive pulmonary disease (COPD)
- pulmonary embolism
- Rarer causes:
  - CHD
  - atrial myxoma
  - pericardial effusion.

Who

AF is the most common persistent arrhythmia. Prevalence in general population 1%. Increased prevalence with age.

Affects 5–10% of those >65 years, >20% of those >80 years.

Clinical features

Symptoms

Often asymptomatic. Features of heart failure:
- irregularly irregular pulse
- palpitations

- fatigue
- chest pain
- faintness.

Investigations

Blood tests

U&Es: check for biochemical disturbances.

ECG

See p. 14 for characteristic ECG pattern:

- Absence of P waves with irregular QRS complexes.

Imaging

- CXR: for infection, often a precipitating cause in the older patient

- Echocardiogram: for structural heart disease and evidence of LV dysfunction.

Treatment

Emergency management

Danger of circulatory collapse

Reduce symptoms

By rate or rhythm control:
- Rate control (reduce heart rate), controlling the ventricular response:
  - beta-blockers (first line)

- calcium channel antagonists
- digoxin (effective only at rest)
- Rhythm control (restore heart rhythm):
  - chemically with flecainide, sotalol, amiodarone

- DC cardioversion: if clear onset of AF within 48 h and a normal echocardiogram, otherwise anticoagulation for 4 weeks, cardiovert and continue anticoagulation for 4 weeks after (reduce risk of embolic stroke). Favourable in younger patients with fewer risk factors for stroke.

Reduce risk of embolic stroke
Anticoagulation with warfarin to reduce risk of stroke. Use CHA2DS2VASC score – if score of 1 point or above should consider anticoagulation. Caveat: being female alone is not enough.
C – cardiac failure, LVEF<45% (1 point)
H – hypertension (1 point)
A – age >65 (1 point), age >75 (2 points)

D – diabetes (1 point)
S – stroke/TIA (2 points)
VASC – vascular disease (coronary artery, peripheral vascular or cerebrovascular disease (1 point) + female (1 point). Also need to consider bleeding risk – use the HASBLED score to weight up benefit vs risk. www.chadsvasc.org for further information.

Poor rate control (with tachy and brady episodes) and symptoms

Pace and ablate strategy: iatrogenic ablation to cause complete heart block and insertion of a pacemaker. Radiofrequency AF ablation – percutaneous technique to cauterise signals in the 4 pulmonary veins to definitely treat and remove the AF altogether. Risk of complications 5% (tamponade, stroke, death). Most patients require >1–2 procedures to completely remove the AF.

Prognosis and complications

Prognosis

Annual stroke risk according to CHA2DS2VASC score:
- 0 points: 0.78%
- 1 point 2%
- 2 points 3.7%
- 3 points 5.9%
- 4 points 9.3%
- 5 points 15.3%
- 6 points 19.7%
- 7 points 21.5%
- 8 points 22%
- 9 points 24%

Once baseline investigations such as ECG, Holter monitor and echocardiogram have been performed, some patients will have an EPS (electrophysiology study) to demonstrate any conduction abnormalities. During this, if accessory pathways or abnormal circuits are found they can be removed with cautery using radiofrequency ablation.

VALVULAR HEART DISEASE

GENERAL FEATURES

Outline

Heart valves facilitate the forward flow of blood through the heart and prevent backflow. There are four heart valves:
- Mitral valve: left side between atria and ventricles
- Tricuspid valve: right side between atria and ventricles
- Aortic and pulmonary valves: in the aorta and pulmonary artery.

There are four heart sounds:
- S1: closure of mitral and tricuspid valve
- S2: closure of aortic valve and pulmonary valve
- S3: rapid ventricular filling. Can be normal
- S4: atrial constriction from blood against a stiff ventricle. Always pathological.

For a full description of the heart sounds and types of murmur see table 15.2 Visual representation of heart sounds in Clinical examinations, p. 638.
Pathology:
Can present with abnormal flow (heard as murmurs on auscultation) or as a clinical syndrome such as pulmonary oedema 2° to heart failure.

Pathogenesis/aetiology

Pathogenesis

- Turbulent flow from stenosis, regurgitation or prolapse can produce abnormal sounds heard on auscultation and thrills (palpable murmurs)
- Stenosis is 'failure of opening' in that there is narrowing of the valve orifice, limiting forward flow
- Regurgitation is 'failure of closing' in that incompetent valves allow blood flow in the wrong direction (regurgitant jets). The regurgitant jet may cause a build up of back pressure or volume
- Not all murmurs are pathological (e.g. a hyperdynamic circulation in pregnancy)

Who

Often the elderly and those with connective tissue diseases.

Clinical features

- Arrhythmias
- Features of heart failure
- Impaired coronary perfusion: chest pain
- Impaired cerebral perfusion: presyncope/syncope.

Investigations

Imaging

CXR:
- May show left atrial or left ventricular enlargement
- Can show valve calcification for example in long-term rheumatic or bicuspid aortic valve disease.
- May show evidence of complications in severe disease e.g. heart failure, pulmonary oedema or pulmonary hypertension

Echocardiogram:
- TTE, including Doppler flow to assess pressure gradients and severity of disease
- TOE: superior imaging of the LA and mitral valves (useful for the diagnosis of mitral valve endocarditis).

Other tests

- Cardiac catheterisation: to measure chamber pressures and gradients.

Treatment

Medical

- Regular monitoring of deterioration in symptoms and serial echocardiography to monitor valve severity.
- Treat arrhythmias and features of heart failure.

Procedure options

- Valvuloplasty:
  - percutaneous, a balloon catheter is inserted across the valve and inflated
- Valvotomy: surgical, stenotic valve separated
- Valve repair or replacement, surgical:

  - tissue: normally porcine (pig), but can be from humans; lasts ~10 years with no need for long-term anticoagulation
  - mechanical: ball and cage (e.g. Starr–Edwards, tilting disc/double tilting disc); these last longer than tissue valves and require lifelong anticoagulation.

Prognosis and complications

Complications

- Can lead to heart failure.
- Of prosthetic valves:
  - infection: almost all cases of infective endocarditis of prosthetic valves need urgent surgical replacement
  - haemolysis and anaemia

  - insufficient anticoagulation: embolic stroke, valve failure
  - over anticoagulation: bleeding
  - valve dehiscence and para-valvular leak causing heart failure.

MITRAL STENOSIS

Outline

Mitral valve is between the LA and LV. Narrowing of the valve orifice limits forward flow:
- Flow obstruction causes increased left atrial pressure, hypertrophy and dilatation, often leading to AF and right heart failure.

- A chronic and progressive disease: fully developed mitral stenosis takes many decades to develop, e.g. rheumatic fever in teens with slowly progressive symptoms in 30 s and causing death (without treatment) in 40–50 s.

Pathogenesis/aetiology

Causes

- Rheumatic heart disease in almost all cases
- Senile calcification
- Congenital (e.g. Lutembacher syndrome: mitral stenosis and ASD)

- Carcinoid: malignant
- Functionally mimicked by atrial myxoma: produces similar clinical picture but the valve is not actually stenotic.

Pathogenesis/aetiology

Pathogenesis

- Back pressure increases pulmonary venous pressure and leads to gradual exertional SOB through reduced pulmonary compliance. This leads to pulmonary hypertension causing RV failure.
- RV failure leads to progressive congestive biventricular failure.

- Onset of AF further reduces ventricular filling through loss of atrial systole and often leads to failure and pulmonary oedema.
- A stenotic mitral valve with AF produces a very high risk of thrombus generation and embolic stroke.

Who

♀ > ♂

Clinical features

Symptoms

Symptoms and signs of pulmonary hypertension and right heart failure with disease progression:
- insidious onset
- dyspnoea

- ↓ exercise tolerance
- cough
- haemoptysis
- palpitations: AF.

Signs

- Murmur features (Fig. 2.20):
  - opening snap in early diastole
  - mid-diastolic murmur (rumbling)
  - presystolic accentuation corresponding to atrial systole (only if in sinus rhythm)

  - loudest with patient on left lateral side, in expiration radiates to axilla
- Sound: loud S1
- Pulse: irregular (AF), low volume
- Apex beat: tapping, not displaced.

Other signs
- ↑ JVP
- Malar flush
- RV heave on palpation
- Also pan-systolic murmur of tricuspid regurgitation (TR is a common complication of mitral stenosis owing to RV dilatation)
- Loud 2nd heart sound (P2) and early diastolic murmur of pulmonary regurgitation (called Graham–Steell murmur in context of right heart failure from mitral stenosis).

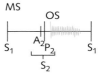

Fig. 2.20 Signs seen in mitral stenosis.

Investigations

ECG

- AF
- P mitrale (bifid M-shaped P waves) suggesting LA enlargement if sinus rhythm

- Evidence of right heart failure: right axis deviation, RV failure.

Imaging

Echocardiogram:
- TTE:
  - to calculate mitral valve orifice area to grade severity <1 cm² is severe.
  - calcification can be visualised
  - gradient can be calculated.

CXR:
- Large LA straightens left heart border, double shadow on right and increases (splays) the angle at the carina
- Kerley B lines showing interstitial oedema
- Pulmonary venous hypertension
- Pleural effusions
- Calcified mitral valve may be radioopaque.

Treatment

Symptom control

- Treat AF: rate control and anticoagulation
- Diuretics for symptomatic pulmonary and peripheral oedema

- Antibiotic prophylaxis before surgery or dental procedures.

Definitive treatment

- Balloon valvotomy: percutaneous procedure to inflate balloon across the valve; suitable for patients with non-calcified pliable valves
- Closed valvotomy: surgical procedure to manually dilate the stenotic valves through LV puncture

- Open valvotomy: surgical procedure with cardiopulmonary bypass
- Valve replacement: more often undertaken than the other surgical procedures.

Prognosis and complications

Complications

- Pulmonary hypertension
- AF
- Emboli: stroke
- Infective endocarditis

- Right heart failure
- Tricuspid regurgitation: through RV dilatation
- Pressure from large LA on local structures (e.g. hoarse, dysphagia, bronchial obstruction).

MITRAL REGURGITATION (MR)

Outline

Mitral valve (bicuspid valve): is between LA and LV. Regurgitation: incompetent valves allow blood flow in the wrong direction (regurgitant jets) causing a build up of back pressure and volume into the LA:

- chronic regurgitation (most commonly): gradual rise in left atrial pressure as the volume overload is gradually accommodated.
- acute (e.g. post MI): rapid rise in left atrial pressure causing raised pulmonary pressures and pulmonary oedema.

Pathogenesis/aetiology

Causes

Leaflet abnormality:
- infective endocarditis
- mitral valve prolapse, myxomatous degeneration
- rheumatic fever: causes both regurgitation and stenosis
- connective tissue disorders (e.g. Marfan, Ehlers–Danlos)
- congenital (e.g. Down's)
- post MI

- trauma
- ischaemic fibrosis.
- Left ventricular abnormality
- Secondary MR from LV dilatation and failure of leaflets to coapt.

Who

♀ < ♂

Clinical features

Symptoms

Symptoms of heart failure resulting from poor forward flow and increased backflow:
- pulmonary oedema
- SOB

- palpitations
- syncope/presyncope
- chest pain.

Signs

- Murmur features:
  - pan-systolic at apex
  - radiates: to axilla
- Sounds (Fig. 2.21):
  - S1: soft
  - S2: often obliterated by murmur; widely split owing to premature aortic valve closure
  - S3: often present because of rapid ventricular filling
- Apex beat: inferolateral displacement, thrusting.

NB: patients can have coexistent MR and mitral stenosis (mixed mitral valve disease). Clinical signs help to determine which is the predominant lesion:

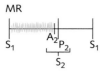

Fig. 2.21 Signs seen in mitral regurgitation.

- MR predominates: soft S1, post-systolic motion with S3 and displaced apex
- MS predominates: loud S1, tapping undisplaced apex.

ECG

- P mitrale: LA enlargement
- P pulmonale: RA enlargement

- LV hypertrophy: hypertension
- AF: common in chronic mitral valve disease.

Imaging

CXR:
- Enlarged LA and ventricle
- Evidence of heart failure.

Echocardiogram:
- TTE
  - dilated LA

- Doppler to quantify degree of MR
- assess LV function
- confirm diagnosis, may indicate cause.
- TOE:
  - better than TTE for visualising the left side of the heart
  - used prior to surgery.

Asymptomatic

Serial echocardiograms.

Symptomatic

Medical
- Treat AF and heart failure

- Vasodilators: reduce regurgitant volume by reducing afterload.

Surgical
Indications: Severe MR with a dilated, impaired LV
- with a dilated LV (usually with impaired function)

Surgical options:
- valve repair; preferable if technically possible.
- valve replacement.

New developments

A percutaneous technique (MitraClip) to repair the mitral valve without open heart surgery.

Prognosis

Severe symptomatic MR: poor prognosis (70% mortality in 7 years).

Complications

- Heart failure
- AF and its complications (e.g. embolic stroke)

- Infective endocarditis: more common than in mitral stenosis.

MITRAL VALVE PROLAPSE

Outline

Mitral valve (bicuspid valve): found between the LA and LV.
Prolapse of the valve during systole: the valve flaps into the LA:

- commonest congenital cause of mitral regurgitation.
- tricuspid involved in 20–40%
- ↑ incidence of arrhythmias.

Pathogenesis/aetiology

Causes

- 1° or idiopathic: commonest
- 2°: dilated cardiomyopathy (e.g. due to IHD)
- rheumatic heart disease

- connective tissue disorders, e.g. Marfan, Ehlers–Danlos, pseudoxanthoma elasticum, osteogenesis imperfecta.

Pathogenesis

- Myxomatous degeneration causes ballooning of valve leaflets

- Posterior leaflet most commonly affected
- Associated MR due to valve prolapse.

Who

Common: ~3% adults affected.

Association

- ASD (secundum): 20% of cases
- Wolff–Parkinson–White syndrome

- Turner syndrome
- Connective tissue disorders.

Clinical features

Symptoms

- Usually asymptomatic
- Atypical chest pain

- Palpitations.

Signs

Mid-systolic click (tension of chordae tendinae) followed by late systolic murmur over the apex.

Murmur can become pan-systolic as the prolapse worsens.

Investigations

ECG

Non-specific ST or T wave changes.

Imaging

Echocardiogram:
- TTE:
  - displacement of leaflets into the LA.

Treatment

- Reassurance
- Investigate and treat associated arrhythmias
- Treat associated MR as above

- Treat AF
- Endocarditis prophylaxis no longer recommended (NICE guidelines).

Prognosis and complications

Prognosis

Most patients lead a normal life.

Complications

- MR
- Infective endocarditis

- Chordae rupture: acute MR
- Fatal arrhythmias and sudden death (uncommon).

AORTIC STENOSIS

Outline

- Aortic valve lies between LV and the aorta
- Stenosis: narrowing of the valve orifice, limiting forward flow
- Narrowed valve reduces outflow and increases back pressure on the LV. This results in LV hypertrophy to maintain cardiac output, leading to elevated end-diastolic pressures and reduced coronary perfusion
- Eventually decompensation or LV failure occurs (often from LV dilatation)
- Chronic, progressive.

Aortic sclerosis

Aortic valve leaflet thickening without obstruction to cardiac output (mild sclerosis found in 25% population >65 years).

Murmur similar to aortic stenosis but no features of haemodynamic effect.

Pathogenesis/aetiology

Causes

- Valvular:
  - degenerative calcification (senile): commonest
  - congenital bicuspid valve: early onset of aortic stenosis aged 30–50
  - rheumatic heart disease
- Supravalvular: William syndrome: elf-like face, hypercalcaemia, aortic stenosis.

Who

- Commonest valve lesion in the UK
- Present in 2% of those >65 years
- Bicuspid aortic valve in 1–2% population.

Associations

- GI bleeding: angiodysplasia (Heyde's syndrome)
- Turner syndrome: bicuspid valve.

Clinical features

Signs

SAD: **s**yncope, **a**ngina, **d**yspnoea
Symptoms of heart failure

Signs

- Murmur features:
  - ejection systolic murmur
  - crescendo–decrescendo
  - ejection click before the murmur from deformed valve (only if mobile)
  - radiates to carotids
- Sounds:
  - S2: soft, reversed splitting and absent entirely if severe
  - S4: apex defining a stiff-walled LV
  - systolic thrill over aortic region (palpable) (Fig. 2.22).
- Pulse:
  - narrow pulse pressure
  - slow rising at carotids

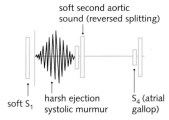

Fig. 2.22 Signs seen in mitral regurgitation.

- Apex beat: sustained (heaving), displaced only with LV dilatation and decompensation.

Investigations

ECG

- LV hypertrophy
- Left axis deviation
- P mitrale from LA enlargement

- AV block: common as calcific degeneration of the valve occurs in close proximity to the AV node.

Imaging

Echocardiogram:
- TTE:
  - calcified non-mobile valve
  - Doppler to assess gradient across valve as well as any coexistent aortic regurgitation
  - LV function

- severe aortic stenosis: aortic valve area <1 cm^2 or gradient >60 mmHg.

CXR:
- Prominence of ascending aorta (post-stenotic dilatation)
- Valvular calcification.

Treatment

Asymptomatic

Serial echocardiograms.

Symptomatic

- Patients should be assessed for suitability for aortic valve surgery which is the treatment of choice in symptomatic patients.

Medical therapy may temporarily treat symptoms but is relatively futile.

- Beta-blockers: ↓ myocardial demand
- Diuretics: for symptoms of heart failure (caution, avoid causing hypovolaemia)
- Avoid drugs which reduce afterload, e.g. nitrates, ACE inhibitors.

Surgical

Assessed for definitive treatment:
- surgical aortic valve replacement: 1–2% operative mortality, patients often require bypass surgery at the same time

- balloon valvuloplasty: in children with congenital lesions or as a palliative procedure in those patients being considered for a TAVI.

New developments

Transcatheter aortic valve implantation (TAVI): alternative to open heart surgery in those deemed unsuitable for surgical aortic valve replacement; uses a transfemoral or transapical approach. Likely to become more mainstream for a larger proportion of patients in the next decade.

Prognosis and complications

Prognosis

Symptomatic aortic stenosis has a very poor prognosis owing to fatal arrhythmias and pump failure:
- 2-year mortality for those with symptoms 50%.

AORTIC REGURGITATION

Outline

Aortic valve lies between LV and the aorta:
- Incompetent valves allow blood flow in the wrong direction (regurgitant jets) causing a build up of back pressure or volume
- Aortic valve allows back flow of blood into the LV
- Higher volumes in the LV causes increased stretch and contractility (Starling principle), thus requiring increased stroke volume to compensate

- Over time the LV dilates and cardiac output becomes compromised
- Left ventricular failure ensues with symptoms of heart failure.

Acute aortic regurgitation

May be caused by trauma, type A aortic dissection, resulting in pulmonary oedema.

Pathogenesis/aetiology

Causes

Leaflet abnormality:
- infective endocarditis
- degenerative mixed aortic valve disease
- rheumatic fever

Aortic root abnormality (dilatation leading to functional aortic regurgitation):
- connective tissue disorders, e.g. Marfan, Ehlers–Danlos
- infection, e.g. syphilis
- inflammatory, e.g. HLA-B27 spondyloarthropathies
- aortic dissection.

Who

Associations

Connective tissue disease.

Clinical features

Symptoms

- Symptoms of heart failure:
  - Dyspnoea
  - Orthopnoea
  - Paroxysmal nocturnal dyspnoea
  - Leg swelling
  - Palpitations

- Fatigue
- Angina (↓ coronary perfusion)
- Symptoms of aortic dissection:
  - Tearing chest pain
  - Pain radiating to the back.

Signs

- Murmur features:
  - Early diastolic murmur (loudest at the left lower sternal edge in expiration, sitting forward)
  - Murmur: the longer the murmur, the more severe the jet of aortic regurgitation
  - Ejection systolic murmur may be heard (coexistent aortic stenosis or high-turbulent flow)
  - Austin–Flint murmur: murmur of functional mitral stenosis caused by a large regurgitant jet pushing the mitral valve leaflet backwards
- Sounds:
  - S1 normal
  - S2 soft (leaflets never meet)
  - S3 present if LV dilated
- Pulse:
  - Collapsing
  - Wide pulse pressure (water hammer pulse)
- *Apex beat*: inferoaterally displaced, hyperdynamic (↑ SV)
- Signs related to the wide pulse pressure:
  - Quincke's: capillary pulsation in nailbed

- De Musset's: head bobbing
- Corrigan's: carotid pulsation visible at ears
- Durozier's: femoral artery bruit
- Traub's: pistol shot heard at the femoral artery
- Muller's: pulsating uvula (Fig. 2.23).

Fig. 2.23   Signs seen in aortic regurgitation.

Investigations

ECG

LV hypertrophy.

Imaging

Echocardiogram
- TTE:
  - Doppler to estimate severity
  - LV function.

CXR:
- Cardiomegaly
- Dilated ascending aorta
- Pulmonary venous congestion.

Treatment

Asymptomatic and normal LV

Serial echocardiograms.

Symptomatic or evidence of LV dysfunction

- Surgical aortic valve replacement, with root replacement if the aortic root is dilated
- Treat heart failure:
  - diuretics for fluid overload

- vasodilators, e.g. ACE inhibitors
- Rate control agents for tachyarrhythmias: caution with beta-blockers if LV function is very poor
- Anti-anginals.

Prognosis and complications

Prognosis

- Chronic aortic regurgitation tolerated for many years
- Acute aortic regurgitation has a high mortality

- Asymptomatic and with a normal LV function: 5 year mortality 25%.

Complications

- Infective endocarditis
- Heart failure

- Fatal arrhythmias.

TRICUSPID STENOSIS

Outline

- Tricuspid valve: between RA and RV
- Stenosis: narrowing of the valve orifice, limiting forward flow

- Narrowed valve causes reduced outflow into the RV.

Pathogenesis/aetiology

Causes

- Rheumatic fever
- CHD

- Carcinoid (but regurgitation is more common)
- Obstructing pacemaker lead.

Who

Uncommon.

Clinical features

Symptoms

- Leg swelling

- Fatigue.

Signs

- JVP: raised, prominent 'a' waves
- Mid-diastolic murmur: loudest in inspiration at the left lower sternal edge

- Hepatomegaly and ascites.

Investigations

ECG

- P pulmonale: right atrial enlargement

- Often features of left atrial enlargement (P mitrale) if coexistent mitral stenosis.

Imaging

Echocardiogram:
- TTE:
  - stenotic leaflet
  - coexistent mitral stenosis.

CXR:
- Enlarged RA.

Treatment

- Salt restriction and diuretics for peripheral oedema
- Valvuloplasty if undergoing mitral valve surgery; tricuspid valve rarely replaced

- Percutaneous balloon valvuloplasty can be performed in some cases.

Prognosis and complications

Prognosis

Related to underlying disease.

TRICUSPID REGURGITATION

Outline

- Tricuspid valve: between RA and RV
- Regurgitation: incompetent valves allow blood flow in the wrong direction (regurgitant jets) causing a build up of back pressure or volume

- Valve allows backflow of blood into the RA.

Pathogenesis/aetiology

Causes

- Functional from RV dilatation: most common
- RV infarction
- CHD (↑ right-sided volumes)
- Pulmonary hypertension
- Infective endocarditis: IDU (often *Staphylococcus aureus*)

- Rheumatic fever
- Carcinoid
- Ebstein's malformation: atrialisation of RV due to maternal lithium therapy.

Who

Uncommon.

Clinical features

Symptoms

- Right heart failure:
  - peripheral oedema
  - fatigue

- Anorexia, nausea
- Abdominal pain.

Signs

- JVP: raised, giant 'v' waves
- RV parasternal heave
- Often in AF
- Pan-systolic murmur at the left lower sternal edge, loudest on inspiration

- S3 common
- Pulsatile, tender hepatomegaly
- Ascites
- Peripheral oedema.

Investigations

ECG

Non-specific abnormalities often with features of right heart pathology e.g right axis deviation, conduction delay.

Imaging

Echocardiogram:
- TTE:
  - estimate pulmonary pressures by calculating velocity of TR jet.

CXR:
- Cardiomegaly.

Treatment

Treatment depends on cause:
- Salt restriction and diuretics for right heart failure
- Coexistent IHD, coronary revascularisation may be indicated

- 2° to mitral stenosis, may improve following surgery on the mitral valve.

Prognosis and complications

Prognosis

Depends on cause.

PULMONARY STENOSIS

Outline

- Pulmonary valve: between the RV and the pulmonary artery
- Stenosis: narrowing of the valve orifice, limiting forward flow

- Narrowed valve causes ↓ outflow and ↑ back pressure on the RV.

Pathogenesis/aetiology

Causes

- Usually congenital, e.g. Noonan syndrome
- Carcinoid

- Rheumatic fever.

Who

Uncommon.

Association

CHD.

Clinical features

Symptoms

Dyspnoea.

Signs

- RV heave
- JVP: raised, prominent 'a' wave

- Widely split S2 (P2 closure delayed).

Investigations

ECG

- Right axis deviation

- RV hypertrophy.

Imaging

CXR:
- Post-stenotic pulmonary artery dilatation.

Echocardiogram
- TTE:
  - demonstrates gradient and level of obstruction
  - shows associated structural abnormalities.

Treatment

- Salt restriction and diuretics for right heart failure
- Balloon valvuloplasty for gradients >50 mmHg

- Surgical valvotomy (open procedure): higher risk of subsequent pulmonary regurgitation
- Surgical pulmonary valve replacement.

Prognosis and complications

Prognosis

Depends on cause.

PULMONARY REGURGITATION

Outline

- Pulmonary valve: between the RV and the pulmonary artery
- Regurgitation: incompetent valves allow blood flow in the wrong direction (regurgitant jets) causing a build up of back pressure or volume

- Valve allows backflow of blood into the RV.

Pathogenesis/aetiology

Causes

Any cause of raised pulmonary pressures causing cor pulmonale (e.g. COPD):
- Pulmonary hypertension

- Infective endocarditis: IDU
- Carcinoid
- Post-pulmonary valvotomy.

Who

Uncommon.

Clinical features

Symptoms

- Usually asymptomatic

- Symptoms with right heart failure (as for TR).

Signs

- RV heave
- JVP raised
- Delayed P2 (↑ stroke volume)

- Loud P2: pulmonary hypertension
- Early-diastolic murmur: loudest at the upper left sternal edge on inspiration (Graham Steell murmur).

Investigations

ECG

RV hypertrophy, often with right bundle branch block.

Imaging

CXR:
- Large pulmonary trunk.

Echocardiogram
- TTE:
  - large RV chamber size
  - RV function
  - associated tricuspid regurgitation.

Treatment

- Salt restriction and diuretics for right heart failure
- Treat pulmonary hypertension
- Surgical pulmonary valve. Percutaneous pulmonary valve implantation (PPVI) is used in patients with

congenital tetralogy of Fallot. Replacement may be needed in severe RV failure.

Prognosis and complications

Prognosis

Depends on cause.

INFECTIVE ENDOCARDITIS

Outline

- Infection of the endocardium of the heart
- Bacteraemia precipitates the adherence of microorganisms to heart valves
- Any cause of bacteraemia or valvular abnormality ↑ the risk of developing endocarditis.

Causes of bacteraemia:
- IVDU: right-sided valves affected owing to venous injection of drugs
- Poor oral hygiene and dental cavities
- Any instrumentation, e.g. surgery, recent central line, catheterisation
- Immunosuppressive conditions, e.g. diabetes mellitus, alcohol excess, chronic renal failure (CRF).

Abnormal valves:
- Turbulent flow makes valves more vulnerable to vegetation adhesion:
  - Stratified according to risk:
    - High: prosthetic valves, mixed mitral valve disease, AV disease, cyanotic CHD
    - Moderate: isolated mitral stenosis, mitral valve prolapse with MR, bicuspid aortic valve, hypertrophic obstructive cardiomyopathy
    - Low: mitral valve prolapse without MR, tricuspid regurgitation, isolated ASD.

Pathogenesis/aetiology

Pathogenesis

- 'Vegetations' comprising fibrin, platelets and microorganisms attach to and can destroy the valve
- This causes valve prolapse and regurgitation and acute cardiac decompensation in some cases

- The immune response can lead to immune complex deposition, which is responsible for many of the features
- Emboli may be dislodged from the vegetation causing embolic phenomena.

Infective agents

- *Streptoccocus viridans*:
  - Commonest, 50–60%
  - Commensal of the upper respiratory tract
- *Staphylococcus* (25%): those with central lines, prosthetic valves and IDUs
  - *Staphylococcus aureus* (coagulase positive)
  - *Staphylococcus epidermidis* (coagulase negative)
- *Enterococcus faecalis* (10%): urogenital or bowel surgery

- Culture-negative group (all are Gram negative)
  - HACEK (5%) (*Haemophilus, Actinobacillus actinomycetencomitans, Cardiobacterium hominis, Eikenella, Kingella*)
- Mycobacteria
- Chlamydia
- *Coxiella* (Q fever)
- Fungi.

Non-infective causes

- Marantic: non-bacterial thrombotic endocarditis; sterile vegetations associated with adenocarcinoma

- Lupus: Libman–Sacks endocarditis has small vegetations of inflammation and sterile thrombi.

Who

- Incidence: 7/10 000 per year in the UK
- Commonest aged 50–60 years
- ♀2:♂3

- Presentation of IE is highly variable therefore have a high index of suspicion in any patient with a fever and a new murmur. Symptoms in the elderly may be non-specific.

Valves affected

- Aortic > mitral > > tricuspid
- Aortic, mitral 80%

- In IVDUs the tricuspid valve is most often affected.

A typical patient

A 55-year-old man develops a fever, night sweats and a new murmur. He had a prosthetic heart valve inserted 5 years ago.

Clinical features

Features of infection

General:
- Fever
- Night sweats
- Malaise
- Fatigue
- Anaemia
- Anorexia
- Weight loss

- Splenomegaly (25%)
- Clubbing.

Cardiac:
- Valve destruction leading to a *new* murmur (90%)
- Heart failure
- Arrhythmias, conduction delay (AV node block from aortic valve abscess)
- Pericarditis.

Immune complex deposition

- Skin:
  - petechiae (common)
  - Osler's nodes: painful pulp nodules of the digits (rare)
  - Janeway lesions: painless palmar lesions (rare)

  - splinter haemorrhages (non-specific)
- Eye: Roth spots (retinal haemorrhages with pale centre)
- Kidney: microscopic haematuria, glomerulonephritis and acute kidney injury.

Embolic phenomena

Septic emboli causing:
- Stroke
- Acute limb ischaemia

- Acute kidney injury
- Most common with *Staphylococcus*, fungal and Gram-negative infections.

Investigations

Blood tests

- FBC
- U&E
- LFTs

- Clotting
- CRP.

Infection screen

As many blood cultures as possible from different sites at least 1–2 h apart; need two positive blood cultures.

Urine

- Dipstick: haematuria

- Microscopy and culture.

Other swabs

From any wounds, cavities.

ECG

Conduction delay (PR interval), AV node block (aortic root abscess in AV endocarditis).

Imaging

Echocardiogram:
- TTE:
  - to look for vegetations, abscess, congenital lesions, LV function. Often TTE cannot exclude endocarditis and a transoesophageal echo is needed to provide higher resolution imaging of the heart valves to look for vegetations.

CXR:
- Pulmonary venous congestions, pulmonary infarcts from emboli in right-sided endocarditis.

Modified Duke's criteria for diagnosis

Requires: 2 major *or* 1 major and 3 minor *or* all 5 minor:
- Major:
  - Positive blood cultures: typical organism in 2 separate cultures
  - Positive echocardiogram (vegetation, abscess)
  - New valvular regurgitation
- Minor:
  - Predisposition e.g poor dental hygiene, recent instrumentation, IDU

- Fever >38 °C
- Vascular phenomena, e.g. embolic stroke
- Immunological phenomena, e.g. glomerulonephritis, Roth spots, positive blood cultures not meeting major criteria
- Positive echocardiogram not meeting major criteria.

Treatment

Management

- >3 blood cultures before starting treatment
- Discuss with microbiology as local protocols differ
- If patient has a prosthetic valve endocarditis, medical therapy is more aggressive and threshold for surgery is lower
- Treatment may change with sensitivity results.

Regimen examples

Often, at least 4 weeks of IV therapy; may require peripherally inserted central catheter (PICC line):
- *Streptococcus viridans*: 4 weeks of IV benzylpenicillin and gentamicin then 2 weeks of oral penicillin
- *Staphylococcus aureus*: flucloxacillin and gentamicin (methicillin-sensitive *Staphylococcus aureus* (MSSA)),

or vancomycin and gentamicin (methicillin-resistant *Staphylococcus aureus* (MRSA)) plus rifampicin if prosthetic valve
- *Enterococci*: amoxicillin and gentamicin.

Monitoring progress

- Review of clinical symptoms, particularly worsening heart failure and new embolic phenomena
- Repeat cultures
- Biochemistry: trends in WBC, CRP, renal and liver function
- Change cannulae every 72 h (or consider PICC line)
- Regular ECG: looking for new-onset conduction delay or AV node block
- Serial echocardiograms
- Discuss with cardiothoracic centre.

Indications for surgery

- Prosthetic valve dehiscence
- Fungal endocarditis
- Poor clinical response after antibiotics
- Severe heart failure
- Secondary valvular regurgitation
- Aortic root abscess with heart block.

Prophylaxis

NICE no longer recommends routine prophylactic antibiotics to all, only a select proportion in the higher anatomical risk category.

Prognosis and complications

Prognosis

- 30% mortality with *Staphylococcus*
- 6% mortality with *Streptococcus*.

Complications

- Acute heart failure
- Valve dysfunction, regurgitation
- Septic shock
- Septic thromboemboli and infarcts: commonest cause of death (via stroke and acute kidney injury)
- Glomerulonephritis.

RHEUMATIC FEVER

Outline

Post-infectious syndrome: sequelae of infection with group A beta haemolytic *Streptococcus pyogenes*:
- Caused by antigenic mimicry
- Multisystem involvement: heart, joints, skin, brain
- If untreated progresses to rheumatic heart disease causing valvular dysfunction (primarily through stenoses) over an insidious period.

Rheumatic heart disease

- Average lag time of 20 years between acute rheumatic fever and chronic manifestations of cardiac involvement
- Fibrosis leads to retraction of heart valves by shortening and thickening chordae; this leads to regurgitation and stenosis
- Regurgitation: occurs as the leaflets are unable to close properly
- Stenosis: occurs through commissural fusion and surrounding fibrosis
- Proportion of valves affected:
  - Most commonly affects the mitral and aortic valves, far less frequently involving the right side of the heart.

Pathogenesis/aetiology

Pathogenesis

- Usually 2–4 weeks after a pharyngitis

- Caused by autoimmune cross-reaction of antibodies made to the cell wall of *Streptococcus pyogenes* and proteins on cardiac valves.

Characteristic lesions

- Aschoff bodies: granulomatous nodules with central necrosis and fibrinoid degeneration, surrounded by macrophages

- Anitschkow cells: altered macrophages within Aschoff body showing nuclei with a ribbon-like chromatin pattern.

Who

- Rare in developed world (use of antibiotics to treat *Streptococcus* throat infection)
- Common in developing world (prevalence 1%)
- Mostly children: 5–15 years

- ♂ ♀
- Higher in lower socioeconomic classes
- Higher in overcrowding.

A typical patient

A 15-year-old girl presents to hospital with a pink rash over her body and recent-onset joint pain in her hands, knees and elbows. She says that she has recently recovered from a sore throat.

Clinical features

Clinical presentation – assessed with Jones criteria:
- Diagnosis confirmed with evidence of recent group A streptococcal infection plus either 2 major criteria or 1 major *and* 2 minor criteria:
  - Major:
    - Joint: polyarthritis (80%): typically flitting (<3 weeks per joint) and mainly affecting large joints; starting in the lower limbs
    - Obviously, cardiac (40–50%): pancarditis (inflammation of all heart layers: peri, myo, endocardium) with valvular dysfunction and heart failure
    - Nodule (rare): subcutaneous nodules over bony prominences

- Erythema marginatum (5%): pink rash with central clearing, persistent fading and reappearing hours afterwards
- Sydenham chorea (10%): jerky involuntary movement affecting: head/face/limbs; sudden movements resulting in prolonged posture, indicating CNS involvement.
- Minor:
  - Inflammatory cells: ↑ WBC
  - Temperature: fever
  - ESR/CRP: elevated
  - PR interval prolonged
  - Previous history of rheumatic fever
  - Arthralgia.

Signs of recent *Streptococcus* infection

- History of scarlet fever
- Positive throat swab

- ↑ Anti-streptolysin O titre, serology tests 2 weeks apart
- ↑ DNase B titre.

Investigations

As per Jones criteria.

Cardiac investigation

- ECG: any conduction delay and arrhythmias

- TTE to assess for valvular and LV dysfunction.

Treatment

Management

- Bed rest and cardiac monitoring if cardiac involvement
- IM benzylpenicillin (single dose) for acute infection or oral penicillin for 10 days (macrolide if penicillin allergic). Treat heart failure if evident.

Sequelae

- Pancarditis: anti-inflammatory agents, e.g. aspirin, NSAIDs for arthritis, steroids although NSAIDs can be harmful in exacerbating heart failure through water retention therefore use with caution.

- Chorea: haloperidol or diazepam
- Heart failure: diuretics, ACE inhibitors, beta blockers, mineralocorticoid antagonists (MRA).

Treatment

Secondary prophylaxis

Penicillin to prevent relapse.

Prognosis and complications

Prognosis

- Acute attack lasts 3 months

- Initial mortality: 1%.

Complications

60% of those with carditis develop chronic rheumatic heart disease, valve disease, stenosis and regurgitation.

MYOCARDIAL DISEASE

Cardiomyopathy: disorder of the heart muscle.
Important causes of sudden cardiac death in the young adult:
- Classified as:
  - 1°: intrinsic HARD:
    - **H**ypertrophic obstructive cardiomyopathy
    - **A**rrhythmogenic RV cardiomyopathy
    - **R**estrictive cardiomyopathy
    - **D**ilated cardiomyopathy

- 2° to:
  - Systemic disease (far more common)
  - Ischaemic (commonest)
  - Hypertension
  - Valvular disorder
  - Inflammatory.

DILATED CARDIOMYOPATHY

Outline

- Dilated flabby heart that contracts poorly
- There is LV hypertrophy and dilatation and increase in heart weight

- Dilatation causes a globular heart shape and may mask hypertrophy
- Leads to heart failure and can lead to fatal arrhythmias.

Pathogenesis/aetiology

Causes

Multifactorial and numerous:
- Commonest, idiopathic
  - hypertension
  - alcohol excess
  - chemotherapy e.g anthracycline

- Less common:
  - inherited myopathy
  - peripartum
  - thyrotoxicosis
  - haemochromatosis
  - nutritional deficiency (thiamine, beri beri)
  - autoimmune.

Pathology

Biopsy demonstrates:
- Haphazard architecture with myocyte and nuclear enlargement

- T lymphocyte infiltration and fibrosis.

Who

Commonest form of cardiomyopathy.

Clinical features

Features of heart failure:
- SOB
- Fatigue

- Nausea
- Oedema
- Ascites.

Signs

- Tachycardia
- Tachynpoea
- Peripheral cyanosis
- S3 heart sound
- Mitral regurgitation

- Basal crepitations
- Pleural effusions
- ↑ JVP
- Hepatomegaly.

Investigations

Investigations for an underlying cause and patient risk stratification.

Blood tests

- U&Es, LFTs, TFTs
- Iron studies
- Autoimmune screen

- Infection screen (to include relevant serology)
- Genetic screening for inherited cardiomyopathies (in specialist centres).

ECG

- To look for a potential cause e.g prior MI, small QRS complexes in infiltrative cardiomyopathy. Most other findings are non specific abnormalities indicative of pathology e.g T wave changes, poor R wave progression

- 24-h ECG for tachyarrhythmias
- Exercise testing to assess functional capacity.

Imaging

CXR:
- To look for features of heart failure

Echocardiogram:
- Dilated chamber size
- Thrombus in LV
- Valve dysfunction
- Ejection fraction.

Cardiac MRI:
- Exquisite image quality to exclude ischaemia (IHD) and demonstrate potential causes.

Cardiac biopsy:
- Percutaneous procedure rarely required due to excellent diagnostic utility of cardiac MRI.

Treatment

- Treat heart failure and arrhythmias (see p. 30)
- Treat underlying cause
- Consider cardiac resynchronisation therapy: percutaneous procedure, a lead is placed at the back of the LV (via coronary sinus) and standard 2 pacemaker leads to the RA and RV to enable

resynchronisation of the ventricles and to improve pump function this reduces mortality
- Anticoagulation: if evidence of thrombus
- Cardiac transplantation can be considered if refractory to above treatment measures, however, only 100/year in UK, therefore rarely available.

Prognosis and complications

Prognosis

- See heart failure

- 50% mortality in 2 years.

Complications 2° to ventricular dilatation

- Tachyarrhythmias causing sudden cardiac death
- LV thrombus, with embolism causing stroke

- Valve dysfunction or regurgitation as leaflets cannot meet, causing reduced flow and heart failure.

HYPERTROPHIC CARDIOMYOPATHY

Outline

- Hypertrophy or enlargement of the LV walls, particularly the interventricular septum

- Stiff ventricular walls limit diastolic filling and impair cardiac output
- Can lead to sudden cardiac death in the young.

Pathogenesis/aetiology

Cause

- Mostly familial, autosomal dominant from mutations in genes encoding cardiac contractile proteins:
  - Beta-myosin heavy chain
  - Troponin T
  - Troponin I
  - α-Tropomyosin

  - Myosin-binding protein C
  - Myosin light chains
  - >10 genes identified
- Variable penetrance of disease
- Phenotypical variability.

Pathology

- Disorganised myocyte architecture (disarray)
- Interstitial fibrosis and whirling of myocytes around central focus of collagen

- Abnormal tissue focused around the septum, causing hypertrophy (usually asymmetrical) leading to LV outflow tract obstruction.

Who

- Prevalence: 1.5%
- 50% autosomal dominant form

- Commonest cause of sudden cardiac death in young athletes (through ventricular arrhythmia).

Associations

- Wolff–Parkinson–White syndrome

- Friedreich's ataxia.

A typical patient

A young man is brought in by ambulance having collapsed while running the marathon. His mother says that he has always been healthy but that his father died suddenly when young.

Clinical features

Symptoms

- Often asymptomatic and incidentally picked up through murmur or ECG/echocardiogram
- SOB
- Palpitations

- Syncope/pre-syncope on exercise
- Angina
- Sudden death: may be first presentation of the disease.

Signs

- Jerky apex beat: from LV outflow tract obstruction on systole

- Harsh ejection systolic murmur, mid-systole at left sternal edge (LV outflow tract obstruction) and a palpable thrill
- Murmur is louder during the Valsalva manoeuvre

Investigations

Clinical diagnosis based on factors below. Also need to stratify risk of sudden cardiac death and decide on whether requires primary prevention ICD. Confirm the diagnosis and stratify risk of sudden cardiac death.

ECG

- Deep T wave inversion and ST segment depression
- May be normal
- 24-h ECG for tachyarrhythmias

- Exercise testing to assess functional capacity, look for haemodynamic response to exercise and any ventricular arrhythmias.

Imaging

Echocardiogram:
- Asymmetric septal hypertrophy
- Systolic anterior movement of the mitral valve
- Small LV cavity size.

- Hyperdynamic LV systolic function
- Impaired diastolic function
- Dilated atria

Genetic testing

- With family screening.

Other tests

MRI:
Cardiac MRI very helpful here and can show areas of scar which may be important in risk stratification cardiac catheterisation to demonstrate outflow tract gradients at rest and during pharmacological stress and to show coronary arteries and exclude IHD.

Treatment

- Patient education

- Controlled exercise: >50% of sudden cardiac deaths occur during strenuous activity.

Treatment

Treatment to reduce incidence of sudden cardiac death

Decreasing heart rate directly decreases tachyarrhythmias. Medical:
- Beta-blockers: improved diastolic filing and ↓ myocardial O_2 demand, negatively inotropic
- Calcium channel antagonists: negatively inotropic, ↓ heart rate during activity
- Disopyramide: reduces the obstructive symptoms of HCM
- Sotalol/amiodarone: for atrial tachyarrhythmias

Other:
- Alcohol septal ablation: percutaneous treatment to cause focal necrosis of hypertrophied septum (can cause complete heart block necessitating a pacemaker in 10%)

- Pacemaker: to reduce LV outflow tract gradient
- Implantable cardiac defibrillators: considered in those who have already survived cardiac arrest (secondary prevention) or in those with high risk of SCD (primary prevention)
- Myomectomy: surgical procedure to debulk the septum.

Prognosis and complications

Prognosis

- Depends on clinical manifestation

- Compatible with normal lifespan.

Complications

- Heart failure

- Sudden death.

Risk factors for sudden cardiac death (SCD)

- Young age at diagnosis
- Family history of SCD
- Certain genes

- Non-sustained ventricular tachycardia on 24-h ECG
- Poor BP response on exercise.

RESTRICTIVE CARDIOMYOPATHY

Outline

- Rigid myocardium leading to poor diastolic filling and impaired cardiac output
- Unable to increase cardiac output owing to a fixed stroke volume

- Main differential diagnosis: constrictive pericarditis.

Pathogenesis/aetiology

Causes

- Idiopathic
- Familial
- Systemic sclerosis
- Infiltration: amyloid, sarcoid, haemachromatosis, storage diseases (lysosomal storage diseases, e.g. Fabry or Gaucher, glycogen storage disease)

- Endomyocardial fibrosis (Loeffler's eosinophilia)
- Malignancy
- Carcinoid
- Iatrogenic (anthracyclines, radiation).

Who

- Rare but commonest cause in UK is infiltration from amyloid

- Commoner in developing world because of increased incidence of endocardial fibrosis from infection.

Clinical features

Cannot be distinguished clinically from constrictive pericarditis, requires cardiac catheterisation (left and right side) for this.

Symptoms

- Exertional SOB and ↓ exercise tolerance
- Fatigue

- Hepatomegaly.

Clinical features

Signs

- Oedema
- Ascites
- Palpable apex
- Loud S3 and/or S4

- ↑ JVP
- Prominent 'x' and 'y' descents
- Kussmaul sign: paradoxical rising of the JVP on inspiration.

Investigations

ECG

P mitrale and P pulmonale revealing atrial dilation. Conduction delay.

Imaging

Echocardiogram:
- LV systolic function often normal
- Infiltration may be seen with speckled myocardium (e.g. amyloid)

- Doppler flow shows restrictive filling (impaired relaxation).

Other tests

- Cardiac biopsy: rarely required due to cardiac MRI
- Serum amyloid protein scan (SAP) if amyloid suspected / bone marrow to look for plasma cells.

Cardiac catheterisation:
- To exclude constrictive pericarditis
- At the end of expiration, LV and RV end-diastolic pressures *differ* in restrictive cardiomyopathy but are the same in constrictive pericarditis.

Treatment

- Treat heart failure

- Rate control any arrhythmias.

Prognosis and complications

Prognosis

Poor, most die within 1 year but dependent on cause

Complications

- Thromboembolic complications
- Pulmonary hypertension

- RV hypertrophy and failure.

MYOCARDITIS

Outline

- Inflammation of the myocardium

- Usually viral infection but rarely identified.

Pathogenesis/aetiology

Causes

Viral
- Cardioselective: coxsackievirus B (commonest in Western world), adenovirus, echoviruses

Non-viral:
- Chlamydia
- Rickettsiae (typhus fever)
- Bacteria: diphtheria (*Corynebacterium diphtheriae*), Lyme disease (*Borrelia* spp.), meningococcus (*Neisseria meningitidis*)

Non-infectious:
- Immune reactions: postviral, rheumatic fever, lupus, drug hypersensitivity, transplant rejection, radiation injury

- Non-selective: any systemic viral infection: HIV, rubella, mumps, cytomegalovirus (CMV), poliovirus.

- Fungi: *Candida*, *Aspergillus*
- Protozoa: *Trypanosoma*, toxoplasmosis (*Toxoplasma gondii*)
- Helminths.

- Unknown aetiology: sarcoidosis, giant cell myocarditis.

Who

All ages affected.

Clinical features

Range of symptoms from asymptomatic to fulminant heart failure:
- Fever
- Fatigue
- SOB
- Chest pain
- Palpitations

- Tachycardia
- Risk of sudden cardiac death in a small proportion therefore require risk stratification in hospital, kept under observation until deemed safe for discharge.

Investigations

Prove the presence of systemic infection and concordant cardiac disease.

Bloods tests

Serology for infectious agents.

ECG

Non-specific T and ST changes.

Imaging

CXR: feature of heart failure.

Treatment

- Supportive therapy
- Appropriate antimicrobial agents

- Treatment of heart failure

Prognosis and complications

Prognosis

Ranges from complete recovery to fulminant heart failure and death (tiny proportion).

PERICARDIAL DISEASE

ACUTE PERICARDITIS

Outline

- Acute inflammation of the pericardium (sac surrounding the heart)
- Can be 1° or 2° to systemic disease

- The inflamed pericardium may be infiltrated by white cells and develop adhesions. Fluid accumulation causes a pericardial effusion.

Pathogenesis/aetiology

Causes

CARDIAC:
- **C**onnective tissue disease: lupus, scleroderma
- **A**utoimmune
- **R**adiation
- **D**rugs: hydralazine
- **I**nfections: coxsackie virus, also streptococcal, TB; bacteria lead to purulent pericarditis

- **I**diopathic
- **I**njury: trauma (bleed) or after surgery
- **I**nfiltrative: neoplasms
- **A**cute renal failure: uraemia
- **C**ardiac: MI, Dressler syndrome: post MI, rheumatic fever.

Who

- ♀ < ♂
- More common in adults than children

- Infection is the commonest cause.

A typical patient

A 45-year-old man complains of chest pain that is relieved on sitting forward. He describes a recent flu-like illness. On auscultation a pericardial friction rub is heard.

Symptoms

- Central chest pain
- Pain worse on lying flat
- Sharp pain on movement, relieved on sitting forward
- Radiates to neck and shoulders

- Symptoms relate to underlying cause, e.g. fever
- Pain may be pleuritic in nature: worsens on inspiration and so causes the patient to catch their breath.

Signs

- Pericardial friction rub: pathognomonic of disease; heard best at the left lower sternal edge.

Infection screen

Blood culture.

ECG

Global, concave (saddle-shaped) ST elevation. PR segment depression is a highly sensitive sign but present infrequently (Fig. 2.24).

Imaging

CXR:
- Signs of pneumonia as differential diagnosis including pleurisy.

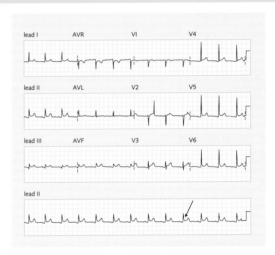

Fig. 2.24 ECG showing saddle-shaped ST elevation typical of pericarditis.

- Treat cause
- Analgesia

- NSAIDs (high dose) and proton pump inhibitor cover
- Steroids/colchicine in resistant disease.

Prognosis

- 15–40% recur (these relapses have a worse outcome)

- Otherwise good prognosis

Complications

- Recurrence
- Pericardial effusion

- Cardiac tamponade
- Constrictive pericarditis.

CONSTRICTIVE PERICARDITIS

Pericardium (sac around the heart) becomes rigid and prevents adequate diastolic filling of the ventricles.

Causes

- TB (commonest worldwide cause)
- Radiation

- Prior trauma
- Sequelae of pericarditis (most often relapsing type).

Pathogenesis

Fibrinous inflammatory exudates become calcified over time; as a result, the heart is unable to properly expand and fill.

Who

Most commonly caused by TB or radiation.

Clinical features

Presents usually with right heart failure:
- Ascites
- Hepatosplenomegaly

- Oedema
- ↑ JVP
- Kussmaul's sign: JVP rises on inspiration.

Other

- Low volume pulse
- Prominent 'x'/'y' descents of the JVP
- Pulsus paradoxus: exaggerated fall in systolic BP on inspiration
- Hypotension

- Impalpable apex beat
- Quiet heart sounds
- Pericardial knock (at time of S3) on auscultation; caused by the abrupt end of ventricular filling.

Investigations

ECG

Small QRS complexes.

Imaging

CXR:
- Normal heart size

Echocardiogram:
- Restrictive filling pattern.

CT/MRI:
- Pericardial thickening and calcification.

- Pericardial calcification common.

Other tests

Cardiac catheterisation:

- For diagnosis: elevation and equalisation of LV and RV end-diastolic pressures (differing right and left pressures in restrictive cardiomyopathy).

Treatment

Surgical excision of the pericardium – a long and difficult procedure with an accompanying peri-operative mortality of 10%. Even post operatively, many patients do badly.

Prognosis and complications

Complications

AF common in chronic stage of the disease due to atrial enlargement.

PERICARDIAL EFFUSION AND TAMPONADE

Outline

Pericardial effusion

Fluid in the pericardium (sac around the heart) restricting ventricular filling and impairing cardiac output.

Cardiac tamponade

Occurs when an effusion is sufficiently large enough to impair cardiac filling and cause a reduction in stroke volume (a clinical diagnosis)

A **medical emergency** can present:
- Acutely, e.g. from trauma (haemorrhagic effusion)
- Chronically/subacutely: with a serous or purulent effusion.

Pathogenesis/aetiology

Causes

- Trauma
- Pericarditis
- Aortic dissection (type A)
- CKD, Uraemia
- Post procedural – cardiac surgery, RF ablation, PCI
- MI (cardiac rupture into pericardium, often fatal)
- TB
- Malignancy
- Myxoedema
- Cardiomyopathy (decompensated heart failure).

Who

Affects all ages: tamponade caused by malignancy or renal failure occurs more in elderly patients while that caused by trauma is more common in younger people.

Clinical features

Symptoms

- Central chest pain
- SOB
- Fatigue.

Signs

- Tachycardia
- Pulsus paradoxus: exaggerated fall in systolic BP on inspiration
- Beck's triad for tamponade, DDD:
  - **D**istant heart sounds
  - **D**istended jugular veins, ↑ JVP with Kussmaul's sign
  - **D**ecreased arterial pressure, hypotension.

Investigations

ECG

- Low-voltage QRS
- Non-specific T wave changes
- Electrical alternans.

Imaging

CXR:
- Large globular heart

Echocardiogram:
- Fluid around the heart:
  - accumulation often starts posteriorly and spreads around the heart
- RA systolic and RV diastolic collapse.

Treatment

- Treat underlying cause if not haemodynamically compromised
- Tamponade requires urgent pericardiocentesis, performed in a catheter laboratory
- Recurrent inflammatory pericardial effusions may necessitate surgery (pericardial window to allow drainage into the peritoneum or pericardectomy in some cases): pericardectomy.

Prognosis and complications

Complications

Cardiorespiratory arrest from restriction of blood outflow.

CONGENITAL HEART DISEASE (CHD)

GENERAL FEATURES

Outline

- CHD is one of the commonest congenital defects.
- Progressively better outcomes for infants means there are now more adults alive than children with CHD.

- Often involves complex cardiac surgery when a child and regular follow-up under an adult cardiologist (grown up CHD (GUCH))
- Some patients only first present in adulthood.

Main classification

Acyanotic (left-to-right shunt)
- Atrial septal defect (ASD)
- Ventricular septal defect (VSD)
- Atrioventricular (AV) septal defect

- Patent ductus arteriosus (PDA)
- Coarctation of the aorta.

Cyanotic (right-to-left shunt)
- Transposition of the great vessels
- Tetralogy of Fallot.

NB: left-to-right shunts such as VSD/ASD, which are classified as acyanotic, can develop into right-to-left shunts

(becoming cyanotic), if untreated. This occurs through persistently high right-sided volumes leading to ↑ pulmonary pressures, which overcome left-sided pressures causing shunt reversal (Eisenmenger syndrome).

Pathogenesis/aetiology

Causes

Teratogens:
- Congenital rubella: PDA, pulmonary stenosis
- Alcohol: ASD, VSD.

Associated with genetic disease:
- Down syndrome: AV septal defect

- Turner syndrome: aortic coarctation, bicuspid aortic valve
- Williams syndrome: supravalvar aortic stenosis.

Who

Commonest group of structural malformations: 6–8/1000 liveborn infants.

Clinical features

Auscultation of these patients is very difficult as many of their congenital defects have been partially or completely corrected.

Symptoms

- Exertional SOB
- ↓ Exercise tolerance
- Chest pain

- Palpitations
- Syncope/pre-syncope. Failure to thrive.

Signs

- Syndromic phenotype, e.g. Down syndrome
- Cyanosis
- Finger clubbing
- Previous cardiac surgery: sternotomy, thoracotomy

- Features of congestive heart failure: evidence of RV overload such as ↑ JVP, RV heave, loud P2
- Radiofemoral delay in coarctation.

Investigations

ECG

- Assess for conduction delay or block and tachyarrhythmias
- Exercise testing: to establish change in function.

Imaging

Echocardiogram:
- Must be done in specialist centres as anatomy is complex
- Cardiac MRI often used to delineate anatomy.

CXR:
Examine pulmonary vascular markings for unusual blood volume through the right side of the heart:
$\uparrow$: ASD/VSD
$\downarrow$: pulmonary stenosis.

Other tests

Cardiac catheterisation:
- To show step up/down gradients and O_2 saturations in different chambers
- To show the location and size of intra-/extra-cardiac shunts.

Treatment

Patient education

- Lifestyle modifications, patient education
- Managed under a specialist centre (13 in the UK).

Procedures

- Usually palliative or reparative
- Blalock–Taussig shunt for cyanotic conditions: systemic to pulmonary circulation shunt to improve pulmonary blood flow and oxygenation
- Percutaneous valvuloplasty to widen a stenotic lesion, e.g. pulmonary stenosis
- Percutaneous closure of secundum ASD
- New development: percutaneous pulmonary valve insertion is a trans-catheter valve implantation for those with RV outflow tract dysfunction, avoiding the need for open-heart surgical correction in patients with pulmonary regurgitation.

Prognosis and complications

Prognosis

80–85% survive to adulthood.

Complications

- Arrhythmias
- Heart failure
- Renal failure
- Chronic hypoxia leading to polycythaemia
- Stroke (paradoxical emboli through shunt)
- Eisenmenger syndrome (very high mortality).

Eisenmenger syndrome:
- Large left-to-right shunt leads to increased flow through the pulmonary vasculature. This leads to pulmonary hypertension and increased pressures on the right side of the heart, reversing the flow to a right-to-left shunt and introducing cyanosis.

Pregnancy:
- Care must be delivered in a specialist centre for pregnant patients with CHD.

ACYANOTIC CHD: ATRIAL SEPTAL DEFECT

Outline

- Connection between the RA and LA
- As left-sided pressures are greater than right, blood shunts from LA to RA across the defect in the interatrial septum (throughout systole and diastole).

Patent foramen ovale

- Occurs in up to 25% of people.
- The foramen ovale allows blood to bypass the lungs (going from RA to LA) while the fetus is developing; it should close at birth following the rise in left-sided pressures.
- A patent foramen ovale is more of a channel, which is usually of no clinical significance. Unlike an ASD, blood

only flows through it when RA pressure > LA pressure transiently e.g isometric exercise – weight lifting or raised right-sided pressures for another reason.
- It can, however, cause a paradoxical embolism, where a thrombus from a DVT can cross to the arterial system, embolise and causing a stroke.

Types of ASD

- Secundum (commonest, 75%)
- Primum (associated with mitral or tricuspid valve abnormalities)
- Sinus venosus defect.
(Fig. 2.25).

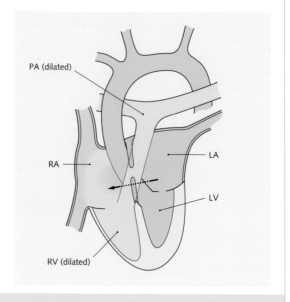

Fig. 2.25 Atrial septal defect.

Who

- May present in adult life (secundum)
- Primum defects are often picked up earlier.

Associations

- Mitral valve prolapse
- Lutembacher syndrome: mitral stenosis and an ASD.

Clinical features

Symptoms

- Recurrent chest infections (as a child)
- Exertional SOB
- Palpitations (new-onset AF/flutter).

Signs

- Features of right-sided volume/pressure increases
- ↑ JVP
- Systolic thrill over pulmonary area
- Ejection systolic murmur in pulmonary area
- Wide fixed splitting of S2 heart sound
- Adults with established untreated ASD may have very high right-sided pressures with:
  - RV heave
  - loud P2
  - end-diastolic murmur.

Investigations

ECG

- Right axis deviation and right bundle branch block (may be incomplete)
- Conduction delay in those with primum ASD (defect near the AV node).

Imaging

CXR:
- Pulmonary plethora (↑ pulmonary vascular markings 2° to raised RV volumes)
- Enlarged RA.

Echocardiogram:
- Identify location and size of defect.

Other tests

- Cardiac catheterisation.

Treatment

- Closure indicated if symptomatic and/or shunt saturations between left and right atria are 2:1 or more:
  - secundum ASD: often closed percutaneously with transcatheter Amplatzer device
- primum/sinus venosus ASD: often requires surgery in childhood, as often associated with valvular dysfunction
- Regular follow-up under specialist cardiac centre to manage arrhythmias, and monitor for features of RV dilatation and dysfunction.

Prognosis and complications

Prognosis

- Good once defects corrected
- Eisenmenger syndrome, if established, has a very bad prognosis but is uncommon with ASD.

Complications

- Atrial arrhythmias are a common, recurrent problem in these patients
- ASD is not high risk for infective endocarditis.

ACYANOTIC CHD: VENTRICULAR SEPTAL DEFECT

Outline

- Connection between two ventricles causing a left-to-right shunt
- Commonest CHD defect
- Smaller the lesion, louder the murmur (maladie de Roger)
- Small lesions self close during childhood (up to 50%)
- Larger lesions with significant shunting need surgical closure.

Atroventricular septal defect (shunt)

- Endocardial cushion defect
- Common in Down syndrome
- Eisenmenger syndrome develops without treatment
- Patients often have mixed mitral valve dysfunction.

Pathogenesis/aetiology

Types of lesion

- Membranous (commonest): may close spontaneously
- Muscular, e.g. acquired after septal MI
- AV defect
- Infundibular (high VSD beneath pulmonary valve), does not close spontaneously, e.g. as part of tetralogy of Fallot (Fig. 2.26).

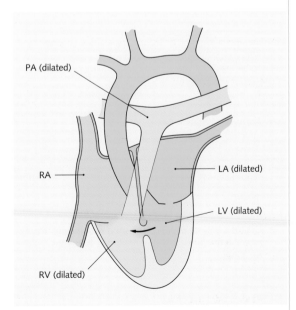

PA (dilated)

RA

LA (dilated)

LV (dilated)

RV (dilated)

Fig. 2.26 Ventricular septal defect.

- Often picked up in infancy childhood as heart failure
- Incidence: 2/1000 live births.

Associated with

- Aortic regurgitation
- PDA (10%).

Clinical features

Features of heart failure in infancy

- Failure to thrive
- Sweating on feeding
- Shortness of breath
- Intercostal recession
- Hepatomegaly.

Signs

- Pan-systolic murmur at left sternal edge (variable depending on type and size)
- Signs of RV overload if large VSD
- S2 may be obscured by a pan-systolic murmur.

Investigations

ECG

- Often normal
- May demonstrate evidence of biventricular hypertrophy with large defects.

Imaging

CXR:
- Pulmonary plethora.

Echocardiogram:
- To identify defect.

Other tests

- Cardiac catheterisation.

Treatment

- Treat heart failure in infancy
- If worsening symptoms or large defect: surgical closure in infancy
- If medical therapy successful, delay closure until age 3–5 years.

Prognosis and complications

Prognosis

Eisenmenger syndrome is a life-threatening complication: all treatment plans aim to reduce pulmonary hypertension and prevent it occurring.

Complications

- Aortic regurgitation (5%)
- Infective endocarditis
- Pulmonary hypertension and Eisenmenger syndrome.

ACYANOTIC CHD: PATENT DUCTUS ARTERIOSUS

Outline

Patent ductus arteriosus (shunt)

- Ductus arteriosus connects the aorta with the pulmonary artery in the fetus, allowing the blood to bypass the lungs.
- Failed closure of this link at birth causes a left-to-right shunt.

Pathogenesis/aetiology

Increased risk of PDA

- Premature babies (up to 50%)
- Down syndrome
- High altitudes
- Maternal rubella (Fig. 2.27)

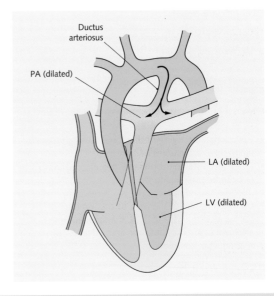

Fig. 2.27   Patent ductus arteriosus.

Who

Associations

- VSD
- Pulmonary stenosis

- Coarctation of the aorta.

Clinical features

- Most are asymptomatic
- Those with larger shunts have symptoms of volume overload or heart failure in infancy (very few)

- Continuous machinery-like murmur (over pulmonary region).

Investigations

ECG

- Usually normal.

Imaging

- CXR: usually normal, may have pulmonary plethora.

Other tests

- Cardiac catheterisation.

Treatment

Treatment

- NSAIDs: indomethacin used for pharmacologically facilitated closure in infancy (side effects: renal dysfunction)

- Close early (<3 months if large, <1 year if smaller) to avoid raised pulmonary pressures and provoking Eisenmenger syndrome.

Prognosis and complications

Prognosis

Excellent once closed.

Complications

- Infective endocarditis

- Pulmonary hypertension and Eisenmenger syndrome if untreated.

ACYANOTIC CHD: COARCTATION OF THE AORTA

Outline

- Congenital narrowing of the aorta causing reduced blood flow in the aorta
- Often just distal to the origin of the left subclavian artery but can be proximal to it
- Infantile and adult forms
- Classified by the relationship to the remnant of the ductus ateriosus (see above), the ligamentum arteriosum, insertion into the aorta (Fig. 2.28):
  - preductal: commonest
  - postductal: 5%
  - ductal: at the duct.

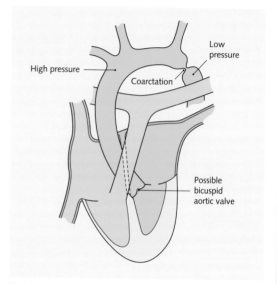

Fig. 2.28 Coarctation of aorta.

Pathogenesis/aetiology

Pathology

Only a small amount of blood can pass the stricture.

Infantile form:
- May present soon after birth as heart failure
- Postductal lesions may be missed in childhood.

Adult form:
- Develops more gradually and presents later
- Associated with a bicuspid aortic valve

- Collateral vessels develop over many years to bypass the obstruction. These can be felt as posterior intercostal arteries and they may cause notching of the ribs that can sometimes be visible on a CXR.

Who

- Uncommon
- 1♀:4♂

- 6% of CHD.

Associations

- Berry aneurysm

- Other congenital abnormalities: transposition of the great arteries, bicuspid aortic valve, Turner syndrome, PDA, circle of Willis aneurysms.

Clinical features

Symptoms

Infantile form:
- Failure to thrive
- Symptoms of heart failure
- Severe heart failure.

Adult type:
- Often asymptomatic
- Dyspnoea on exertion

- Headaches and nose bleeds from high BP in the upper body
- Claudication and cool legs from poor circulation in the lower limbs.

Signs

Adult type:
- Hypertension
- Ejection systolic murmur that radiates to the intrascapular region
- Radiofemoral delay: delay in the femoral pulse compared with the radial pulse, with upper limb hypertension and lower limb hypotension

- Systolic BP difference between left and right arms if cooarctation is between the origin of the left subclavian and the brachiocephalic arteries (also seen with aortic dissection)
- LV hypertrophy.

Investigations

Clinical examination

Radiofemoral delay.

ECG

LV hypertrophy (from increased back pressure on LV) and right bundle branch block.

Imaging

CXR:
- Dilated aorta
- Notching of the ribs from erosion by collaterals.

Echocardiogram:
- Coarctation and associated anastomoses.

Other tests

- Cardiac catheterisation:
  - demonstrates other complex lesions.

Treatment

- Percutaneous transcatheter balloon dilatation and stenting or surgical correction
- Preductal lesions require surgery in infancy to prevent heart failure

- Postductal lesions can often wait until childhood
- Medical management of hypertension in adulthood and risk stratify for IHD (may occur prematurely).

Prognosis and complications

Prognosis

Poor without surgery.

Complications

- Stroke
- Subarachnoid haemorrhage
- Aortic rupture
- Infective endocarditis

- Uncontrolled hypertension: persists in 70% because of renal damage
- Atherosclerosis
- Heart failure.

CYANOTIC CHD: TETRALOGY OF FALLOT

Outline

- Combination of shunt and obstructive lesion.
- Failure of bulbus cordis (becomes part of the ventricle in the developing heart) to rotate, causing misalignment of heart structures.
- Four main features:
  - large venous septal defect
  - over-riding aorta (across septum)
  - pulmonary stenosis (RV outflow tract obstruction)
  - RV hypertrophy
- Adults would have undergone previous partial/full correction.

Pathogenesis/aetiology

Pathogenesis

- Main problem relates to RV outflow obstruction, causing lack of flow to the lungs and poor oxygenation of blood
- Patients often have the obstruction corrected in childhood
- Later problems relate to pulmonary valve dysfunction (pulmonary regurgitation) and arrhythmias (Fig. 2.29).

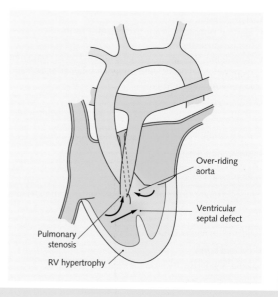

Fig. 2.29   Tetralogy of Fallot.

Who

- 6–10% of CHD
- Commonest cause of cyanotic CHD presenting beyond infancy.

Clinical features

Symptoms

- Babies not cyanotic at birth
- Cyanosis appears at 2–6 months with cyanotic spells (with feeding, crying)
- Failure to thrive
- Squatting in older children (increases pulmonary flow, reduces shunting).

Signs

- Clubbing
- Polycythaemia
- Hypoxia
- RV heave
- Loud, single S2 heart sound
- Loud ejection systolic murmur of pulmonary stenosis
- VSD inaudible as very large.

Investigations

ECG

- Right axis deviation
- RV hypertrophy

- Right bundle branch block.

Imaging

CXR:
- Boot shaped heart (apex not touching diaphragm)
- Oligaemic lung fields because of small pulmonary vessels.

Echocardiogram:
- Right ventricle dimensions.

Other tests

Cardiac catheterisation
- Visualises size and flow across pulmonary arteries

- Examines step down saturations.

Treatment

Children

- Under specialist paediatric cardiologists
- May need palliative Blalock–Taussig shunt in infancy if severe hypoxaemia

- Definitive surgical repair in early childhood (may need numerous operations).

When adult

- Management under specialist team
- Investigate and treat arrhythmias
- Monitor for pulmonary regurgitation

- Implantable cardiac defibrillator if dangerous arrhythmias develops.

Prognosis and complications

Prognosis

Used to be fatal, now most patients live until adulthood.

Complications

- Arrhythmias
- Pulmonary regurgitation as a consequence of RV outflow tract surgery

- Heart failure (right sided)
- Infective endocarditis.

CYANOTIC CHD: TRANSPOSITION OF THE GREAT VESSELS

Outline

- Aorta rises from RV
- Pulmonary artery arises from LV.
- See Fig. 2.30

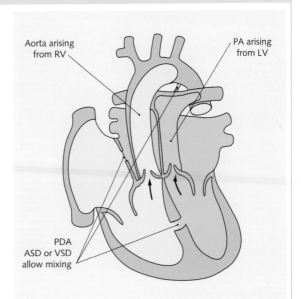

Aorta arising from RV

PA arising from LV

PDA
ASD or VSD
allow mixing

Fig. 2.30   Transposition of the great arteries.

Pathogenesis

Unless there is a shunt (ASD, VSD, PDA) allowing mixing of the two circulations, this defect is lethal at birth when the ductus arteriosus closes.

Who

- 5% of CHD
- 1♀:3♂

- Commonest cyanotic CHD presenting in first few days of life.

Clinical features

- Hyperdynamic circulation

- Cyanosis.

Investigations

ECG

Variable axis deviation.

Imaging

CXR:
- Pulmonary plethora (opposite to tetralogy of Fallot)
- Heart looks egg shaped.

Echocardiogram:
- Diagnostic
- Looks for additional defects.

Other tests

- Cardiac catheterisation:

  - dye injected into the RV fills the aorta.

Treatment

- Prostaglandin IV infusion for newborns (to keep ductus arteriosus open until an iatrogenic shunt can be created)
- Therapeutic balloon atrial septostomy: life-saving palliative procedure

- Definitive surgical correction of pulmonary and systemic connections to the heart often within 1 year.

Prognosis and complications

Prognosis

- Fatal unless treated

- Significant comorbidity into adulthood.

Complications

- Arrhythmias
- Heart failure (right sided)

- Infective endocarditis.

HYPERTENSION AND CARDIOVASCULAR CHANGES

PULMONARY HYPERTENSION

Outline

- Mean pulmonary arterial pressure >25 mmHg
- Can be primary or secondary to other conditions
- In primary disease, hypertrophy of small pulmonary vessels leads to vascular obstruction

- Over time, pulmonary hypertension develops into right heart failure (main cause of morbidity, mortality): cor pulmonale
- Cor pulmonale: right heart failure caused by chronic pulmonary hypertension.

Pathogenesis/aetiology

Causes

- Primary pulmonary hypertension (PPH): unknown aetiology.
- Secondary: most common:
  - chronic hypoxia: COPD, obstructive sleep apnoea, living at high altitude
  - ↑ pulmonary blood flow from shunts: ASD, VSD, PDA

- left-sided heart disease, e.g. mitral stenosis and LV failure
- recurrent pulmonary emboli
- miscellaneous: appetite stimulants, fenfluramine, sarcoid.

Who

- ♀ > ♂
- PPH: rare, Afro-Caribbean women
- Incidence: 2 per million.

Clinical features

Symptoms

- Chest pain
- Fatigue
- SOB
- Syncope
- Related to underlying condition, e.g. haemoptysis with chronic mitral stenosis.

Signs

- Peripheral oedema
- ↑ JVP: dominant a wave
- Loud S2 heart sound (from loud P2); widely split S2
- Pulmonary regurgitation
- Tricuspid regurgitation
- Parasternal or RV heave.

Investigations

To identify an underlying cause.

Blood tests

- Autoimmune screen
- HIV
- B-type natriuretic peptide: useful for monitoring progression
- ABG.

Imaging

CXR:
- Enlarged pulmonary trunk.

CT:
- High-resolution CT and CT pulmonary angiography (CTPA)
    V/Q scan.

Echocardiogram:
- Estimate pulmonary pressures
- Exclude causative cardiac disease.

ECG

- RV hypertrophy
- P pulmonale
- Right axis deviation.

Other tests

- Cardiac catheterisation:
    - **gold standard** for diagnosis and quantifies severity
    - vasoreactive testing: if administration of nitric oxide to the pulmonary artery causes fall in BP >10 mmHg, calcium channel antagonists are indicated.
- Cardiac investigations:
    - nocturnal and exercise oximetry
    - 6-min walk test.
- Pulmonary function tests.

Treatment

Advice

- Avoid strenuous exercise
- Explain risks of pregnancy: advise contraception
- Support groups

- Referral to specialist centres: if likely PPH
- Treat secondary causes.

Medical therapy

- Anticoagulation: with RV dilatation, high risk of thrombus and pulmonary embolism, mainly in PPH
- Digoxin: may improve EF
- Diuretics: for heart failure
- Ambulatory O_2: if secondary to hypoxaemia
- Vasodilator therapy *(after vasoreactive testing)*

- Prostanoids: IV infusion
- Endothelin receptor antagonists
- Calcium channel antagonists
- Nitric oxide
- Adenosine
- Phosphodiesterase inhibitors.

Surgical

Heart–lung transplant:
- Definitive treatment but patient needs to be fit for surgery

- Usually only for younger patients with PPH, without heart failure.

Prognosis and complications

Prognosis

50% mortality within 3 years.

Complications

Cor pulmonale: death from heart failure, fatal arrhythmias.

SYSTEMIC HYPERTENSION

Outline

- BP > 140/90 mmHg based on 2 readings at 2 separate occasions
- High cause of morbidity/mortality through IHD, renal failure, stroke, peripheral vascular disease

- Continuous increase in risk linking rising BP and cardiovascular risk.

Malignant hypertension

- Severe hypertension >200/130 mmHg and grade III–IV retinopathy

- Often headache with visual disturbance
- **Medical emergency.**

End-organ damage

Retinopathy:
- Leads to papilloedema (grade IV retinopathy)

Cardiac disease:
- Contributes to IHD
- LV hypertrophy with decompensation and LV dilatation (untreated) leading to dilated cardiomyopathy and heart failure.

Kidney disease:
- One of the commonest causes of chronic kidney failure in adults (particularly Afro-Caribbeans)

Cerebrovascular disease and peripheral vascular disease:
- Independent risk factors for atherosclerosis of carotid vessels causing TIA and cerebrovascular attack and iliac/femoral vessels causing peripheral vascular disease.

Pathogenesis/aetiology

Causes

Essential primary hypertension: 90% cases:
- Multifactorial
- Genetics
- Obesity
- Sedentary lifestyle
- Alcohol
- Smoking
- Diet: high salt intake
- Insulin resistance.

Secondary hypertension: 5%:
- Renal disease 75%, e.g. glomerulonephritis, polycystic disease
- Renovascular disease 25%, renal artery stenosis
- Endocrine disease: Cushing, Conn, phaeochromocytoma, acromegaly, hyperparathyroidism
- Coarctation of the aorta
- Pre-eclampsia in pregnancy
- Drugs: steroids, amphetamines.

Who

Epidemiology

20% of UK adult population.

Clinical features

Symptoms

- Usually asymptomatic
- Occasional headache
- Visual disturbance.

Signs

- High BP
- Related to cause, e.g. delayed femoral pulses, cushingoid features
- Fundoscopy – signs of hypertensive retinopathy:
  - grade 1: mild arteriolar narrowing
- grade 2: definite narrowing
- grade 3: cotton wool spots, flame haemorrhages
- grade 4: swelling of optic disc (papilloedema) and silver wiring.

Investigations

Investigations focus on stratifying cardiovascular risk (most important), looking for end-organ damage and finding an underlying cause.

Clinical examination

Evidence of end-organ involvement:
- Cardiovascular
- Peripheral vascular disease in limbs
- Retinopathy (fundoscopy).

Blood tests

- Fasting lipids
- Fasting glucose
- U&Es.

Urine

Blood/protein.

ECG

- LV hypertrophy
- Left axis deviation.

Imaging

CXR: pulmonary venous congestion.

Suspected secondary hypertension

- Primary aldosteronism: renin:aldosterone ratio, adrenal CT
- Renal parenchymal disease: renal US/biopsy
- Renovascular disease: renal angiogram/MRI angiogram (MRA)
- Phaeochromocytoma: 24-h urinary catecholamines
- Cushing syndrome: 24-h urinary cortisol, dexamethasone suppression tests
- Coarctation: CXR, BP in arms and legs, transthoracic echo
- Younger patients are more thoroughly investigated to exclude a secondary cause.

Treatment

Hypertensive emergencies

- Control BP: rapid reduction is dangerous, causing cerebral hypoperfusion and stroke
- Aim to reduce BP by 25% over 4 h (more aggressive if aortic dissection or MI)

- Oral therapy if alert and well, e.g. beta-blocker, calcium channel antagonist
- HDU/ICU if unwell or encephalopathic needing central venous and arterial line monitoring with IV therapy, e.g. labetalol, nitroprusside, glyceryl trinitrate, hydralazine.

Chronic treatment

Aim for systolic BP <140 mmHg, <130 mmHg in diabetic patients:
- Lifestyle measures:
  - ↓ Weight: regular exercise, diet
  - Diet: ↓ alcohol, ↑ fruit, ↑ vegetables
  - top smoking
- Indications for pharmacological treatment:
  - Malignant hypertension
  - BP >160/100 when already on lifestyle measures
  - BP >140/90 with clinical evidence of atherosclerosis (angina, claudication) or with evidence of end-organ damage (e.g. LV hypertrophy, proteinuria) or with a 10-year cardiovascular risk >20%.

Medical

The British Hypertensive Society guidelines for lowering hypertension are illustrated in Figure. 2.31.

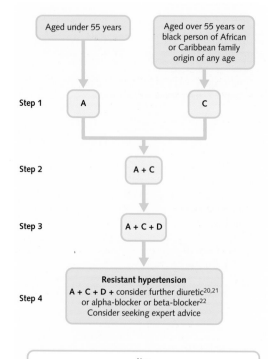

18 Choose a low-cost ARB.
19 A CCB is preferred but consider a thiazide-like diuretic if a CCB is not tolerated or the person has oedema, evidence of heart failure or a high risk of heart failure.
20 Consider a low dose of spironolactone[21] or higher doses of a thiazide-like diuretic.
21 At the time of publication spironolactone did not have a UK marketing authorisation for this indication. Informed consent should be obtained and documented.
22 Consider an alpha-blocker or beta-blocker if further diuretic therapy is not tolerated, or is contraindicated or ineffective.

Fig. 2.31 British Hypertensive Society guidelines for lowering hypertension.

Prognosis and complications

Prognosis

- Malignant hypertension untreated: 90% mortality in 1 year

- Those with hypertension die younger through cardiovascular morbidity/mortality.

Complications

- Atheroscleosis leading to multisystem disease as described

- Hypertension is also a risk factor for aortic aneurysmal development and aortic dissection.

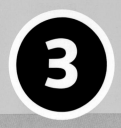

Respiratory system

Faculty Contributor: Anita Jayadev

Types of ventilation aids

- Hand-controlled bag-valve mask: used to force air (i.e. positive pressure) into the airway of a patient in respiratory arrest or where they are hypoventilating.
- Mechanical non-invasive ventilation: a tight-fitting mask is placed over the patient's face and a ventilator pushes air into the respiratory tract. Not all patients can tolerate this intervention due to claustrophobia and there is a risk of aspiration in those who are very drowsy:
  - continuous positive airway pressure (CPAP) the ventilator delivers air or O_2 at a constant pressure; used for obstructive sleep apnoea, acute lung injury, heart failure with pulmonary oedema
  - bilevel positive airway pressure: the ventilator administers pressures at two levels to mimic inspiration and expiration. The machine can sense a patient's inspiratory effort and provides higher pressures in inspiration before returning to a lower setting in expiration. The constant background pressure maintains the patency of the airways. Useful for respiratory failure secondary to COPD exacerbations or neuromuscular disease.
- Invasive: endotracheal tube or tracheostomy attached to a ventilator.

Investigations

Bedside tests

- Pulse oximetry: assesses arterial O_2 saturations, non-invasive

- Sputum, colour:
  - green: infection/inflammation
  - black: tar stained
  - red: blood
- Peak flow:
  - maximum forced expiratory flow through a peak flow meter
  - correlates with forced expiratory volume in 1 second (FEV1), see below
  - good in asthmatics to monitor disease control and therapy.

Blood tests

- FBC: useful to measure anaemia and polycythaemia (a disorder of a raised haematocrit, p. 363), which can be caused by chronic hypoxia
- WBC and CRP: useful to suggest respiratory tract infection.

Arterial blood gas

A sample of heparinised (to prevent clotting) arterial blood is taken from a peripheral artery. On this pH, partial pressures of O_2 and CO_2 (PaO_2 and $PaCO_2$), base excess and bicarbonate levels can be measured. Most also report basic electrolytes and lactate: useful where the patient:

- unexpectedly deteriorates
- has impaired consciousness
- has impaired respiratory effort
- has an exacerbation of a chronic chest condition
- shows signs of CO_2 retention.

Table 3.1 summarises findings of an ABG assessment and their interpretation (see also Figure 12.1).

Table 3.1 Arterial blood gases

Test	Normal values	Diagnostic inference	
		Increased	Decreased
pH	7.35–7.45	Alkalosis, hyperventilation	Acidosis, CO_2 retention
PaO_2	11–13 kPa.		Hypoxia
$PaCO_2$	4.7–6.0 kPa	Respiratory acidosis (if pH decreased)	Respiratory alkalosis (if pH increased)
Base excess	±2 mmol/L	Metabolic alkalosis	Metabolic acidosis
Standardised bicarbonate	22–26 mEq/L	Metabolic alkalosis	Metabolic acidosis

Lung function tests: spirometry

Spirometry is the measurement of the volume of air in the lungs and its speed of expiration. The patient first breathes in to maximum inspiration and then breathes out completely as fast as they can:

- Used to estimate vital capacity, forced vital capacity (FVC) and FEV1: volume exhaled in the first second
- FEV1 can be expressed as a percentage of the FVC; this is useful to diagnose restrictive (e.g. fibrosis) or obstructive patterns (COPD) of airway disease:
  - normal: 70–80%
  - obstructive defect: <70%
  - restrictive defect: both FEV1 and FVC are reduced but the ratio is little changed, being >80% predicted.

Lung volumes

Figure 3.1 illustrates tidal breathing and lung volumes.
   Important terms:

IRV: inspiratory reserve volume
ERV: expiratory reserve volume
TV: tidal volume (measured using spirometry)
RV: residual volume (TLC−VC)
IC: inspiratory capacity
FRC: functional residual capacity
VC: vital capacity (measured using spirometry)
TLC: total lung capacity (measured using helium dilution)
FEV1: volume exhaled in the first second
FVC: total volume exhaled.

Chest radiography

Ionising X-rays are used to generate an image of the chest (Fig. 3.2A). Specific landmarks (Fig. 3.3B) are very useful in determining respiratory conditions such as consolidation, pleural effusion, pneumothoraces or lung tumours.

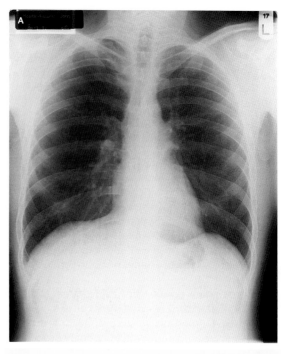

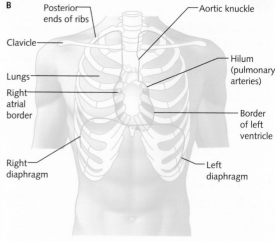

Fig. 3.2   CXR: (A) normal (from Swash 2007 with permission); (B) landmarks.

Bronchoscopy

Bronchi are directly visualised using an endoscopic camera:

- Can use flexible or rigid (general anaesthetic) bronchoscope, through the nose or mouth (rigid)
- Can sample tissues with brushings, lavage or biopsy
- Useful in the diagnosis and staging of lung cancer, diffuse lung disease and infection

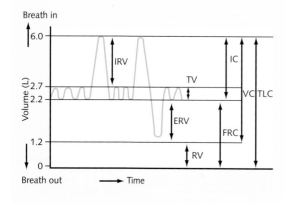

Fig. 3.1   Typical spirometer trace showing lung volumes.

- Bronchoalveolar lavage: sterile saline delivered through the bronchoscope and aspirated for diagnosing malignancy or infection
- Can be combined with ultrasound (US) to sample lymph nodes (EBUS. EndoBronchial UltraSound)
- Can perform some therapeutic manoeuvres for tumours causing airway obstruction.

Diagnostic pleural fluid aspiration

In a pleural effusion, excess fluid can collect in the pleural space. This can be aspirated, and biochemistry, cytology, microbiology and immunology can be measured for diagnostic purposes.

Historically classified as:

- exudate if >30 g/L protein: normally results from infection, inflammation or malignancy
- transudate if <30 g/L protein: normally results from 'failure' of heart, kidney or liver. If pleural fluid is between 25–35g of protein BTS guidelines recommend you use Light's. Criteria to accurately determine if transudate or exudate. (see p. 102)

Ventilation perfusion (V/Q) scan

Lung ventilation (how well air reaches the airways) and perfusion (how well blood reaches the airway capillaries) can be measured using nuclear imaging (Fig. 3.3); these can then be compared. A ventilation/perfusion mismatch (with reduced perfusion) suggests a pulmonary embolism and can identify its location. CT pulmonary angiography (CTPA; see below) is now used more commonly.

Hard to interpret in the presence of lung disease

CT pulmonary angiography

CT with IV contrast through the pulmonary artery to view filling defects in the pulmonary vasculature: gold standard for diagnosing pulmonary emboli.

Ultrasound

Good for pleural effusions including US-guided taps.

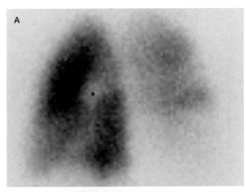

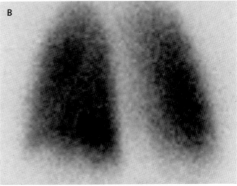

Fig. 3.3 Ventilation (B), perfusion (A) scans.

Lung biopsy

For tissue diagnoses of cancers and suspicious lesions.

Video-assisted thoracoscopic surgery

A camera is passed through the chest wall and surgery can be performed under visual guidance.

Good for mesothelioma diagnosis.

See also

- Biochemistry (Ch. 12): interpreting ABGs
- The patient presents (Ch. 14): SOB, cough, haemoptysis, cyanosis
- Clinical examinations (Ch. 15): respiratory.

UPPER TRACT DISEASE

OBSTRUCTIVE SLEEP APNOEA

Outline

- Obstruction of the upper airway at night (obstructive sleep apnoea) from airway collapse during sleep leading to disturbed sleep and subsequently daytime symptoms (obstructive sleep apnoea syndrome)
- Apnoea: literally means 'no breathing' but here describes pauses in breathing for >10 seconds

- Hypopnea: a 10s event where there is continued breathing but ventilation is reduced by at least 50% from previous baseline, during sleep.
- Apnoea/Hyponea Index (AHI): the frequency of apnoeas and hypopneas hourly, used to assess severity.
- Obstructive sleep apnoea/hypopnoea forms part of a spectrum from snoring to repetitive complete obstruction throughout the night.

Pathogenesis/aetiology

Causes

- Obesity
- Large tonsils
- Abnormal facial shape
- Muscle relaxants, alcohol

- Neuromuscular diseases causing pharyngeal involvement, e.g. Duchenne dystrophy, cerebral vascular accident
- Endocrine: hypothyroidism, acromegaly.

Pathogenesis

- Occurs during sleep when the muscles normally holding the airway open are relaxed
- Terminated by partial arousal as the patient tries to breath

- Arousal can cause transient ↑ in BP, that can ↑ risk of sustained systemic and pulmonary hypertension, cor pulmonale, MI and stroke
- Sleep disturbance can lead to daytime symptoms.

Who

- 1♀:2–3♂
- Prevalence: 2–4% in middle age

- 3rd commonest respiratory condition after asthma/COPD.

Symptoms and signs

Symptoms

At night:
- Snoring
- Partner may describe apnoeic episodes
- Poor sleep quality
- Choking

During the day:
- Morning headache
- Daytime drowsiness
- ↓ concentration and cognitive performance
- ↓ libido
- Irritability
- Personality changes.

Investigations

Diagnosis requires abnormal sleep study plus symptoms. Another test – Epworth Score: a crude measurement of tendency to fall asleep. Max 24 points.

Overnight oximetry

- Shows frequent falls in arterial O_2 saturation

- Can be done as an in/outpatient with airflow, respiratory movement, +/− video. Useful for initial assessment but cannot exclude obstructive sleep apnoea/hypopnoea syndrome.

Polysomnography

- Detailed sleep study in a sleep lab at night
- Includes EEG, ECG, and electromyography (EMG)
- >5 apnoeas of >10 seconds per hour of sleep is abnormal, graded on number, AHI:

- Mild: AHI 5-14/hour
- Moderate: AHI 15-30/hour
- Severe: AHI>30/hour.

Treatment

- Current evidence suggests treatment if AHI $\geq$15 or a 4% O_2 saturation dip rate >10/hour.

Conservative

- ↓ Weight
- Avoid alcohol
- Correct causative factors where possible

Oral devices:
- Gum shields to hold mandible forward for mild/ moderate OSA syndrome.

Ventilation

- for moderate/severe OSA and symptomatic

- CPAP via a mask to keep the airway open. Effective but some patients find it uncomfortable.

Surgical

- Surgical procedures to relieve obstruction, e.g. in facial deformity or tonsilar hypertrophy or bariatric surgery where necessary if other treatments fail.

Prognosis and complications

Complications

- Pulmonary hypertension
- Type II respiratory failure
- Road traffic accidents (falling asleep at the wheel) DVLA recommends Group 1 (licence for normal car) permitted to drive when satisfactory control of symptoms

achieved. Group 2 (HGV/PSA) can be permitted to drive when satisfactory control of symptoms achieved and confirmed specialist opinion.
- Risk of systemic hypertension, heart failure, MI

UPPER TRACT INFECTION

RHINITIS

Outline

- Nasal irritation and inflammation
- Lasts >1 h on most days

- Inflammation results in excessive mucus production.

Classification

- Allergic rhinitis: from IgE allergens similar to those in asthma. Can be seasonal or all year very common. affects 1:4 in UK.

- Non allergic rhinitis
- Infective rhinitis: bacterial or viral cause.

Pathogenesis/aetiology

Causes

Allergic rhinitis:
- Atopy syndrome: allergic hypersensitivity reaction affecting areas not directly in contact with the allergens. Syndrome includes eczema, allergic conjunctivitis and asthma (as well as rhinitis)

Non allergic rhinitis:
- Inflammatory causes

- Hyperreactive causes: from hormonal changes, drugs or irritants

Infective rhinitis:
- Common: rhinoviruses, coronaviruses.
- Less common: respiratory syncytial virus, parainfluenza virus, flu virus, adenovirus, enterovirus.

Who

Hay fever:
- Affects 30% of young British people

Associations:
- Atopy syndrome.

- Commonest allergic disease.

Symptoms

- Coryza (inflammation of mucus membranes lining the nasal cavity)
- Postnasal drip (excessive mucus passing back in to nasopharynx)
- Sneezing
- Anosmia (lack of smell)
- Sleeplessness
- Seasonal rhinitis: itching of the eyes, ears or throat.

Investigations

- Skin prick test
- Serum IgE antibody
- ENT examination: swollen turbinates (bony extensions on the side of the nose into the nasal cavity).

Treatment

Conservative

- Avoid allergens.

Medication

Non allergic:
- Nasal decongestants
- Antihistamines: to ↓ mucus secretion
- Nasal ipratropium bromide
- Above for maximum 3 weeks then high dose nasal steroids: 3 months

Allergic:
- Antihistamine
- Increase dose nasal steroids for at least 3 months.

Other potentially useful treatments:
- leukotriene receptor antagonists, cromoglycate
- immunotherapy (desensitisation). This involves giving graded increases of allergens to which sufferer is sensitive in order to induce allergen tolerance. Subcutaneous or sublingual preparations given regularly by specialists over 3 years.

Surgical

- Severe chronic rhinitis: refer to ENT (possible turbinate reduction).

Prognosis and complications

Complications

- Nasal polyps causing nasal obstruction and anosmia.

INFLUENZA

Outline

- Infectious disease caused by an orthomyxovirus virus
- More serious than the common cold and lasts longer
- Transmitted by respiratory secretions
- Rapidly and easily spread
- Incubation 1–4 days
- Usually lasts 3–7 days.

Classification

Three main types:
- A: main cause of epidemics and pandemics
- B: milder disease
- C: not pathogenic in humans.

Pathogenesis/aetiology

The virus:
- Orthomyxovirus
- RNA virus
- Viral proteins on the surface:
  - Neuraminidase: important in the release of new viruses from infected cells
  - Haemagglutinin mediates binding and entry of the virus into the cell
- The virus can undergo shift or drift:
  - Shift:
    - Major change
    - From genetic preassortment of RNA segments during replication
    - Causes pandemics
  - Drift:
    - Minor change
    - Spontaneous point mutations of the haemagglutinin protein
    - Causes epidemics.

Who

- May affect healthy people
- Risk factors:
  - COPD
- Immuno-compromised
- Elderly.

A typical patient

A woman presenting with myalgia, fever and a blocked nose that develops over 36 h.

Symptoms and signs

Symptoms

- Fever
- Chills, shivering
- Myalgia
- Malaise
- Headache
- Coryza
- Sneezing

- Non productive cough
- Sore throat
- Hoarseness.

Postviral syndrome:
- Prolonged debility and depression lasting weeks or months.

Investigations

- Usually none
- Nasopharyngeal secretions or throat swabs: viral culture, antigen detection, nucleic acid detection
- Antibody tests.

Treatment

Conservative

- Bed rest
- Fluids.

Medication

- Analgesia: aspirin/paracetamol
- Antibiotics if with chronic bronchitis, heart or renal disease
- Within 48 h of symptoms: zanamivir, oseltamivir (neuraminidase inhibitors).

Prevention:
- Inactivated vaccine for those at risk: elderly >65, health workers, pregnant women, diabetes mellitus, chronic respiratory, heart or renal disease
- Oseltamivir for prophylaxis.

Prognosis and complications

Complications

Usually in infants, elderly or immunosuppressed:
- 1° influenzal pneumonia
- 2° bacterial pneumonia:
  - *Staphylococcus aureus* (most severe), *Streptococcus pneumonia*, *Haemophilus influenzae*

- Reye's syndrome:
  - Mostly in children
  - Predisposed by aspirin treatment
  - Leads to cerebral oedema and fatty liver change.

PHARYNGITIS

Outline

- Painful inflammation of the pharynx
- Due to infection, usually viral.

Pathogenesis/aetiology

Causes

Common:
- Adenovirus, parainfluenza virus, influenza virus, HSV, EBV (glandular fever)

Less common:
- Respiratory syncytial virus, rhinovirus, adenovirus, CMV, streptococcal A.

Who

Associations:
- Tonsillitis

- Glandular fever (80% of cases).

Symptoms and signs

Symptoms

- Sore throat
- Fever
- Malaise

- Headache
- Nausea and vomiting.

Investigations

- Throat swab for acute bacterial pharyngitis
- Test for glandular fever: monospot or Paul Bunnell test.

Treatment

Conservative

- Usually symptomatic.

Medication

- If 2° bacterial invasion: antibiotics but avoid amoxicillin as it causes a rash with glandular fever.

Surgical

- If abscess develops may require drainage.

Prognosis and complications

Prognosis

- Mostly self-limiting.

Complications

- 2° bacterial invasion
- Retropharyngeal abscess: very rare.

LOWER TRACT INFECTION

ACUTE BRONCHITIS/TRACHEITIS/TRACHEO-BRONCHITIS

Outline

- Inflammation of the bronchi causing airway obstruction
- Mostly due to infection

- Terminology depends on anatomical site
- Acute bronchitis is very different from chronic bronchitis (part of the COPD syndrome see p. 91).

Pathogenesis/aetiology

Causes

- Healthy individuals usually have a viral cause
- Smokers or COPD patients usually have a bacterial cause.

Who

Risk factors:
- Smokers
- COPD.

Symptoms and signs

Symptoms

- Cough: at first unproductive
- Sputum production: yellow/green
- Retrosternal discomfort if tracheitis
- Chest tightness
- Wheeze.

Investigations

- Diagnosis usually based on the history
- Sputum microbiology
- CXR is normal.

Treatment

Conservative

- ↓ smoking.

Medication

- No specific treatment necessary in most cases
- Antibiotics: if bacterial
- Bronchodilators: to ease obstruction.

Prognosis and complications

Prognosis

- Usually lasts a few days without serious complications.

PNEUMONIA

Outline

- Inflammation of the lung parenchyma with symptoms and signs of consolidation.
- Usually caused by a bacterial infection
- Major cause of death worldwide, particularly in children and the elderly
- Severity is commonly assessed using the CURB65 score (see page 83).

Classification

1. Hospital-acquired pneumonia vs. community-acquired pneumonia: most commonly used classification. Hospital-acquired pneumonia is defined as pneumonia occurring >48 h after admission or 7–10 days after hospital discharge
2. Typical or atypical: symptoms differ in atypical patients: extrapulmonary involvement is more common, e.g. hepatitis, skin/joint involvement, neurological signs, hyponatraemia
3. By location: lobar (affecting a lung lobe) or bronchopneumonia (patchy affecting bronchi and surrounding alveoli).

Aspiration pneumonia:
- Pneumonia caused by the Inhalation of oropharyngeal anaerobes
- Commonly occurs in stroke patients, alcoholics, those with decreased consciousness.

Pneumocystis jiroveci (was *carinii*) pneumonia (PCP):
- Pneumonia commonly affecting HIV patients or the immunosuppressed
- Caused by a fungus
- Presents as SOB, dry cough and characteristic desaturation on exercise
- Typical radiological features and diagnosed on bronchoscopy, with silver staining of bronchoalveolar lavage.

Pathogenesis/aetiology

Causative organisms

Community-acquired pneumonia:

- Typical:
  - *Streptococcus pneumoniae*
  - *Haemophilus influenzae*
  - *Staphylococcus aureus*
  - *Moraxella catarrhalis*
- Atypical:
  - *Legionella pneumophila*
  - *Coxiella burnetti*
  - *Chlamydia psittaci*
  - *Mycoplasma pneumoniae*

Hospital-acquired pneumonia:

- *Streptococcus pneumoniae*
- *Staphylococcus aureus*
- *Pseudomonas*
- *Bacteroides*
- *Gram −ve (Escherichia coli, Klebsiella, Proteus)*

Aspiration pneumonia:

- *Streptococcus pneumoniae*
- Anaerobes

Opportunist pneumonia (in immunosuppressed):

- *Pneumocystis jiroveci*

- *Mycobacterium tuberculosis*
- *Aspergillus fumigatus*
- *Mycobacterium avium-intracellulare*
- CMV

'Typical presentation':

- Pleuritic chest pain, SOB, cough and:
  - rusty sputum: *Streptoccocus pneumoniae*
  - foreign travel/air conditioning: *Legionella*
  - working with animals: *Coxiella burnetti*
  - had contact with birds, particularly parrots: *Chlamydia psittaci*
  - COPD: *S. pneumoniae, H. influenzae, Moraxella catarrhalis*
  - cystic fibrosis: *Pseudomonas aeruginosa*
  - young patient: mycoplasma
  - smoker: *Haemophilus influenzae*
  - immunocompromised/IVDU: *Staphylococcus aureus, Mycobacterium tuberculosis*
  - homeless or alcoholic: *Klebsiella, Mycobacterium tuberculosis*
  - HIV patient: *Streptococcus pneumoniae, Pneumocystis jiroveci, Mycobacterium tuberculosis.*

Who

- Incidence: 0.1–0.3%
- Pneumonia is the fourth commonest cause of death worldwide

Risk factors:

- Elderly
- Children <2 years

- Flu patients
- Smokers/alcoholics
- HIV
- Lung disease
- Immunosuppressed

A typical patient

A 65-year-old man presents with fever and left-sided pleuritic chest pain. He is coughing up rusty sputum. On the left side, percussion is dull and there is bronchial breathing.

Symptoms and signs

- Symptoms and signs vary according to cause. The history is often short.

Symptoms

- Fevers/sweats
- Purulent sputum: green or rusty
- Dyspnoea

- Pleuritic chest pain
- Cough
- Haemoptysis.

Symptoms and signs

Signs

- Consolidation: hallmark:
  - Dull percussion
  - ↑ vocal fremitus
  - Coarse crepitations
  - Bronchial breathing
  - ↓ chest expansion
- Pyrexia
- Tachycardia, tachypnoea
- Small effusion
- Pleural rub

Atypical presentation:
- Confusion, e.g. particularly in the elderly or if cause is legionella
- Myalgia, arthralgia
- Headache
- Vomiting/diarrhoea
- Non-productive cough
- Abdominal pain

Severity assessment:

CURB65:
- **C**onfusion (New AMTS ≤ 8)
- **U**rea >7 mmol/L
- **R**espiratory rate >30/min
- **B**P <60 mmHg diastolic/or <90 mmHg systolic
- >**65** age

- score of 0 = low risk, may be suitable for home treatment
- score 1-2 = consider hospital referral/admission
- score ≥ 3 = Ideally admit for IV antibiotics
- score 4 = 83% mortality - use with caution alongside clinical judgement of individual patient.

Features of concern:
- CURB65 score >3 in community-acquired pneumonia
- Saturations <92%
- PO_2 <8 kPa
- New AF
- WBC <4 or >20 × 10^9/L
- Albumin <35 g/L
- Bilateral/multilobar consolidation
- Septicaemia: mortality 20% (non-septicaemia is 5%).

Investigations

Blood tests

- FBC:
  - WBC ↑ or ↓
  - Hb: haemolytic anaemia caused by mycoplasma
- U&Es:
  - Hyponatraemia: a complication in legionella
  - ↑ urea: a sign of severity

ECG

- Differential diagnoses, complications.

Additional tests for infection

- Serology: antibodies to specific bacteria
- Sputum and blood: microscopy and culture (prior to antibiotics)
- Urine: pneumococcal antigen and legionella
- Nasopharyngeal aspirates: viruses

- LFTs:
  - can be deranged with atypical pneumonia
- ↑ CRP
- Blood gases:
  - O_2 saturations: assess severity.

- Aspirate pleural effusion: send for microscopy, culture and sensitivity, pH (to exclude an empyema, pH <7.2).
- Bronchoalveolar lavage e.g. for mycoplasma: rarely necessary.

Imaging

CXR: the gold standard test (Fig. 3.4).
Shows:
- Infiltrates
- Cavitation with certain causative microorganisms: *Staphylococcus aureus, Pseudomonas, Klebsiella, Legionella, Mycobacterium tuberculosis,* fungi, enteric Gram –ve bacilli
- Pleural effusion
- Hilar lymphadenopathy
- Air space shadowing
- Air bronchograms

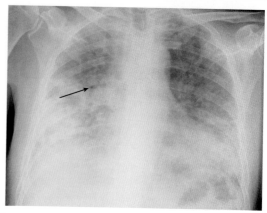

Fig. 3.4 CXR showing typical consolidation and air bronchograms (arrowed).

On admission: if severe:
- High flow O_2: consider CPAP if hypoxia not responding to O_2 therapy
- IV fluid resuscitation
- IV antibiotics

- ICU if severe
- Aspirate or drain pleural effusion if necessary
- If presenting with severe sepsis follow the 'sepsis six' within 1 h (see p. 486)

Conservative

- Chest physiotherapy +/− suctioning to aid bringing up of sputum.

Medical

- Analgesics
- Fluids
- Antibiotics: always consult local guidelines
Community-acquired pneumonia:
- Typically amoxicillin to target *Streptococcus* and/or a macrolide to target atypicals e.g. clarithromycin (clarithromycin alone if penicillin allergy) for 5–7 days
- Severe: coamoxiclav or cefuroxime and macrolide IV 10–14 days

- Legionnaires: clarithromycin, rifampicin
- *Chlamydia*: tetracycline e.g. doxycycline
- *Mycoplasma pneumoniae*: clarithromycin
- *Pneumocystis jiroveci* pneumonia: O_2, steroids, cotrimoxazole (trimethoprim and sulfamethoxazole)
Hospital-acquired pneumonia:
- Aminoglycoside antipseudomonal penicillin or third generation cephalosporin. IV
Aspiration pneumonia:
- Cefuroxime and metronidazole

Follow-up and Prevention

- Any abnormal CXR should be repeated at 6 weeks to ensure resolution

- Influenza and *Streptococcus pneumoniae* vaccines if high risk

Prognosis

- Proportion of adults who require hospital admission in UK is between 22 and 42%.
- Mortality of adults hospitalised is between 5.7 and 14%.

Estimated mortality from CURB65:
- 4 points = 83%
- 3 points = 33%
- 2 points = 23%
- 1 point = 8%
- 0 points = 2.4%

Complications

- Lung abscess
- Empyema
- Pleural effusion
- Respiratory failure

- AF
- Acute renal failure
- Healing by scar formation
- Septicaemia.

TUBERCULOSIS

Outline

- Chronic granulomatous disease from an infection with mycobacteria, usually *Mycobacterium tuberculosis*
- Tuberculosis (TB) has typically caseating granulomas: with necrotic debris

- The body establishes a cell mediated immune response to the bacteria causing the formation of tubercles in the tissues and leads to many of the symptoms and signs
- TB usually affects the upper lung lobes

Classification

Active TB:
- Positive skin tests, e.g. Mantoux and smear or culture positive. Symptomatic and likely abnormal CXR

Latent TB:
- Disease is not active, they are not infectious but it may become active. Positive skin tests, but no symptoms and normal CXR. Potential candidates for chemoprophylaxis

Pulmonary:
- TB mostly affects the lungs
- Primary: initial infection with bacilli
- Postprimary: also called reactivation or secondary TB

Extrapulmonary:
- In 30% of patients.
- If TB spreads to the blood it is called miliary TB as the multiple blood spread tubercles have a distinctive appearance on CXR with multiple small opacities across the lung fields which are about the same size as 'millet seeds' (Fig. 3.5)
- Miliary TB can cause 2° lesions affecting the CNS, lymphatic, circulatory, genitourinary and musculoskeletal systems

Granuloma:
- A cluster of modified macrophages surrounded by lymphoid cells in response to indigestible matter within the macrophages (see also sarcoidosis below).

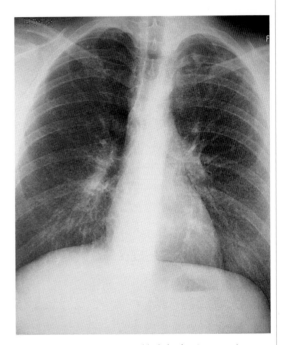

Fig. 3.5   CXR showing speckled shadowing seen in miliary TB.

Pathogenesis/aetiology

Pathology

- *Mycobacterium tuberculosis* is a rod shaped bacteria that is stained and cannot be decolourised by acid alcohol (acid-alcohol fast bacilli)
- Transmission: airborne droplets that are inhaled into the lungs

Primary TB:
- The initial infection is normally solitary and occurs in the middle or upper lung zones
- In the lungs the bacteria are phagocytosed by alveolar macrophages where the infection can be contained or leads to primary TB
- The first site of infection, a small area of granulomatous inflammation is called the ghon focus. If this involves inflammation in surrounding lymph nodes, it is called the primary complex

- After 3–8 weeks the *Mycobacterium tuberculosis* surrounded by macrophage becomes a tubercle, a granulomatous form of inflammation
- The granulomatous lesion necroses through a process called caseation
- The caseous tissue can liquefy, empty into an airway and be transmitted to other parts of the lung
- Most patients do not progress further than primary TB; the rate of relapse to postprimary is small except with immunosuppression

Postprimary pulmonary (2°) TB:
- Reactivation of latent infection or preinfection
- Usually due to immunocompromise
- often localised to apical and posterior parts of upper lobes
- Tubercle follicles develop and lesions enlarge
- Lesions are usually bilateral and show evidence of cavities.

- Leading cause of death worldwide from single infectious disease
- >30% are carriers
- Worldwide incidence ↑ due to HIV and drug resistance
- Highest incidence in sub-Saharan Africa, high in Asia
- Initial infection normally is at childhood

Risk factors:
- Immunocompromised
- Young or old
- Socially deprived
- Immigrants
- Alcoholics
- HIV (coinfection).

A typical patient

A 30-year-old immigrant from Zimbabwe presents with weight loss, fever and night sweats. His blood cultures are positive on a Ziehl Neelsen stain.

Symptoms and signs

Primary TB

- Normally asymptomatic
- May have mild fever

- Erythema nodosum (tender shin nodules)

Progressive TB

Symptoms
- Cough
- Fever
- Night sweats
- Haemoptysis

- Weight loss
- Sputum: purulent or blood stained
- Malaise.

Signs
- Cervical lymphadenopathy

Extra-pulmonary disease

- TB meningitis
- Pericardial TB: can lead to tamponade
- Pott's disease: TB of the spine may need surgery
- Joints: any joint may be affected

- Scrofula: TB lymphadenitis affecting neck lymph nodes
- Genitourinary disease: classically gives a sterile pyuria (urine with pus).

Investigations

Stain and culture

- Stain and culture from:
  - Sputum
  - Urine, usually three samples
  - Pleural fluid (if effusion)
  - CSF if meningitis suspected
  - Bone biopsy if spinal involvement
  - Lymph nodes: fine node aspiration
- Ziehl Neelsen stain for acid–alcohol fast bacilli

- Cultured on Lowenstein–Jensen medium (specific for mycobacterium). Takes 4–6 weeks, identifies resistance
- Results from stain and culture:
  - 'Smear +ve' for acid-alcohol fast bacilli from sputum: patients are highly infectious, **must be isolated**
  - 'Culture +ve': acid–alcohol fast bacilli not seen but TB grown on culture: less infectious
  - Rapid sputum identification test: also predicts resistance.

Imaging

- CXR: patchy or nodular shadows in upper zones (cavitation), loss of volume, fibrosis, calcification, miliary TB.

Other tests

Special tests:
- Bronchoscopy with biopsy
- Bronchoalvolar lavage
- CT
- Lymph node biopsy

Tests to determine exposure:
- Mantoux test:
  - Intradermal injection of tuberculin (extract of tubercule), diameter measured 48–72 h later. Immune response if patient exposed to infection or vaccination, a large response suggests active infection (>15 mm strongly +ve)
- Heaf test:
  - Six simultaneous injections of tuberculin. Less used than Mantoux

- New interferon-gamma tests:
  - WBC release interferon-gamma in response to contact with TB antibodies
  - Interferon-can be detected
  - Good as little cross-reactivity with other mycobacteria, results available quickly, but only available in specialist centres.
  - T-Spot TB (Elispot): counts individual T-cells producing interferon-gamma
  - Enzyme-linked immunosorbent assay (ELISA; e.g. QuantiFERON): measures level of interferon-gamma in supernatant.

Treatment

Medical

'4 (medications) for 2 (months) and 2 for 4'.
Initial phase: **RIPE** for 2 months:
- **R**ifampicin: (side effect orange discoloured urine, hepatitis)
- **I**soniazid: (side effect peripheral neuropathy, psychosis, hepatitis)
- **P**yrazinamide: (side effect gout, hepatotoxic)
- **E**thambutol: (side effect optic neuritis)
- + Pyridoxine (vitamin B_6 prevents CNS and peripheral nervous system effects of isoniazid)
- Steroids may be indicated
Continuation phase: 4 months:
- Rifampicin and isoniazid

- If CNS is involved: 12 months treatment minimum
- Advise HIV testing

All TB patients need referral to regional TB clinic:
- To monitor side effects and screen at baseline e.g. bloods, including LFTs and visual acuity for side effect of medication
- Arrange directly observed therapy (DOT as recommended by WHO) if needed
- Contact tracing
- TB is a notifiable disease and must be reported to the consultant in communicable disease control through the local Health Protection Unit www.hpa.org.uk

Prevention

- BCG (Bacille Calmette, Guerin) vaccination prevents TB in 70% of cases

Contacts

- Screened with tuberculin test: Heaf/Mantoux and chest X-ray
- +ve result and +ve X-ray: start standard treatment

- +ve result with normal X-ray: start TB chemoprophylaxis: isoniazid for 6 months or isoniazid and rifampicin for 3 months
- Test is −ve: give BCG.

Prognosis and complications

Prognosis

- Usually good with complete treatment

- Can recur.

Complications

- Side effects from drugs, e.g. hepatitis
- Bronchiectasis
- Pleural disease
- Pneumothorax: rare but can lead to broncho-pleural fistula
- Abscess formation

- Right middle lobe syndrome: collapse 2° to compression of bronchus by hilar nodes
- Multidrug-resistant (MDR) TB and extensively drug resistant (XDR) either acquired (rare in UK) or through poor compliance with medication. Needs specialist advice.

OBSTRUCTIVE AIRWAY DISEASE

Pathogenesis/aetiology

Causes

- Acute: foreign body, bronchiolitis
- Recurrent acute: asthma

- Chronic: COPD, bronchiectasis.

ASTHMA

Outline

- A chronic inflammatory condition with acute, reversible airway narrowing
- From airway hyperresponsiveness to different stimuli or precipitating factors
- Leads to wheeze, cough and SOB
- Most patients are well between attacks but may have mild symptoms
- Status asthmaticus: severe asthma which can be life threatening.

Classification

- Extrinsic asthma (atopy): increased IgE production in response to environmental antigens
- Intrinsic asthma: precipitated by infections but not other identifiable agents.

Table 3.2 compares asthma and COPD

NB: 'cardiac asthma' sometimes used to describe wheeze caused by left ventricular failure.

Table 3.2 Comparison between asthma and COPD

COPD	Asthma
Mostly smokers	Possibly smokers, history of atopy +/− eczema
Middle aged–old	Any age
Chronic productive cough	Cough usually dry
SOB: persistent and progressive	SOB: variable
Diurnal variability: uncommon	Diurnal variability: common
FEV/FVC remains abnormal despite treatment	Often returns to normal

Pathogenesis/aetiology

Precipitating factors for attack:
- **DIPLOMATs**:
  - **D**rugs: beta-blockers aspirin, NSAIDs
  - **I**nfections: rhinovirus
  - **P**ollutants
  - **L**aughter (emotion)
- **O**esophageal reflux: nocturnal asthma
- **M**ites
- **A**llergens, **a**ctivity
- **T**emperature (cold)
- **s**ome exercise

Pathogenesis

Three causes of airway narrowing:
1. **Bronchoconstriction** due to airway hyper responsiveness
2. Mucosal **inflammation**
3. ↑ **mucus production**

Airway narrowing in an attack:
- Acute response: precipitating factor leads to release of preformed mediators causing smooth muscle constriction and mucosal oedema
- Late phase reaction: further constriction and inflammation 3–24 h later. From ↑ inflammatory cells and mediators leading to epithelial damage, inflammation and mucous production.
- Chronic phase from repetition of attacks: mucous gland hyperplasia, smooth muscle hypertrophy, basement membrane thickening.

Who

- Typical age: commonest in childhood
- ♀ < ♂ in children
- Prevalence: 10% of population
- Genetic associations

Associated diseases:
- Atopy syndromes (see rhinitis)
- Acid reflux
- Churg–Strauss (asthma, eosinophilia, vasculitis)
- Allergic bronchopulmonary aspergillosis: response of the immune system to the fungus aspergillus. Presents like asthma but with eosinophilia.

A typical patient

An 8-year-old boy presents with intermittent breathlessness and wheeze, provoked by exercise, cold air and colds.

Symptoms and signs

Well controlled

- Symptom-free, exacerbation free. This is the aim of treatment for most patients

Exacerbations

Symptoms
- Wheeze
- Dyspnoea
- Cough (often nocturnal)

Signs
In attack:
- Tachycardia
- Tachypnoea
- Hyperinflated chest
- ↓ chest wall movement
- Resonant percussion.

Initial assessment on acute admission

- Table 3.3 gives the important classification for determining treatment
- Beware of the asthma patient with normal or high CO_2 in an attack: indicates a medical emergency; CO_2 should be low in response to hypoxia and airway narrowing.

- May have diurnal variation: symptoms worse at night (e.g. peak expiratory flow rate (PEFR), lowest at 2–3 am)

Table 3.3 Classification of shock to determine treatment

	Severe	Life threatening: SHOCK
Respiratory rate	>25 bpm	Silent
Blood Pressure	>110 bpm	Hypotension
Peak expiratory flow rate	30–50% of normal	One third of normal
SaO_2 and Blood gas if <92%	Normal or low CO_2, hypoxic	Cyanosis ↑ CO_2, acidotic
General	Anxious, cannot complete sentences	Konfusion

Investigations

Tests for an acute admission

- Heart rate
- BP
- Pulse oximetry

- Peak expiratory flow rate
- ECG.

Blood tests

- FBC (look for eosinophilia for allergic bronchopulmonary aspergillosis):
  - U&Es
  - CRP

- Infection screen
- Blood gas if saturations <92% (CO_2 levels important).

Imaging

- CXR: not routinely recommended unless life-threatening asthma or suspect complications, e.g. hyper-inflation or pneumothorax, Although do not delay treatment waiting for a CXR in emergency situation.

Further tests

- PEFR diary.
- Blood tests: IgE levels, aspergillus titres
- Lung function tests: spirometry to look for an obstructive defect. Check reversibility with a bronchodilator: >15% ↑ after using a bronchodilator suggests asthma

- Skin prick: detect allergens
- Bronchial challenge tests: for occupational exposure. Measure fall in FEV1.

Ask about

- Precipitants: cold, air, exercise
- Diurnal variation
- Nocturnal cough
- Exercise

- Smoking history
- Other atopic disease
- Home environment: pets, carpet
- Occupation

Management and lifestyle
- Who manages your asthma?
- Does it stop your daily activities of living?
- What is your best PEFR?
- Days off per week for attacks?
- Recent change in medication?

- What medication: inhalers, tablets, steroids
- Compliance with medication and check inhaler technique
- When was the last time you were ventilated?
- Have you ever been admitted to ITU?

Treatment

Acute admissions

British Thoracic Society Guidelines (Table 3.4) on acute admission:
- ABC approach (see p. 2)
- O_2: maintain saturations at >94%
- Salbutamol: 5 mg nebulised with O_2 (Can give 3 doses back to back initially). Then nebulisers every 15 min if needed. If not responding: continuous nebuliser or IV salbutamol
- Ipratropium bromide 0.5 mg 4–6 h with salbutamol nebuliser if severe or life threatening
- Steroids: hydrocortisone 100 mg IV (if unable to take orally) or 30 mg prednisolone. Prednisolone continued daily for >5 days after acute attack
- Life threatening: IV $MgSO_4$ max 2 g over 20 min
- Not responding: aminophylline: 5 mg/kg IV over 20 min (ensure not on theophylline)
- Call ICU if requiring ventilation or if not responding to therapy

NB: different guidelines for children.

Discharge plan:
- Modify treatment
- Ensure patient is stable (PEFR >50%)
- Assess triggers
- Educate inhaler technique
- Self management plan: measurement with peak flow
- Follow-up: at GP within 1 week, brittle/severe asthma also followed up with specialist in 4 weeks

Non acute treatment

- Conservative:
  - stop smoking, avoid precipitants

Medications

Beta-2 agonists:
- Relax bronchial muscle by ↑ cAMP in smooth muscle: bronchodilator
- Salbutamol (blue inhaler): short acting (4 h), salmeterol: long acting (12 h)
- Side effect: hypokalaemia, tachycardia, arrhythmias

Corticosteroids (brown inhaler):
- ↓ inflammation
- Beclomethasone: inhaled (side effect oral candida/hoarseness)
- Prednisolone: orally

Methylxanthines:
- Inhibit phosphodiesterase and block adenosine receptors leading to bronchodilation

Table 3.4 British Thoracic Society Guidelines: stepwise management

1. Mild intermittent asthma: short-acting beta-2 agonist taken when needed e.g. salbutamol

2. Regular preventer therapy: add regular inhaled steroid e.g. beclomethasone

3. Initial add on therapy: add long-acting beta-2 agonist e.g. salmeterol

4. Persistent poor control: ↑ inhaled steroids, add leukotriene antagonists, theophyllines

5. Continuous or frequent use of oral steroids: add oral steroids: e.g. high dose prednisolone. Short courses <21 days

- Medical:
  - patients start treatment at a step appropriate for them and move up or down depending on control.

- Aminophylline, theophyllin

Leukotriene antagonists:
- Block leukotriene receptors on inflammatory and smooth muscle cells: both bronchodilator and anti-inflammatory role
- For prophylaxis in mild/exercise induced asthma, and for children
- Montelukast

Anticholinergenics:
- Ipratropium bromide, tiotropium
- For life-threatening asthma or when standard therapy has failed.

Prognosis

- In a severe attack patient may be too exhausted to ventilate: $PaO_2 \downarrow$, $PaCO_2 \uparrow$
- Mortality 1200/year

- Many child sufferers grow out of it or suffer less as adults
- A significant amount get chronic asthma later.

Complications

- Persistent irreversible obstruction
- Bronchiectasis

- Pneumothorax.

CHRONIC OBSTRUCTIVE PULMONARY DISEASE

Outline

- Disease state associated with small airway obstruction that is progressive and not fully reversible. Mostly associated with smoking
- Obstruction from narrowing of small airways by inflammation and airway collapse during expiration due to loss of elastic recoil
- A disease that consists of chronic bronchitis, emphysema and small airways inflammation in varying degrees

Chronic bronchitis:

- Defined clinically: a cough with productive sputum for most days for 3 months over 2 consecutive years

Emphysema:

- Defined histologically: permanent distension of the distal air spaces with destruction of alveolar walls without fibrosis

Global Initiative for Chronic Obstructive Lung Disease (GOLD) classification of COPD severity:

- Classified by degree of impairment of lung function
- FEV1/FVC ratio <70% and post-bronchodilator FEV1 values:
  - Mild: FEV1: $\geq$80% predicted
  - Moderate: FEV1 <80%
  - Severe: FEV1 <50%
  - Very severe: FEV1 <30%.

Pathogenesis/aetiology

Causes

- Smoking: main cause in developed world
- α1 antitrypsin deficiency: uncommon, illustrates importance of protease damage
- Pollution: indoor pollution from biomass fuels in low income countries

- Occupation: dusts, fumes
- Infection: 50% bacteria, 50% viral. Important in acute exacerbations and may be a factor in progression

Pathology

- Chronic bronchitis:
  - Hyperplasia and hypertrophy of the mucus glands causing $\uparrow$ mucus production and airway narrowing
  - Eventually leads to squamous metaplasia of respiratory epithelium (replaces columnar epithelium) and fibrosis
- Emphysema:
  - From an imbalance between protease (which destroys the lungs) and anti-protease and oxidants/antioxidants
  - α1 antitrypsin is the most important anti-protease

- α1 antitrypsin is inhibited by proteases from neutrophils attracted to the lung by cigarette smoke ($\downarrow$ production can also be inherited)
- Leads to $\downarrow$ surface area for gaseous exchange and loss of elastic recoil leading to airflow collapse in expiration and air trapping
- Emphysema can be:
  - *Centriacinar*: destruction limited to respiratory bronchioles. Found in the upper lobes and associated with smoking and chronic bronchitis
  - *Panacinar*: involves central and peripheral parts of alveoli and so $\downarrow$ gas exchange. Typically affects the lower lobes and associated with α1 antitrypsin deficiency.

Who

- Common
- 5–10% of all UK deaths
- Third commonest death by 2020

Chronic bronchitis:

- In old terminology classified as blue bloaters as they are cyanosed (blue) not breathless. Patients are chronically hypoxic with right heart failure

Emphysema:

- Old terminology: pink puffers as they are breathless not cyanosed (pink). Patients maintain O_2 by $\uparrow$ ventilation.

A typical patient

A 68-year-old smoker presents with cough, wheeze and breathlessness on exertion which has been getting steadily worse for the last 3 years.

Symptoms and signs

Stable COPD

- Dyspnoea
- Sputum
- Cough
- Wheeze

Exacerbation of COPD

Symptoms

As above but worse with green and purulent sputum.

Signs

Hands:
- Tar staining
- CO_2 flap
- Peripheral cyanosis

Face:
- Central cyanosis

Chest and neck:
- Barrel chested – hyper-inflated
- ↓ chest expansion
- ↑ respiratory rate (unless there is CO_2 retention)
- Percussion: resonant
- Auscultation: wheeze, ↓ breath sounds, early inspiratory crackles.

Investigations

Blood tests

FBC:
- ↑ Hb and packed cell volume due to hypoxaemia leading to secondary polycythaemia
- WBC, CRP: infection
- α1 antitrypsin measurement (once only to rule out deficiency)

ABG:
- Hypoxia and hypercapnia in advanced disease

Imaging

CXR:

Features (Fig. 3.6) include:
- hyperinflation (can count >7 ribs anteriorly)
- flat diaphragm because of over inflation
- heart: appears long and slim in relation to chest cavity
- bullae (pockets of air) seen in emphysema
- consolidation if active infection
- lungs appear blacker and larger in volume than normal.

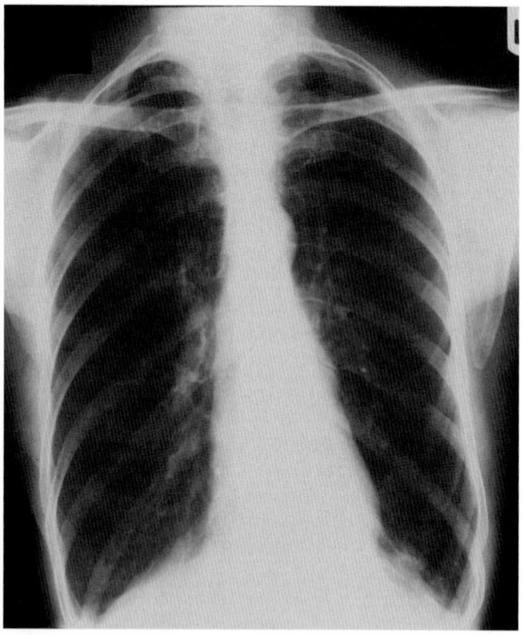

Fig. 3.6 Features of COPD.

Other tests

Sputum:
- Culture if present

Peak expiratory flow rate:
- ↓, but not best test for COPD

Lung function tests:
- Most important: spirometry: ratio of FEV to FVC is decreased (<70%).

Treatment

Acute exacerbation

- O_2: to ↓ hypoxia. Give cautiously as in severe COPD, hypoxia, rather than CO_2, may drive ventilation. Give 24–28%, then aim to maintain saturations at 88–92%. Monitor with repeat ABGs
- Salbutamol and ipratropium bromide nebulised on room air

- Oral steroids: high dose for 7–14 days
- Broad spectrum antibiotics: amoxicillin
- Consider IV aminophylline if no improvement
- Non or invasive ventilation/intubation: if type II respiratory failure or no response
- Later: physio for sputum clearance

Stable COPD: NICE Guidelines

- Smoking cessation.

Inhaled therapy
- Short-acting beta-2 agonist (e.g. salbutamol) or short-acting muscarinic antagonist (e.g. ipratropium)
- If exacerbations persist: long-acting beta-2 agonist (e.g. salmeterol) and long-acting muscarinic agonist. (e.g. tiotropium) Add inhaled corticosteroid in a combination inhaler with the long-acting beta-2 agonist if FEV1 <50%
- If persistent exacerbations: combine long-acting muscarinic agonist + long-acting beta-2 agonist + inhaled corticosteroid

Oral therapy
- Long-term oral steroids not recommended, can use short term after exacerbation
- Theophylline

- Mucolytics: may benefit some patients with chronic sputum production

O_2 therapy
- Long-term O_2 therapy, home O_2 if PaO_2 <7.3 kPa. Only factor to reduce mortality if given >15 h/day
- Before treatment consider: 2 blood gases, 3, weeks apart, 4 weeks after infection

Follow-up
- At least once a year, twice if severe
- Multidisciplinary working
- Prevent infection: vaccinations
- Nutrition, exercise
- Education and inhaler technique
- Severe end-stage COPD, refer to palliative care

Surgery

- For recurrent pneumothoraces, bullous disease
- Bullectomy: for large bullae

- Lung volume reduction
- Transplant: 50% 5 year survival.

Prognosis and complications

Prognosis

- 50% in hospital will die within 2 years

Lung transplants:
- Patients considered for lung transplant if they have end-stage lung disease and are functionally disabled from the condition (i.e. poor prognosis).

Complications

- Respiratory failure
- Cor pulmonale
- Pneumonia

- Polycythaemia
- Pneumothorax.

BRONCHIECTASIS

Outline

- Permanent dilatation and thickening of bronchi leading to mucus pooling, obstruction and often subsequent infection
- Disease can be localised to a lobe or to the whole bronchial tree

Congenital links:
- Certain congenital diseases are associated with bronchiectasis:
  - Cystic fibrosis (main cause in developed countries): thick viscus mucus
  - Kartagener syndrome: affects motility of lung cilia
  - Young syndrome: abnormally viscous mucus.

Pathogenesis/aetiology

Causes

- Idiopathic: in 50%
- Postinfective: pneumonia, TB, influenza
- Obstruction: inhaled foreign body, enlarged lymph nodes, bronchial obstruction, tumour, allergic bronchopulmonary aspergillosis: (airway damage, producing proximal bronchiectasis)

- Congenital predisposition: cystic fibrosis, Kartagener syndrome.

Pathogenesis

Propagating cycle of bronchiectasis (Fig. 3.7):
- Dilated bronchi are inflamed, and collapsible
- This results in airflow obstruction and impaired secretion clearance
- Infection damages the lung tissue causing inelasticity and further dilation of bronchi propagating the cycle.

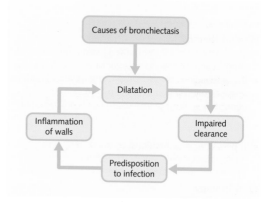

Fig. 3.7 Propagating vicious cycle of bronchiectasis.

Who

- Typical age: more in adults (unless cystic fibrosis is the cause)
- Prevalence of severe bronchiectasis falling (probably due to antibiotic treatment and vaccinations)
- More common in less developed countries

Associations:
- Connective tissue disease, e.g. lupus, inflammatory bowel disease (IBD); yellow nail syndrome, $\alpha 1$ antitrypsin deficiency.

A typical patient

A 42-year-old woman presents with a history of SOB, digital clubbing and daily green sputum production. On auscultation there are coarse crackles.

Symptoms and signs

Symptoms

- Sputum: thick, purulent, green, may be large quantities (>2 cups/day)
- Haemoptysis: blood stained or haemorrhage

- Breathlessness: from airflow limitation
- Cough
- Foetor (bad breath).

Signs

- Clubbing
- Coarse crackles: in affected area

- Patients usually present with a chronic history of months–years.

Investigations

1. Confirm the diagnosis

- Pulmonary function tests
- Immunoglubulins.

Imaging

CXR:
- Dilated bronchi with thick walls
- Tram-lining and ring shadowing: both from dilated bronchi (Fig. 3.8)

High resolution CT:
- Investigation of choice: shows airway dilatation, bronchial wall thickening and cystic change.

2. Find the cause

- E.g. genotyping, sweat test for cystic fibrosis, bronchoscopy, foreign body; saccharin test for nasal mucociliary clearance, α1 antitrypsin, aspergillus IgE antibodies

3. Consider treatment

- Which organisms are present? (whether cause or effect of disease): sputum cultures, acid fast bacilli.

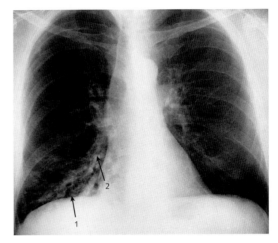

Fig. 3.8   CXR of bronchiectasis with ring shadows (1) and tramline shadowing (2).

Treatment

- Treat the cause.

Conservative

- Physiotherapy: postural drainage, twice a day
- Sputum clearance techniques
- Breathing exercises
- Nutrition
- Stop smoking.

Medical

- Bronchodilators: nebulised salbutamol if there is an airflow limitation
- Inhaled N-acetylcysteine: for mucolytic therapy*
- Antibiotics: to control infection
- Steroids*
- O_2 therapy: for severe and end-stage disease
- Annual influenza and pneumococcal vaccine. Discuss self management plan with patients.

Surgical

- Surgery for localised disease or severe haemoptysis
- May need transplant.

*Little evidence for these. There are very few studies that have researched treatment of non-CF bronchiectasis. Refer to BTS Guidelines published 2010 for guide on antibiotics management.

Prognosis and complications

Prognosis

- Permanent condition
- May develop severe complications such as respiratory failure.

Complications

- Haemoptysis
- Pneumonia
- May develop respiratory failure
- Recurrent infective exacerbations.

RESTRICTIVE AIRWAY DISEASE

GENERAL FEATURES

Outline

- An umbrella term for a group of diseases characterised by inflammation and fibrosis of the lung parenchyma (alveoli and interstitium) leading to loss of function
- Defined by lung function tests as having a 'restrictive pattern' due to ↓ lung compliance and gas exchange

- Also called 'diffuse parenchymal lung disease' or 'interstitial lung disease'
- Mostly caused by immune mechanisms.

Typical distribution of fibrosis by cause

- **BREAST SCAR**:

Upper lobe:
- **B**eryliosis
- **R**adiation
- **E**xtrinsic allergic alveolitis/employment e.g. coal worker
- **A**nkylosing spondylitis
- **S**arcoidosis
- **TB**

Lower lobe:
- **S**ystemic sclerosis
- **C**ryptogenic fibrosing alveolitis (idiopathic interstitial pneumonia)
- **A**sbestosis
- **R**adiation.

Pathogenesis/aetiology

Classification

British Thoracic Society classification based on cause:
1. Acute (<3 weeks): e.g. 2° to infection, allergy, toxin or haemorrhage
2. Episodic: e.g. eosinophilic pneumonia, cryptogenic organising pneumonia, vasculitis, Churg–Strauss syndrome
3. Chronic due to occupational or environmental agents or drugs: e.g. pneumonoconiosis (see below) extrinsic allergic alveolitis (see below), asbestosis, drug induced (antibiotics, or anti-inflammatory agents)

4. Chronic 2° to systemic disease: typically connective tissue disease, e.g. lupus, systemic sclerosis, Sjögren syndrome, rheumatoid arthritis, ankylosing spondylitis
5. Chronic with no evidence of systemic disease: includes idiopathic interstitial pneumonia (see below).

Who

- 15% of respiratory problems in clinical practice.

Symptoms and signs

Symptoms

- Dyspnoea on exertion
- Non productive cough

- Haemoptysis (rare)
- Weight loss.

Signs

- Cyanosis
- Clubbing
- Crackles

- Look for extra pulmonary disease, e.g. rheumatoid arthritis, lupus

Investigations

Blood tests

- FBC, ESR, CRP, U&Es, LFTs, autoantibodies, serum precipitins, anti-basement membrane, serum ACE (although non-specific).

Imaging

- CXR: fibrosis, loss of lung volume
- High resolution CT (HRCT): diagnostic and prognostic information, shows fibrosis.

Other tests

- Bronchoalveolar lavage esp. for TB
- Lung biopsy: to differentiate subtypes. could be transbronchial, open lung biopsy or video-assisted thoracoscopic surgery. Although now,with HRCT, rarely indicated. As fibrosis may be patchy, with poor yield and relatively higher risk than HRCT, value is under review
- Spirometry: restrictive FEV1/FVC >80%, ↓ transfer factor of the lung for carbon monoxide, ↓ lung volumes.

Treatment

- Treatment and management of individual cause:
  - Remove offending agent
  - Treat infections
  - Stop offending drugs
- Often require high dose steroids, nebulisers, antibiotics, O_2 therapy and possible non-invasive ventilation acutely
- When stable, attempt to wean steroids gradually, and consider steroid sparing agents e.g. azathioprine. Other possible treatments: N acetylcysteine, pirfenidone
- Often patients require ambulatory O_2 at home or long-term O_2 therapy in advanced disease
- May need specialist input, e.g. rheumatology, ICU, depending on how acute and unwell the patient is.

Prognosis and complications

Prognosis

- Depends on cause and coexisting lung disease, e.g. COPD

Complications

- Includes irreversible lung fibrosis which is progressive leading to cor pulmonale and pulmonary hypertension
- Lung cancer.

PNEUMONOCONIOSES

Outline

- Group of disorders caused by occupational inhalation of dust that builds up in the lungs
Coal workers' pneumoconiosis:
- Main cause of pneumoconiosis
- Characterised by rounded opacities on CXR +/− emphysema
- Can be simple (small opacities in upper lobes), or complicated (progressive massive fibrosis: upper lobe fibrosis and mass formation that can cavitate)
Caplan syndrome:
- Coal workers' pneumoconiosis with rheumatoid arthritis
Silicosis:
- Due to silica (silicon dioxide) inhalation.

Pathogenesis/aetiology

Pathogenesis

- Due to dust exposure over many years
- Dust <5 μm can reach distal alveoli
- Larger dust particles remain in the airways and alveoli
Lung damage:
- The lung tissue reacts to the dust
- Phagocytes ingest the dust particles and drain to the lymphatic system
- Over time, phagocytes can accumulate in the alveoli and lead to fibrosis
- Smoking can confound the effects of pneumoconiosis.

Who

- ↓ in number of cases due to improved working conditions
- Silicosis occurs in stonemasons and sand-blasters.

A typical patient

An 80-year-old retired coal minor presents with SOB. He has opacities on CXR.

Symptoms and signs

- Depends on type of pneumoconioses.

Symptoms

- Progressive SOB
- Cough.

Signs

- May have fine crackles and ↓ breath sounds on chest auscultation.

Investigations

- Take full occupational and exposure history

Blood tests

- FBC, ESR, CRP, U&Es: exclude infective process.

Imaging

- CXR: opacities visible, mostly in upper lobe
- High resolution CT: for evaluation of fibrosis

Other tests

Pleural fluid aspiration:
- Send for WBC, MC + S, amylase, LDH, protein, cytology

Lung function test:
- Shows restrictive lung defect with ↓ transfer factor of the lung for carbon monoxide, and decreased lung volumes

Treatment

Treatment

- Mainly supportive, little effective treatment
- Smoking cessation
- Both coal workers' pneumoconiosis and silicosis may be entitled to compensation

Prevention

- Prevent exposure, e.g. protective masks at work
- Remove exposure if still exposed.

Prognosis and complications

Prognosis

- Depends on time course of exposure
- Damage once done is irreversible
- Progressive massive fibrosis has a poor prognosis.

Complications

- Cor pulmonale
- Lung cancer.

EXTRINSIC ALLERGIC ALVEOLITIS

Outline

- Widespread inflammation of the alveoli and small airways from hypersensitivity to inhaled organic dusts in sensitive people
- Also called hypersensitivity pneumonitis
- Exposure is often at work
- Hypersensitivity is from an IgG reaction to an offending allergen: type III hypersensitivity reaction
- With chronic exposure granulomas, bronchiolitis and fibrosis may occur.

Pathogenesis/aetiology

Pathogenesis

- Response to an allergen leads to accumulation of acute inflammatory cells and immune complexes within the airways

- Over time there is granuloma formation, and fibrosis from long-term exposure.

Causes

- Farmer's lung disease: from fungi contaminating damp hay, most common cause *Micropolyspora faeni*
- Bird fancier's: from dander release particularly from pigeons

- Bagassosis: sugar cane fibres, *Thermoactinomyces sacchari*
- Malt workers lung: *Aspergillus fumigatus*
- Mushroom workers lung: *Thermactinomyces vulgaris.*

Who

- Farmer's lung disease is commonest.

A typical patient

A 45-year-old farmer with repeated fever, SOB and a dry cough precipitated by working in his barn. On auscultation there are inspiratory bibasal crackles.

Symptoms and signs

Acute allergen exposure:
- Cough
- Dyspnoea
- Crackles
- Fever
- Rigors
- Myalgia
- Occurs a few hours after exposure and generally settles in a few days, may progress if antigen not removed

Chronic:
- ↑ dyspnoea
- Weight loss
- Type 1 respiratory failure
- Cor pulmonale.

Investigations

Blood tests

- ↑ WBC, ↑ ESR
- Serum precipitins

- Specific serum antibodies: only supportive, not diagnostic.

Imaging

- CXR: nodular shadowing, consolidation particularly in the upper and middle zones. Chronic disease may show honeycombing

Other tests

Spirometry:
- Restrictive defect
- ↓ lung volume
- ↓ transfer factor of the lungs for carbon monoxide

Bronchoalveolar lavage:
- ↑ T lymphocytes and granulocytes.

Treatment

Conservative

- Avoid allergen exposure

Medical

- O_2 for an acute attack. If poor recovery: may need ambulatory or long-term home O_2 therapy

- Oral prednisolone: if chronic, trial long-term steroids and review after 1 month
- May be entitled to compensation.

Prognosis and complications

Prognosis

- Variable
- Usually good when antigen exposure is removed.

Complications

- Respiratory failure and death can rarely occur if high exposure
- Chronic condition can lead to cor pulmonale.

IDIOPATHIC INTERSTITIAL PNEUMONIAS

Outline

- A group of diffuse lung diseases that mainly involve the lung interstitium where the cause is unknown.

Classification

1. Idiopathic pulmonary fibrosis/usual interstitial pneumonia:
   - Previously called cryptogenic fibrosing alveolitis
   - High-resolution CT: little ground-glass shadowing, basal sub-pleural fibrosis, honeycombing
   - No benefit from steroids
2. Non-specific interstitial pneumonia:
   - High-resolution CT: diffuse ground glass shadowing
   - Responds to steroids
3. Cryptogenic organising pneumonia:
   - Previously called bronchiolitis obliterans organising pneumonia
   - High-resolution CT: consolidation, some honeycombing
4. Acute interstitial pneumonia/Hamman Rich syndrome:
   - Like acute respiratory distress syndrome (ARDS). Poor prognosis
5. Respiratory bronchiolitis associated interstitial lung disease:
   - Rare, occurs in smokers. Good prognosis
6. Desquamative interstitial pneumonia:
   - Usually smoking related
7. Lymphoid interstitial pneumonia.

Pathogenesis/aetiology

Pathogenesis

- Varies between types, with a spectrum from inflammation to fibrosis:
  - Inflammation from various causes leads to neutrophil migration, desquamation of alveolar cells and ↑ fibroblasts
  - This leads to cellular infiltration and thickening of the interstitium between the alveoli from collagen deposition
- Fibroblasts proliferate and this leads to further fibroblast proliferation
- Fibrosis follows in chronic disease.

Who

- Typical age: >60 years
- Rare

Associations:
- Autoimmune diseases.

A typical patient

A 62-year-old non-smoking female with a history of progressively worsening SOB and a dry cough. On examination she has finger clubbing and inspiratory bilateral basal crackles.

Symptoms and signs

Symptoms

- Non productive, dry cough
- Exertional dyspnoea
- Malaise
- Arthralgia
- Weight loss.

Signs

- Clubbing
- Cyanosis
- Fine end inspiratory basal crackles.

Investigations

- A diagnosis of exclusion so all causes must be excluded.

BTS Guidelines for Diagnosis, adapted from ATS/ERS criteria:
Major criteria:
1. Exclusion of other known causes of ILD, e.g. drugs
2. Restriction and impaired gas exchange on PFTs (pulmonary function tests)
3. Bibasilar reticular abnormalities with minimal ground-glass opacities on HRCT scans
4. Transbronchial lung biopsy or BAL showing no features to support alternative diagnosis.

Minor criteria:
1. Age > 50 years
2. Bibasilar inspiratory crackles
3. Insidious onset, unexplained dyspnoea on exertion
4. Duration > 3 months.

MDT approach to diagnosing Interstitial disease is considered the gold standard. Consideration given to all of the above. Note: the role of biopsy is currently under review.
(Adapted from Wells A U et al. Interstitial Lung Disease Guideline: The British Thoracic Society in collaboration with The Thoracic Society of Australia and New Zealand and Irish Thoracic Society. Thorax 2008;63 (supp v):V1-V58.)

Blood tests

- FBC, ESR, CRP, U&Es, LFTs

Serology:
- Autoantibodies useful in distinguishing differential diagnosis and for prognosis: ANA (30%), rheumatoid factor 10%

Imaging

CXR:
- Fibrotic shadowing: ground glass appearance or streaks of fibrosis (Fig. 3.9)

High-resolution CT
- Helps to differentiate types of idiopathic interstitial pneumonia. Honeycomb lung mostly in lower zones: dilated airspaces between areas of collagenous thickening appears like honeycomb
- Most idiopathic interstitial pneumonia diagnosed on high-resolution CT alone

Other tests

- Lung function tests: restrictive defect
- Biopsy: for confirmation and prognosis if uncertain
- Bronchoalveolar lavage: lymphocytes > neutrophils indicates better response to steroids.

- Acute phase response with polyclonal hypergammaglobinemia.

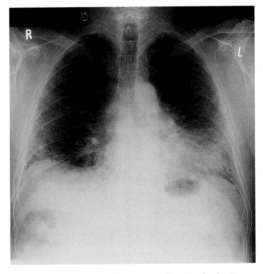

Fig. 3.9 CXR showing lower zone fibrotic shadowing.

Treatment

Conservative

- Avoid allergen exposure if relevant.

Medical

- Prednisolone for 1 year, reducing dose slowly
- Immunosuppressants: azathioprine, cyclophosphamide
- Always treat superadded infection aggressively

- New treatments such as perfenidone showing some promise of slowing progression.

Surgical

- Lung transplantation.

Prognosis and complications

Prognosis

- 50% mortality at 2 years
- Usual interstitial pneumonia: poor, similar to lung cancer. Usually progressive over years

- Non specific interstitial pneumonia: better than for Usual interstitial pneumonia
- Cryptogenic organising pneumonia: good response to corticosteroids.

Complications

- Respiratory failure: type 1
- Pulmonary hypertension

- Cor pulmonale
- Lung cancer.

PLEURAL DISEASE

PLEURAL EFFUSION

Outline

- Excess fluid in the pleural space
- Special types of effusion include collections of:
  - Blood: haemothorax
  - Pus: empyema (see below)
  - Lymph: chylothorax
- Important to distinguish between transudate and exudate:
  - Transudate if <30 g/L protein:
    - Pressure problem: often bilateral
    - From oedema from high hydrostatic pressure or low oncotic pressure
    - Usually from systemic problem: from 'failure': heart, kidney, liver

- Exudate if >30 g/L protein:
  - Local problem: often unilateral
  - High protein, usually from malignancy, inflammation or infection which ↑ leakiness of the lung capillaries

Light's criteria:
- If the protein amount is borderline, counted as exudative if:
  1. Ratio of pleural fluid protein: serum protein >0.5
  2. Ratio of pleural fluid LDH and serum LDH >0.6
  3. Pleural fluid LDH is >2/3 normal upper limit for serum.

Pathogenesis/aetiology

Causes

Transudates:
- *High hydrostatic pressure:*
  - ↑ venous pressure
  - Left ventricular failure
  - Fluid overload
- *Low oncotic pressure*
  - Hypoalbuminia
  - Nephrotic syndrome
  - Chronic liver disease
  - Malnutrition/absorption
Exudates:
- Malignancy
- Infection, e.g. TB, bacterial pneumonia (some pneumonias are associated with pleural effusion)

- Inflammation
- Connective tissue disease
Chylothorax:
- Follows disruption of the thoracic duct
- Fluid appears turbid/milky
- Measure pleural fluid triglyceride and cholesterol. If triglyceride is >1.10 g/L chylothorax. Causes include malignancy (particularly lymphoma), trauma, following thoracotomy
Pseudochylothorax:
- Chronic effusion appears milky secondary to cell wall breakdown, found in TB or rheumatoid arthritis. Cholesterol >200 g/L.

Who

- Common in many conditions.

A typical patient

A 53-year-old woman with a history of breast carcinoma presents with right pleuritic chest pain and worsening breathlessness. On examination her breath sounds are diminished and her lungs are stony dull to percussion over the lower half of the right lung,

Symptoms and signs

Symptoms

- Depends on size of effusion
- Asymptomatic

- Dyspnoea
- Pleuritic chest pain.

Signs

On side of effusion:
- ↓ Chest expansion
- Stony dull percussion
- ↓ Breath sounds

- Bronchial breathing above level of effusion.
- ↓ Tactile fremitus
- Mediastinal shifts away from large effusion.

Investigations

Imaging

CXR:
- Small effusions: blunt costophrenic angle
- Large: dense homogeneous opacity from base (Fig. 3.10)

US:
- To show presence of pleural fluid

Contrast-enhanced thoracic CT scan:
- Identifies pleural nodularity

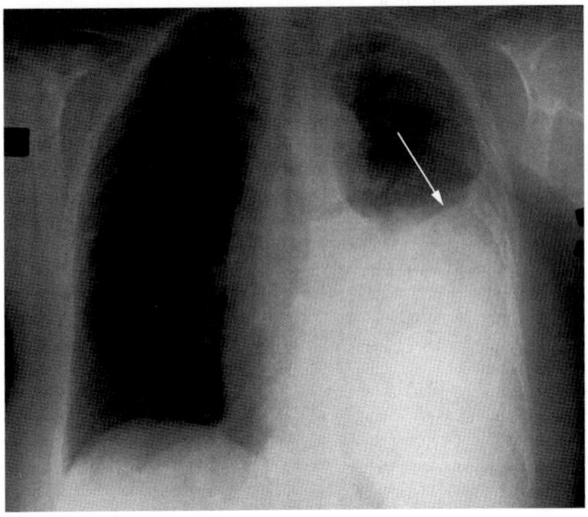

Other tests

Pleural fluid aspiration:
- Current guidelines recommend US guidance
- Analyse sample for pH, protein, glucose, amylase, LDH, microbiology, cytology, immunology. Need to send paired serum for LDH, glucose, protein

Pleural biopsy:
- Do if pleural fluid analysis is inconclusive
- CT guided is best.

Fig. 3.10   CXR showing a left pleural effusion (arrowed).

Treatment

- Asymptomatic small effusions: leave
- Drainage: using aspiration or drain
- Identify and treat cause

Pleurodesis:
- For repeated effusions
- Artificially obliterate the pleural space to prevent recurrence of a pneumothorax or pleural effusion.

Chemically or surgically:
- Chemicals: bleomycin, tetracycline, talc introduced into the pleural space causing irritation between the pleural layers and preventing accumulation of more fluid
- Surgical pleurodesis: via thoracotomy or thoracoscopy. Mechanically irritates the parietal pleura.

Prognosis and complications

Prognosis

- Depends on the cause.

EMPYEMA

Outline

- Pus in the pleural cavity due to an infected pleural effusion.

Pathogenesis/aetiology

Causes

- Secondary to pneumonia: commonest cause
- Rupture of lung abscess into pleural cavity

- Iatrogenic.

Who

A typical patient

A 62-year-old woman with resolving pneumonia develops a recurrent fever.

Symptoms and signs

Symptoms

- High fever
- Malaise
- Weight loss
- Cough.

Investigations

Imaging

- CXR: shows pleural effusion

Other tests

Bacterial investigation:
- Pleural tap: Pleural fluid pH <7.2

- Diagnosis and indication for chest drain include:
  - Positive pleural microscopy and culture and sensitivity
  - large effusion/symptomatic.

Treatment

- Drainage:
  - Normally with US or CT guidance
  - Larger-bore drain as thick fluid blocks small lumens, flush regularly
  - Guidelines recommend written consent
- Antibiotics: discuss with microbiologist (depends on source)

- Consider referral to cardiothoracic surgeons for consideration of video-assisted thoracoscopic surgery, thoracotomy and decortication or open thoracic drainage
- Trials currently evaluating use of intrapleural fibrinolytics

Prognosis and complications

Prognosis

- 15% mortality within 1 year.

PNEUMOTHORAX

Outline

- Air in the pleural cavity breaking the pleural seal allowing lung collapse

- Caused by a breach in the lung surface or chest wall
- Spontaneous, or from a 2° cause.

Classification

- Primary pneumothorax: occurs in apparently normal lungs
- Secondary pneumothorax: occurs in the presence of underlying lung disease or from an iatrogenic cause

Remember:
- Aspirate: 2nd intercostal space in mid-clavicular line (or 4th to 6th intercostal space mid-axillary line)
- Drain: 4th to 6th intercostal space anterior to mid-axillary line = 'safe triangle'. See BTS guidelines for illustration.

Pathogenesis/aetiology

Cause

Primary pneumothorax:
- Trauma: common
- Normally apical from rupture of sub-pleural bleb (blister on lung surface, a congenital defect in the connective tissue of the alveolar wall)

Secondary pneumothorax:
- Infection: with *Pneumocystis jiroveci* (previously PCP) in the acquired immunodeficiency syndrome (AIDS)
- Obstructive lung disease: asthma, COPD

- Carcinoma
- Congenital: cystic fibrosis
- Connective tissue disorders: Marfan syndrome, Ehler's Danlos
- Catamenial pneumothorax: occurs at same time as menstruation (may be related to endometriosis, where endometrial lining found around lung tissue)
- Iatrogenic: inserting a central line, pleural biopsy, pleural aspiration.

- ♀ < ♂
- Spontaneous pneumothorax often affects tall, thin, young males

Risk factors:
- Smokers
- ↑ height
- ↑ age
- Underlying lung disease.

A typical patient

A 21-year-old smoker with sudden onset of right sided chest pain and breathlessness that partially resolves over a few minutes.

Symptoms

- Asymptomatic
- Sudden onset of pleuritic pain

- Dyspnoea
- Deterioration in conditions like asthma or COPD.

Signs

- ↓ chest expansion and breath sounds
- Tracheal deviation away from pneumothorax: in tension pneumothorax
- Hyper-resonant chest

- Absent vocal fremitus
- Hamman's sign: a 'click' or 'crunch' on auscultation in time with heart sounds due to movement of pleural surfaces with left sided pneumothorax.

- ABG

Imaging

CXR:
- Line of visceral pleura with no lung markings outside the line. Can be total so that the whole lung cavity appears to have no markings
- Mediastinal shift away from affected side, in tension pneumothorax (Fig. 3.11).

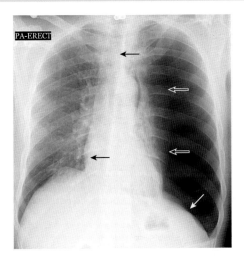

Fig. 3.11   CXR showing a tension pneumothorax (white arrows) with tracheal deviation (black arrows).

Treatment

Treatment depends on:
- The size, severity, if it is primary or secondary.

British Thoracic Society Guidelines

Primary pneumothorax:
- Small (<2 cm on CXR): consider discharge with follow up (2 cm equates to approximately 50% lung volume)
- Bigger (>2 cm on CXR):
  - Needle aspiration
  - Repeat if unsuccessful
  - Chest drain if still unsuccessful
  - Refer to chest physician within 48 h and consider suction if still unsuccessful.

Secondary pneumothorax:
- <2 cm and <50 years and not breathless: aspirate and admit for 24 h. If unsuccessful: drain
- If >2 cm, >50 and breathless:
  - Aspirate
  - If unsuccessful: chest drain
  - If unsuccessful refer to chest physician and consider suction.

Surgical

- Pleurodesis or sealing the lung
Considered if:
- Pneumothorax is bilateral
- Spontaneous haemothorax

- The lung fails to expand after a chest drain, i.e. persistent air leak or 5–7 days of drainage
- Recurrent pneumothorax.

Prognosis and complications

Prognosis

- 10% mortality in secondary pneumothorax

- 30% of primary spontaneous pneumothoraces will recur.

Complications

- Recurrent pneumothoraces
- Re-expansion pulmonary oedema: occurs in 14%. Presents as cough and SOB/desaturation. It is precipitated by late presentation of large pneumothoraces or very early use of suction.

- Surgical emphysema: (air in the subcutaneous layer) particularly if there is a large air leak. This is usually harmless although can cause acute respiratory compromise.

TENSION PNEUMOTHORAX

Outline

- A pneumothorax where the pleural tear acts like a valve: air enters the pleural space but can not leave
- Positive pressure builds up and causes the lung to collapse

- Medical emergency: can be minutes before death.

Pathogenesis/aetiology

Cause

- Trauma, e.g. stab wound or rib fracture

- Positive pressure ventilation

Sequelae

- ↑ air in the pleural space impairs venous return to the heart. This ↓ cardiac output

- The mediastinum is pushed to the contralateral hemithorax which can compress the great veins.

Who

- As before.

Symptoms

- Respiratory distress
- Tachycardia

- Hypotension
- Fever.

Signs

- Cyanosis
- ↓ air entry on affected side
- Trachea deviated away from pneumothorax

- Hyper-resonance
- BP ↓ on inspiration.

- If it is suspected, do not delay for investigations

- CXR *not* done before procedure due to urgency of treatment.

- Immediate decompression: large bore needle inserted to second intercostal space, mid-clavicular line on affected side
- Wait for hiss

- Then chest drain inserted immediately: sixth intercostal space mid-axillary line with underwater seal drainage.

Prognosis

- Can kill

Complications:
- ↑ pleural pressure can lead to hypotension and cardiac arrest.

VASCULAR LUNG DISEASES

PULMONARY EMBOLISM (PE)

Outline

- Obstruction of the pulmonary artery or one of its branches by an embolus
- An embolus is an abnormal mass of material (blood, clot, air, fat or tumour cells) transported in the blood from one area to the other

- Commonest cause: a dislodged thrombus, usually from a deep vein thrombosis (DVT), passing through the right heart and into the pulmonary arteries
- Always suspect in a patient suffering from a collapse or cardiac arrest in the first few weeks following surgery

Pulmonary embolism and DVT

- A pulmonary embolism and a DVT are aspects of the same disease

- In 90%, a pulmonary embolism is caused by a DVT
- 70% of those with a pulmonary embolism have a DVT.

Pathogenesis/aetiology

Cause

- DVT
- Various risk factors

- May be caused by an underlying malignancy, consider investigation if additional symptoms or signs suggest malignancy.

Pathogenesis

- Following a pulmonary embolism an area of lung is not perfused but remains well ventilated resulting in impaired gas exchange, hypoxia and circulatory collapse
- Large pulmonary embolism: obstructs right ventricular outflow causing ↑ pulmonary vascular resistance and acute heart failure. Present with signs of shock and is a medical

emergency. More than 50% of the pulmonary vascular bed must be occluded for a fatal pulmonary embolism
- Small pulmonary embolism: block peripheral vessels. Often asymptomatic unless causing an infarction
- Multiple pulmonary embolisms: can present with pulmonary hypertension.

- Incidence: 0.02–0.06%
Risk factors (**6 H's**):
- **H**ereditary (e.g. factor V Leyden, protein C or S deficiency)
- **H**ypercoagulability (smoking, malignancy, prothrombotic)

- **H**istory: DVT, pulmonary embolism, surgery, stroke
- **H**ypomobility (fracture, cerebral vascular accident, severe illness, obesity, long travel)
- **H**ypovolaemia (nephrotic syndrome, dehydration)
- **H**ormones (oestrogens, oral contraceptive pill).

A typical patient

A 30-year-old woman presents a week after a knee operation with haemoptysis and pleuritic chest pain. CXR is normal.

Symptoms

- Asymptomatic in most
- Dyspnoea*
- Chest pain: pleuritic

- Cough
- Haemoptysis

Signs

- Hypoxic
- Pyrexia
- Tachypnoea
- Tachycardia
- Pleural rub
- Clear chest on auscultation

- Signs of right ventricular failure (third heart sound), pleural effusion or DVT
- Cyanosis*
- Hypotension/shock*
- Collapse.*

*symptoms and signs of a massive pulmonary embolism

Blood tests

- ABG: ↓ PaO_2

- D dimers: Fibrinogen degradation products released when a clot dissolves. Not the only cause of ↑ d dimer but a –ve result makes pulmonary embolism unlikely.

ECG

- Normal or sinus tachycardia is commonest change

- May show features of right ventricular hypertrophy: peaked P waves, right axis deviation, right bundle branch block, **S1, Q3**, T3 (deep S in lead 1, Q waves and inverted T waves in lead 3).

Imaging

CXR:
- May be normal
- Translucency if severe
- Linear, wedge shaped opacities
- Pleural effusions
Ventilation/perfusion scan (V/Q) scan:
- See recap pages
CTPA:
- CTPA is now used more commonly.
- Gold standard of non-massive pulmonary embolism

Echo:
- Acute right ventricular dysfunction
US lower limbs:
- To find DVT or clot
- Search for underlying cause
Consider:
- malignancy
- thrombophilia: protein C, S, antithrombin, antiphospholipid syndrome,
- paroxysmal nocturnal haemoglobinuria (see haematology chapter).

Treatment

- ABC approach
- O$_2$, fluids, analgesia
- If systolic BP <90 mmHg:
  - Colloid infusion
  - Dobutamine and noradrenaline if BP is still low

See NICE guidance (May 2011)

Mechanical interventions:
- Graduated elastic stockings for post thrombotic syndrome (if DVT present)
- Inferior vena cava filler if contraindication for medical coagulation

Pharmacological interventions:
- LMWH: continued until warfarin treatment is begun and the therapeutic target INR is attained. Unless due to malignancy when LMWH is continued instead of warfarin
- Vitamin K antagonist e.g. Warfarin: Target INR 2–3 (with regular monitoring). Anticoagulated for 3–6 months if there is a definite trigger that has been eliminated and this is the 1st event. Ongoing treatment if there are persistent multiple risk factors or this is the second episode
  - Factor Xa inhibitors, e.g. fondaparinux, rivaroxaban.

Thrombolysis:
- Consider if haemodynamic instability

Surgical

- Necessary for severe cases
- Pulmonary embolectomy

- Vena cava filter if prone to DVTs or cannot anticoagulate

Prevention

- Heparin for all immobile patients
- Antiembolism compression stockings
- Stop hormone replacement therapy or the pill preoperatively

British Thoracic Society guidelines for flying:
- Low to moderate risk: antiembolism compression stockings +/- low dose aspirin before flight

- High risk (previous VTE, within 6 weeks of surgery, current malignancy): low dose aspirin, LMWH or formal anti-coagulation (INR 2–3) before flying.

Prognosis and complications

Prognosis

- Can be fatal
- Many die within 1 h

- Likelihood of relapse: 7% annually

Complications

- Haemorrhage
- Infarction

- Pulmonary hypertension (mean pulmonary arterial pressure >25 mmHg, see Ch. 2)
- Death

LUNG CANCER

MALIGNANT LUNG CANCERS

Outline

- Malignant cancers of the lung
- Most are centrally located

- Can be peripheral (mainly adenocarcinomas).

Classification

- Bronchogenic carcinomas (90% of 1° lung cancers)
  - Small cell (oat cell)
  - Non small cell (75% of bronchogenic)
    - Squamous
    - Adenocarcioma
    - Large cell

- Carcinoid tumours 5% (see surgery Ch. 13)
- Mesotheliomas (see below)
- Lung metastases (see below)

Pathogenesis/aetiology

Causes

- A number of risk factors, particularly smoking (95% of lung cancers are linked to smoking)

Other factors ↑ risk:

- ↑ age

- Chemicals: asbestos
- Radiation
- Industrial hazards
- Air pollution
- Genetics.

Paraneoplastic syndromes (including pathogenesis)

- Syndromes in lung cancer patients from secretory products released from the tumour that mimic hormones and modulators
- Occurs in 20% of lung cancers

Endocrine:

- Cushing syndrome: ectopic ACTH secretion
- Excess antidiuretic hormone (ADH; vasopressin), leading to syndrome of inappropriate ADH secretion (SIADH): ectopic ADH secretion: hyponatraemia

- Hypercalcaemia: PTH or PTH-related peptide (PTHrp)
- Hypocalcaemia: calcitonin secretion

Non endocrine:

- Hypertrophic pulmonary osteoarthropathy, causing wrist pain
- Weakness: Eaton Lambert syndrome (see neurology section)
- Trousseau syndrome: migratory thrombophlembitis.

Who

- Typical age: 50–70 years
- 1♀:3♂: (incidence ↑ in women)
- Commonest fatal cancer in western world

- In UK 40 000 new cases per year
- 20% of all cancers, 30% of cancer deaths.

A typical patient

- A 74-year-old woman presents with weight loss, cough, SOB and haemoptysis. On examination she has clubbing

- Pancoast tumour: 70-year-old man with weight loss and haemoptysis comes in with right-sided chest pain. His right eyelid is drooping.

Symptoms and signs

From growth into the lung

- **B**reathlessness
- **C**ough: mucosal irritation
- **C**hest pain
- **W**heeze

- Haemoptysis: vascular destruction
- Infection, e.g. pneumonia
- Airway obstruction.

Signs

- Consolidation/collapse
- Pleural effusion

- Hilar and mediastinal lymphadeopathy
- Clubbing

From regional spread

- Rib fractures, bone pain
- Oesophageal compression: dysphagia
- Vocal cord palsy (left recurrent laryngeal nerve) hoarse voice
- Phrenic nerve paralysis: breathlessness
- Superior vena cava obstruction: plethoric face, distended neck veins
- Extension to the heart: pericardial effusion or tamponade

- Horner syndrome: sympathetic ganglion invasion. **MAP** (usually from Pancoast tumour at pulmonary apex, superior sulcus):
  - **M**iosis: constricted pupil
  - **A**nhidrosis: ipsilateral loss of sweating
  - **P**tosis: drooping eyelid

Common signs of cancer

- Cachexia, anorexia, weight loss, anaemia.

- Aim to confirm the diagnosis, the type of cancer and then to assess the staging.

Blood tests

- FBC: anaemia
- U&E: ↓ sodium from inappropriate ADH secretion
- LFTs: metastasis
- Bone profile: metastasis.

Imaging

CXR:
- Most important initial test to confirm diagnosis
- Tumour: round shadow with a fluffy, spiked or a smooth (coin lesion) edge (Fig. 3.12)
- May show: pleural effusion, collapse, pneumonia, cavitation

CT/US/positron emission tomography (PET):
- To stage and assess metastases

Other tests

Histology and cytology:
- Sputum cytology: for malignant cells
- Pleural fluid cytology
- Bronchoscopy: washings/brushings (cytology) with biopsy at endoscopy or percutaneously (histology)
- Transthoracic fine needle aspiration biopsy with CT guidance: patient must be able to tolerate procedure. There is a risk of pneumothorax. Good for tissue diagnosis of peripheral lesions
- Resection: enables true grading and staging.

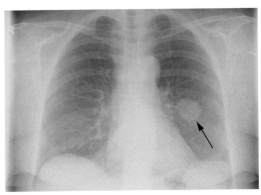

Fig. 3.12 Coin lesion (arrowed) typical of lung cancer.

Treatment depends on cell type/stage/grade/fitness/patient's wishes. All patients with a suspected diagnosis of lung cancer should be discussed at lung cancer MDT.

Palliation

- Analgesia
- Radiotherapy: for bone pain, superior vena cava obstruction and cerebral metastases
- Pleurodesis for repeated pleural effusions
- Also: stenting, laser, brachytherapy.

Prognosis

- 80% inoperable at presentation

Complications

- **SPEECH:**
  - **S**uperior vena cava syndrome
  - **P**aralysis of diaphragm (**Ph**renic nerve palsy)
  - P**e**ricarditis
  - **E**ctopic hormones
  - **E**aton–Lambert syndrome
  - **C**ollapse of lung
  - **H**orner syndrome/
  - **H**oarseness
- SPEECH: recurrent laryngeal nerve palsy
- Metastases to BLAB:
  - B: bone
  - L: liver
  - A: adrenals
  - B: brain

SMALL CELL CANCER

Outline

- Also called oat cell carcinoma
- 25% of bronchogenic carcinomas
- Rapid growth, so generally present late
- Most are metastatic at time of presentation.

Pathogenesis/aetiology

Pathology

- From neuroendocrine cells
- Poorly circumscribed small mass from the bronchial wall
- Usually central tumours
- Called 'oat cell' due to the shape: little cytoplasm, cells have an ovoid shape.

Classification

- Limited: Cancer within one lung +/− lymph nodes in mediastinum. (i.e. stage I, II or II disease). approx. 1/3 of patients.
- Extensive: Spread to other lung or distant metastasis. Not curable, surgery not an option.

Who

- ♀ < ♂
- Associations:
  - Smoking.

Symptoms and signs

- As for lung cancer
- Varied presentation due to paraneoplastic syndromes:
- ACTH, PTH, ADH leading to Cushing's, SIADH and Eaton–Lambert syndrome

Investigations

- As for lung cancer.

Treatment

- Quality statement by NICE in 2011 recommends that treatment should be started within 2 weeks of histological diagnosis for small cell lung cancer (SCLC).
- This is because it is very chemosensitive and without treatment survival is usually weeks.
- Resection rarely performed as most are metastatic at presentation (< 5% of patients)
- Responds well initially to chemotherapy, usually cisplatin and etoposide
- Radiotherapy may be added. Prophylactic brain irradiation is usually offered to all.

Prognosis and complications

Prognosis

- Poor prognosis
- 1–1.5 years treated (2–4 months if not)
- Present late
- Generally good response to treatments but short lived.

NON-SMALL CELL: SQUAMOUS CELL CARCINOMA

Outline

- 40% of bronchogenic carcinomas
- From the large airways
- Commonest cause of Pancoast tumour: 60% from squamous cell

Pancoast tumour

- Any lung cancer infiltrating the brachial plexus
- As it enlarges it affects nearby structures causing characteristic features:
- Cervical sympathetic plexus compression. **Horner** syndrome
- Brachial plexus involvement: shoulder and arm pain in an ulnar distribution
- Subclavian artery and vein compression
- Laryngeal nerve palsy: hoarseness.

Pathology

- Central tumour from the squamous epithelium in the large bronchi
- Grows slowly, spreads late.

- ♀ < ♂

Associations:
- Smoking.

- As for lung cancer
- Often presents with obstructive lesion

Paraneoplastic syndromes

- Hypercalcaemia commonest paraneoplastic syndrome from production of substance similar to PTH (PTH-related peptide)
- Hypertrophic pulmonary osteoarthropathy.

- As for lung cancer.

As for non small cell lung cancer

- Stage 1 and 2 – resectable. Options are surgery (10–20%) or radiotherapy
- Stage 3 – Occasionally surgery an option, may be offered neoadjuvant treatment. Offered chemotherapy and sometimes both chemotherapy and radiotherapy.
- Stage 4 – chemotherapy or radiotherapy or targeted therapy
- Undergo resection where possible chemo before or after surgery = neoadjuvant chemotherapy

- Curative radiotherapy is possible CHART – Continuous Hyperfractionated Accelerated Radiotherapy. For patients with stage 1 and 2 disease that can't be operated on (occasionally for stage 3 disease if not fit enough for chemotherapy and radiotherapy)
- Chemotherapy produces response but rarely cures in non-small-cell lung cancer.
- Examples of chemotherapy for adenoca and large cell lung ca = cisplatin and pemetrexed. Examples of chemo for squamous cell are cisplatin and gemcitabine.

Targeted anti-cancer treatments

- Erlotinib (Tarceva): A tyrosine kinase inhibitor, test EGFR status first. Licensed for first-line treatment in metastatic NSCLC
- Gefitinib (Iressa): A tyrosine kinase inhibitor. Only works if EGFR-positive mutation.
- Note, most likely to be EGFR positive if female; never smokers; adenocarcinoma and Asian origin

Prognosis

- Least likely to metastasize
- Local spread common.

Complications

- Obstruction of lumen
- Prone to cavities, infection and necrosis.

NON-SMALL CELL: ADENOCARCINOMA

Outline

- 10% of bronchogenic carcinomas
- Includes bronchoalveolar cell carcinoma.

Pathogenesis/aetiology

Pathology

- Arise from glandular cells: mucus goblet cells, type II pneumocytes
- Poorly circumscribed
- Mainly peripherally located so tends to be clinically silent as there are rarely obstructive symptoms.

Who

- 1♀<1♂

Associations:
- Asbestos exposure
- Smoking less of a risk
- Diffuse pulmonary fibrosis
- Occupational factors.

Symptoms and signs

- 15 years to presentation
- Paraneoplastic syndromes rare

- Hypertrophic pulmonary osteoarthropathy.

Investigations

As for lung cancer.

Treatment

As for non-small cell cancer.

Prognosis and complications

Complications

- Metastases at intermediate rate to pleura, lymph nodes and brain

- Leads to thrombophlebitis.

NON-SMALL CELL: LARGE CELL CARCINOMA

Outline

- 25% of bronchogenic carcinomas

- Also called anaplastic carcinoma.

Pathogenesis/aetiology

Pathology

- Poorly circumscribed large tumour
- Arises centrally so tends to present earlier than peripheral lesions due to obstruction

- Often with cavitation
- Large cells with marked cytotypical abnormalities.

Who

- ♀<♂

Associations:
- Smoking.

Symptoms and signs

- Paraneoplastic phenomena rare

- Can be ectopic excretion of gonadotrophins: leads to gynaecomastia and testicular atrophy.

Investigations

As for lung cancer.

Treatment

As for non-small cell cancer.

Prognosis and complications

Prognosis

- Poor prognosis

- Metastasises early.

LUNG METASTASIS

Outline

- Metastases from another location to the lung
- Commonly from the kidney, prostate, breast, bone, GI tract, cervix and ovary.

Pathogenesis/aetiology

Pathology

- Adenocarcinoma commonest histological type.

Who

- Depends on primary cancer.

Symptoms and signs

- Symptoms mainly related to space occupation within the lung.

Investigations

- Identify primary cancer.

Imaging

CXR:
- Cannonball metastases: multiple, well-circumscribed nodules of various sizes in the lungs seen on CXR. Classically from primary renal tumours (Fig. 3.13)

CT:
- Of chest, abdomen and pelvis for staging.

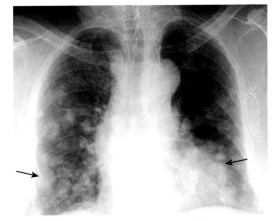

Fig. 3.13 CXR showing typical cannonball metastases (some arrowed).

Treatment

- Mostly palliative
- Solitary metastases can be resected if primary tumour is treatable
- Treat underlying cancer.

Prognosis and complications

Prognosis

- Poor
- Depends on primary tumour.

MESOTHELIOMA

Outline

- Malignant tumour of the mesothelium, the protective lining covering the internal organs
- Most common site is the pleura, where it begins as nodules and then obliterates the pleural cavity
- Spreads extensively
- Rarely affects peritoneum (including scrotal sac) and pericardium.

Pathogenesis/aetiology

Causes

Asbestos exposure:
- Most common cause: 90%
- 10% risk with heavy exposure

- Up to 40 years latency
- Important as patients can claim compensation if proven.

Metastases

- Aggressive direct invasion to lung and mediastinum.

Who

- Rare

- 1000 cases per year.

A typical patient

A 68-year-old retired builder presents with SOB, weight loss and pleuritic chest pain. A CT of the chest shows right pleural effusion and nodular pleural thickening.

Symptoms and signs

Symptoms

- Chest pain
- Dyspnoea

- Weight loss.

Signs

- Cachexia
- Clubbing

- Pleural effusions
- Lymphadenopathy.

Investigations

- Take full occupational and exposure history.

Imaging

- CXR (Fig. 3.14).
- CT: including staging CT scan – to assess spread.

Other tests

- Pleural biopsy, usually referred for video-assisted thoracoscopic surgery, biopsy and pleurodesis.

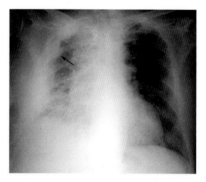

Fig. 3.14 CXR of mesothelioma with thickened, irregular margins (arrowed).

Treatment

- Often supportive and palliative measure only, little effective treatment
- Poor response to chemotherapy or radiotherapy

- Usually irradiation of biopsy track required as mesothelioma cells seed along the track
- Surgery rarely possible
- Eligible for industrial injuries benefit.

Prevention

- Prevent exposure, e.g. protective masks at work (buildings now screened for asbestos before building work occurs)

- Remove exposure if still exposed.

Prognosis and complications

Prognosis

- Poor
- Damage once done is irreversible
- 50% dead within 1 year, most in 2

- If asbestos is the cause: refer to a coroner
- Prognosis is worse if peritoneal involvement.

Complications

- Metastases, commonly to lymph nodes.

SYSTEMIC DISEASE AFFECTING THE RESPIRATORY SYSTEM

SARCOIDOSIS

Outline

- Systemic, chronic, multisystem granulomatous disease characterised by non-caseating granulomas (inflammatory nodules) which mostly appear in the lung (90%) or lymph nodes
- The skin, eye, bone, liver, kidney, CNS and heart also often affected
- The granulomas in sarcoidosis differ from those in TB because the granulomas are non-caseating and non-necrosing

Clinical course:
- Either the earlier stages are asymptomatic and resolve spontaneously or persistent progressive infiltrative lung disease

Stages of lung disease:
- *Stage 1*: bilateral hilar lymphadenopathy
- *Stage 2*: bilateral hilar lymphadenopathy and peripheral pulmonary infiltrates
- *Stage 3*: peripheral pulmonary infiltrates
- *Stage 4*: progressive pulmonary fibrosis, bullae, pleural involvement

Lofgren syndrome:
- Triad of bilateral hilar lymphadenopathy, arthralgia, erythema nodosum
- An acute form of sarcoidosis, good prognosis.

Pathogenesis/aetiology

Causes

- Unknown

- Probable response to unidentified antigen.

Pathogenesis

- Sarcoidosis is a granulomatous disease
- A granuloma is a cluster of modified macrophages surrounded by lymphoid cells in response to indigestible matter within the macrophages
- The granulomas usually heal, but in 20% the disease progresses and interstitial pulmonary fibrosis develops. This is due to ↑ local fibroblast production by macrophages which stimulates the fibrosis

- The macrophages cause an ↑ in ACE levels and may cause hypercalcaemia through activation of vitamin D
- Untreated, the disease can lead to life-threatening complications.

Who

- Typical age: 20–40 years
- ♀ > ♂
- Prevalence: 0.015%
- Black > > white > > Asian

- Genetic predisposition: siblings of affected persons have 5 × ↑ risk of sarcoid

Associations:
- Coeliac disease.

A typical patient

A 30-year-old black man presents with a dry cough but no other symptoms. On CXR he had bilateral hilar lymphadenopathy. He also has a bruise-like rash on his shins.

Symptoms and signs

- Asymptomatic in approximately 1/3: often discovered incidentally on routine CXR

Pulmonary

Symptoms
- Dry cough
- Dyspnoea

Signs
- Lung fibrosis

Non pulmonary

- Skin: erythema nodosum (tender shin nodules), lupus pernio (purplish raised lesions of the skin particularly the face
- Eyes: anterior uveitis, conjunctivitis, glaucoma
- CNS: Bell's palsy, cranial nerve palsies, meningitis, space occupying lesion

- Gradual onset:
  - General features of fever, malaise
- Pulmonary (90%).

- Chest pain
- ↓ exercise tolerance.

- Bilateral hilar lymphadenopathy

- Metabolic: hypercalcaemia leading to renal stones, hypothalamic involvement, diabetes insipidus
- Bones: arthralgia, bone cysts
- Heart: conduction defects, ventricular arrhythmias, cardiomyopathy, cor pulmonale
- Liver: hepatosplenomegaly, granulomatous hepatitis.

Investigations

Blood tests

- ESR ↑
- Hypercalcaemia

Urine

- Hypercalciuria.

Imaging

- CXR: bilateral hilar lymphadenopathy (in 90%) with fibrosis (in 10% of those) (Fig. 3.15)
- Differential diagnosis of bilateral hilar lymphadenopathy: TB, bronchial carcinoma, lymphoma
- High resolution CT: gold standard, can be diagnostic Nodules along septae and broncho-vascular bundles
- Bone X-rays: lesions in the terminal phalanges
- US: nephrocalcinosis, hepatosplenomegaly
- CT/MRI: assess severity, for neurosarcoidosis

Other tests

- ECG
- Lung function tests: show a restrictive defect, ↓ FVC, ↓ transfer factor of the lung for carbon monoxide
- Tissue biopsy: non-caseating granulomata, diagnostic test
- Broncho-alveolar lavage fluid cytology shows ↑ CD4 T-cells macrophages, lymphocytes and neutrophils
- Mantoux reactions: usually negative, even after BCG.

- ACE ↑
- Immunoglobulins ↑.

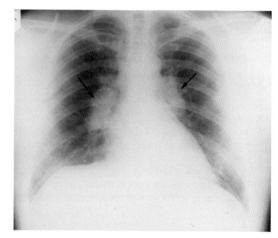

Fig. 3.15 CXR showing bilateral hilar lymphadenopathy (arrows).

Treatment

Conservative

- Leave to resolve.

Medical

Acute attack:
- Bed rest, NSAIDs

Chronic:
- Moderate dose steroids for 6 weeks (reducing dose slowly over 6–12 months) if:
  - Parenchymal lung disease (↑ symptoms, deteriorating lung function or CXR changes)
  - Hypercalcaemia

- CNS sarcoid
- Cardiac problems
- Lupus pernio
- Uveitis
- Splenic/hepatic or renal sarcoid
- Add immunosuppressants or anti-malarials for severe disease

Surgical

- Consider lung transplant if end-stage lung disease or rapidly progressive. Granulomata can recur in transplanted lung.

Prognosis and complications

Prognosis

- Most resolve spontaneously, and many with addition of steroid therapy
- Mortality is 5–10%

- Prognosis best in those with bilateral hilar lymphadenopathy and no chest infiltration on CXR
- Prognosis poorer in those with cardiac and CNS disease.

Complications

- Pulmonary fibrosis
- Cor pulmonale

- Respiratory failure
- Renal failure from hypercalciuria.

CYSTIC FIBROSIS

Outline

- Inherited disease where there is a defect in a transmembrane protein responsible for chloride transport across epithelial membranes, which affects water and sodium transmembrane transport

- Leads to viscous secretions and destruction of exocrine glands including:
  - pancreas
  - respiratory system
  - GI
  - reproductive tracts.

Pathogenesis/aetiology

Pathogenesis

- Autosomal recessive
- Due to mutation of the gene on chromosome 7 encoding the cystic fibrosis transmembrane conductance regulator (CFTR), which regulates chloride and water movement across the cell membrane
- Heterozygotes have an advantage as they are resistant to *Escherichia coli* diarrhoea and cholera
- Changes in composition of airway surface liquid predisposes to chronic pulmonary infections and bronchiectasis

- Airway colonisation ↑ with age and time
- Colonisation with pseudomonas worsens lung function
- Other organisms:
  - *Stentrophomonas maltophilia*
  - *Burkholderia cepacia complex*
  - Both are highly resistant to antibiotics.

Who

- Incidence: 0.05% of births
- Usually presents in childhood

- Common in Caucasians (1/25 are carriers).

A typical patient

A 1-year-old child with recurrent chest infections and failure to thrive. On examination she has clubbed fingers.

Symptoms

- Respiratory: usually presenting symptoms. Thick mucus leads to recurrent infection, airway can be obstructed by mucus leading to: cough, wheeze, pneumothorax, bronchiectasis
- GI: ↓ secretion of pancreatic enzymes from pancreatic duct obstruction leading to: diabetes, gallstones, greasy stool (from malabsorption), failure to thrive

- Other: male infertility, osteoarthropathy, nasal polyps, sinusitis, meconium ileus (earliest stool of infant are thickened and obstruct the ileum, common presenting symptom in newborns).

Signs

- Underweight
- Cyanosis

- Clubbing
- Crackles on auscultation of the lungs.

- Sweat test: sweat sodium and Cl measured. ↑ levels of Cl in sweat (two +ve results of high Cl on two separate days
- Lung function tests: FEV1 is best marker of disease progression
- Faecal elastase for exocrine pancreatic dysfunction
- Genetic testing

Screening:
- In the UK there is a national screening programme: neonatal heel-prick for immunoreactive trypsinogen

Diagnosis:
- Is made based on clinical findings and biochemical or genetic confirmation.

- Multidisciplinary team
- Fertility advice and psychosocial support
- Vaccinations: influenza and pneumococcus

Chest:
- Physiotherapy, postural drainage, bronchodilators, antibiotics
- Advanced disease: O_2 (long-term O_2 therapy) diuretics, hypertonic saline, short course steroids, immunisation non-invasive ventilation

GI:
- Pancreatic enzyme replacement, nutritional support

Gene therapy:
- Human DNAase has been cloned, can be given nebulised if FEV >40% predicted

Annual screening for:
- Biliary cirrhosis
- Portal hypertension
- Cystic fibrosis-related diabetes;
- Osteoporosis

Surgical

- Lung or heart transplantation
- Consider if prognosis <2 years or very poor quality of life.

Prognosis

- Predicted life span ~40 years

- Death mainly from respiratory complications.

Complications

- Pulmonary infection is a recurrent problem: in childhood *Staphylococcus* infection predominates. *Pseudomonas aeruginosa* is a common later infection.

CRITICAL CARE MEDICINE

PULMONARY OEDEMA

Outline

- Accumulation of fluid in the lungs
- Impaired gas exchange leads to ↑ work of breathing and respiratory failure

- Medical emergency: life threatening.

Classification

- Cardiogenic pulmonary oedema: usually from left ventricular failure, mitral stenosis, arrhythmias, MI, malignancy, hypertension

- Non-cardiogenic pulmonary oedema: due to acute lung injury, acute respiratory distress syndrome (see below), fluid overload.

Pathogenesis/aetiology

Pathogenesis

- Cardiogenic (high pressure): elevation of left atrial pressure causes ↑ pulmonary capillary pressure and ↑ transudation of fluid into the pulmonary interstitium and alveoli. Occurs only after lymphatic drainage capacity has been exceeded so if there is blockage e.g. from a tumour, it will occur more readily

- Non-cardiogenic (low pressure): damage from trauma, burns or other causes increases vascular permeability from the release of inflammatory mediators.

Who

A typical patient

An 80-year-old patient presenting with pink frothy sputum and SOB, particularly at night.

Symptoms and signs

Symptoms

- Acute extreme dyspnoea
- Cough: white or pink (blood tinged) sputum
- Wheeze (cardiac asthma)

- Sweating
- Symptoms secondary to initial disorders such as cardiac failure.

Signs

- Tachypnoea
- Pallor
- Cyanosis
- Low O_2 saturations

- Tachycardia
- Raised JVP
- Crackles: bilateral bibasally on auscultation
- Paroxysmal nocturnal dyspnoea.

Investigations

Blood tests

- FBC, U&Es, cardiac enzymes, ABG.

ECG

- May help identify precipitating cause, e.g. MI.

Imaging

CXR: ABCDE
1. **A**lveolar oedema: bats wing appearance of lung fields from bilateral perihilar patchy shadowing from alveolar fluid
2. Kerley **B** lines: short horizontal opacities seen at the lung periphery representing fluid in thickened interlobular septa

3. **C**ardiomegaly
4. **D**ilated prominent upper lobe vessels: from ↑ pulmonary venous pressure
5. Pleural **e**ffusion
See heart failure p. 22 and Fig. 2.18, p. 23.
Echocardiogram

Treatment

Acute management:
- Sit the patient up
- O$_2$
- IV morphine 2.5–10 mg: relieves dyspnoea (give with antiemetic)
- Furosemide 80 mg IV: vasodilate, reduce preload and water removal
- Glyceryl trinitrate: to reduce the preload, use spray first, infusion if systolic BP >100 mmHg

- IV aminophylline or inhaled B blockers can be considered for bronchospasm
- Investigate and treat cause
- Mechanical ventilation if needed
- Monitor progress regularly: specifically fluid balance, renal function and arrhythmias
- Treat underlying cause.

Prognosis and complications

Prognosis

- Depends on the cause.

ACUTE RESPIRATORY DISTRESS SYNDROME/ACUTE LUNG INJURY

Outline

Acute respiratory distress syndrome (ARDS):
- Severe respiratory failure precipitated by lung injury or an indirect systemic illness, causing a pulmonary inflammatory response leading to non-cardiogenic pulmonary oedema, pulmonary hypertension, fibrosis, stiffening of the lungs and multiorgan failure
- Life-threatening condition

- Three phases of ARDS:
  1. Early period of alveolar damage/pulmonary infiltrates
  2. 1 week later infiltrates resolve. Early collagen formation
  3. If patient survives: fibrotic stage. Residual lung cysts/fibrosis
- Acute lung injury (ALI) is a less severe form
- Transfusion-related lung injury (TRALI):
  - Occurs within a few hours of blood transfusion.

Pathogenesis/aetiology

Causes

General:
- Sepsis, trauma, burns, drug overdose, haemorrhage, pancreatitis, disseminated intravascular coagulation, blood transfusion

Pulmonary:
- Pneumonia
- Aspiration
- Inhalation injury

Pathophysiology

Damage to alveolar capillary wall from precipitating cause
↓
Inflammatory mediators released
↓
Vascular permeability
↓
Non cardiogenic pulmonary oedema
↓
Acute respiratory failure
↓
Vasoconstriction as blood is redirected to better areas of oxygenation
↓
Pulmonary hypertension
↓
Within days new epithelial lining forms, causing fibroblasts to gather. This leads to lung fibrosis and lung stiffening
↓
Multiorgan failure can follow.

Who

- Depends on the cause.

A typical patient

A road traffic accident patient with a broken leg arrives in A&E hypotensive and has a blood transfusion. The next day he is more breathless and this is not corrected with O_2. He deteriorates further the following few days.

Symptoms and signs

Symptoms

- Respiratory distress normally 12–48 h after initial event
- Dyspnoea
- Signs and symptoms of pulmonary oedema
- Symptoms of precipitating event.

Signs

- Cyanosis
- Tachypnoea
- Tachycardia
- Hypoxia
- Bilateral basal crackles on auscultation

Investigations

Blood tests

- FBC
- U&Es
- LFTs
- Amylase
- Clotting
- Cultures
- ABG.

Imaging

- CXR: bilateral diffuse infiltrates
- Echo

Other tests

Pulmonary artery catheter:
- For pulmonary capillary wedge pressure measurement.

ARDS: diagnostic criteria

- **A**cute onset
- **R**atio (PaO_2/FiO_2 <40 kPa)
- **D**iffuse infiltration: bilateral basal infiltrates on CXR
- **S**wan-Ganz wedge pressure <19 mmHg on CXR (excludes cardiogenic pulmonary oedema). ARDS: As above but ratio $PaO_2/FiO_2 < 26.7$kPa).

Treatment

Admit to ICU:
- Find and treat underlying condition
- Mechanical ventilation: needed in most patients. Extracorporeal oxygenation/CO_2 removal (ECMO) is very specialist and expensive, but may 'buy time'
- Fluid balance: careful fluid monitoring and management
- For pulmonary oedema: fluid restriction and diuretics

Other treatments:
- Antibiotics if septic
- Nitrous oxide to vasodilate and increase lung perfusion
- Nutritional support
- Prone positioning may help.

Prognosis and complications

Prognosis

- Poor, particularly in the elderly
- Varies with cause, age, and organ involvement
- Mortality ~40%
- 90% if there is sepsis and most die from this
- Worse with fibrosis
- Those surviving often have residual lung damage.

Complications

- Barotrauma from high ventilation pressure: pneumothorax, emphysema
- Infection in 50%
- Myopathy: from steroid and neuromuscular blockade

- DVT
- Poor nutrition
- GI bleed.

RESPIRATORY FAILURE

Outline

Pulmonary gas exchange is impaired, causing hypoxia.

Classification

Type 1:
- Hypoxia (<8 kPa) with normal or low Pa_{CO_2}
- Type 1: '1 gas changed'
- Due to any of the following:
  - Diffusion defect in gas exchange in part of the lung
  - Ventilation/perfusion mismatch
  - Right-to-left shunting of blood in the heart, e.g. cyanotic CHD
  - Low inspired O_2, e.g. high altitude

Type 2:
- Hypoxia (<8 kPa) with hypercapnia (>7 kPa)
- Type 2: '2 gases changed'
- Due to hypoventilation, with or without ventilation/ perfusion mismatch.

Pathogenesis/aetiology

Causes

Type 1 causes:
- Lung disease
  - Pulmonary oedema, pneumonia, asthma, COPD, pulmonary embolism, lung fibrosis, ARDS, tension pneumothorax
- General causes:
  - High altitude, cardiogenic shock, cyanotic CHD

Type 2 causes:
- Lung disease:
  - COPD, asthma, restrictive lung disease
- Neuromuscular disorders:
  - Spinal cord lesion, Guillain-Barre, polio, myasthenia gravis, kyphoscoliosis
- ↓ Central respiratory drive:
  - Trauma, CNS tumour, brain stem disease, drugs (opiates, barbiturates).

Who

Depends on cause.

A typical patient

Type 1:
A patient with a pulmonary embolism is acutely breathless, tachycardic and tachypnoeic.
Type 2:
A patient with a history of COPD and obesity is cyanosed, sleeps all day and snores.

Symptoms and signs

Symptoms

Hypoxia:
- Dyspnoea
- Restlessness
- Confusion
- Cyanosis

Hypercapnia:
- Confusion
- Headache
- Drowsiness
- ↓ Consciousness
- Coma.

Signs

- Tachycardia
- Bounding pulse
- Tremor of outstretched hands

- Papilloedema
- 2° polycythaemia.

Investigations

- Pulse oximetry.

Blood tests

- FBC, U&Es, CRP, ABG, microscopy, culture and sensitivity

Normal values:
- O_2: 10–13.3 kPa
- CO_2: 4.7–6 kPa

Imaging

- CXR.

Other tests

- Lung function tests
- Spirometry: FVC can guide deterioration

- Specific tests to investigate suspected underlying causes.

TREATMENT

- General supportive measures
- Treat underlying condition

Type 1:
- O_2
- Mechanical ventilation, e.g. CPAP if refractory hypoxia. Consult ICU

Type 2:
- O_2 but give cautiously as respiratory centre may be driven by hypoxia due to CO_2 retention: begin at 24% with a Venturi mask and adjust according to blood gas concentration
- Mechanical ventilation if needed, e.g. non-invasive positive-pressure ventilation
- Consider intubation if no success.

Prognosis and complications

Prognosis

- Depends on cause
- Worse if requiring ventilation: 30% 1 year survival.

Complications

- Type 2 can cause cor pulmonale and pulmonary hypertension.

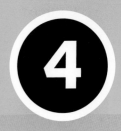
Sections of the gut

Foregut: mouth to second part of duodenum, blood supply from coeliac artery

Midgut: second part of the duodenum to proximal two thirds of the transverse colon, blood supply from superior mesenteric artery

Hindgut: distal third of the transverse colon to the anus, blood supply from the inferior mesenteric artery.

Abdominal pain

- Visceral pain: originates from internal organs and visceral peritoneum (inner layer around the internal organs). It is a dull pain and poorly localised.
- Parietal pain: originates from the abdominal wall of parietal peritoneum (outer layer attached to the abdominal wall). Pain is sharper and better localised.

Investigations

Blood tests

- *LFTs*: see hepatology (Ch. 5).
- *Vitamin levels*: particularly as different vitamins are absorbed in different parts of the gut, e.g. vitamin B_{12}
- *Amylase*: very high levels suggests pancreatic disease but may be raised in anyone presenting with an 'acute abdomen'.

Abdominal radiography (AXR)

Useful for investigating:

- obstruction (dilated bowel loops)
- perforation (air under the diaphragm)
- calcification (e.g. in the pancreas).

Normal AXR shown in Figure 4.1.

Abdominal US

Good first-line investigation. Indications include abdominal pain, abdominal masses, hepatomegaly, identifying ascites, liver disease.

Abdominal CT

Good for imaging the pancreas and staging all GI tumours.

CT pneumocolon now replacing Barium enema as an alternative to colonoscopy, or if colonoscopy fails.

Abdominal MRI

- CT is preferable as movement of abdomen affects the quality of MRI. MRI images becoming better and, therefore, increasingly used.
- Small bowel MRI is very useful for investigating small bowel Crohn's disease.
- Abdominal MRI is also better than CT or USS for detecting gallstone disease.

Barium studies

Barium is given orally and X-rays used to visualise the GI tract:

- Useful for investigating strictures, intraluminal abnormalities and motility disorders
- Largely replaced by endoscopy which allows direct views and biopsies, however, still useful as a non-invasive investigation for upper GI symptoms
- Types:
  - barium swallow to investigate dysphagia and motility disorders
  - barium meal to investigate epigastric pain and vomiting
  - small bowel follow through for diarrhoea and abdominal pain
  - barium enema for change in bowel habit and lower abdominal pain (rarely used). Now largely replaced for this purpose by MR/CT enterography and capsule.

Oesophageal pH monitoring

Invasive monitoring using a pH probe via the nose into the lower oesophagus for a 24 hour period.

Allows monitoring of reflux. Often performed in conjunction with oesophageal manometry.

Manometry

Monitors the motor function of the oesophageal sphincter by measuring pressures in the oesophagus, thus recording peristaltic swallow waves.

A catheter is inserted via the nose in patients with dysphagia or reflux to determine the cause.

Endoscopy

Direct visualisation of the GI tract with a video endoscope:

- Can be upper GI (oesophagogastroduodenoscopy (OGD)) or lower (colonoscopy or sigmoidoscopy)

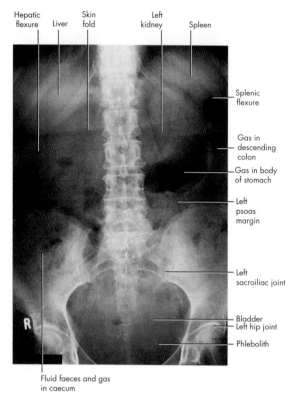

Hepatic flexure Liver Skin fold Left kidney Spleen

Splenic flexure

Gas in descending colon

Gas in body of stomach

Left psoas margin

Left sacroiliac joint

Bladder
Left hip joint

Phlebolith

R

Fluid faeces and gas in caecum

Fig. 4.1 The abdominal X-ray and its features.

- Good for detecting polyps, inflammatory bowel disease, ulcers, tumours, diverticular disease, angiodysplasia (vascular abnormalities of the gut mucosa)
- Therapeutic procedures at endoscopy include:
  - polypectomy: excision of polyps
  - endoscopic retrograde cholangiopancreatography (ERCP): see hepatology
  - management of variceal bleeds and ulcers.

Wireless capsule endoscopy: ingestion of a pill which contains a camera. Images uploaded and viewed digitally. Useful for investigation of small bowel pathology.

Preparation for an endoscopy
- Gastroscopy (oesophagogastroduodenoscopy, OGD) and ERCP: must be nil by mouth for 6 h
- Colonoscopy: bowel preparation involves taking laxatives the day before and again 12 h before the test. Only clear fluid intake for 24 h before the test
- OGD: the pharynx is sprayed with local anaesthetic and sedation is sometimes given; the flexible endoscope is inserted through the mouth.
- Colonoscopy: the colonoscope is advanced via the anus.
- Usually after intravenous analgesia and/or sedation.

Complications of endoscopy
- Transient sore throat (upper)
- Aspiration (upper)
- Amnesia of sedation
- Perforation (risk in OGD 1 in 3000–5000 and colonoscopy 1 in 1000–2000)
- Cardiac arrest (<0.1%)
- Abdominal discomfort and haemorrhage.

See also
- Hepatology (Ch. 5): oesophageal and gastric varices surgery (Ch. 13): malignancy of the GI tract
- The patient presents (Ch. 14): dysphagia, nausea and vomiting, constipation, diarrhoea, dyspepsia, GI bleeding, pruritus ani, abdominal pain, abdominal masses, hepatomegaly, hyposplenism
- Clinical examinations (Ch. 15): GI system.

OESOPHAGEAL DISORDERS

ACHALASIA

Outline

- Aperistalsis of the muscular wall of the oesophagus

- Non-propulsive contraction of the oesophagus and failure of relaxation of the lower oesophageal sphincter (LOS) on swallowing.

Pathogenesis/aetiology

Causes

- Majority: aetiology unknown

- Occasionally: *Trypanosoma cruzi* (Chagas' disease) can result in mega-oesophagus.

Pathogenesis

- Reduction in ganglionic cells in the nerve plexus of the oesophageal wall

- Results in failure of relaxation of LOS and uncoordinated, weak or absent peristalsis.

Who

- Rare in childhood
- Typical age: 35–60 years

- 1♀:1♂
- Incidence: 0.001%.

Clinical features

- Dysphagia: difficulty in swallowing
- Chest pain: severe and retrosternal (due to non-peristaltic muscle contraction)

- Fluid regurgitation: often worse at night.

Investigations

Imaging

CXR:
- Dilated oesophagus or fluid level behind the heart may be seen.

Barium swallow
- Demonstrates a dilated oesophagus above a tapered section (bird's beak sign) and reduced peristalsis.

CT chest
- To rule out other causes of pseudoachalasia such as malignancy.

Other tests

Oesophageal manometry
- Measurement of intra-oesophageal pressure which demonstrates non-relaxation of the LOS and aperistalsis.

Endoscopy
- To exclude malignancy, which may mimic achalasia (pseudoachalasia) and eosinophilic oesophagitis.

Treatment

Endoscopic

- Endoscopic dilatation of LOS

- Endoscopic injection of botulinum toxin into LOS. Temporary benefit only.

Medical

- Calcium antagonists, e.g. nifedipine, where surgery is not possible. Reduces LOS pressure.

Surgical

- Heller's cardiotomy with anti-reflux procedure: surgical splitting of the LOS muscular ring (performed laparoscopically).

- Increasingly performed as a primary procedure rather than if dilatations fail

Prognosis and complications

Complications

- Gastro-oesophageal reflux disease (GORD): with all treatments
- Aspiration pneumonia
- Squamous cell carcinoma of oesophagus (3–5%).

GASTRO-OESOPHAGEAL REFLUX DISEASE

Outline

- Gastric contents reflux back up into the lower oesophagus
- A small amount of reflux is normal
- Symptoms occur where there is prolonged exposure to gastric contents
- Symptomatic only in a few people

Oesophagitis

- Inflammation of the oesophagus
- Results in damage to the oesophageal mucosa
- Predisposes to Barrett's oesophagus.

Pathogenesis/aetiology

Predisposing factors

- Increased abdominal pressure:
  - Pregnancy
  - Obesity
  - Vomiting
- Incompetence of lower oesophageal sphincter:
  - Smoking
- Alcohol
- Hiatus hernia
- Systemic sclerosis
- Reduced mucosal protection:
  - NSAIDs

Causes of oesophagitis

- GORD
- Infection: *Candida*, HSV, CMV
- Chemicals: NSAIDs, toxins, alcohol, radiation therapy
- Inflammation: Crohn's disease, eosinophilic oesophagitis.

Who

- ↑ with age
- Prevalence: 10%
Risk factors:
- Smoking
- Alcohol
- Hiatus hernia
- Pregnancy
- Obesity
- Tight clothes
- Big meals
- Drugs, e.g. anticholinergics, nitrates, tricyclics antidepressants
- Systemic sclerosis
- Also certain foods, typically caffeine, acidic foods, fatty foods.

A typical patient

An obese man presents with a history of retrosternal burning pain worse on lying flat and after meals.

Clinical features

- Heart burn after eating, when lying/stooping, relieved by antacids
- Odynophagia: pain on swallowing
- Retrosternal chest pain: due to muscular spasm (the commonest cause of non-cardiac chest pain)
- Regurgitation of acid/bile

Other symptoms

- Nocturnal cough from microaspiration
- Morning hoarseness
- Water brash: accumulation of saliva in the mouth due to excess acid.

Investigations

Imaging

- Upper GI endoscopy to exclude a sinister cause if:
  - age is >40 years
  - symptoms persist >4 weeks despite treatment
  - weight loss

Other tests

Special tests:
- 24 h oesophageal pH monitoring
- Oesophageal manometry.

Treatment

Conservative

- Lifestyle: ↓ weight and smoking, avoid eating at bedtime, review medication predisposing to GORD.
- Dietary modification

Medical

- Antacids: magnesium trisilicate mixture or alginates, e.g. Gaviscon
- H_2 receptor antagonists, e.g. ranitidine
- Proton pump inhibitors (PPIs), e.g. omeprazole
- Prokinetics, e.g. metoclopramide (promotes gastric emptying and reduces nausea and vomiting).

Surgical

- Nissen fundoplication: wrapping the upper part of the stomach around the oesophagus. Not really for severe symptoms. Consider fundoplication in established reflux despite lifestyle modification and patient does not wish to continue long-term acid suppression. Patients with symptoms which are resistant to high dose PPIs may not do well from fundoplication.

Prognosis and complications

Complications

- Oesophagitis
- Oesophageal stricture and dysphagia
- Barrett's oesophagus (10%)
- Ulceration
- Anaemia
- Mucosal erosions
- Bleeding: haematemesis/melaena
- Adenocarcinoma
- Aspiration pneumonitis

BARRETT'S OESOPHAGUS

Outline

- Abnormal change (metaplasia) in the cells of the lower part of the oesophagus
- Due to cellular damage from chronic acid exposure, or reflux oesophagitis
- A premalignant condition: increased risk of oesophageal cancer

Pathogenesis/aetiology

Pathology

- Squamous epithelium replaced with glandular epithelium (also called columnar-lined oesophagus)
- 40% of gastro-oesophageal strictures are associated with Barrett's oesophagus.

Who

- 4♀:7♂
- 15% of GORD patients

Risk factors:
- Obesity
- High fat intake
- Smoking/alcohol

Clinical features

- As for GORD
- Also dysphagia as an alarm symptom, particularly in patients with Barrett's oesophagus.

Investigations

Endoscopy

- Columnar lined oesophagus visible >3 cm above the gastric folds. Anything less than 3 cm is colloquially referred to as short-segment Barrett's oesophagus.

Treatment

Endoscopic:
- Surveillance: regular endoscopy with biopsies to detect dysplastic changes before progression to cancer.
- Locally ablative therapies or surgery if dysplasia develops.

Medical

- Proton pump inhibitor lifelong, e.g. omeprazole.

Prognosis and complications

Complications

- Oesophageal cancer (30–40× increased risk).

OESOPHAGEAL STRICTURE

Outline

- Narrowing of the oesophagus.

Pathogenesis/aetiology

Causes

- Chronic acid reflux
- Malignancy
- Ulceration: can cause stenosis
- Radiotherapy.

Who

- Lower prevalence of benign stricture due to widespread proton pump inhibitor use.

Clinical features

- Dysphagia: difficulty swallowing (solid foods more than fluids)
- Odynophagia (pain on swallowing)
- Weight loss
- Regurgitation/vomiting.

Investigations

- Endoscopy with mandatory biopsies to exclude malignancy
- Barium swallow.

Treatment

For benign stricture:
- Treat underlying cause

Medical

- Lifelong proton pump inhibitors.

Surgical

- Endoscopic dilatation
- Oesophageal resection
- Also sometimes temporary stent placement

Prognosis and complications

Prognosis

- Remains lifelong once formed but can be managed with regular dilatations.

MALLORY–WEISS TEAR

Outline

- Tearing of the oesophageal lining around the gastro-oesophageal junction
- Due to violent or repeated vomiting or retching.

Pathogenesis/aetiology

Causes

- Pressure on the gastro-oesophageal junction mucosa from raised intragastric pressure during vomiting results in tearing and bleeding.

Who

- Young people
- Binge drinkers.

Clinical features

- Haematemesis usually after initial history of vomiting or retching
- Melaena: if severe.

Investigations

Blood tests

- FBC
- Clotting.

Treatment

- Antiemetics
- Treat cause of vomiting
- Endoscopy to rule out other causes of GI bleed and rarely for therapeutic intervention if there is a large tear.

Prognosis and complications

Prognosis

- Good.

STOMACH DISORDERS

PEPTIC ULCER DISEASE

Outline

- Ulcer: severe mucosal defect extending through the muscularis mucosa into the submucosa.

Found in

- Stomach
- Proximal duodenum
- Oesophagus
- Gastro-oesophageal junction
- Jejunum: in Zollinger–Ellison syndrome (gastrinoma). Also a cause of recurrent ulceration proximal to the jejunum

Pathogenesis/aetiology

Causes

Multiple factors are additive:
- *Helicobacter pylori (H. pylori)*:
  - Commonest cause
  - Colonisation present in 90% with duodenal ulcers, 50% with gastric ulcers
  - 10% of those with *H. pylori* will progress to ulcer disease
  - Causes ulcer from:
    1. Toxins released by bacteria and the inflammatory response of the body result in direct injury of the mucosa
    2. Excess acid due to increased parietal cell mass and gastrin secretion

- NSAIDs: 2nd commonest cause
- Smoking
- Hypercalcaemia
- Stress: 5–10% of ITU admissions develop acute ulcers
- Chemical poisoning
- Hyperparathyroidism
- Gastric acid hypersecretion, e.g. Zollinger–Ellison syndrome rare disorder of excessive gastrin secretion
- Primary gastric cancer presenting with the features of an ulcer.

Pathogenesis

- Imbalance between mucosal defences and harmful effects of acid
- Normally hydrochloric acid is secreted by the parietal cells in the stomach on the stimuli of gastrin, acetylcholine and histamine

- Protective factors: mucus, bicarbonate and prostaglandins.

Who

Lifetime risk:
- ♀ 5%, ♂ 10%

Risk factors:
- *H. pylori*
- NSAIDs

- Elderly
- Smoking
- Stress
- Steroids

A typical patient

- A middle aged man with long-standing epigastric pain presents with melaena.

Clinical features

- Epigastric pain: worse at night and soon after eating. Pain radiates to chest, neck or back. Relieved by antacids
- Nausea/vomiting
- Haematemesis/melaena: if the patient is bleeding acutely see 'patient presents' chapter for investigations and management

- Weight loss
- Anaemia
- May be asymptomatic.

Investigations

Screen for *H. pylori*

- Invasive tests
  - Rapid urease test (also known as the CLO (campylobacter-like organism) test): biopsy containing *H. pylori* causes a colour change on the indicator due to the breakdown of urea to ammonia by *H. pylori*
  - Histology
  - Cultures

- Non-invasive tests
  - Stool test
  - Serology
  - Urea breath test: radiolabelled carbon 13 is given orally, it can be detected in the breath in a positive test

Endoscopy

- Investigation of choice as can exclude malignancy with direct vision and biopsies

- Used in high-risk groups vs. a test-and-treat strategy in low-risk groups.

Treatment

Conservative

- Avoid foods that worsen symptoms
- Stop smoking
- Stop NSAIDs

Medical

- Acid suppressing drugs:
  - Proton pump inhibitors, e.g. lansoprazole, omeprazole
  - H$_2$ receptor antagonists, e.g. ranitidine
- *H. pylori* eradication therapy: (if *H. pylori* +ve) triple therapy of proton pump inhibitor and two antibiotics for 7 days.

Surgical

- Rarely required, unless complications occur
- Partial gastrectomy: excision of ulcer and antrum of the stomach while retaining continuity of stomach and duodenum
- Vagotomy: resection of the vagus nerve to reduce gastric acid secretion (vagus nerve stimulates the parietal cells to secrete gastric acid)
- Repeat endoscopy to assess healing for gastric ulcers.

Treatment of complications

- Haemorrhage:
  - first line: endoscopic intervention with thermal methods, adrenaline or clips, or more recently with haemostatic powder application, e.g. Hemospray
  - second line: surgical excision
- Perforation:
  - Surgical laparoscopic repair
- Pyloric stenosis:
  - Endoscopic balloon dilation or stent insertion or partial gastrectomy.

Prognosis and complications

Prognosis

- Good with medical treatment
- May recur.

Complications

- Malignancy: particularly gastric ulcers
- Haemorrhage (15–20%)
- Anaemia
- Perforation (5%). More with duodenal ulcers
- Gastric outlet obstruction (2%)
- Pyloric stenosis: due to scarring

Complications of peptic ulcer surgery:
- Post-op complications (see surgery chapter)
- Dumping syndrome: rapid emptying of the stomach after a meal causing a fall in blood sugar, nausea and weakness
- Post-vagotomy diarrhoea.

GASTRITIS

Outline

- Inflammation of the gastric mucosa
- Histological diagnosis.

Classification

Acute:
- Transient acute inflammatory response to gastric mucosal damage
- Superficial and self-limiting

Chronic:
- Chronic inflammation of mucosa.

Pathogenesis/aetiology

Causes

Acute:
- Chemicals: alcohol, smoking, NSAIDs, chemotherapy, bile reflux
- Stress
- Infections: HSV, CMV
- Inflammation

Chronic:
- *H. pylori*: commonest cause
- Crohn's
- Autoimmune gastritis. Immune mediated destruction of gastric glands with chronic inflammation. Causes pernicious anaemia in 10%. Autoantibodies are directed against either parietal cells (found in gastric glands that secrete acid) or intrinsic factor (required for absorption of vitamin B_{12})
- Radiation
- Smoking
- Alcohol.

Who

- Very common

Associations:
- Chronic autoimmune gastritis is associated with other autoimmune diseases.

Clinical features

- Usually asymptomatic

Acute:
- Epigastric burning
- Nausea/vomiting
- Indigestion
- If severe may result in mucosal erosion, ulceration, bleeding, acute necrotising gastritis with severe pain, haematemesis, melaena or shock

Chronic:
- Few symptoms
- Pain
- Nausea/vomiting.

Investigations

Blood tests

Auto-antibodies:
- Intrinsic factor
- Anti-parietal cell

Schilling test:
- Test to assess if symptoms are due to vitamin B_{12} or intrinsic factor deficiency
- See vitamin B_{12} deficiency in haematology chapter for details.

Other tests

Endoscopy:
- Erythematous mucosa

- Atrophic mucosa in chronic inflammation.

Treatment

- No specific treatment required
- Eradicate *H. pylori* if present

- Acid suppression therapy
- Vitamin B_{12} injections in chronic autoimmune gastritis.

Prognosis and complications

Prognosis

- Good.

Complications

- Anaemia: megaloblastic in vitamin B_{12} deficiency unless treated

- Ulceration
- Gastric carcinoma.

BOWEL DISORDERS

IRRITABLE BOWEL SYNDROME

Outline

- Chronic abdominal pain, change in bowel habit and bloating mostly due to disorders of intestinal motility
- Exact cause unclear
- Symptoms are chronic lasting >6 months
- No weight loss, blood loss, abdominal mass, anaemia or raised inflammatory markers

- Diagnosis based on symptom based criteria
- Important to identify red flags that may signal alternative diagnosis
- Classified by predominant system.

Classification

- Constipation

- Diarrhoea

Pathogenesis/aetiology

Causes

- Aetiology unknown
- Linked to psychological stress and may be exacerbated by stress or menstruation

Theories of aetiology include:
- Postinfection
- Altered GI motility

- GI hypersensitivity
- Psychological factors
- Associated with serotonin which:
  - May stimulate intestinal secretion and peristalsis
  - Stimulate visceral pain receptors
  - Is a target of new therapies.

Who

- Typical age: 20–40
- 7♀:3♂
- Common. Prevalence: 3–22% worldwide

- 40% of gastroenterological consultations
Associations:
- Stressful situations and events.

Clinical features

Main symptoms

- Constipation
- Diarrhoea

- Pain: possibly due to bowel spasm and visceral hypersensitivity. Often relieved by flatulence and defecation

Other symptoms

- Abdominal bloating
- Rectal dissatisfaction (sensation of incomplete defecation)
- Nausea

- Anxiety or depression
- Bleeding or weight loss should prompt a search for an alternative diagnosis

Several diagnostic criteria (not always helpful)

- Rome criteria:
  - >12 weeks per year with abdominal pain and discomfort
  - Continuous or recurrent
  - Associated nausea and bloating

- At least 2 of:
  - Pain relieved by defecation
  - Change in stool frequency
  - Change in stool form/appearance.

Investigations

- Mainly to exclude other diagnoses.

Blood tests

- Inflammatory markers (CRP, ESR, WBC)
- Haematinics: ferritin, folate, vitamin B_{12}
- Thyroid function

- Coeliac serology
- Ca-125 for women where ovarian cancer is suspected and consider a pelvic US.

Imaging

- Abdominal US

Other tests

- Stool culture (if diarrhoea)
- Faecal calprotectin – a marker of inflammation of the bowel

- Urinalysis
- Invasive tests are not usually indicated if the diagnosis can be made confidently with normal bloods and a good history.

Treatment

Exclude other diagnoses:
- Conservative:
  - Reassurance
  - Dietary fibre: some improve, others worsen
  - Limit: alcohol, caffeine, fat, known exacerbators, dairy products, yeast, wheat
  - Avoiding fermentable foods, e.g. a low-FODMAP diet.
- For diarrhoea:
  - Loperamide (an opioid agonist, trade name: Imodium)
  - Cholestyramine
- For constipation if bile salt malabsorption a possibility:
  - Fibre. Soluble fibre such as psyllium, sterculia, ispaghula. NOT insoluble such as bran, which will cause fermentation, gas and pain

- Gentle laxatives. Osmotic laxatives for long term use and only occasionally stimulant laxatives. Newer treatments for constipation e.g. prucalopride or linaclotide
- For pain:
  - Antispasmodics: mebeverine/ merbentyl (antimuscarinic)
  - Peppermint oil or dimethicone
  - Antimuscarinics: propantheline
- Psychological therapy:
  - Identify associated factors and treat, e.g. anxiety/ stress/social phobia/depression/dysthymia/panic disorder/substance abuse
  - Psychotherapy
  - Antidepressants: amitriptyline at a low dose or SSRIs if amitryptiline has too many side effects or ineffective.

Prognosis and complications

Prognosis

- Usually excellent but can significantly impact on quality of life

- 50% improve after 1 year
- <5% worsen.

INFLAMMATORY BOWEL DISEASE

General features

Outline

- Chronic relapsing inflammatory disorders of obscure origin

- Two main forms: ulcerative colitis and Crohn's disease (Table 4.1).

Table 4.1 Main features of ulcerative colitis (UC) and Crohn's disease

UC	Crohn's
Colon and rectum only	Whole GI tract
Continuous lesion	Skip lesions
Normal bowel thickness	Thick bowel wall
No fistula	Fistulae due to transmural nature of disease
Mucosal inflammation	Transmural inflammation: this makes the outside of the serosa sticky and encourages fat wrapping
Crypt abscess and goblet cell depletion	No crypt abscesses
No granulomas	Granulomas sometimes seen
Common bleeding	Uncommon bleeding
Uncommon abdominal pain	Common abdominal pain
Majority have rectal disease	Rectal disease 20%
Worse in non-smokers	Worse in smokers

Pathogenesis/aetiology

Causes

- Multifactorial aetiology (genetic predisposition and environmental triggers) but precise cause unknown.

Who

- Typical age: 20–40
- Family history
- Genetics: NOD2 and Card15 genes in Crohn's

Associations:
- HLA-B27.

Clinical features

Extraintestinal manifestations

- Eyes: uveitis (5%), episcleritis, conjunctivitis
- Joints: arthritis (20% of patients with IBD have arthritis), ankylosing spondylitis, sacroileitis, enteropathic arthritis
- Skin: erythema nodosum (tender bruise-like swelling on shins), pyoderma gangrenosum (ulcerated deep skin lesion), vasculitis, clubbing

- Liver: fatty changes, sclerosing cholangitis, with subsequent cirrhosis or cholangiocarcinoma (cancer of the bile ducts)
- Calculi in Crohn's: urinary tract or gallbladder (oxalate stones).

Investigations

Imaging

Endoscopy
- sigmoidoscopy with biopsies
- colonoscopy with biopsies
- Imaging: small bowel follow through, CT or MRI

- Barium follow through: largely replaced by MRI or capsule endoscopy
- Small bowel ultrasound.

Treatment

- Aminosalicylates (5ASA): act on distal small bowel and large bowel. A topical anti-inflammatory which inhibits prostaglandin production. More effective in UC. Side effects: hepatitis, pancreatitis, pancytopenia.
- 5ASA more useful in UC than Crohn's

- Topical steroids (e.g. suppositories or enemas)
- Systemic steroids for short periods only
- Immunosuppression, e.g. azathioprine
- Biological agents, e.g. anti-tumour necrosis factor (TNF) (infliximab) or adalimumab
- Surgery

Support

- IBD clinics
- Bone clinics

- Rheumatology/dermatology/ophthalmology

Managing complications

- Collitis and colorectal cancer risk:
  - Colonoscopic surveillance 10 years after diagnosis with repeat procedures depending on risk stratification

- In-patient admissions:
  - LMWH to reduce risk of VTE
- Out-patient:
  - Vitamin D and calcium supplementation for patients on steroids/DEXA.

Prognosis and complications

Prognosis

- Usually a lifelong remitting and relapsing disease
- UC 'cured' with colectomy

- 65% of Crohn's patients will require surgery at some time during their life.

Complications

- Colonic cancer
- Short bowel (Crohn's)

- Fistulating disease (Crohn's)
- Malnutrition, mostly in Crohn's.

ULCERATIVE COLITIS

Outline

- See 'inflammatory bowel disease' on page 000 for general features
- Inflammation of the colonic mucosa, characterised by relapses and remissions
- Affects only colon and rectum: but in severe pancolitis 10% can develop mild inflammation in the distal ileum due to 'backwash ileitis'
- Begins in rectum extends proximally.

Pathogenesis/aetiology

Causes

- Aetiology unknown
- Can be precipitated by infection or stress.

Associations

- Link with HLA-B27 and ankylosing spondylitis
- Primary sclerosing cholangitis
- Non-smokers.

Pathology

- T-helper type 2-mediated response
- Can lead to cancer.

Macroscopic features:
- Continuous lesion (no gaps)
- Ulcers
- Pseudopolyps: ulceration leaves islands of residual mucosa that look like polyps.

Microscopic features:
- Inflammation limited to the mucosa
- Goblet cells depleted
- Crypt abscess from inflammatory cells accumulating in the lamina propria.

Who

- Typical age: 15–30
- 1♀:1.2♂
- Prevalence: 0.1%
- More common in whites
- p-ANCA found in 60%.

Clinical features

- Insidious onset but can be rapid
- Diarrhoea: mixed with blood and accompanied by urgency. Often continues during the night (unlike irritable bowel syndrome)
- Cramping abdominal discomfort: urge to defecate
- Abdominal distension
- Malaise
- Anorexia
- Severe colitis: fever, weight loss, haemodynamic compromise

Extraintestinal manifestations

- As above

Associated diseases

- Sclerosing cholangitis: scarring and inflammation of the bile ducts.

Investigations

Blood tests

- FBC: ↓ Hb
- ↑ ESR/CRP
- U&Es
- LFTs: ↑ biliary enzymes suggests primary sclerosing cholangitis

Stool

- Culture
- *Clostridium difficile* toxin.
- Faecal calprotectin

Imaging

- AXR: no faecal shadows, mucosal thickening. Loss of colonic markings on X-ray giving the appearance of 'lead piping'. There may be toxic dilatation (toxic megacolon)
- Abdominal US & MRCP/ERCP if LFTs show an obstructive picture.

Endoscopy
- Flexible sigmoidoscopy / colonoscopy: mucosa is inflamed and friable with bleeding and ulceration. Full colonoscopy contraindicated in severe exacerbation due to risk of perforation so perform a limited flexible sigmoidoscopy.

Treatment

Medical

Introducing remission:
- >85% medically managed
- Mild to moderate: prednisolone, aminosalicylate, e.g. mesalazine, steroid enemas
- Severe: IV hydration, IV hydrocortisone. If no improvement consider infliximab or ciclosporin before surgery, but involve the surgeons early

Surgical

- 20% require surgery which may be curative
- Total colectomy and ileostomy

Screening

- Colonoscopy after 10 years of disease with repeat examinations dependent on risk stratification

Maintaining remission (steroid-sparing agents):
- 5-Aminosalicylates: mesalazine, reduce relapse rates from 80% to 20% at 1 year
- High dose oral mesalazine is the mainstay of mild-moderate UC management
- Azathioprine/mercaptopurine (immunosuppressants)
- Don't give anti-diarrhoeals.

- Indications: CHOP
  - **C**arcinoma
  - **H**aemorrhage
  - **O**bstruction
  - **P**erforation

- Regular colonoscopy with dye spray to target biopsies to exclude dysplasia.

Prognosis and complications

Prognosis

- Variable
- Relapsing-remitting: most common
- Proctitis (inflammation of the rectal and anal lining) alone: good prognosis
- In severe fulminating disease: mortality up to 25%.

Complications

- Perforation
- Bleeding
- Toxic megacolon: toxic damage to the muscle wall and neural plexus results in the shutdown of neuromuscular function. Colon can distend, perforate and become gangrenous (Fig. 4.2)
- Colonic cancer risk: 30% risk at 35 years after diagnosis.
- Risk of CRC dependent on time elapsed since diagnosis, extent of disease, severity and frequency of flares.

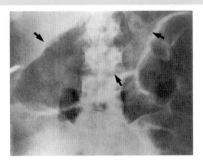

Fig. 4.2   Toxic megacolon (colonic wall arrowed).

CROHN'S DISEASE

Outline

- See 'inflammatory bowel disease: General features' p. 138
- Chronic inflammatory disease of the bowel
- Affects any part of the gut: mostly affects terminal ileum and proximal colon
- Shows classic string sign and skip lesions on imaging (Fig. 4.3).

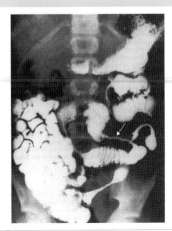

Fig. 4.3   Abdominal X-ray of small bowel showing characteristic skip areas and string sign (white arrow) in Crohn's disease.

Pathogenesis/aetiology

Causes

- Aetiology unknown
- Mutation in NOD2/CARD15 gene

Associations

- Ankylosing spondylitis/sacroiliitis
- Bronchiectasis
- Fibrosing alveolitis
- Fistula in-ano

Pathology

- Skip lesions: unaffected bowel between areas of active disease
- Transmural inflammation: entire gut wall affected which encourages ulcer formation and fat wrapping due to inflammation of the external serosa which makes it sticky. This also contributes to fistula formation as adjacent structures stick
- Fistula formation: tracts form between structures resulting in pneumaturia and faeces in urine, or through the vagina
- Deep ulcers: through the mucosa (rose thorn ulcers). This also encourages fistula formation. Endoscopically a cobble stone appearance due to fissuring ulcers around residual mucosa
- Granulomata may be present
- T-helper type 1 response.

Who

- Prevalence: 0.03–0.05%
- Associations:
  - Smokers
  - High sugar, low fibre diet.

Clinical features

- Diarrhoea: often non-bloody and continues during the night (unlike irritable bowel syndrome)
- Abdominal pain: in right iliac fossa (RIF)/suprapubic region (more common in Crohn's than UC)
- RIF mass
- Weight loss
- Fever
- Malaise
- Anorexia
- Ulceration: mouth
- Perianal abscesses, fistulae, skin tags, anal and rectal strictures
- Terminal ileum disease (common): can impair vitamin B_{12} absorption and lead to general signs of malabsorption
- Protein losing enteropathy

Extraintestinal manifestations

- As above

Investigations

Blood tests

- FBC: ↓ Hb, ↑ platelets
- ↑ ESR/CRP
- U&Es
- LFTs: ↓ albumin

Microbiology

- Faecal calprotectin
- Stool microscopy and culture.

Imaging

- AXR with oral contrast: shows string sign (severe narrowing of bowel seen as a thin stripe of contrast or string like on X-ray)
- Small bowel barium meal (less common now)
- CT enterography: large quantity of oral contrast ingested to stretch small bowel for optimal imaging. Avoid CT in young patients due to radiation dose
- Small bowel MRI: investigation of choice for imaging small bowel Crohn's disease
- Video capsule endoscopy.

Endoscopy

- OGD (if upper GI symptoms or young patient)
- Colonoscopy with ileo-colonic biopsies

Treatment

- Stop smoking.

Medical

Introducing remission:
- >85% medically managed
- Mild to moderate disease: prednisolone, aminosalicylates, e.g. mesalazine, steroid or salicylate enemas
- Severe disease: IV hydration, IV hydrocortisone. If not improving consider surgery

Maintaining remission:
- 5-Aminosalicylates: sulfasalazine, mesalazine, olsalazine
- 5-ASA has a minor role in Crohn's unlike UC. Most do not use it to maintain or induce remission now

- Azathioprine or mercaptopurine

Alternative agents:
- Azathioprine or mercaptopurine if side effects from steroids
- Methotrexate: second line after azathioprine
- Metronidazole: an antimicrobial drug against anaerobic bacteria indicated to treat peri-anal disease
- Anti-TNF, e.g. infliximab, adalimumab. Useful for disease resistant to standard treatment. Expensive, increased infection and lymphoma risk, can reactivate TB and HBV. Need to check varicella zoster immune status and vaccinate if required

Surgery

- 65% will need surgery
- Surgery is not curative
- Aim to remove as little bowel as possible
- Indications: failure of medical therapy, intestinal obstruction, intestinal perforation, local complications

- Small bowel: stricturoplasties or resect diseased bowel
- Large bowel: panproctocolectomy (removal of the entire colon, rectum and anal canal) and ileostomy

Prognosis and complications

Prognosis

- Lifelong relapsing–remitting course.

- Aim to maximise quality of life and minimise need for surgery

Complications

- Malabsorption
- Small intestinal obstruction
- Short gut syndrome postsurgery
- Stricture formation
- Abscess formation
- Fistulae

- Fissures
- Toxic dilation with perforation
- Colonic carcinoma
- Post-terminal ileal resection: oxalate renal calculi.

COLONIC POLYPS

Outline

- Polyp is an elevation of tissue projecting from a mucous membrane
- Colonic polyps project into the colonic lumen

- May be multiple
- Malignant potential in adenomatous polyps.

Classification

Adenomatous polyps:
- 70–80% of polyps
- Benign tumours of neoplastic epithelium
- Sporadic or familial (e.g. Gardner syndrome or familial adenomatous polyposis)

Types:
1. Tubular adenoma:
   - Multiple in 25% cases
   - Most are <2 cm diameter
   - Malignant risk is <5% but they account for most colorectal carcinomas
2. Villous adenoma:
   - Large, occur in recto-sigmoid colon
   - Fibrovascular stalks, covered by neoplastic epithelium

- 40% contain invasive carcinoma
3. Mixed:
- Hamartomatous polyps:
  - Benign tumours
- Inflammatory polyps:
  - In inflammatory bowel conditions e.g. pseudopolyps in ulcerative colitis
- Metaplastic (or hyperplastic) polyps:
  - Normally small, multiple, slightly raised
  - Not malignant
  - No treatment needed.
4. Serrated polyps:
  - Often sessile (flat) in the right colon
  - Malignant potential

Pathogenesis/aetiology

Causes

- No definite cause
- Genetic associations (see below)

Polyposis syndromes

- Familial adenomatous polyposis (FAP):
  - autosomal dominant
  - gene mutation on *APC* (adenomatous polyposis coli) gene on long arm of chromosome 5
  - hundreds of adenomatous polyps throughout gut at an early age
  - commonly present in teens
  - leads to colon cancer unless large bowel is removed
  - many also have congenital hypertrophy of the retinal pigment epithelium (CHRPE; pigmented lesions of the retina)
- Gardner syndrome:
  - autosomal dominant
  - multiple colonic adenomas with bony osteomas and epidermoid cysts
  - variant of FAP
  - mutation in *APC*
- Type 1: juvenile polyps:
  - low malignant potential
  - dominantly inherited
  - in children and teens
- Type 2: Peutz–Jeghers syndrome:
  - rare, autosomal dominant
  - polyps throughout tract
  - pigmentation of skin around lips, gums, palms and soles
  - malignant potential <3%.

Who

- Adenomatous polyps in 10% of population
- Most colonic carcinomas originate from polyps.

Clinical features

- Usually asymptomatic: most found incidentally on colonoscopy
- Obstruction (rarely)
- Diarrhoea: if large secretory villous adenoma
- Bleeding and anaemia
- Tenesmus (sensation of incomplete defecation).

Investigations

Stool

- Faecal occult blood as part of national Bowel Cancer Screening Programme: detects hidden blood in the faeces

Colonoscopy

- With biopsy and polypectomy.

Other tests

Genetic studies:
- If familial syndrome suspected.

Treatment

- Endoscopic polypectomy (removal of polyp)
- Surgical polypectomy: for some large polyps
- Screening: for at-risk patients
- Post polypectomy surveillance dependent upon size and number of polyps endoscopically excised

Familial adenomatous polyposis

- Counsel carriers
- Prophylactic total colectomy
- After colectomy they remain at risk of small bowel cancer.

Prognosis and complications

Prognosis

- After removal of adenomatous polyp, 50% recur.

Complications

- Malignancy: 5% of polyps removed are found to have invasive carcinoma
- Bleeding
- Obstruction
- Intussusception (telescoping of one part of the bowel into the other, see surgical chapter): can act as an apex.

MALABSORPTION

General features

Outline

- Reduced absorption of nutrients in the small intestine
- Leads to symptoms and signs caused by lack of essential nutrients and steatorrhoea from fat malabsorption.

Pathogenesis/aetiology

Causes

Anything affecting the digestive process:
- Failure of digestive enzymes
- Increased small bowel transit time
- Inflammation, e.g. Crohn's
- Structural abnormalities: blind loops, diverticulae, fistulae, malignancy, arterial insufficiency, intestinal resections
- Pancreatic disease: cystic fibrosis, chronic pancreatitis, cancer

- Impaired absorption of nutrients by intestinal wall: malignancy, coeliac disease, intestinal resection, tropical sprue, Whipple's
- After surgery: decreased stomach and gut transit time, reduced bile concentrations
- Infection by damage to the mucosa
- Bacterial overgrowth.

Who

- Depends on cause.

Clinical features

- Diarrhoea
- Weight loss
- Failure to thrive
- Lethargy
- Flatus
- Ascites and oedema: due to ↓ protein
- Unabsorbed substances in gut: steatorrhea, abdominal pain, distension

- Vitamin deficiency: specific signs and symptoms:
  - Osteomalacia: ↓ vitamin D
  - Anaemia: ↓ iron/folate/B_{12}
  - Bleeding disorders and bruising: ↓ vitamin K
  - Peripheral neuropathies: ↓ vitamins A/B_1/B_{12}
  - Mouth ulcers, glossitis, stomatitis: ↓ vitamin B/vitamin C/folate/iron.

Investigations

Blood tests

- FBC: ↓ Hb
- Iron studies: ferritin, folate, vitamin B_{12}, iron
- LFTs: albumin

- Clotting: PT
- Coeliac serology.

Other tests

Specific tests:
- Faecal calprotectin
- Stool appearance and faecal fat collected over 3 days: >18 mmol/24 h indicates malabsorption

- Enzyme deficiency test: faecal elastase
- Brush border enzyme assays (rarely)
- Endoscopy: for direct visualisation and biopsies
- Video capsule endoscopy.

Treatment

- Supplement malnutrition: enterally, parenterally or total parenteral nutrition (TPN)
- Bacterial overgrowth: metronidazole, oral tetracyline

- Treat cause, e.g. pancreatic supplements for pancreatic insufficiency or gluten-free diet for coeliac.

Prognosis and complications

Complications

Deficiency states including:
- ↓ Calcium: paraesthesia, tetany (see hypocalaemia p. 424)
- ↓ Magnesium: fits and paraesthesia
- ↓ Phosphate: osteoporosis
- ↓ Vitamin A: xerophthalmia (eyes unable to produce tears) leading to blindness
- ↓ Vitamin B_1 (thiamine): wet beri-beri (heart failure and oedema) or dry beri-beri (neuropathy)

- ↓ Vitamin C: scurvy with poor healing and gum disease
- ↓ Nicotinic acid: pellagra. Triad of DDD: diarrhoea, dermatitis, dementia. May develop neurological sequalae, e.g. neuropathy, fits and depression.
- ↓ Zinc: poor wound healing, depressed growth
- ↓ Copper: kinky hair
- ↓ Selenium: cardiomyopathy

COELIAC DISEASE

Outline

- Gluten intolerance
- An autoimmune condition where the small intestine fails to digest and absorb food due to permanent sensitivity of small bowel lining to the gliadin protein of gluten
- Villous atrophy of the small bowel causes malabsorption

- Sensitive to: rye, wheat and barley (all contain gliadin) and sometimes oats but this can usually be reintroduced
- Underdiagnosed – 1% of UK population prevalence
- Should be considered in a case of unexplained iron-deficiency anaemia.
- See also 'malabsorption' on page 000 for general features

Pathogenesis/aetiology

Pathogenesis

- Immune system abnormally activated by gluten
- Toxic part is α-gliadin in wheat, rye, barley and sometimes oats
- Inappropriate T-cell response in genetically predisposed people
- Leads to small bowel villous atrophy: absent villi, hyperplastic crypts

- Inflammation and plasma cell infiltrate in lamina propria
- Increase in lymphocytes (predominantly T-cells) in the epithelium
- Results in malabsorption
- Changes more prominent on proximal than distal small intestine

Associated conditions

- Dermatitis herpetiformis: intensely itchy pruritic papulovesicular lesions occurring symmetrically over extensor surfaces (often the elbows), buttocks, trunk, neck and scalp. Patients respond to gluten-free diet or can try dapsone, 30% have coeliac disease.
- Diabetes mellitus type 1

- Autoimmune thyroiditis
- Seizure disorder
- IgA deficiency
- Sjögren syndrome
- Rheumatoid arthritis
- Collagen disorders
- Down syndrome.

Who

- Presents at any age, with 2 peaks: infancy and 30–40 (more common)
- ♀ > ♂
- Up to 1% of European population – most are undiagnosed
- High prevalence: Irish, India, S. USA, N. Africa

- Low prevalence in China, Japan Afro-Caribbean
- Associations: HLA-DQ2, HLA-DQ8
Genetics:
- 75% concordance identical twins, 5–20% first-degree relatives
- HLA-DQ in 95%
- Family history (10% among first-degree relatives).

Clinical features

- Diarrhoea: in 50%
- Frothy foul smelling stools: steatorrhoea may be absent, particularly if disease is proximal small bowel
- Weight loss
- Failure to thrive: common in children

- Flatulence
- Distended abdomen
- Abdominal pain
- Mouth ulcers
- Asymptomatic: 30%

Extraintestinal manifestations from mineral and vitamin deficiency

- Iron-deficiency anaemia: commonest presentation
- Folate or vitamin B_{12} deficiency: glossitis, anaemia, peripheral neuropathy
- Vitamin K deficiency: deranged coagulation and purpura
- Vitamin D deficiency: hypocalcaemia and tetany, osteomalacias
- Vitamin A deficiency: night blindness

- Osteoporosis
- Hypocalcaemia
- Pruritus
- Malaise
- Hyposplenism
- Neuropsychiatric symptoms.

Investigations

Blood tests

- FBC: ↓ Hb, often iron deficient
- LFTs: ↑ ALT, ↑ ALP, ↓ albumin

- Vitamin and mineral levels: to confirm malabsorption
- IgA levels ↓ in 2–3%

Auto-antibodies

- Anti-endomysial antibodies: but note that patients with IgA deficiency will lack IgA antibodies and will require an IgG based test
- Tissue transglutamase: most reliable marker if the patient is not IgA deficient, 90% sensitivity

- Reticulin
- Gliadin

If antibody positive confirm diagnosis with biopsy (while on a gluten diet). Diet:
- Monitor for clinical improvement with gluten-free diet

Other tests

Endoscopy:
- Duodenal biopsy is diagnostic with flattening of intestinal villi and elongation of crypts

DEXA: all patients have ↑ risk of osteoporosis.
Genetics: HLA testing

Treatment

- Strict gluten-free diet for life
- Vitamin supplementation initially
- Vitamin D and calcium supplements if osteoporotic
- Avoid oats: can be reintroduced later in most cases

- Repeat biopsy after gluten free diet to confirm return of normal villous architecture
- Steroids and immunosuppression for refractory disease.

Prognosis and complications

Prognosis

- 70% improve within 2 weeks of a gluten-free diet
- Full resolution of histology, more common in children: 2–3 months after diet

- Disease does not improve in 5% despite strict gluten-free diet.

Complications

- Susceptibility to GI malignancy
- Ulcerative jejunitis
- T-cell lymphoma of bowel
- Severe malnutrition
- Anaemia

- Secondary lactose intolerance
- Myopathies
- Neuropathies
- Osteoporosis.

TROPICAL SPRUE

Outline

- Malabsorptive disease found in the tropics.
- See also 'malabsorption' on page 000 for general features

Pathogenesis/aetiology

Causes

- Aetiology unknown
- Likely to be an infective agent
- Many have a preceding enteric infection.

Pathogenesis

- Entire small intestine affected
- Microscopic appearances variable
- Inflammation and villous flattening.

Who

- Tropics: Asia, S. America, Caribbean.

Clinical features

- Anaemia
- Anorexia
- Weight loss
- Diarrhoea with malabsorption and nutritional deficiencies.

Investigations

Stool
- Culture: exclude infectious causes of diarrhoea

Endoscopy
- Jejunal biopsy: partial villous atrophy.

Treatment

- Antibiotics (e.g. tetracycline) for up to 6 months.
- Folic acid and vitamin supplements.

Prognosis and complications

Complications

- Folate deficiency (common)
- Vitamin deficiencies.

WHIPPLE'S DISEASE

Outline

- A rare systemic disease caused by the Gram+ve actinomycete *Tropheryma whippelii*
- Reduced intestinal absorption of digested food
- Can affect any body organ: primarily intestine, CNS, joints.

Pathogenesis/aetiology

Pathology

- Causes minimal villous atrophy
- Exact mechanism of destruction unknown.

Who

- Typical age >40
- 1♀:10♂
- Rare.

Clinical features

- Steatorrhoea
- Hyperpigmentation
- Anorexia
- Weight loss
- Lymphadenopathy
- Diarrhoea
- Arthritis
- Abdominal pain.

Investigations

Endoscopy:
- Jejunal biopsy: macrophages contain rod-shaped bacilli which stain positive with periodic acid-Schiff stain within the lamina propria.

Treatment

- Antibiotics: penicillin, tetracycline, chloramphenicol
- Vitamin and mineral supplements: for severe malabsorption.

Prognosis and complications

Complications

- Encephalitis.

GUT INFECTION

GASTROENTERITIS: BACTERIAL

Outline

- Infection of the bowel by bacteria
- 50% of food infections linked to chicken

Types

1. Food poisoners:
   - The food consumed is contaminated with bacterial toxins
2. Toxin mediated:
   - Organism binds to receptors in the tract and secretes toxins, which disrupt enterocyte cell signalling leading to loss of cell NaCl and water

3. Cell invaders:
   - Organism multiplies in the GI tract and invades the epithelium leading to inflammation, cell necrosis and apoptosis
   - Cause erosion, ulceration and diarrhoea

GI defences:
- Acid in stomach
- Bacterial flora of intestines.

Pathogenesis/aetiology

Causes

- Bacterial causes of gastroenteritis are shown in Table 4.2.

Table 4.2 Bacterial causes of gastroenteritis

Bacteria	Source	Symptoms
Food poisoners		
Staphylococcus aureus	Cream, cold meat	Vomiting
Bacillus cereus	Rice	Vomiting, diarrhoea
Clostridium botulinum	Canned food, yogurts	Paralysis
Toxin-producing bacteria		
Vibrio cholerae	Water	Cholera: loss of fluid rapid dehydration, 'rice water stool'
Clostridium perfringens	Meat stews	Abdominal pain, diarrhoea
Enterotoxigenic *Escherichia coli* (ETEC)	Poorly cooked meat	Watery diarrhoea, cramps
Cell invaders		
Shigella spp.	Faeco–oral spread	Dysentery (bloody diarrhoea)
Enterohaemorrhagic *Escherichia coli* (EHEC)	Raw meat and milk	Dysentery
Campylobacter jejuni	Chicken	Dysentery
Salmonella enteritidis	Meat, eggs	Dysentery, diarrhoea

Who

At risk:
- Infants
- Children
- Elderly
- Travellers
- Antibiotic-associated colitis
- Immunocompromised.

Clinical features

- Diarrhoea ± vomiting
- Dysentery: severe bloody diarrhoea with mucus
- Symptoms 1–4 h after a meal is indicative of food poisoners
- Symptoms 12–48 h after a meal are suggestive of cell invaders or toxin-mediated invaders.

Investigations

Blood tests

- FBC: ↑ WBC: CRP

Culture

- Food source
- Stool: at least three specimens
- *Clostridium difficile* toxin in stool
- Blood

ELISA and electron microscopy

- Viral detection

Sigmoidoscopy

- If symptoms persistent.

Treatment

- Rehydrate
- Most cases are self limiting
- Antiemetics
- Avoid antidiarrhoeals/opiates
- Antibiotics only if systemically unwell/immunosuppressed/old
- Cholera: tetracycline
- *Salmonella* and typhoid fever, *Shigella*, *Campylobacter*: ciprofloxacin
- *Clostridium difficile*: oral metronidazole, oral vancomycin
- If food-related infection: notify local health authority

Prevention

- Hygiene
- Abroad: avoid water/peel fruit/no salads
- Safe water supplies
- Good sewage disposal
- Vaccination: typhoid.

Prognosis and complications

Prognosis

- Good once over the acute episode.

Complications

- Haemolytic uraemic syndrome from *Escherichia coli* serotype O157:H7 (see Haematology [Ch. 8]).

GI INFECTIONS: VIRAL

Outline

Gastroenteritis caused by:
- norovirus (Norwalk agent): causes ∼50% of gastroenteritis cases worldwide
- rotavirus: young patients
- adenovirus
- astrovirus
- small round-structured viruses (SRSVs)
- CMV: immunocompromised
- HIV: causes a diarrhoeal illness in 30–60%.

Pathogenesis/aetiology

Transmission:
- Faeco–oral route: commonest
- Contaminated food/water

- Vomitus is source of infection in SRSV-associated gastroenteritis.

Who

- Typical age: mostly in children, rarer in adults

- ↑ in areas of overcrowding, poor sanitation and poverty.

Clinical features

- Diarrhoea
- Vomiting
- Abdominal cramps

- Fever
- Dehydration
- Hyponatraemia.

Investigations

- Electron microscopy of stool samples: useful for outbreaks

- Antigen detection in stool: ELISA/Latex agglutination.

Treatment

Treatment is symptomatic:
- Rehydration
- Correct sodium loss
- Prevention
- High standards of hygiene

- Clean water supply
- Efficient sewage disposal
- Hospitals: source isolation, hand washing
- Vaccines: hep A, rotavirus.

Prognosis and complications

Prognosis

- Usually excellent

- Developing countries have a high mortality.

Complications

- Can be life threatening in young.

GI INFECTION: PROTOZOA

Outline

Gastroenteritis caused by:
- *Giardia*: intestinal parasite from contaminated water.

- *Entamoeba histolytica*: spread by faeco–oral route. Can spread to the lungs/heart/kidneys/brain and liver (leading to hepatic abscesses, see Hepatology section).

Pathogenesis/aetiology

Pathogenesis

- *Giardia*: attaches to small intestine mucosa blunting the vili. Leads to malabsorptive diarrhoea

- *Entamoeba*: amoebas burrow into the colonic mucosa leading to characteristic flask-shaped ulcer production and acute dysentery.

Who

- Transmission mainly via water

- Rare in the West but common in developing countries.

Clinical features

- Watery diarrhoea
- Nausea
- Abdominal pain
- Distension

- Malabsorption
- *Entamoeba histolytica*: causes dysentery and can lead to fulminating colitis.

Investigations

Blood tests

- LFTs: for liver abscesses

- Serology: FAT test (amoebic fluorescent antibody test).

Other tests

Stool:
- Microscopic examination

Biopsies:
- To look for entamoeba and giardia.

Treatment

Giardia:
- Metronidazole for 3 days or stat dose of tinidazole

Entamoeba histolytica:
- Metronidazole for 5 days, 10–14 if liver abscess
- Diloxanide at end of course to kill gut ova.

Prognosis and complications

Prognosis

- Usually excellent once spotted and treated.

Complications

- *Entamoeba histolytica*: inflammatory fibrotic mass (amoeboma) (10%) can cause bleeding, obstruction, intussusception

- Amoebic liver abscess and rupture

Liver function

- Synthesis of albumin, clotting factors, cholesterol
- Metabolism of drugs, toxins and bilirubin
- Synthesis and metabolism of carbohydrates, proteins.

Liver anatomy

- The liver has two major lobes (right and left) and two minor lobes (caudate and quadrate). Functionally it can be divided into eight segments.
- Blood supply to the liver is from the portal vein (which comes from the small intestine, 75%) and the hepatic artery (directly from the aorta, 25%). The liver is drained by the hepatic vein which leads to the inferior vena cava.
- The functional unit of the liver is the hepatic lobule, which consists of a central vein fringed by a portal triad consisting of a branch of the portal vein, a branch of the hepatic artery and the bile duct (Fig. 5.1). Blood flows from the portal triad to the central vein through a specialised endothelium (sinusoid) to supply the hepatocytes (liver cells). Bile, produced by the hepatocytes, flows in the opposite direction through the canaliculi into the bile duct.

Bilirubin metabolism

Haemoglobin is broken down in the spleen to unconjugated bilirubin. Most of the bilirubin is carried in blood bound to albumin. It is subsequently conjugated in the liver making it soluble, then:

- a small amount is excreted by the kidneys as urobilinogen
- the rest is excreted from the liver as bile into the gall bladder and then to the small intestine where:
  - some is reabsorbed (10%) back to the liver to be re-processed
  - most is converted to stercobilinogen and excreted in faeces (90%).

This is summarised in Figure 5.2.

Acute and chronic liver injury

Liver disease can be caused by acute and chronic liver injury, both with different causes and presentations (Fig. 5.3).

The gallbladder

The relationship of the gall bladder with the hepatic duct, bile duct, duodenum and pancreatic duct can be seen in Figure 5.4.

Important terms

Cholelithiasis: gallstones in the gallbladder

Choledocholithiasis: gallstone passes into the bile ducts leading to clinical symptoms

Cholestasis: build up of bile within the liver often due to a blockage of the bile ducts

Cholecystitis: inflammation of the gall bladder

Cholangitis: infection of the bile ducts

Biliary colic: severe pain from obstruction of the gall bladder or common bile duct normally by a stone; a misnomer as it is more often prolonged episodes of pain than colicky (waves of spasm)

Mucocoele: overextended gall bladder caused by a mucus build up after the neck of gall bladder has been blocked by an impacted stone; can lead to infection

Liver tumours

Benign primary tumours

Haemangiomas: commonest benign cause, needs no treatment

Hepatic adenomas: less common, associated with oral contraceptives, may present as haemoperitoneum and shock; resection is required if symptomatic (pain/bleeding); small risk of turning malignant

Follicular nodular hyperplasia: mesenchymal, nodules form in the liver, no malignant potential, related to oral contraceptive pill; 50% become symptomatic with pain in right upper quartile.

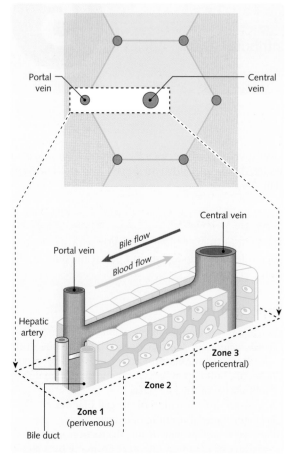

Fig. 5.1 Functional unit of the liver, illustrating the portal triad.

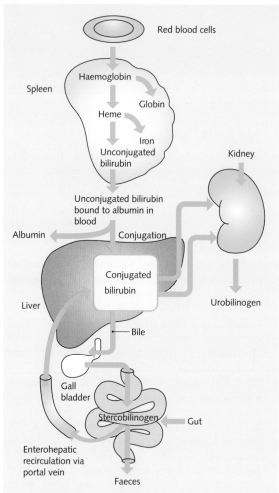

Fig. 5.2 Metabolism of bile.

Malignant primary tumours

Hepatocellular carcinoma (HCC): tumour of the hepatocytes; causes 90% of primary liver tumours
Cholangiocarcinoma: malignant tumour of the bile ducts
Angiosarcoma: from exposure to arsenic/vinyl chloride
Hepatoblastoma: rare tumour of children
Lymphoma/sarcoma: can affect the liver, often confined to one lobe.

Secondary tumour: metastases

Most common cause of cancer of the liver; from GI, breast, bronchus, thyroid.

Investigations

Blood tests

- 'Liver screen' (specific blood tests performed when liver disease is suspected). These include:
- FBC: platelets may be reduced with splenomegaly

- Albumin: made by the liver; therefore, low levels are a marker of disease severity but may also be low in malnutrition or chronic inflammatory states
- Liver function tests (LFTs):
  - AST (normally 10–40 U/L) and alanine aminotransferase (ALT) (normally 5–40 U/L): enzymes found within hepatocytes that are released when the liver is damaged. Levels are high in liver disease (e.g. acute hepatitis). ALT is fairly specific for liver disease, but AST is also found in cardiac and skeletal muscle and so may be high for other reasons. An ALT >1000 U/L is likely caused by one of three things: viral hepatitis, ischaemia or toxins (e.g. paracetamol)
  - Alkaline phosphatase (ALP) (normally 25–115 U/L): an enzyme found particularly within the bile ducts so commonly high in cholestatic liver disease. Non-specific as also found in the

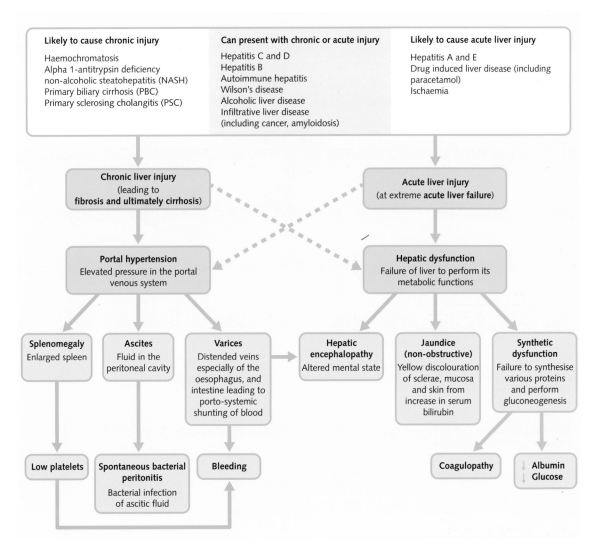

Fig. 5.3 Summary of liver disease.

placenta and bone so may also get raised values in Paget's disease, osteomalacia, pregnancy and bone metastases

- Gamma-glutamyl transpeptidase (GGT): high in cholestatic liver disease or in alcohol abuse as it is induced by alcohol
- Bilirubin (normally <17 μmol/L): high levels cause yellowing of the skin and sclera. May be high in pre-hepatic, hepatic or post-hepatic liver disease. Very high levels in biliary tract obstruction.
- International normalized ratio (INR) or prothrombin time (PT): measures of clotting function. Markers of synthetic impairment and hence severity of liver disease

- Copper studies and caeruloplasmin: for investigation of Wilson's disease
- Iron studies: ↑ iron, ↑ ferritin and ↓ total iron-binding capacity in haemachromatosis
- α_1-Antitrypsin: serum levels ↓ in α_1-antitrypsin deficiency
- α-Fetoprotein: ↑ in HCC
- Viral screen: for hepatitis viruses A, B, C, D and E (HAV, HBV, HCV, HDV, HEV, respectively); CMV; Epstein-Barr virus (EBV)
- Autoimmune screen and immunoglobulins (Table 5.1): useful if suspecting autoimmune liver disease, e.g. autoimmune hepatitis, primary biliary cirrhosis or primary sclerosing cholangitis.

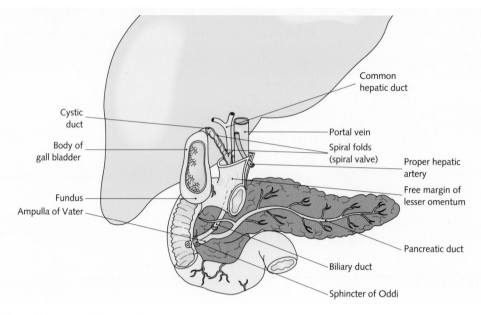

Fig. 5.4 The gall bladder and its connections.

Table 5.1 Autoimmune screen for liver disease	
Disease	**Antibodies**
Autoimmune hepatitis	Anti-nuclear (ANA) Anti-smooth muscle (Type 1) Anti-liver/kidney microsomal (Type 2) IgG↑
Primary biliary cirrhosis	Anti-mitochondrial antibodies (AMA), M2 subtype IgM↑
Primary sclerosis cholangitis	ANA Anti-neutrophil cytoplasmic antibodies (ANCA)
Alcoholic liver disease	IgA↑

Ultrasound

First-line investigation. Look for:

- architecture of liver: nodular/small/enlarged
- echotexture: heterogeneous in cirrhosis, bright with fat infiltration
- vasculature: is there flow in portal and hepatic veins?
- direction of flow: reversal suggests portal hypertension, absence of flow suggests thrombosis
- splenomegaly or varices: in portal hypertension

- ascites?
- Gallstones and common bile duct dilatation.

Transient elastography

A scan that assesses the 'stiffness' of the liver to sound waves. The stiffer the liver the more fibrosis. Two main methods: using a Fibroscan (R) machine or performing Acoustic Radiation Force Impulse (ARFI) during ultrasound. Most useful to identify the extremes (ie. either no fibrosis or cirrhosis).

CT

Gives better views of liver architecture.

A triple phase (arterial, venous and non-contrast) CT is useful for investigating the vasculature and visualising thromboses as well as staging cancers.

MRI

Is useful for the identification of cancers if CT is inconclusive.

Magnetic resonance cholangiopancreatography

Magnetic resonance cholangiopancreatography (MRCP) visualises the bile and pancreatic ducts using MRI.

It is a non-invasive diagnostic method for biliary problems (particularly primary sclerosing cholangitis).

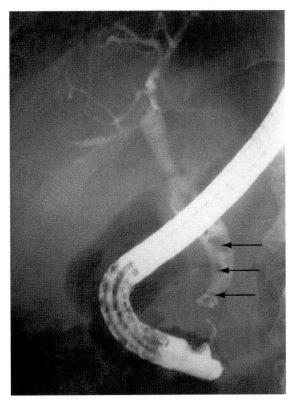

Fig. 5.5 ERCP showing dilated bile duct and filling defects compatible with gall stones.

Endoscopic retrograde cholangiopancreatography

Endoscopic retrograde cholangiopancreatography (ERCP) is endoscopy followed by cannulation of the ampulla of Vater in the duodenum (the entrance to the pancreatic and bile ducts):

- Dye is injected and X-rays used to visualise the ducts (Fig. 5.5)
- Indications (mainly therapeutic) include: treatment of obstructive jaundice (e.g. stenting in primary sclerosing cholangitis or removal of gallstones) and obtaining brushings for cytology.
- Complications include pancreatitis (2%), bleeding but mortality of <0.2%.

Percutaneous transhepatic cholangiography

A procedure where contrast medium is injected with a needle through the skin directly into the bile duct to allow radiographic visualisation of the biliary system. Also allows therapeutic intervention such as drainage of infected bile or extraction of gallstones. It is useful if there is a dilated biliary tree and ERCP is contraindicated or cannot be performed.

Liver biopsy

Percutaneous or transjugular approaches for obtaining tissue for diagnosis of cirrhosis or to assess severity for treatment and prognosis:

- Side effects: bleeding, shoulder tip pain, bile leak, infection.

See also

The patient presents (Ch. 14): hepatomegaly, hepatosplenomegaly, abdominal masses, abdominal pain, GI bleeding.

COMPLICATIONS OF LIVER DISEASE

CIRRHOSIS

Outline

- Liver fibrosis and the conversion of normal cell architecture into abnormal nodules resulting in irreversible impairment of liver cell function
- A histological diagnosis
- A cause of portal hypotension (see below)
- A risk factor for hepatocellular carcinoma (HCC) so screening is necessary

Compensated cirrhosis

- Cirrhosis without clinical manifestations

Decompensated cirrhosis

- Cirrhosis with the development of at least one of ABC:
  - **A**scites
- **B**leeding: massive GI bleed from oesophageal or gastric varices in 30%
- **C**onscious level ↓: hepatic encephalopathy

Acute-on-chronic liver failure

- Cirrhotic patient who develops an acute deterioration in liver function and clinical condition which results in organ failure.

Classification

Micro or macronodular cirrhosis:
- Micronodular: nodules <3 mm
- Macronodular: nodules >3 mm
- Mixed: macro and micronodular

Scores to assess severity and prognosis

Child-Pugh(-Turcotte) score (CP):
- Made up of bilirubin, albumin, PT, ascites and encephalopathy (BAPAE)
- Each variable has value 1–3 therefore total score ranges from 5 to 15
- CP class A: 5–6, CP class B: 7–9, CP class C: 10–15

MELD: Model for End-stage Liver Disease (US):
- Uses bilirubin, INR, creatinine
MELD-Na:
- MELD with sodium
UKELD: United Kingdom End-stage Liver Disease
- Uses INR, creatinine, bilirubin and sodium.

Pathogenesis/aetiology

Causes

Common: ABC:
- Alcohol (25%)
- Chronic hep B
- Chronic hep C
Others:
- Non-alcoholic steatohepatitis/fatty liver disease (NASH)
- Autoimmune: autoimmune hepatitis, primary biliary cirrhosis, primary sclerosing cholangitis, Overlap syndromes

- Genetic: adult: haemochromatosis, Wilson's disease, α1-antitrypsin deficiency childhood: glycogen storage diseases, cystic fibrosis
- Vascular: chronic Budd–Chiari syndrome, veno-occlusive disease
- Drugs: methotrexate
- Cryptogenic
- Congenital: biliary atresia (see jaundice)
- Infectious: schistosomiasis
- Rare: familial intrahepatic cholestasis, hepatic sarcoidosis.

Pathogenesis

- Liver cell damage, then fibrosis and regeneration with formation of nodules, disrupting normal architecture.

Who

- Any age or sex
Risk factors:
- Alcohol abuse
- Blood borne: viruses, IVDUs, blood transfusion, tattoos, healthcare professionals

- Sexually transmitted
- Ethnicity: Asia and Africa for viral hepatitis
- Past medical history: IBD, autoimmune disease, chronic medication use
- Family history of liver disease: genetic or autoimmune.

Clinical features

- Well compensated cirrhosis may be entirely asymptomatic with no clinical signs
- Symptoms and signs from 1° disease or 2° complications

Hand signs:
- Clubbing
- Leuconychia: white nails from hypoalbuminaemia
- Palmar erythema
- Dupuytren's contracture (fibrosis in palms)

Face:
- Jaundice
- Cyanosis (from hepatopulmonary syndrome)
- Raised JVP

Chest and abdomen:
- Spider naevi: in the distribution of superior vena cava drainage
- Splenomegaly
- Ascites
- Caput medusae: distension and dilation of umbilicus veins
- Enlarged or shrunken (advanced) liver

Other symptoms and signs:
- Malnutrition (muscle loss)
- Bruising
- Pruritus
- Oedema
- Confusion and drowsiness
- ↑ oestrogen in liver disease leads to: testicular atrophy, hair loss, gynaecomastia, palmar erythema.

Investigations

Blood tests

General:
- FBC: ↓ WBC and platelets (from hypersplenism)
- U&Es: ↓ sodium and possibly high creatinine in severe liver disease
- Clotting: ↑ INR with severe disease
- LFTs:
  - ↑ ALT, AST (may only be modest)
  - ↑ ALP, GGT (particularly in cholestatic aetiologies)
  - ↑ bilirubin
  - ↑ albumin
- ↑ α-fetoprotein in HCC

Aetiology specific tests:
- Immunoglobulins:
  - IgA ↑ in alcoholic cause
  - IgM ↑ in primary biliary cirrhosis
  - IgG ↑ in autoimmune hepatitis
- Raised autoantibodies
- Chronic viral hepatitis screen
- Genetics for haemachromatosis
- α1-antitrypsin level
- Copper studies for Wilson's.

Imaging

- Liver US
- Liver CT
- MRCP or ERCP in primary sclerosing cholangitis
- Transient elastography.

Other tests

- Liver biopsy
- Diagnostic paracentesis (ascitic tap).

Treatment

- Treat underlying cause
- Adequate nutrition
- Alcohol abstention.

Medical

- Avoid NSAIDs, sedatives, opiates or hepatotoxic drugs
- Cholestyramine for pruritus
- Urso-deoxycholic acid in primary biliary cirrhosis and sclerosis cholangitis.

Surgical

- Shunt procedure for uncontrolled portal hypertension with complications
- Liver transplantation is definitive treatment. Used for end-stage cirrhosis and HCC

Treat complications

- Ascites
- Spontaneous bacterial peritonitis
- Varices
- Hepatic encephalopathy
- Infections (spontaneous bacterial peritonitis)
- Hepato-renal syndrome

Treatment

Screening

- Screen for HCC every 6 months with α-fetoprotein and liver US. May require contrast CT or MRI
- Regular endoscopy to screen for varices and treat with banding and/or beta-blockers
- Monitor renal function.

Prognosis and complications

Prognosis

- Depends on cause and complications
- Rate of change from compensated to decompensated cirrhosis: 5–7% per year
- Median survival compensated cirrhosis: >12 years
- Median survival decompensated cirrhosis: 2 years
- 2 year survival from Child-Pugh score:
  - class A 90%
  - class B 70%
  - class C 38%.

Complications

- Portal hypertension:
  - Variceal haemorrhage
  - Ascites
  - Hepatic encephalopathy
- HCC
- Infections: particularly enteric organisms
- Renal failure (hepato-renal syndrome)
- Respiratory failure (hepato-pulmonary syndrome)
- Pulmonary hypertension (porto-pulmonary syndrome).

PORTAL HYPERTENSION

Outline

- ↑ BP in the portal vein
- The portal vein carries blood from the gut and spleen to the liver contributing to 75% of hepatic blood flow
- Portal hypertension is defined as a hepatic vein pressure gradient (HVPG) >5 mmHg (but ≥10 is clinically significant)
- Causes can be *hepatic*: blood can not flow easily due to disrupted hepatic anatomy or *pre- or post-hepatic*: normal liver but mechanical obstruction to flow of blood in portal system
- Back pressure leads to splenomegaly, ascites (fluid in the peritoneal cavity), and varices which may rupture and lead to further complications.
- Also leads to hepatic encephalopathy (see below).

Pathogenesis/aetiology

Causes

Pre-hepatic:
- Portal/mesenteric/splenic vein thrombosis
- Extrinsic compression

Hepatic:
- Cirrhosis (90%): from fibrosis and portal vein compression
- Stiff liver of other cause: acute liver failure (ALF), hepatitis
- Polycystic liver disease
- Schistosomiasis (a parasite)
- Sarcoidosis

Post-hepatic:
- Hepatic vein thrombosis (Budd–Chiari syndrome)
- Cardiac failure: constrictive pericarditis, right heart failure.

Pathogenesis

- Obstruction to portal flow or hepatic outflow leads to high pressure in the portal vein
- To relieve pressure, portosytemic collaterals (varices) open up into which blood is diverted back towards the heart, e.g. gastro-oesophageal, umbilicus (caput medusae), ileocaecal, rectum, and splenic collaterals
- Where vessels are superficial and thin, e.g. oesophageal varices, they may rupture causing complications (see gastroenterology chapter)
- Shunting of blood from the portal to systemic system leads to hepatic encephalopathy as blood bypasses the liver so is not 'detoxified'
- Through complex mechanisms ascites is formed with ↑ total body sodium and water.

Who

Risk factors:
- Chronic liver disease from any cause
- Following acute hepatic failure

- Pro-thrombotic tendency, ask for family history.

Clinical features

- ABC:
  - A: ascites

- B: bleeding. Massive GI bleeding from oesophageal or gastric varices in 30%
- C: ↓ conscious level (Hepatic encephalopathy).

Investigations

Blood tests

- FBC
- Biochemistry
- Clotting

- Liver screen
- Thrombophilia screen (for thromboses).

Imaging

- US: with vascular doppler to diagnose hepatic or portal vein thrombosis
- CT: to diagnose mesenteric thrombosis and assess intra-abdominal varices.

Transient elastography to assess liver stiffness

Other tests

Invasive:
- Portal pressure studies: radiological study where a transducer is introduced (usually transjugular) to measure hepatic vein pressure and then inflating an

attached balloon (wedging) as an estimate of portal pressure
- Liver biopsy if unsure about aetiology.

Treatment

Treat cause:
- Anti-coagulation for thrombosis

- Liver transplant for end-stage cirrhosis.

Medical

- Beta-blockers (most common propranolol) to help lower portal pressure

- Transjugular intrahepatic portosystemic shunt (TIPS) (a radiological procedure where an artificial channel linking the portal and hepatic veins is established to ↓ pressure in the portal vein and so ↓ portal hypertension).

Surgical

- Surgical shunt.

Prognosis and complications

Prognosis

- Depends on underlying cause.

Complications

Due to back pressure in portal vascular bed:
- Varices

- Ascites
- Splenomegaly.

OESOPHAGEAL AND GASTRIC VARICES

Outline

- Distended veins due to portal hypertension p 160
- When there is portal hypertension, portosystemic collaterals open up (varices) to relieve this pressure
- Common anatomical sites for varices (Fig. 5.6) are the oesophagus and stomach
- Can also be rectal, ileocecal and umbilical varices and internal (eg spleno-renal) (Fig. 5.6 for location of all varices)
- These can rupture resulting in life-threatening haemorrhage: **a medical emergency**.

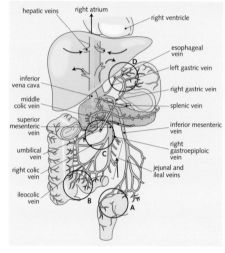

Fig. 5.6 Location of varices: rectal (A), ileocecal (B), umbilical (C), gastro-oesophageal (D).

Pathogenesis/aetiology

Causes

- Any cause of portal hypertension
- Liver cirrhosis: 70% develop varices
- Non-cirrhotic portal hypertension e.g. portal/mesenteric vein thrombosis
- Budd–Chiari syndrome.

Who

- See cirrhosis section for epidemiology and risks.

A typical patient

An alcoholic man with known liver disease presents with large volume haematemesis and melaena.

Clinical features

- Unwell patient
- Haematemesis (vomiting blood)
- Melaena (black, sticky, smelly, tar-like stool caused by digestion and oxidation of Hb as it passes through the gut, usually from an upper GI bleed)

Haemodynamically unstable due to massive blood loss:
- Pale
- Low BP
- Tachycardic
- Shock: if large haemorrhage

Other signs of chronic liver disease:
- Such as jaundice, ascites and encephalopathy.

Investigations

Blood tests

- FBC: particularly Hb
- Biochemistry: evidence of liver disease
- Clotting: particularly INR
- Cross match blood
- Order platelets and clotting products
- Blood cultures
- ABG.

Endoscopy

- To treat and confirm diagnosis
- Seen as bulges into the lumen of the oesophagus on endoscopy.

Treatment

Treatment of acute, bleeding varices:
- General:
  - ABC approach: treat as any GI bleed chapter 14. Low threshold for airway protection/ICU
  - Fluid resuscitate: blood transfusion
  - Correct clotting/platelets: vitamin K, fresh frozen plasma
  - Prophylactic broad spectrum antibiotics as high risk patients
- 1st line interventions:
  - Endoscopy: as soon as stable. 'Banding' to tie off oesophageal vessels or sclerotherapy (injecting glue) of gastric varices (stops bleed in 80%)
  - IV terlipressin to vasoconstrict portal system

- If unable to obtain endoscopic control can place a Sengstaken Blakemore tube (a rubber tube with a balloon to tamponade oesophageal bleeds) up to 24 h until endoscopic control or TIPS
- 2nd line interventions:
  - TIPS to relieve portal vein pressure (see portal hypertension)
- Follow-up:
  - Need repeat OGD at ~10 days to ensure variceal obliteration

Treatment of chronic varices
- Endoscopic banding regularly until resolved
- Treat portal hypertension, e.g. propranolol.

Prognosis and complications

Prognosis

- 30% of those with varices have an acute bleed
- 50% mortality from 1st variceal bleed
- High risk of re-bleed, 80% at 2 years
- Prognosis depends on Childs-Pugh score (see cirrhosis above)
- 30–50% of cirrhotics will have variceal bleed

Prevention:
- Any cirrhotic should be screened regularly with an OGD for the development of varices.

Complications

- GI bleeds with high mortality.

ASCITES

Outline

- Fluid in the peritoneal cavity
- Causes can be divided into transudate or exudate depending on the protein content of the fluid. However the serum ascitic albumin gradient (SAAG) is a better guide as to whether the cause is due to portal hypertension or not.

- Most common cause is portal hypertension ($\uparrow$ BP in the portal vein, see above) leading to $\uparrow$ renal sodium and water retention (activation of renin–angiotensin system).

Pathogenesis/aetiology

Causes

Transudate: protein content: <25 g/L:
- Liver failure (75%): cirrhosis with portal hypertension (common causes of ascites), ALF, Budd–Chiari (hepatic vein occlusion)
- Renal failure: hypoalbuminaemia, e.g. nephrotic syndrome

Exudate: >25 g/L:
- Malignancy (10%)
- Infection (2%)
- Inflammation
- Pancreatitis (1%)
- Lymphatic obstruction

Cardiac failure (3%) can cause either.

Who

- 50% of cirrhotics after 10 years

Clinical features

- Abdominal distension
- Fullness in flanks
- Shifting dullness on percussion

- Fluid thrill
- Other associated effusions: pleural, pericardial.

Blood and urine tests

- FBC (platelets)
- U&Es
- Coagulation

- LFTs
- Urine for sodium and potassium.

Tests on the aspirated fluid

- Inspection:
  - Normal: clear, straw-coloured
  - ↑ bilirubin: orange
  - Infection: turbid
  - Malignancy: blood stained

- Cell count, Gram stain, culture
- Protein content to determine transudate or exudates
- Serum-ascites albumin gradient if >11 g/L then likely to be due to portal hypertension.

Imaging

- Abdominal US
- Abdominal CT

- Echocardiogram.

Treatment

Conservative

- Treat underlying cause
- Reduce sodium intake

- Fluid restriction
- Monitor fluid balance.

Medical

- Diuretics: spironolactone, furosemide

Invasive

- Paracentesis: draining fluid for immediate relief. Give albumin replacement depending on the amount drained

- TIPS (see portal hypertension).

Prognosis and complications

Prognosis

- 40% 2 year survival in hospitalised patients.

Complications

- Spontaneous bacterial peritonitis (spontaneous infection of ascites, see below): in 8% of cirrhotic patients with ascites

- Hyponatraemia (due to drugs and advanced liver disease)
- Pleural effusion and respiratory distress
- Overdiuresis: dehydration, uraemia.

SPONTANEOUS BACTERIAL PERITONITIS

Outline

- Spontaneous infection of ascites
- Due to a single organism
- High risk if:
  - ascitic protein low (<15 g/L)
  - previous episode

2° bacterial peritonitis:
- Caused by multiple organisms after recent intra-abdominal instrumentation.

Pathogenesis/aetiology

Pathogenesis

- Thought to be due to translocation of bacteria from the gut due to increased permeability and reduced immune function

Causative organisms:
- *Escherichia coli*
- *Klebsiella*
- *Streptococcus.*

Who

- Consider in any patient with ascites with sudden deterioration

- Occurs in ∼10% of hospitalised patients who have an ascitic tap.

Clinical features

- Ranges from asymptomatic to severe sepsis
- Abdominal pain
- Clinically relevant change in bowel habit

- Signs of systemic infection
- Hepatic encephalopathy
- Oliguria/renal dysfunction with no apparent cause.

Investigations

- As for ascites above

- Diagnose spontaneous bacterial peritonitis if:
  - polymorphonuclear leucocytes (PMN) >250/μl
  - Gram stain positive
  - growth of organism.

Treatment

- Broad spectrum IV antibiotics (cefotaxime or Tazocin) for 5 days

Prophylaxis:
- Usually norfloxacin in high-risk patients.

Prognosis and complications

Prognosis

- 1 year survival: 30–50%

- 2 year survival: 25–30%.

Complications

- Renal failure

- Sepsis and multi-organ failure.

ACUTE LIVER FAILURE

Outline

Acute liver injury:
- Rapid deterioration in hepatic function (<6 months) in a previously healthy liver
- Due to hepatocellular cell death
- Elevated transaminases and jaundice seen

Acute liver failure:
- Acute liver injury which progresses causing an elevated INR (>1.5) and hepatic encephalopathy (see below)

- Time from development of jaundice to encephalopathy used to categorise it as:
  - hyper-acute: <7 days
  - acute: 8–28 days
  - sub-acute: 4–12 weeks.

Pathogenesis/aetiology

Causes

Infection:
- Hepatitis A, B, E
- Immunocompromised patient, e.g. Epstein–Barr virus (EBV), CMV
- Foreign travel: dengue fever
- Leptospirosis leading to Weil's disease.

Drugs / Toxins:
- Paracetamol (commonest cause in UK)
- Cocaine/amphetamines
- Iron overdose
- Drug-induced liver injury: idiosyncratic drug reaction (e.g. amoxicillin, rifampicin, isoniazid, phenytoin, valproate, sulphonamides)
- Death cap mushroom *Amanita phalloides*

Malignancy:
- Lymphoma, melanoma, breast cancer

Other:
- Autoimmune hepatitis
- Wilsons' disease
- Budd–Chiari
- Ischaemia: particularly in right heart failure
- Pregnancy related:
  - Acute fatty liver of pregnancy
  - HELLP (heaemolysis, elevated liver enzymes, low platelets) syndrome
- Sero-negative (15%): no cause found. Could be unknown virus or autoimmune with no antibodies.

Who

Ask the patient:
- Recent new medication
- Recent foreign travel

- Unprotected sexual contact
- IVDUs
- Prodromal illness.

Who

A typical patient

A young girl impulsively took many tablets a couple of days ago. History of depression and self harm. She did not tell anyone at the time but now is feeling nauseous with epigastric pain. She regrets taking the tablets.

Clinical features

- Jaundice
- Abdominal discomfort
- Bruising from coagulopathy

- Hyper-acute: patient may be profoundly unwell with circulatory collapse, low Glasgow Coma Scale and anuria
- Patients must be monitored closely as hepatic encephalopathy can develop quickly.

Investigations

Blood tests

- INR*
- LFTs*
- U&Es*
- FBC*
- Creatine kinase
- Coagulation
- ABG*: pH, lactate, ammonia
- Glucose.*
- Group and save

- Blood culture
- Paracetamol level
- Drug screen
- Hepatitis screen
- Auto-antibodies/immunoglobulins
- Copper studies

*Need to be repeated regularly.

Imaging

- US liver: review hepatic vasculature. Any evidence of chronic liver disease?

- CT scan: vasculature, hepatic size, any evidence of malignancy

Other tests

- Transjugular biopsy if diagnosis is uncertain, however often will not change management.

Treatment

General:
- ABC approach
- Early IV access and fluid resuscitation
- Low threshold for antibiotics
- N-acetylcysteine IV
- Can give vitamin supplement such as vitamin K or thiamine
- Discuss early with local transplant centre
- Transfer to ICU for early organ support if needed.

Monitor:
- Nurse in a closely monitored environment
- Regularly for hepatic encephalopathy: any affected patient should be transferred to ICU, intubate if grade 3 or 4
- INR 6 hourly: no fresh frozen plasma unless actively bleeding
- Urine output and creatinine
Treat underlying cause.

Prognosis and complications

Prognosis

Prior to liver transplantation:
- 80–85% mortality overall
King's College Hospital Criteria for Liver Transplantation (i.e. poor prognosis):
- Paracetamol:
  - pH <7.3 after adequate resuscitation or concurrent findings of:
    - Hepatic encephalopathy grade 3
    - Creatinine >300
    - INR >6.5

- Non-paracetamol:
  - INR >6 or any three of the following:
    - Age <10 or >40
    - Unfavourable aetiology (seronegative, drug-induced liver injury)
    - Not hyper-ALF
    - INR >3.5
    - Bilirubin >300.

Prognosis and complications

Complications

- Multi-organ failure
- Sepsis: commonest mode of death
- Cerebral oedema and intracranial hypertension: particularly if young, hyper-acute, or renal failure.

HEPATIC ENCEPHALOPATHY

Outline

- A syndrome of global brain dysfunction ranging from mild psychiatric, cognitive and motor dysfunction to coma due to liver disease of any cause
- From the accumulation of toxic substances in the peripheral blood, normally 'detoxified' or removed by the liver, that impair the function of brain cells
- Nitrogenous metabolites particularly implicated (especially ammonia)

Fulminant hepatic failure:
- Sudden onset liver failure with hepatic encephalopathy within 2 weeks in a person with no previous underlying liver pathology.

Pathogenesis/aetiology

Causes

- Presence of a porto-systemic shunt (i.e. a link between the portal venous and peripheral circulation such as large varices)
- Any cause of liver failure: acute, chronic
- Often triggered by a precipitating event

Precipitating event:
- Infection (e.g. Spontaneous bacterial peritonitis)
- High protein absorption from GI tract: GI bleed, constipation
- Dehydration
- Drugs: sedatives, alcoholic binge
- Metabolic disarray: hyponatraemia, hypokalaemia, renal dysfunction
- Following TIPS (see portal hypertension).

Who

- Rule out any other causes of acute confusion or coma.

Clinical features

Grades of hepatic encephalopathy:
0. No impairment
1. Altered mood or behaviour
2. Drowsy. Inappropriate behaviour. 'Liver flap' (asterixis)
3. Inarticulate speech. Marked confusion
4. Comatose, may be aroused by painful stimuli

Precipitating event:
- Signs of infection/sepsis
- Evidence of GI bleed
- Faecal impaction
- General signs of chronic liver disease.

Investigations

Blood tests

- FBC, LFTs, U&Es, CRP, Coag
- Glucose
- ABG
- Arterial ammonia

Microbiology

- Blood culture
- Ascitic tap
- Urine culture.

Imaging

- CXR
- Abdominal/liver US
- CT: abdomen

Other tests

Consider:
- OGD/colonoscopy
- Electroencephalography (EEG)
- CT head
- Lumbar puncture.

- ABC approach: intubation and ICU if airway at risk or grade 4 disease
- Antibiotics
- IV fluids
- Lactulose/enemas: thought to release toxins from the bowels

Treat precipitating event:
- Treat infection
- Control GI bleed
- Stop sedating medication
- Transplantation if due to TIPS or recurrent and not controlled by medical therapy.

Prognosis

- Depends on grade and cause

- Rifaximin (a non-absorbable antibiotic) reduces re-admission rates to hospital in patients with cirrhosis who previously were admitted for encephalopathy.

JAUNDICE (ICTERUS)

Outline

- Yellowing of the skin, eyes and mucosa from ↑ serum bilirubin
- Normal levels of bilirubin 5–17 mmol/L

- Clinically detectable when bilirubin >50 μmol/L
- See p. 152 to understand 'the liver in bilirubin metabolism'.

Classification

Pre-hepatic (unconjugated):
- Due to ↑ bilirubin being produced or ↓ conjugation
- As the bilirubin has not yet reached the liver it is not conjugated (therefore insoluble) so it is excreted directly in the faeces making them darker. If there is normal liver function, there is also ↑ urobilinogen and stercobilinogen, as there is ↑ build up through the normal excretory pathway

Hepatic:
- Hepatocyte dysfunction leads to altered bilirubin metabolism. Usually mixed but predominantly conjugated picture

Post-hepatic (conjugated/obstructed):
- Bilirubin has been conjugated by normal hepatocytes, but cannot drain into the gut due to biliary tree obstruction. The conjugated bilirubin therefore leaks into the blood. Since it is soluble the urine becomes dark, with less excreted in the faeces so these are light. Pruritus can occur from irritation by bile salts deposited in the skin.

NB: often mixed picture.

Pathogenesis/aetiology

Causes

Unconjugated:
- Congenital: Crigler–Najjar (affects metabolism of bilirubin)
- Gilbert syndrome: affects 5% causing an isolated ↑ unconjugated serum bilirubin
- Haemolysis: ↑ break down of RBCs.

Predominantly conjugated:
- Congenital: biliary atresia (absent or blocked bile duct), Alagille syndrome
- Infection: acute viral hepatitis

- Drugs: paracetamol, antibiotics, anti-TB drugs, OC pill, antimalarials, phenytoin
- Intra-hepatic or extra-hepatic cholestasis: primary biliary cirrhosis, primary sclerosing cholangitis, sepsis, gallstones, pancreatic cancer, chronic pancreatitis (pseudocyst/stricture), cholangiocarcinoma
- Cancer: liver metastases, pancreatic cancer
- Acute alcoholic hepatitis
- End-stage cirrhosis of any cause
- Autoimmune liver disease
- Budd–Chiari (hepatic vein obstruction).

Who

Ask the patient:
- Age at onset
- Duration
- Urine and stool colour
- Pruritus
- Associated symptoms: chills, fever, weight loss, anorexia, abdominal pain
- Previous attacks
- Full drug history

- Family history
- Infection risk
- Blood transfusion
- Contact with other people with jaundice
- Occupation
- Alcohol
- Travel
- Sexual history
- Recent surgery.

Clinical features

- Yellow discoloration of the skin, conjunctiva and mucous membranes
- Abdominal mass
- Splenomegaly
- Enlarged gall bladder – Courvoisier's rule: if a patient presents with painless, obstructive jaundice, and a palpable gallbladder, it is not due to gallstones (i.e. suggests cancer of the head of pancreas)
- Signs of right heart failure

- Lymphadenopathy.

Unconjugated (pre-hepatic):
- Urine: normal
- Faeces: dark

Conjugated (hepatic, post-hepatic):
- Urine dark
- Faeces: pale
- Pruritus/scratch marks

Signs of chronic liver disease

- Evidence of hepatic encephalopathy
- Spider naevi

Hands:
- Palmar erythema
- Clubbing
- Leukonychia
- Dupuytren's contracture

Chest, abdomen, groin:
- Gynaecomastia
- Ascites
- Testicular atrophy

Investigations

Blood tests

- FBCs, U&Es, coagulation
- LFTs: ↑ ALT/AST liver cell damage, ↑ ALP/γGT obstructive/cholestatic
- 'Split bilirubin': unconjugated and conjugated bilirubin levels
- Haemolysis screen (Coombs' test), reticulocyte count haptoglobins (bind free Hb, blood film)
- Tumour screen: α-fetoprotein, CA 199

- Autoimmune screen:
  - Anti-smooth muscle: primary sclerosis cholangitis
  - AMA: primary biliary cirrhosis
  - ANA
  - ANCA
- Viral hepatitis screen
- Iron studies: haemochromatosis
- Serum caeruloplasmin and copper: Wilson's.

Imaging

US: first line:
- Dilatation of bile ducts
- Gallstones
- Pancreatic tumour
- Liver metastases
- Hepatic and portal vein Dopplers

ERCP/MRCP:
- If dilation of the bile ducts.

CT/MRI:
- Malignancy.

Other tests

Histology:
- ERCP: brushings for cholangiocarcinoma (cancer of the bile ducts)

- Liver biopsy: for other causes of liver disease.

Treatment

Treat cause:
- Stop incriminating drugs
- Decompress obstruction

Treat symptoms:
- Itch: cholestyramine (bile acid sequestrant), chlorphenamine (antihistamine).

Prognosis and complications

Complications

Complications of obstructive jaundice:
- Infection (cholangitis)
- Coagulopathy: failure to absorb vitamin K, give IV vitamin K

- Renal failure
- Malnutrition.

AUTOIMMUNE LIVER DISEASE

AUTOIMMUNE HEPATITIS

Outline

- Inflammation of the liver from an immune response against the liver cells

- **Ultimately leads to acute liver injury and/or chronic liver injury**
- Often progresses to cirrhosis.

Classification

Type 1:
- Occurs in: adults and children
- Autoantibodies: anti-smooth and ANA

Type 2:
- Occurs in: children
- Autoantibodies: type 1 anti-liver/kidney microsomal antibodies, anti-liver cytosol
- Progression to cirrhosis: 80%

Type 3:
- Occurs in: adults
- Autoantibodies: soluble liver kidney antigen
- Progression to cirrhosis: 75%.

Pathogenesis/aetiology

Causes

- Unknown cause
- Genetic disposition with association with other autoimmune diseases

- May be environmental triggers.

Pathogenesis

- Immune mediated: raised autoantibodies, IgG and cytotoxic T-cells and regulatory T-cell dysfunction

- Sometimes referred to as seronegative if no antibodies found.

Who

- Typical age: bimodal:
  - 3–15 years
  - 40–60 years
- 6♀:1♂

Associations:
- Other autoimmune diseases: SLE, thyroid disease, pernicious anaemia
- HLA-A1, HLA-B8, HLA-DR3.

A typical patient

A middle-aged woman with history of thyroid disease and pernicious anaemia, presents with fever, right upper quadrant pain and abnormal LFTs.

Clinical features

- May present with acute or chronic liver disease
- Jaundice
- Symptoms and complications of cirrhosis

- Autoimmune features: fever, malaise, fatigue, nausea, arthritis, rash.

Investigations

Blood tests

- FBC: leukopenia, low platelets
- LFTs: ↑ bilirubin, ↑ ALT/AST, hypoalbuminaemia
- INR
- ↑ IgG
- Autoantibodies: varies with type 1 and type 2 disease:
  - Anti-smooth muscle: 70% (type 1)

- ANA 80% (type 1)
- AMA: 25%
- Type 1 anti-liver/kidney microsomal antibodies (type 2)
- Anti-liver cytosol (type 2)
- Exclude other causes of liver disease

Diagnosis

- Based upon scoring system considering:
  - LFTs
  - presence of autoantibodies
  - lack of other diagnosis

- consistent histology
- genetic factors
- response to therapy

Investigations

Liver biopsy

- Plasma cell infiltrate
- Cirrhosis
- Interface hepatitis

- Overlaps with primary sclerotic cholangitis and primary biliary cirrhosis.

Treatment

Medical management

- Effective in 80%
- Relapse rate 80% at 3 years if treatment stopped

Ist line:
- Prednisolone for 2–3 weeks: reduces inflammation

- Azathioprine (suppresses the immune system): for maintenance and allows steroid sparing

2nd line immunosuppressive agents:
- Tacrolimus, cyclosporin, mycophenolate.

Surgical

- Liver transplant for end-stage liver disease or if sub-ALF fulfilling transplant criteria.

Prognosis and complications

Prognosis

- 5 year survival without treatment: 50%
- 10 year survival with treatment: 90%

- Can re-occur after transplant
- Worse if there is cirrhosis.

Complications

- 15% progress to sub-ALF

- Complications of cirrhosis and portal hypertension.

PRIMARY BILIARY CIRRHOSIS

Outline

- Autoimmune liver disease where there is slow progressive destruction of the intralobular ducts

- See also Table 5.2 below for the differences between primary biliary cirrhosis and primary sclerosis cholangitis.

Secondary biliary cirrhosis

- Cirrhosis from prolonged large duct biliary obstruction caused by another 1° cause.

Pathogenesis/aetiology

Causes

- Exact cause unclear

- Autoimmune disorder: autoantibodies found, particularly AMA M2

Pathogenesis

- Unknown event leads to build up of antibodies and sensitisation of T cells to bile duct epithelium
- Trigger may be an environmental event in a genetically susceptible person
- Leads to inflammation, fibrosis and loss of small bile ducts.

- This leads to cholestasis (blockage of bile transport to the gut) as bile can not flow out of the liver
- Failure of biliary secretion leads to retention of toxic substances leading to further hepatocyte damage and inflammation
- This chronic inflammation and fibrosis leads to cirrhosis.

Who

- Typical age: 40–65 years
- ♀10:♂1
- Prevalence 4/100 000

Genetics:
- HLA-DR8
- IL12 polymorphisms

Associations:
- Other autoimmune disease:
  - Rheumatoid arthritis
  - Sjögren syndrome
  - Scleroderma
  - Thyroid disease.

Who

A typical patient

A middle-aged woman presents to her GP with itch and lethargy. She has xanthelasmata. Blood tests show ↑ ALP, GGT, bilirubin, cholesterol but only slightly ↑ ALT and AST.

Clinical features

- Often asymptomatic
- Fatigue
- Arthralgia
- Skin pigmentation
- Xanthelasma: due to 2° hypercholesterolaemia (fat absorption impaired by build up of bile)
- Abdominal pain
- Dry eyes and mouth as AMA is also specific for these sites

Symptoms and signs of cholestasis:
- Pruritus: commonest complaint (from bile salts under the skin)
- Cholestatic jaundice: cholestatic: dark urine pale stools (see jaundice above)
- Steatorrhea
- Gallstones

Signs of chronic liver disease:
- Jaundice
- Hepatomegaly: late
- Clubbing

Signs of portal hypertension:
- Ascites
- Variceal bleeding
- Hepatosplenomegaly.

Investigations

Blood tests

- LFTs: ↑↑ ALP (v high), ↑↑ GGT, ↑ AST/ALT, ↑ bilirubin
- ↓ albumin
- ↑ serum cholesterol: from cholestasis
- ↑ IgM: primary biliary cirrhosis
- Exclude other causes of chronic liver disease

Autoantibodies:
- 98% are AMA specific (M2)

Other antibodies: ANA, anti-RO, anti-thyroid, anit-acetylcholine, anti-smooth muscle.

Imaging

- US and MRCP to exclude extrahepatic cholestatsis.

Other tests

Histology:
- Loss of bile ducts, lymphocyte infiltration of portal tracts, granuloma formation, fibrosis and cirrhosis.

Treatment

For disease process:
- Ursodeoxycholic acid: improves biochemistry but not prognosis
- Not steroids

For complications:
- Pruritus:
  - Cholestyramine (bile acid sequestrant)
  - Rifampicin
- Single-pass albumin dialysis (SPAD): dialysis using albumin to bind bile salts/bilirubin
- Fat-soluble vitamin deficiencies:
  - Vitamins A, D and K
- Cirrhosis and portal hypertension:
  - Treat as above
- End-stage:
  - Transplantation for end-stage disease.

Prognosis and complications

Prognosis

- From diagnosis 40–60% will develop symptoms within 5–7 years
- Median survival in symptomatic patients: 7.5 years from diagnosis
- Median survival if asymptomatic: 16 years from diagnosis
- After transplant: 5 year survival ↑ to >70%
- Death is from chronic liver disease and its complications.

Complications

- Malabsorption of fat-soluble vitamins (A, D, K) from decreased bile salts leads to: osteomalacia, osteoporosis, steatorrhoea and coagulopathy
- As for cirrhosis and portal hypertension of any aetiology.

PRIMARY SCLEROSING CHOLANGITIS

Outline

Chronic liver disease from chronic inflammation and fibrosis of the bile ducts leading to cholestasis (blockage of bile transport to the gut) and cirrhosis:

- may lead to complications such as ascending cholangitis (infection in the biliary tract) and cholangiocarcinoma
- affects extrahepatic +/− intrahepatic bile ducts
- cause unknown but thought to be autoimmune
- **ultimately leads to chronic liver injury**.

Table 5.2 shows the differences between primary biliary cirrhosis and primary sclerosing cholangitis.

Table 5.2 Differences between primary biliary cirrhosis and primary sclerosing cholangitis

	Primary biliary cirrhosis	Primary sclerosing cholangitis
Bile duct changes	Intrahepatic	Intra- and extrahepatic
Autoimmune disease association	Yes	Possibly
Those affected	Mainly women	Mainly men
Associated with IBD	No	Yes
Age affected	Older adults	All ages
Antibodies detected	AMA (M2)	p-ANCA

Pathogenesis/aetiology

Causes

- Exact cause unknown
- Autoimmune cause is probable
- Association with autoantibodies in 80%:
  - p-ANCA found in 60%
- ANA
- Anti-smooth muscle
- Some antigens associated with a worse outcome.

Who

- Typical age of onset: 40 years
- 1♀:3♂

Associations:
- IBD, mainly ulcerative colitis (UC) in 75–90%
- Halotypes HLA: a1, B8, DR3.

A typical patient

40-year-old man with a long history of UC presents with fatigue, pruritus and jaundice. His GP performs blood tests which show abnormal LFTs.

Clinical features

- May be asymptomatic.

Symptoms

- Right upper quadrant pain
- Fatigue
- Pruritus.

Signs

- Jaundice
- Excoriations
- Hepato-splenomegaly
- Symptoms and complications of cirrhosis and portal hypertension.

Investigations

Blood tests

- Liver biochemistry: ↑ bilirubin and ALP
- Autoantibodies, p-ANCA
- ↑ IgG and/or IgM
- Exclude other causes of chronic liver disease.

Imaging

- US liver: look for any evidence of cirrhosis or portal hypertension or any obvious ductal pathology
- MRCP: MRI to image ducts, non-invasive but can not perform interventions

Other tests

- Endoscopic retrograde cholangiopancreatography (ERCP): shows characteristic beading (Fig. 5.7) of bile ducts from intermittent strictures. Can obtain brushings for cytology or place stent for any dominant strictures. NB: risk of pancreatitis
- Liver biopsy: to confirm diagnosis and assess extent of liver damage.

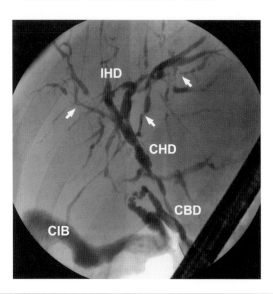

Fig. 5.7 ERCP showing typical beading of primary sclerosing cholangitis. IHD, intrahepatic ducts; CBD, common bile duct; CHD, common hepatic duct.

Treatment

For disease process:
- No curative medical therapy
- Ursodeoxycholic acid
- Immunosuppression: steroids/azathioprine, etc. Not much evidence that helps

Pruritus:
- Cholestyramine

Treat complications:
- e.g. ascending cholangitis

Liver transplantation:
- For end-stage disease or if refractory recurrent cholangitis. Recurrence in 5–20% at 1 year.

Prognosis and complications

Prognosis

- Mostly runs a benign course
- Mean survival is 12 years.

Complications

- As for cirrhosis and portal hypertension of any aetiology
- Cholangiocarcinoma: bile duct cancer 15–30% lifetime risk. Think of this in any patient with primary sclerosing cholangitis who has sudden worsening of clinical state, such as weight loss or jaundice. Should have screening US 1–2x/year
- Ascending cholangitis
- 2° biliary cirrhosis
- Fat-soluble vitamin deficiency (bile normally ↑ fat absorption).
- Risk of gallbladder cancer: Screen with regular abdominal US and refer for surgery if any gallbladder polyps seen.

METABOLIC AND DRUG-CAUSED LIVER DISEASE

ALCOHOLIC LIVER DISEASE

Outline

- Liver disease caused by excessive consumption of alcohol
- Maximum weekly alcohol recommendations: 21 units for males, 14 for females
- **Ultimately leads to chronic liver injury, although can present in an 'acute' fashion**

Disease can take three forms:

- Alcoholic fatty liver: histological or radiological diagnosis similar to non-alcoholic fatty liver disease, reversible on abstinence
- Acute alcoholic hepatitis (AAH): clinical diagnosis in a chronic alcohol abuser who acutely develops severe jaundice, fever, marked impairment of liver synthetic function and manifestations of portal hypertension. Frequently accompanied by steatosis (depositing of fat in the hepatocytes) and cirrhosis. Characterised by systemic inflammation and pro-inflammatory cytokines
- Alcoholic cirrhosis (AC): histological or radiological diagnosis in a patient with a background of heavy alcohol use. The final stage of alcoholic liver disease. Cirrhosis occurs in only 10–20% of long-term alcoholics. Presentation as for other causes of cirrhosis.

Pathogenesis/aetiology

Pathogenesis

- Alcohol metabolism occurs in the liver and involves either alcohol dehydrogenase or the microsomal ethanol oxidising system
- Both lead to increased reduced nicotinamide adenine dinucleotide (↑ NADH/NAD ratio), changing the redox potential
- The change in redox potential causes a ↓ in fatty acid oxidation and an ↑ in hepatic fatty acid synthesis leading to steatosis and to fatty liver disease (alcoholic fatty liver)
- When a florid immunological response to this occurs, this leads to AAH
- Chronic inflammatory reaction to these events leads to fibrosis and eventual AC

Scoring systems for AAH

- Glasgow Alcoholic Hepatitis Score: based upon age, bilirubin, urea, WBC, INR. Score ≥9 benefit from steroids
- Maddrey's Discriminant Function: based upon PT and bilirubin. Score of >32 suggests poor outcome, may benefit from steroids.

Who

- Typical age: 40–50s, but getting younger
- ♂ > ♀, but ↑ more women
- Was commonest cause of chronic liver disease in Western world (now NALFD catching up)
- 1% of population is alcohol dependent: 20–30% of them develop alcoholic liver disease.

A typical patient

A middle-aged publican who presents with fevers, malaise and profound jaundice.

Clinical features

Alcohol misuse

- Drink driving offences
- Relationship difficulties
- Poor social situation
- Occupational risk
- Not able to hold down employment
- 'CAGE' screen (have you felt you should **C**ut down, do you get **A**ngry at people criticising your drinking, have you ever feel **G**uilty about the amount you drink, do you ever need an '**E**ye opener' (drink first thing in the morning))
- Malnourished
- Parotid enlargement
- Peripheral neuropathy
- Multiple bruises/injuries
- Cardiomyopathy

Acute alcoholic hepatitis

- Jaundice
- Hepatic encephalopathy
- Nausea and vomiting
- Fatigue
- Anorexia
- Diarrhoea
- Abdominal pain
- Often with cirrhosis and signs of decompensated liver disease

Clinical features

Alcoholic cirrhosis

- Symptoms and signs of cirrhosis and portal hypertension.

Investigations

Blood tests

FBC:
- Macrocytic anaemia
- Thrombocytopenia: alcohol is toxic to megakaryoctes, also if splenomegaly
- AAH: leucocytosis

LFTs:
- Drinking alcohol ↑ GGT
- AST, ALT (ratio >2 in AAH), usually only moderate elevation
- ↑ bilirubin in late cirrhosis

Synthetic dysfunction:
- ↑ INR, ↓ albumin
- In AAH, extremely high bilirubin (>100) and more profound synthetic dysfunction

Other:
- ↑ IgA
- Renal function particularly in AAH
- Alcohol level
- Exclude other causes of chronic liver disease.

Imaging

- US: fatty acid change, cirrhosis and portal hypertension. Rule out gallstone disease.

Other tests

Liver biopsy:
- Steatosis and steatohepatitis, Mallory bodies (dense eosinophilic cytoplasmic inclusion bodies found in hepatocytes, typical, but not exclusive, also occur in NASH). In AAH: neutrophil infiltrate and features of cirrhosis.

Treatment

General:
- Stop drinking: often develop alcohol withdrawal. Treat symptoms with benzodiazepines: diazepam, chlordiazepoxide
- Nutrition: supplements, may require NG feed and admission to hospital
- Vitamin replacement: folate, thiamine, vitamins K and B_{12}

Alcoholic cirrhosis:
- As for any patient with cirrhosis (see above)

Acute alcoholic hepatitis:
- Patients range from mild to extremely unwell.

- ABC with support where necessary
- Watch renal function
- High incidence of sepsis: low threshold for antibiotics
- Pharmacological:
  - Pentoxifylline TNF antagonist
  - Corticosteroids: depending on scoring systems criteria

Liver transplantation:
- For end-stage disease
- Very good prognosis following liver transplantation
- In UK require 6 months of abstinence to be considered.

Prognosis and complications

Prognosis

- No cirrhosis: 5 year survival: 60% with no abstinence, 90% with abstinence

- Cirrhotic: Depends on severity of cirrhosis. If no abstinence survival much worse.

Complications

- As for cirrhosis and portal hypertension of any aetiology
- Alcohol withdrawal

- Multi-organ failure in AAH.

NON-ALCOHOLIC FATTY LIVER DISEASE

Outline

- Fatty infiltration of the liver, from a non-alcoholic cause. In up to 5% of people this leads to inflammation (NASH)

- In 10–20% NASH can lead to fibrosis and eventually, cirrhosis:
- **Ultimately leads to chronic liver injury.**

Pathogenesis/aetiology

- Becoming increasingly common due to obesity epidemic and increased incidence of insulin resistance.

Pathogenesis

- Insulin resistance and disregulated free fatty acid metabolism results in lipid droplet accumulation within hepatocytes
- This can provoke an inflammatory response.

Who

- Becoming increasingly common

Risk factors:
- Obesity
- Diabetes
- Hyperlipidaemia
- Drugs/toxins
- Starvation.

A typical patient

An overweight man with diabetes, high cholesterol and high BP is found on routine check up to have ↑ GGT.

Clinical features

- Mainly asymptomatic
- Hepatomegaly
- Symptoms and signs risk factors, e.g. hyperlipidaemia, diabetes
- If progresses, can have symptoms and signs of cirrhosis and portal hypertension.

Investigations

Blood tests

- LFTs: often just ↑ GGT or ALP. AST, ALT ↑ in NASH. AST/ALT < 1
- Lipids
- Glucose tolerance
- Ferritin often high
- Exclude other causes of chronic liver disease.

Imaging

- US: characteristic 'bright liver.' May have features of cirrhosis with portal hypertension

Other tests

- Liver biopsy: Fat droplets within hepatocytes, inflammatory cells in the lobule, Mallory bodies (dense eosinophilic cytoplasmic inclusion bodies found in hepatocytes), and fibrosis.

Treatment

- Treat or control cause

Lifestyle measures:
- Weight reduction
- Exercise
- Low fat and low carbohydrate diet
- Control diabetes
- Treat hyperlipidaemia.

Prognosis and complications

Prognosis

- In non-alcoholic fatty liver disease over 3 years 30% progress, 30% remain stable and 30% improve
- In NASH patients: 10–20% will develop cirrhosis.

Complications

- Associated complications of the metabolic syndrome
- As for cirrhosis and portal hypertension of any aetiology.

PARACETAMOL OVERDOSE

Outline

- Severe overdose of paracetamol >10 g (20 tablets)
- **Leads to severe hepatic necrosis, renal failure and liver failure within 72 h of overdose**
- Lower doses can cause toxicity if liver enzymes are induced, e.g. in alcoholics, certain drugs (CYP450 inducers) or there are reduced glutathione stores available (malnourished, anorexia)
- Renal failure is caused by hepatorenal syndrome or multiple organ dysfunction.

Pathogenesis/aetiology

Pathogenesis

- 95% of paracetamol is normally metabolised in the liver into conjugates which are excreted
- 5% is metabolised by the CYP450 pathways into a toxic metabolite: N-acetyl-p-benzoquinoneimine (NAPQI)
- Glutathione, a derivative of cysteine, can conjugate this toxin into an inactive state in normal individuals
- There is excess NAPQI in:
  - severe overdose, as all the glutathione is used up
  - moderate overdose, where the CYP450 has been induced or there are reduced glutathione stores
- N-acetylcysteine, a glutathione precursor, can be given in these patients to replenish glutathione levels
- It's use is guided by referring to a nomogram (see investigations)
- Side effects: bronchospasm, rash, flushing, hypotension, anaphylaxis, wheeze, angioedema (swelling of dermis and subcutaneous tissue); often overcome by reducing the rate of infusion
- Methionine, taken orally, which is converted to glutathione in the liver, can also be used but is less reliable if there is vomiting.

Who

- Commonest overdose in UK
- Higher risk in malnourished patients.

Clinical features

- Initially asymptomatic
- Nausea and vomiting within 24 h
- Malaise
- Right upper quadrant pain
- Severe transaminitis
- Jaundice if staggered overdose and delayed presentation
- Hepatic encephalopathy.

Investigations

Nomogram:
- A chart of measured plasma paracetamol levels against time used to determine treatment after paracetamol overdose
- To use:
  - Assess time of overdose
  - Take paracetamol plasma level after four hours (those taken before give an unreliable estimate)
  - Check level on nomogram: plot the appropriate plasma paracetamol level at the number of hours after digestion (at least 4 h) and assess if the level is above the normal treatment line (or the high risk treatment line, if appropriate) to determine the appropriate treatment (Fig. 5.8)
  - Give N-acetylcysteine IV if above the treatment line
  - Obese patients should have their dose calculated based upon 110 kg weight

General tests:
- As for ALF above
- Monitor blood glucose hourly

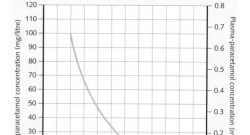

Fig. 5.8 Nomogram used to determine treatment in paracetamol overdose.

Treatment

- ABC approach
- Early IV access and fluid resuscitation
- If worsening clotting, renal failure or hepatic encephalopathy: refer early to liver unit/ITU
- Transfer to ITU for early organ support if needed

Monitor:
- Nurse in a closely monitored environment
- INR 6 hourly: no fresh frozen plasma or vitamin K unless actively bleeding
- Glucose regularly
- pH and lactate
- Urine output, creatinine
- Check for hepatic encephalopathy
- Assess risk: high in those on anti-epileptics, alcoholics, or malnourished

N-acetylcysteine:
- <8 h:
  - Check level on nomogram after 4 h
- >8–24 h:
  - Treat with N-acetylcysteine at once
  - On return of the blood tests refer to the nomogram for decision to continue treating based on blood level
- Unknown or >24 h:
  - Treat with N-acetylcysteine at once
  - Continue for 24 h
- Treatment duration:
  - Continue N-acetylcysteine for 5 days or until INR is <1.5

Other medication:
- Alternative is methionine taken orally <12 h
- Low threshold for antibiotics
- Vitamin supplement such as vitamin K or Pabrinex.

Prognosis and complications

Prognosis

Poor if:
- pH <7.3 after adequate resuscitation or:
- Concurrent findings of: hepatic encephalopathy grade 3, creatinine >300, INR >6.5

Refer patient if:
- Day 2: pH <7.3, INR >3, oliguria, creatinine >200, hypoglycaemia
- Day 3: pH <7.3, INR >4.5, oliguria, creatinine >200, any hepatic encephalopathy
- Day 4: INR >6, progressive rise in INR, oliguria, creatinine >300, any hepatic encephalopathy.

INHERITED METABOLIC DISORDERS

WILSON'S DISEASE

Outline

- An inherited disease causing failure of biliary copper excretion due to a defect in the protein exporting it from the liver to be excreted into bile
- Leads to toxic accumulation of copper in the liver and brain (particularly the basal ganglia) and other tissues

- Also called hepatolenticular degeneration
- **Ultimately leads to chronic liver injury, although can present like an acute liver injury.**

Pathogenesis/aetiology

Causes

- Autosomal recessive genetic disease
- Defect in copper transporting ATPase (ATP7B)

- On chromosome 13: wil3on.

Pathogenesis

- In Wilson's disease there is altered incorporation of copper into caeruloplasmin (main copper carrying protein) and impaired excretion of copper into the bile
- The excess build up of copper in hepatocytes leads to:
  - free radical formation
  - oxidation of lipids and proteins

- This leads to hepatocyte damage
- As hepatic copper builds up it is eventually released into the circulation thereby affecting other organs.

179

Who

- Rare
- High in areas of consanguinity (e.g. India).

A typical patient

A 19-year-old girl presents with tremors and altered mental state. There is a history of liver disease in the family. Her GP notes that LFTs are abnormal.

Clinical features

In children (10–13 years):
- Manifests as chronic liver disease/cirrhosis

In young adults:
- Manifests as neuropsychiatric disorder:

In general:
- Can present with a picture of ALF often with associated 'Coombs' test negative' haemolytic anaemia. The only form of ALF that allows the patient to be cirrhotic

Symptoms and signs:
- Liver disease: symptoms of ALF or cirrhosis and portal hypertension

- Neuropsychiatric: affective symptoms, e.g. labile and depressed; cognitive
- Neurological: tremor very common
- Ophthalmologic: Kayser–Fleischer rings on iris from copper deposition in Descemet's membrane of the eye seen on slit-lamp as green/brown pigment at corneal edge
- Musculo-skeletal: osteoarthritis, osteopenia
- Renal: symptoms of renal failure from renal tubular damage similar to Fanconi syndrome.

Investigations

Blood tests

- ↑ serum copper
- ↓ caeruloplasmin

- Very ↓ ALP unlike other causes of liver disease. Other LFTs may be elevated or normal.
- Haemolytic anaemia (Coombs' test negative).

Urine

- ↑ urinary copper.

Imaging

- US liver: as for all liver disease
- CT liver: as for all liver disease

- CT head: bilateral lesions either small and well defined in basal ganglia or larger lesions including basal ganglia and thalamus
- MRI: basal ganglia degeneration. 'Face of Panda'

Other tests

- Exclude other causes of chronic liver disease
- Molecular genetic testing to confirm diagnosis.

Liver biopsy:
- ↑ copper content

- Steatosis
- Mononuclear cell infiltrates
- Necrosis and fibrosis/cirrhosis (Mallory bodies may be seen)

Treatment

- Avoid high copper foods: liver, chocolate, legumes, shellfish
- Chelating agents that bind to copper and allow it to be excreted: lifelong **penicillamine** (side effect: blood disorders, nausea, rash) and zinc
- Treat as for cirrhosis of any aetiology
- If presenting as ALF: must be transplanted

Screening:
- Screen relatives
- Screen all children presenting with liver disease (as is a treatable cause).

Prognosis and complications

Prognosis

- Pre-cirrhotic liver disease is reversible and treatable with good prognosis
- Cirrhosis and neurological damage are not reversible.

Complications

- Complications of cirrhosis and portal hypertension of any aetiology.

α-1-ANTITRYPSIN (A1-AT) DEFICIENCY

Outline

- Inherited disease leading to lung and liver damage due to deficiency of the protective protease inhibitor: α-1-antitrypsin

- **Ultimately leads to chronic liver injury**

Genetics

- PiMM: normal
- PiMZ/PiSZ: heterozygous for disease (variable type: lower risk of disease)

- PiZZ: homozygous for disease (severe symptoms).

Pathogenesis/aetiology

Causes

- Co-dominant genetic disease

- Gene on chromosome 14.

Pathogenesis

- A1-AT, produced in the liver, is a protease inhibitor (proteases such as elastase destroy tissue during inflammation)
- In A1-AT deficiency the A1-AT is altered so that it can not be released from the hepatocytes

- This results in excess A1-AT in the hepatocytes where it builds up and causes damage
- It also leads to insufficient amounts in the lungs where proteases can cause alveolar destruction over time without protection from A1 to AT. This leads to early-onset emphysema (by 40 years).

Who

- Rare

In children:
- Commonest genetic cause of liver disease (lung disease occurs later after ~30 years)

In adults:
- Causes emphysema (in 75%) with early onset in smokers
- Also causes chronic liver disease and HCC in patients in their 40s.

Clinical features

Liver disease:
- Symptoms and complications of cirrhosis and portal hypertension

- Can present as neonatal jaundice or cholestatic jaundice in infancy

Lung disease:
- Symptoms of emphysema: mainly SOB in adults.

Investigations

Blood tests

- ↓ Serum A1-AT levels
- Genetic phenotyping

- Exclude other causes of chronic liver disease.

Imaging

CXR:
- As for other chronic liver disease

Other tests

Liver biopsy:
- Abnormal enzyme unable to leave hepatocytes shows as pink cytoplasmic globules on periodic acid–Schiff stain. Confirm using immunohistochemistry.

Lung tests:
- Pulmonary function tests

Treatment

- No specific treatment
- Management of emphysema and complications of liver disease

- Stop smoking
- A1-AT supplementation (expensive treatment).

Surgical

- Liver transplantation for patients with end-stage liver cirrhosis.

Prognosis and complications

Prognosis

- Emphysema is main cause of death.

Complications

- Complications of cirrhosis and portal hypertension of any cause
- Respiratory failure.

HAEMOCHROMATOSIS

Outline

- Inherited disease causing abnormal excessive iron absorption from the small intestine
- Leads to iron deposits in multiple organs causing damage and can lead to organ failure
- Affects: the liver, pancreas, skin, joints, pituitary, heart, gonads
- Also called bronze diabetes (due to skin pigmentation and diabetes)
- **Ultimately leads to chronic liver injury**

Secondary haemochromatosis

- Excess iron from too many transfusions. Occurs in those with diseases like thalassaemia or sickle cell.

Pathogenesis/aetiology

Causes

- Autosomal recessive
- Mutations of the HFE gene on chromosome 6: commonest mutations are C282Y and H63D
- Women are protected by menstruation and pregnancy and therefore tend to present later.

Who

- Typical age: middle age
- ♀:5–10♂
- Prevalance: ~0.05–0.5%

Associations:
- North Europeans
- HLA-A3, HLA-B7, HLA-B14
- Alcohol excess significantly worsens disease.

A typical patient

A middle-aged Irish man with family history of liver problems presents with fatigue, arthritis, new-onset diabetes and abnormal LFTs.

Clinical features

- Asymptomatic until iron overload

Liver:
- Cirrhosis, leading to symptoms and complications of cirrhosis and portal hypertension including hepatomegaly and HCC

Skin:
- Bronze/pigmented skin: from iron deposition and melanin

Pancreas:
- Diabetes

Heart:
- Cardiomyopathy and conduction problems

Brain:
- Hypogonadism (loss of libido) from pituitary disease (direct damage to gonads can also occur but is rarer)

Joints:
- Arthritis: from calcium pyrophosphate deposition in joints

Gonads:
- Hypogonadism, impotence.

Investigations

Blood tests

- Exclude other causes of chronic liver disease
- Blood glucose: for diabetes
- ↓ hepcidin (liver hormone involved in iron homeostasis)

Iron studies:
- ↑ serum iron, ↑ ferritin >500, ↑ transferrin saturation
- ↓ total iron-binding capacity

Imaging

- US liver: as for all liver disease
- Echo and ECG
- X-rays: for joints

Investigations

Other tests

Liver biopsy:
- Perls' potassium cyanide stain goes Prussian blue in presence of haemosiderin (an iron storage complex)

- May be features of cirrhosis or fibrosis.

Genetics:
- Phenotyping.

Treatment

- Treatable
- Venesection (remove blood): 1 unit removed weekly for 6–12 months until iron deficient. Continue for life with 2–3 units removed per year
- Chelating agents: desferrioxamine (binds iron), if significant anaemia or severe end organ involvement

- Diet: low iron, limit vitamin C (increases iron absorption), stop alcohol

End-stage disease:
- Liver transplantation

Prevention:
- Screen relatives.

Prognosis and complications

Prognosis

- Survival depends on complications
- Venesection gives excellent prognosis if treated early
- Cirrhosis, gonadal failure: non-reversible

- Cirrhosis is commonest cause of death in haemochromatosis.

Complications

- As for cirrhosis and portal hypertension of any aetiology

- HCC (iron deposition causes genetic defects), so monitor for this.

VENO-OCCLUSIVE LIVER DISEASE

BUDD–CHIARI SYNDROME/HEPATIC VEIN THROMBOSIS

Outline

- Occlusion of hepatic vein by thrombosis
- Prevents outflow of blood from the liver
- Build up of blood leads to a congested liver causing hepatocyte damage and ischaemia and ALF

- Can present acutely or chronically
- **Can cause acute and/or chronic liver injury.**

Pathogenesis/aetiology

Causes

Haematological disorders:
- Polycythaemia, thrombocythaemia (↑ platelets)

Hypercoagulable states:
- Pregnancy, malignancy, chronic inflammatory states
- Congenital causes: protein C and protein S deficiency, factor V Leiden deficiency, anti-phospholipid syndrome

Drugs:
- Oral contraceptive pill

Unknown:
- In 30%.

Who

- Typical age: usually 20–40 years old

- Rare.

A typical patient

A 30-year-old lady on the pill, previously well, presents with abdominal pain, jaundice and ascites.

Clinical features

Acutely:
- Right upper quadrant pain
- Hepatomegaly
- Ascites

- Nausea/vomiting
- Jaundice

Chronically:
- Signs of chronic liver failure.

Investigations

Blood tests

- Exclude other causes of chronic liver disease
- Pro-thrombotic screen: (protein C, protein S, factor V Leiden, anti-phospholipid antibodies)
- JAK-2: mutation implicated in myeloproliferative disorders

Imaging

- US liver with Doppler: no flow in hepatic vein. Signs of portal hypertension
- CT: enlarged caudate lobe, no flow in hepatic vein

Other tests

Liver biopsy:
- Not usually required:
  - Venous congestion and thrombi.

Ascitic tap:
- ↑ protein in ascitic fluid.

Treatment

Medical

- Anticoagulation
- Thrombolysis (acute) although not shown benefit
- Diuretics for ascites

Radiological:
- Angioplasty (acute)
- TIPS (see portal hypertension).

Surgical

- Shunting
- Liver transplantation.

Prognosis and complications

Prognosis

- Mortality over 5 years in chronic form: 50%.

Complications

- Complications of cirrhosis and portal hypertension of any cause
- Related to hyper-coaguable state.

VIRAL HEPATITIS

HEPATITIS A VIRUS

Outline

- **Causes an acute liver injury which is usually self-limiting**
- Single stranded RNA virus
- Enterovirus
- Incubation: 2–6 weeks
- No risk of chronic infection
- Epidemics: associated with overcrowding and poor sanitation as it thrives in areas of poor hygiene
- A 'Notifiable disease'; in the UK.

Pathogenesis/aetiology

Transmission

- Enteric entry: faeco–oral
- From contaminated water or shellfish
- Most infectious before onset of jaundice

Pathogenesis

- 1° multiplication in gut
- Then multiplies in liver hepatocytes.

Who

- Young people most affected
- Occurs world wide

Risk factors:
- Travellers
- Childcare workers.

A typical patient

A young lady returning from India has felt unwell for a week. Her urine went dark and she became jaundiced 4 days later.

Clinical features

- Varies from subclinical to fulminant hepatitis.

Symptoms

- Like gastroenteritis: nausea/vomiting, diarrhoea
- Malaise/fatigue: can last months
- Anorexia

- Headache
- Upper abdominal pain.

Signs

- Jaundice: after 10–14 days, resolves after 14–21 days. May last 3–4 months
- Hepatomegaly
- Splenomegaly: 10%

- Lymphadenopathy
- Rash.

Investigations

Blood and stool tests

- FBC: leucopenia
- ↑ ESR
- ↑ AST, ALT: usually >1000
- ↑ bilirubin
- Exclude other causes of acute liver injury

Diagnosis:
- Detect anti-HAV specific IgM
- Anti-HAV IgG suggests previous infection (immunity) or vaccination

Culture:
- Virus in faeces for 2 weeks before onset of jaundice and a few days after.

Imaging

- US liver: to exclude other pathology.

Treatment

- Mostly conservative with complete resolution
- Supportive

Prophylaxis:
- Immunisation for at-risk patients: leads to lifelong immunity.

Prognosis and complications

Prognosis

- 0.1% mortality
- Most resolve over weeks with no complications

- Can relapse
- <0.1% progress to acute liver failure.

Complications

- Myocarditis
- Arthritis

- Vasculitis
- May trigger autoimmune hepatitis.

HEPATITIS B VIRUS

Outline

Leads to acute and/or chronic liver injury:

- Infection is dynamic and changes over time therefore needs lifelong monitoring
- DNA virus
- Hepadnavirus
- Has an outer envelope and lipid core with associated antigens (see below)
- Incubation: 2–6 months
- Begins as acute infection but can progress to chronic infection in 10% of adults and 90% of infants

HBV antigens

- The surface antigens associated with the viral envelope and core are important in understanding infectivity and serology (Fig. 5.9).

These antigens and resulting antibodies change over the course of an infection and are indicative of the stage (Fig. 5.10):

- *HBV surface antigen (HBsAg)*: the outer lipoprotein envelope
- *HBV core antigen (HBcAg)*: the internal core, which surrounds the viral DNA genome
- *HBV e antigen (HBeAg)*: in the past used as a marker of circulating virus and infectivity

Life cycle of the virus:

- The virus replicates in the hepatocytes
- Uses a reverse transcriptase (like HIV)
- Core antigen incorporated into host genome.

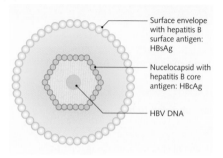

Fig. 5.9 HBV virus and surface antigens.

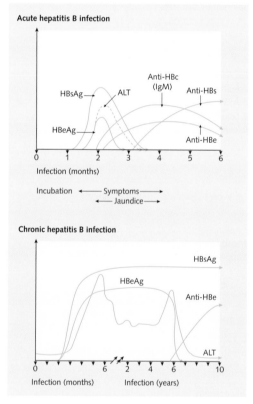

Fig. 5.10 Changes in HBV antigens and antibodies over the disease course.

Pathogenesis/aetiology

Transmission:
- Mother to child peri-natal: commonest cause worldwide
- IV route: contaminated needles or blood products, e.g. IVDU
- Sexual intercourse

Pathology:
- Phases of acute HBV:
  1. Prodrome with unchecked viral replication
  2. Body recognises infection and kills infected liver cells. ↑ ALT/AST, may become jaundiced
  3. If immune competent: virus clears
  4. If not: leads to chronic HBV
- Chronic HBV: terminology:
  - Recently changed. Terms like 'low risk carrier' phased out. Instead reference HBeAg:
  - HBeAg + ve chronic HBV OR HBeAg − ve chronic HBV
- Infectivity is dependent upon viral load
- Viral load is usually higher in HBeAg + ve patients, but can be high in HBeAg − ve patients

- Phases of chronic HBV:
  - There are three ways in which HBV and the body react together:
    1. Immune-tolerant: HBV replicates unchecked and the body acts as if it is unaware of the virus with no immune response, so no liver damage occurs. HBeAg + ve with very high viral load ($>10^8$). Previously called 'high infectivity'
    2. Immune-active: body recognises the virus but mounts an inappropriate immune response so there are fluctuating levels of virus, infectivity and liver inflammation. Can lead to fibrosis, cirrhosis and HCC. HBeAg + ve **or** − ve. Viral load usually high
    3. Immune-control: body recognises the virus and controls it, so there are low levels of virus (<1000), low infectivity and little liver damage. HBeAg –ve. Used to be called 'low risk carrier' or 'inactive'. Low risk for complications

Who

- 350 000 000 chronic carriers world wide
- Prevalent: Africa, Middle and Far East

Risk factors:
- Homosexual men
- Blood recipients
- Injecting drugs

- Health care workers
- Those in high prevalence countries
- Family history
- Piercings or tattoos performed in non-reputable establishments.

A typical patient

Young oriental lady having first child, HBsAg detected on screening bloods.

Young homosexual man discovered to be positive after sexual health check up.

Clinical features

Acute infection:
- In children:
  - Often subclinical
- In adults:
  - Prodrome
  - Malaise/fatigue
  - Anorexia
  - Abdominal discomfort
  - Arthritis/arthralgia

  - Rash
  - Jaundice
  - 0.1% will progress to ALF
Chronic infection:
- Asymptomatic
- Symptoms and complications of cirrhosis and portal hypertension
- Can present with HCC.

Investigations

Blood tests

- ↑ LFTs: AST, ALT high in acute infection (>1000), may be normal or slightly raised in chronic infection
- Viral load (HBV DNA)
- Exclude liver disease of any other cause
- Consider HIV test

Serology:
- Antigens/antibodies are used for diagnostic purposes (Fig. 5.10)

HBsAg:
- Active infection, if present >6 months after acute infection this signifies chronic infection

Anti-HBs (antibody to surface antigen):

- Signifies life long immunity from past infection or vaccination

Anti-HBc (antibody to core antigen) IgM:
- Found in recent acute infection

Anti-HBc IgG:
- Has been infected with HBV virus (and may still be)

HBeAg: pre-core:
- All infections start off with HBeAg detectable

Anti-HBe antibody (Ab):
- In chronic HBV, development of anti-HBeAb leads to clearance of HBeAg called eAb seroconversion.

Investigations

Other tests

Liver biopsy:
• Used to assess degree of inflammation and fibrosis to decide on the phase of disease and so guide treatment.

Treatment

Acute:
• Supportive
• Anti-viral drugs may have a role in ALF
• May require emergency transplant in ALF

Chronic:
• Aim to ↓ inflammation and development of chronic liver disease/HCC
• Minimise aggravators of liver disease (e.g. alcohol).

Medical

Interferon-alpha (pegylated):
• Previously eAg+ve but now can be tried in eAg −ve as well
• To precipitate seroconversion
• PEGylation 'hides' the interferon from the immune system

• Side effect: depression, bone marrow suppression
Nucleos(t)ide analogues:
• Tenofovir or entecavir (previously lamivudine and adefovir)
• Inhibit HBV replication

Surgical

• Transplantation for end-stage cirrhosis or HCC

• Must give HBV Immunoglobulin (HBiG) to prevent recurrence in graft

Prophylaxis

• Immunisation for high risk groups/family members
• Care with handling blood
• Screen donated blood

• Barrier contraception
• Screen health workers.

Prognosis and complications

Prognosis

Acute infection:
• Mortality <1%
• Acute liver failure occurs in 0.1% (mortality of 80% without transplantation)
• Can reactivate if becomes immunosuppressed (e.g. chemotherapy)

Chronic infection:
• Needs lifelong monitoring
• 40% of chronic HBV will go on to develop cirrhosis or HCC
• Likelihood of HCC is increased in HBV even without cirrhosis. Need to screen for HCC.

Complications

• Complications of cirrhosis and portal hypertension
• Can also get: polyarteritis nodosa (vasculitis), glomerulonephritis, cryoglobulinaemia

• Complication: pregnancy with HBV mother:
  • Low risk: (low maternal HBV DNA) immunise newborn child immediately after birth (active vaccination)
  • High risk: (high maternal HBV DNA) give HBiG to child (passive vaccination) as well as active vaccination. Consider giving anti-viral medication in 3rd trimester to ↓ viral load.

HEPATITIS C VIRUS

Outline

• **Leads to acute hepatitis; ultimately progresses to chronic liver injury**
• No current vaccination
• RNA virus
• Flavivirus like
• Incubation period: 2–3 months
• 80% progress to chronic infection
• Alcohol consumption aggravates damage

Genotypes:
• 6 genotypes, genetically diverse (three main ones):
  • Genotype 1: most common particularly in IVDUs, 40–50% of cases
  • Genotype 2 and 3: 40–50%
  • Genotype 4: common in Egypt (vaccination programme for schistosomiasis, a parasite, thought to have spread HCV from contaminated needles) prevalence 22%.

Pathogenesis/aetiology

Transmission:
- Parenteral
- Blood: IVDUs, blood products
- Mother to child
- High risk sexual activity
- Unknown transmission: 20%.

Who

- 170 000 000 cases world wide
- Common: Egypt, S Europe, Africa
- UK 0.01–0.02%

Risk factors:
- Renal dialysis patients
- Haemophiliacs
- Drug users
- Tattoos, piercings
- Family history.

A typical patient

An Egyptian/ex-IVDU presented to her GP with non-specific symptoms. Blood tests showed abnormal LFTs, GP sent HCV antibodies which were positive.

Clinical features

Acute infection:
- Mostly subclinical
- Mild: lethargy, malaise and anorexia
- Jaundice uncommon, 10%

Chronic infection:
- Non-specific: fatigue, malaise
- Complications of cirrhosis, pulmonary hypertension.

Investigations

Blood tests and virology

- Exclude other causes of chronic liver disease
- FBC: need to assess Hb and Plt for treatment
- LFTs: ↑ ALT, AST
- INR
- α-fetoprotein: often mildly ↑
- Consider HIV test

Virology:
- HCV antibody: screening test for HCV, will be positive even if virus has cleared
- HCV RNA: positive in active infection
- HCV genotype.

Imaging

- US/CT liver: as for other causes of chronic liver disease
- Transient elastography: non-invasive testing liver stiffness. Gives estimation of degree of fibrosis.

Other tests

Liver biopsy:
- Shows extent of fibrosis/cirrhosis.

Treatment

Lifestyle:
- ↓ alcohol

Medical

The way HCV is treated is a rapidly changing field. Previously treatment was based upon pegylated interferon alpha and ribavirin but many newer directly acting antiviral agents are, or about to, be licensed. These newer agents have superior cure rates for all genotypes of HCV and in the future pegylated interferon may not be needed.
- Interferon-alpha (usually pegylated) side effects: bone marrow suppression, depression
- Ribavirin (antiviral) side effect: bone marrow suppression

- Treat for 24–48 months
- Monitor treatment with reverse transcriptase-PCR for viral load:
  - Newer agents include: protease inhibitors (currently licensed 1st generation: telaprevir and boceprevir), NS5A inhibitors, polymerase inhibitors. The length of treatment and combination of agents are currently being researched.

Surgical

- Liver transplantation

Prognosis and complications

Prognosis

- Genotype 1 and 4: 30–50% cure rate
- Genotype 2 and 3: 70–80% cure rate
- The above rates are for standard treatment with pegylated interferon and ribavirin. Trials with newer agents are showing >90% cure rates for nearly all genotypes and new data will emerge as the best combinations to use
- 20% of chronic HCV patients will develop cirrhosis over 20 years
- After transplant HCV has high incidence of recurrence.

Complications

- Complications of cirrhosis and portal hypertension of any aetiology

Extrahepatic manifestations (rare):
- Glomerulonephritis
- Cryoglobulinaemia
- Lichen planus
- Aplastic anaemia.

HEPATITIS D VIRUS (DELTA VIRUS)

Outline

- **Leads to acute and/or chronic hepatitis**
- **A virus that cannot replicate alone, being dependent on HBV**
- RNA (delta) virus
- High risk of chronic infection.

Pathogenesis/aetiology

- Parenteral
- Sexual less efficient than HBV
- Vertical transmission form mother to child is rare

Patterns of infection:
- Co-infection: primary HDV infections occur simultaneously with HBV
- Superinfection: primary HDV infection in pre-existing chronic HBV.

Who

- S Italy, N Africa, Middle East

A typical patient

- As for HBV but with IVDU transmission.

Risk factors:
- IVDU.

Clinical features

Symptoms and signs

Acute coinfection:
- In adults indistinguishable from hepatitis B infection
- ALF occurs in 1%
- Chronic coinfection 5%

Superinfection:
- 90% asymptomatic
- Flare of AST/ALT can occur.

Investigations

Investigations:
- As for HBV

Diagnosis:
- Anti-D IgM in acute infection
- Anti-D IgG in chronic infection
- HDV RNA to demonstrate active infection.

Treatment

- Pegylated interferon alpha
- Supportive
- Treat underlying hepatitis B.

Prognosis and complications

Prognosis

- Faster progression to fibrosis and cirrhosis than with hepatitis B alone.

Complications

- Faster progression to liver decompensation than hepatitis B alone. Possibly higher rate of hepatocellular carcinoma.

HEPATITIS E VIRUS

Outline

- **Leads to acute hepatitis**
- Usually self-limiting disease resembling HAV

- Resembles HAV
- Single stranded RNA
- Calicivirus

Pathogenesis/aetiology

- As for HAV

- Spread by faeco–oral route.

Who

- As for HAV

- Endemic in Russia, Indian sub-continent and Africa.

Clinical features

- As for HAV

- Worse clinical course in pregnancy.

Investigations

- As for HAV

Diagnosis:
- Anti-HEV IgM in acute
- Anti-HEV IgG if previous exposure.

Treatment

- As for HAV

- Vaccine being developed.

Prognosis and complications

Prognosis

- 4% overall fatality rate

- 20% mortality in pregnant women.

Complications

- As for HAV.

LIVER LESIONS

HEPATOCELLULAR CARCINOMA

Outline

- Primary tumour of the hepatocytes
- 90% of primary liver tumours

- 60–80% express α-fetoprotein, which can be used to screen for the disease
- For general tumours see recap pages p. 153.

Pathogenesis/aetiology

Causes

- 90% occur on background of cirrhosis from any cause

- Particularly associated with HBV (even without cirrhosis), HCV and haemochromatosis.

Who

- Becoming increasingly common with increased incidence of cirrhosis, and chronic viral hepatitis

- Common in Asia and Africa (high rates of HBV and HCV)

A typical patient

An oriental patient with HBV infection and chronic liver disease that has never been treated presents with new-onset weight loss, jaundice and ascites.

Clinical features

Symptoms

- Weight loss/anorexia
- Right upper quadrant pain
- Malaise.

Signs

Signs of liver disease:
- Ascites
- Jaundice
- Hepatomegaly.

Investigations

Blood tests

- FBC
- Clotting
- LFTs: also ↑ ALP with bone metastases
- Serum α-fetoprotein (for screening)
- Iron studies: to identify haemochromatosis as a cause
- Viral hepatitis screen: link with HBV and HCV.

Imaging

The diagnosis of HCC can be made purely on characteristic radiological findings in a patient with cirrhosis
- US: first line to detect lesion (used for screening)
- CT: characteristic arterialisation, tumour thrombus in the vessels, distant spread. Also important for staging
- MRI: characteristic contrast uptake and 'wash out'

Other tests

Liver biopsy:
- If diagnostic uncertainty. Classically not performed as worry of seeding tumour along the biopsy tract. Newer techniques burn the tract on removal to try to prevent this

Screening:
- Routine screening of cirrhotic patients means patients diagnosed earlier.

Treatment

Chemotherapy (not curative):
- Systemic chemotherapy for liver metastases
- Sorafenib: a new anti-angiogenic and pro-apoptotic agent for advanced HCC

Loco-regional therapy:
- Radiofrequency ablation: conducting needle placed in tumour and current applied
- Transarterial chemoembolisation: tumour identified angiographically and chemotherapy infused through the feeding artery
- Percutaneous ethanol injection.

Surgical

- Resection: possible in <30%
- Depends on degree of cirrhosis and tumour size
- Transplantation: Milan criteria: up to 3 tumours of ≤3 cm or 1 tumour ≤5 cm. Newer criteria being developed. Potentially curative.

Prognosis and complications

Prognosis

- Even if not transplantable, loco-regional therapy able to prolong life
- Resection increases 5 year survival to 40%, but in 60% it recurs
- If within criteria, transplant increases 5 year survival to 75%.

Complications

- Metastases
- Tumours can rupture, causing intraperitoneal haemorrhage.

CHOLANGIOCARCINOMA

Outline

- Malignant tumour of the bile ducts
- Adenocarcinoma
- 10% of primary liver cancers.

Pathogenesis/aetiology

Causes

- Link with primary sclerosing cholangitis: 15–30% lifetime risk

- Chronic infections: flukes (Far East), ascaris.

Pathogenesis

- Can be intra- or extrahepatic.

Who

- Typical age: 60–70 years
- ♀ > ♂
- Highest incidence: Israel and Japan

Associations:
- IBD: link with primary sclerosing cholangitis.

Clinical features

Symptoms

- Jaundice
- Pruritus
- Weight loss
- Abdominal pain (late)

- Extrahepatic tumours: painless obstructive jaundice
- Intrahepatic tumours: present more like primary liver tumours as they invade the liver parenchyma.

Signs

- Palpable gall bladder if distal to cystic duct

- Hepatomegaly (25%).

Investigations

Blood tests

- LFTs: ↑ bilirubin, ↑ ALP
- Tumour markers: non specific but CA19–9 and carcinoembryonic antigen may be raised

Endoscopy

- Endoscopic US: allows visualisation and fine needle aspiration for cytology
- ERCP: allows visualisation and brushing for cytology. Also stenting to relieve obstruction (Fig. 5.11).

Imaging

- US: identify duct dilatation and large tumours
- CT: demonstrate tumour plus any local or distant spread (e.g. lymph nodes)
- MRI/MRCP (angiography): good for vascular invasion and preoperative planning.

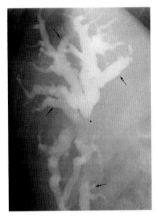

Fig. 5.11 Features of cholangiocarcinoma including dilated intrahepatic biliary tree (barred arrows) and filling defects within the biliary tree (*).

Treatment

- Mostly unresectable: can do radical hepatectomy and bile duct excision which is curative, but rarely possible
- Aggressive recurrence in liver transplantation, may benefit a very selected group of patients

Palliative:
- Stenting can give symptomatic relief

- Radiotherapy or chemotherapy alone are unhelpful. Together they can aid with local control but not affect mortality
- Photodynamic therapy is being trialled (IV administration of photosensitiser, then activate by light illumination).

Prognosis and complications

Prognosis

- 2–8 months if treated palliatively
- About 1 year survival if can tolerate chemoradiation/photodynamic therapy

- If resected, many recur.

Complications

- Cholangitis
- Metastatic complications

- Side effects of treatments.

LIVER ABSCESS

Outline

- Abscess: pus collection in a cavity formed by the tissue as a defence against internal infection.

Pathogenesis/aetiology

Causes

- Pyogenic (80%): *Escherichia coli* and *Klebsiella pneumoniae* commonest pathogens
- Amoebic (10%): *Entamoeba histolytica* that later spreads to the liver via the portovenous system
- Fungal (10%): usually *Candida*

- Biliary tract disease: 60%, due to obstruction such as stones, tumour stricture
- Abdominal infection: 24%, e.g. diverticulitis spread to the liver via the portovenous system
- May be unknown.

Who

- Amoebic in tropics.

A typical patient

A 65-year-old lady with a history of diverticular disease presents with right upper quadrant pain, fevers of unknown origin and weight loss. US shows a lesion in the liver.

Clinical features

- Diarrhoea
- Malaise
- Fever
- Anorexia

- Right upper quadrant pain
- Jaundice
- Hepatomegaly
- Reactive right pleural effusion.

Investigations

Blood tests

- Liver biochemistry
- Blood cultures and stool cultures

- Amoeba serology.

Imaging

- CXR: for pleural effusion
- Liver US: hypoechoic mass with irregularly shaped borders. May show internal septations or cavity debris
- CT: lesions are well-demarcated areas hypodense to surrounding hepatic parenchyma. Peripheral

enhancement is seen when IV contrast is administered. Gas can be seen in 20% of lesions
- Primary site of infection may be seen

Invasive:
- CT or US guided aspiration for culture

Treatment

- Aspirate abscess under US or CT
- Pyogenic: broad spectrum antibiotics

- Amoebic: metronidazole for 2 weeks
- Surgical drainage if large or resistant.

Prognosis and complications

Prognosis

- Multiple abscesses: poorer prognosis

- Good for amoebic cause.

Complications

- Cystic rupture.

GALL BLADDER DISEASE

GALLSTONES

Outline

- Crystalline hard masses formed in the gall bladder made of bile pigments, cholesterol and calcium salts

- Leads to cholelithiasis (gallstones in the gallbladder), choledocholithiasis (gallstone passes into the bile ducts) and cholecystitis (inflammation of the gall bladder)

Classification of gallstones

- Cholesterol gallstones (10%):
  - Large, usually only one with smooth yellow surface
  - Formed mainly from cholesterol
  - Associated with obesity and high oestrogen states
  - Rarely radiopaque: only if enough calcium
- Pigment stones (rare):
  - Many small, irregular stones

- Black, facetted surfaces
- Made of bilirubin polymers such as calcium bilirubinate
- Found in patients with cirrhosis or chronic haemolysis where bilirubin production is ↑ from blood breakdown
- 50–75% radiopaque
- *Mixed (70–80%).*

Pathogenesis/aetiology

Causes

- Infection in gall bladder can precipitate mixed stones

- Incidence increased by the oral contraceptive pill, pregnancy, diuretics, multiparity, rapid weight loss, possibly smoking.

Pathogenesis

- Bile is composed of bile pigments, cholesterol and phospholipid. The concentration variation affects the stone formed
- The gall bladder is shrunken in gallstone disease and often enlarged in pathologies causing obstruction of the biliary tree over a shorter period of time, e.g. pancreatic malignancy

Courvoisier's law:
- If a patient presents with painless, obstructive jaundice and a palpable gallbladder, the cause is not gallstones (suggests cancer).

Who

- Typical age: ↑ with age
- 2♀:1♂
- 20% of population

- More in the Western world
- Rare in Far East and Africa.

A typical patient

40-year-old Caucasian lady who is overweight, presenting with right upper quadrant pain after eating, particularly fatty foods:
- Female, fair, fat, forty, fertile.

Clinical features

- Mostly asymptomatic: 80%
- Symptoms caused by complications of gallstones
- Obstructive jaundice: from choledocholithiasis
- Nausea/vomit
- Positive Murphy's sign from cholestasis (see below)

- Biliary colic:
  - Episodes of continuous acute pain in the right upper quadrant that radiate to the costal margins and back
  - Precipitated by fatty meals when gall bladder contracts
  - Pain leaves patient writhing, sweaty, pale and tachycardic
  - Caused by obstruction of the gall bladder or common bile duct normally by a stone.

Investigations

Blood tests

- May be entirely normal
- FBC: ↑ WBC in cholecystitis

- LFTs:↑ bilirubin, GGT and ALP if obstruction.

Imaging

- X-ray: only 10% of gallstones are radiopaque
- US: shows stones and thickened wall, if there is common bile duct dilatation, an ERCP is needed
- MRCP: non-invasive, better visualisation of biliary tree, used when diagnostic uncertainty

- ERCP: can visualise biliary tree as well as perform interventions e.g. remove stone
- Percutaneous transhepatic cholangiography: if there is a dilated biliary tree and ERCP cannot be performed
- Radioisotope scan: for gallbladder function.

Treatment

- Small stone can pass spontaneously

- Asymptomatic stones found incidentally can be left and treated conservatively.

Medical

- Analgesia for biliary colic: morphine
- Antiemetics
- Antibiotics for cholecystitis

- Urso-deoxycholic acid can help dissolve cholesterol stones

Lithotripsy and endoscopic techniques

- Procedure to break up small stones so that they can be small enough to pass. Not effective, mainly used in inoperable patients

- ERCP.

Surgical

- Laparoscopic cholecystectomy for complications or symptomatic stones

- Open cholecystectomy if felt that laparoscopic will be technically difficult.

Prognosis and complications

Prognosis

- Very good.

Complications

- Cholecystitis
- Cholangitis
- Gallstone illeus
- Empyema of gallbladder
- Mucocoele

- Carcinoma of gall bladder: from chronic inflammation
- Perforation
- Fistulae
- Pancreatitis, if stone obstructs pancreatic duct, even temporarily.

ACUTE CHOLECYSTITIS

Outline

- Inflammation of the gall bladder
- Almost always from gallstones: calculous cholecystitis

- Can be mild and transient or a medical emergency.

Classification

Calculous cholecystitis 90%:
- Impaction of stone leads to bile stasis
- This raises the intralumenal pressure and produces gall bladder distension reducing blood flow to mucosa and compromising defences

Acalculous cholecystitis 10%:
- Mainly from ischaemic mucosal damage.

Pathogenesis/aetiology

Causes

Calculous:
- Gallstones

Acalculous:
- Infection: typhoid, brucellosis
- Complications of parenteral nutrition
- Polyarteritis nodosa (form of vasculitis)
- Abnormality of cystic duct

- After major surgery
- Trauma
- Burns
- Organ failure
- Sepsis
- Postpartum.

Pathogenesis

- Balance between mucosal defences and effects of bile salts is lost
- Mucosa exposed to detergent action of bile salts, so get inflammatory response

- Bacterial infection probably a secondary event (33%): more likely to get complications.

Who

- As for gallstone disease

- Occurs at any age.

A typical patient

A patient becomes feverish and unwell, with right upper quadrant pain. She has previously been told she had gallstones.

Clinical features

Symptoms

- Biliary colic-like pain with addition that:
    - it is referred to the right shoulder
    - it is associated with fever
    - it is worse on inspiration
    - it causes the patient to lie still and take shallow breaths

- it is different from biliary colic as includes an inflammatory component
- it is associated with nausea/vomiting
- it is associated with indigestion
- it is associated with bloating, burping.

Signs

- Tachycardia
- ↑ respiratory rate
- Jaundice uncommon: suggest obstruction
- Mass in the right upper quadrant: not usually gall bladder but inflamed omentum with pus and bowel around the gallbladder

Murphy's sign:
- Two fingers placed on right upper quadrant as patient breathes in. Pain worse on inspiration as inflamed gallbladder moves below the costal margin, but not when the test is repeated on the left
- Typically, +ve in cholecystitis, but −ve in choledocholithiasis and ascending cholangitis.

Investigations

Blood tests

- FBC: ↑ WBC
- U&Es
- LFTs

- Amylase
- ↑ CRP and ESR
- Blood culture.

Imaging

- AXR shows only 10% gallstones
- US: to confirm. Demonstrates thickening and oedema of gall bladder wall, shrinking of gall bladder and stones if present

- Hepatobiliary iminodiacetic acid scan: this nuclear medicine scan can occasionally be used. A radioisotope is taken up by liver to bile, if the duct is patent, the gall bladder will fill excluding cholecystitis.

Treatment

- Initially managed conservatively
- Nil by mouth
- IV fluid

- Broad spectrum antibiotics with aerobic and anaerobic cover: cefotaxime and metronidazole
- Analgesia
- 80–90% will settle over 36 h

Surgical

- Cholecysectomy if significant or complications as relapse occurs in 20% and can lead to additional complications. Best within 72 h, if not, wait 6–12 weeks.

Prognosis and complications

Prognosis

- Untreated: spontaneous resolution in 1–10 days but recurrence is common

- 25% worsen requiring surgery.

Complications

- Sepsis
- Cholangitis

- Peritonitis: from infarction of gall bladder or perforation
- Empyema of gall bladder.

CHRONIC CHOLECYSTITIS

Outline

- Chronic inflammation of the gall bladder
- Stones cause chronic inflammation and colic

- In chronic gallstone disease the stones induce a fibrotic reaction that shrinks the gall bladder. This is relevant for Courvoisier's law (see above)
- Wall is thickened, opaque and stiff.

Pathogenesis/aetiology

Causes

- From recurrent acute attacks

- 90% associated with gallstones.

Who

- As for gallstone disease.

Clinical features

- Often asymptomatic
- Abdominal discomfort
- Fatty food intolerance
- Bloating

- Nausea
- Flatulence
- Chronic right hypochondrial pain.

Investigations

Imaging

- US: shows stones and thickened wall, if there is common bile duct dilatation then perform ERCP
- MRCP: non-invasive, better visualisation of biliary tree, used when diagnostic uncertainty

- ERCP: can visualise biliary tree as well as perform interventions, e.g. remove stone, take brushings for cytology.

Treatment

- Cholecystectomy

- If stone in common bile duct, remove that first by ERCP.

Prognosis and complications

Prognosis

- Good.

Complications

- Cholangitis
- Sepsis
- Perforation
- Abscess formation
- Peritonitis

- Cholecystenteric fistulae with ↑ risk of gallstone ileus
- Bacterial infection
- Bile drainage to adjacent organs
- Can precipitate decompensation in patients with pre-existing renal, hepatic, cardiac, pulmonary disease.

CHOLANGITIS

Outline

- Infection in the biliary tract
- Leads to sepsis
- Treat as an emergency as if left untreated it can have a high mortality

- Rare unless associated with obstruction or retained foreign body (e.g. stent).

Pathogenesis/aetiology

Causes

- Ascending infection: normally bacterial, *Escherichia coli* and *Klebsiella* are the commonest offenders

Precipitated by:
- Iatrogenic, e.g. ERCP
- Obstruction, e.g. neoplasm, patients with biliary strictures (e.g. primary sclerosing cholangitis, gallstones).

Who

- Typical age: 50–60

Risk factors:
- Occurs in those with gallstones

A typical patient

A patient with primary sclerosing cholangitis had a stent placed a few years ago and didn't see the doctor again. Now has new-onset jaundice and feels very unwell.

Clinical features

Charcot's triad (in only 25%):
- Pain (right upper quadrant)
- Rigors/fever
- Jaundice

Features of sepsis:
- ↑ respiratory rate
- ↑ temperature
- ↑ heart rate
- May have signs of septic shock
- ↓ BP
- Altered cognitive state.

Investigations

Blood tests

- Septic screen: ↑ WBC

- Bloods: as for acute cholecystitis.

Treatment

- Treat as an emergency: ABC approach (see Chapter 1)
- Resuscitate with fluid
- IV antibiotics: cefuroxime and metronidazole
- Analgesia

- Relieve obstruction depending on cause: ERCP involving decompression of common bile duct with urgent drainage, stone removal or stenting as necessary.

Prognosis

- Prompt diagnosis and treatment or high mortality.

Complications

- Septic shock
- Multi-organ failure.

GALLSTONE ILEUS

Outline

- Obstruction of the bowel from a gallstone that has eroded the gall bladder and reached the duodenum
- Can obstruct the terminal ileum.
  NB: ileus is a misnomer: ileus is normally the absence of peristalsis. Gall bladder ileus is small bowel obstruction.

Pathogenesis/aetiology

Pathogenesis

- Over a long period a large gallstone can erode through the gall bladder wall to the duodenum which is situated next to the gall bladder
- Once in the duodenum, the stone moves down the intestine by peristalsis and may impact.

Who

- Rare.

Clinical features

- Present with features of small bowel obstruction.

Investigations

Imaging

X-ray:
- A gallstone may be visible
- Air within the biliary tree
- Evidence of small bowel obstruction.

Treatment

Surgical

- Remove through enterotomy: incision in small bowel.

Prognosis and complications

Complications

- As for small bowel obstruction.

GALL BLADDER CANCER

Outline

- Cancer of the gall bladder
- Mostly adenocarcinomas.

Pathogenesis/aetiology

Associations:
- Chronic gallstones
- Anatomical defects: choledochal cysts (congenital bile duct dilatation) or abnormal pancreaticobiliary duct junctions
- Gall bladder polyps (if >1 cm remove gall bladder).

Who

- Typical age: elderly

Rare:

- <1% of all adenocarcinomas

- Found incidentally in 0.5–1% of cholecystectomies.

Clinical features

- Advanced at time of presentation
- Malaise
- Weight loss

- Jaundice
- Right upper quartile mass.

Investigations

Blood tests

- CA19–9 (non-specific, raised in other cancers, e.g. pancreatic cancer)

- LFTs.

Imaging

- US: first line, mass seen in gall bladder, may see hepatic metastases
- CT: as for US

- MRI: assess extension into surrounding tissues, preop planning

Treatment

- Chemotherapy and radiotherapy little value.

Surgical

- Operate if high suspicion.

Prognosis and complications

Prognosis

- Poor, as present late
- Most live ~1 year

- 5 year survival <5%.

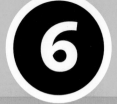
The brain

The brain is organised into four main lobes: frontal, parietal, temporal, occipital. The areas of the brain are labelled in Figure 6.1.

Blood supply to the brain is from the internal carotid and vertebral arteries. These arteries feed into the circle of Willis (Fig. 6.2).

Loss of function to an area of the brain will lead to specific symptoms depending on the location (Fig. 6.3).

The spinal cord

The spinal cord consists of ascending and descending tracts connecting the peripheral nervous system with the brain (Fig. 6.4):

Corticospinal tracts:
- Descending
- Contain motor fibres
- Originate in the cerebral cortex and cross the midline in the medulla above the spinal cord
- The tracts synapse in the anterior horn with the peripheral nervous system; spinal lesions, therefore, cause ipsilateral upper motor neuron (UMN) signs

Spinothalamic tracts:
- Ascending
- Contain sensory fibres carrying pain and temperature information
- Fibres cross the midline almost as soon as they enter the spinal cord; therefore, spinal lesions cause contralateral loss of pain and temperature

Dorsal columns:
- Ascending
- Contain sensory fibres carrying vibration and proprioception information
- Fibres synapse in the brainstem after crossing the midline; therefore, spinal lesions cause ipsilateral loss of vibration and proprioception sense.

Aspects of the spinal cord:
- *Conus medullaris*: the end of the spinal cord, around the level of L1/L2
- *Cauda equina*: the collection of nerve roots coming down from the conus medullaris like a horse's tail (thus the name in Latin)

The motor system

Damage to the motor system causing limb weakness can be caused by damage at any level: including damage to the brain, spinal cord, nerve root, nerve plexus and the peripheral motor nerves. Damage can be divided into upper motor neuron (UMN) or lower motor neuron (LMN) lesions (Table 6.1):

- *UMN lesions*: damage anywhere between the brain and the synapse with the anterior horn cells in the spinal cord
- *LMN lesions*: damage anywhere from the anterior horn cells in the spinal cord to the peripheral nerves.

Table 6.1 Presentation of upper and lower motor neuron defects

	UMN	LMN
Reflexes (Babinski sign)	Hyper-reflexia (upgoing plantars)	Hyporeflexia (down going plantars)
Paralysis	spastic	Flaccid
Tone	↑ (spasticity)	↓
Clonus	yes	No
Fasciculations	no	Yes
Power	Weakness	Weakness
Wasting	No	Yes
Gait	Spastic/scissor	Variable

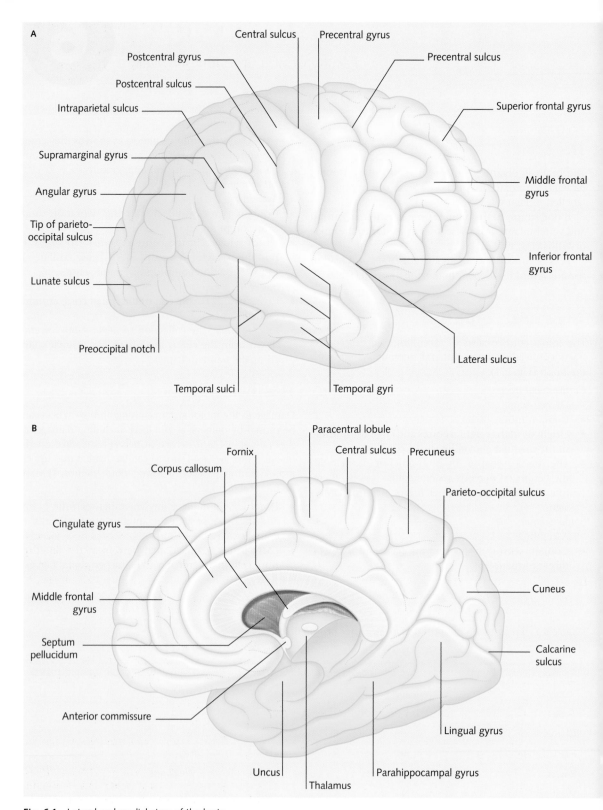

A

Central sulcus

Precentral gyrus

Postcentral gyrus

Precentral sulcus

Postcentral sulcus

Intraparietal sulcus

Superior frontal gyrus

Supramarginal gyrus

Middle frontal gyrus

Angular gyrus

Tip of parieto-occipital sulcus

Inferior frontal gyrus

Lunate sulcus

Preoccipital notch

Lateral sulcus

Temporal sulci

Temporal gyri

B

Paracentral lobule

Fornix

Central sulcus

Precuneus

Corpus callosum

Parieto-occipital sulcus

Cingulate gyrus

Middle frontal gyrus

Cuneus

Septum pellucidum

Calcarine sulcus

Anterior commissure

Lingual gyrus

Uncus

Parahippocampal gyrus

Thalamus

Fig. 6.1 Lateral and medial view of the brain.

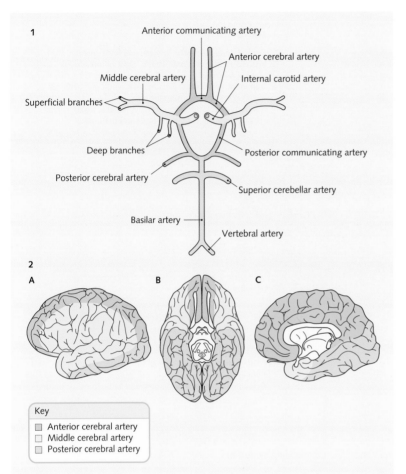

Fig. 6.2 Blood supply to the brain and the territories of the major arteries. (1) Main cerebral arteries forming the circle of Willis. (2) Artery territories in lateral (A) inferior (B) and medial (C) views.

Innervation

Myotome: muscle or group of muscles innervated by a single spinal nerve

Dermatome: area of skin innervated by a single spinal nerve; damage to that nerve will result in loss of sensation in that dermatomal distribution (Fig. 6.5).

Vision and the eyes

The type of visual loss depends on the location of the damage along the visual field pathway (Fig. 6.6).

For the homonymous quadrantanopias remember the order PITS: **p**arietal lobe – **i**nferior homonymous quadrantanopia, **t**emporal lobe – **s**uperior homonymous quadrantanopia.

Innervation of the muscles of the eye

This can be remembered by $(LR_6SO_4)_3$:

- The oculomotor nerve (3rd cranial nerve) supplies all the eye muscles apart from:

- superior oblique (SO) is innervated by the trochlear nerve (4th cranial nerve); remembered by SO_4
- lateral rectus (LR) is innervated by the abducens nerve (6th cranial nerve); remembered by LR_6.

Horner's syndrome: a disruption of the sympathetic nerve supply to the eye that leads to a clinical picture of MAPS:

miosis: constricted pupil
anhydrosis: reduced sweating of the ipsilateral forehead
ptosis (drooping eyelid): partial, can be overcome by voluntary up gaze
sunken eye (enophthalmos).

Caused by damage at a number of levels:

- Central lesions, e.g. multiple sclerosis, brainstem stroke
- Preganglionic fibre damage to the sympathetic chain, e.g. masses (cervical lymph nodes, tumour including Pancoast's tumour, aneurysm, thyroid mass), trauma
- Postganglionic fibre damage, e.g. carotid aneurysm, cavernous sinus disease.

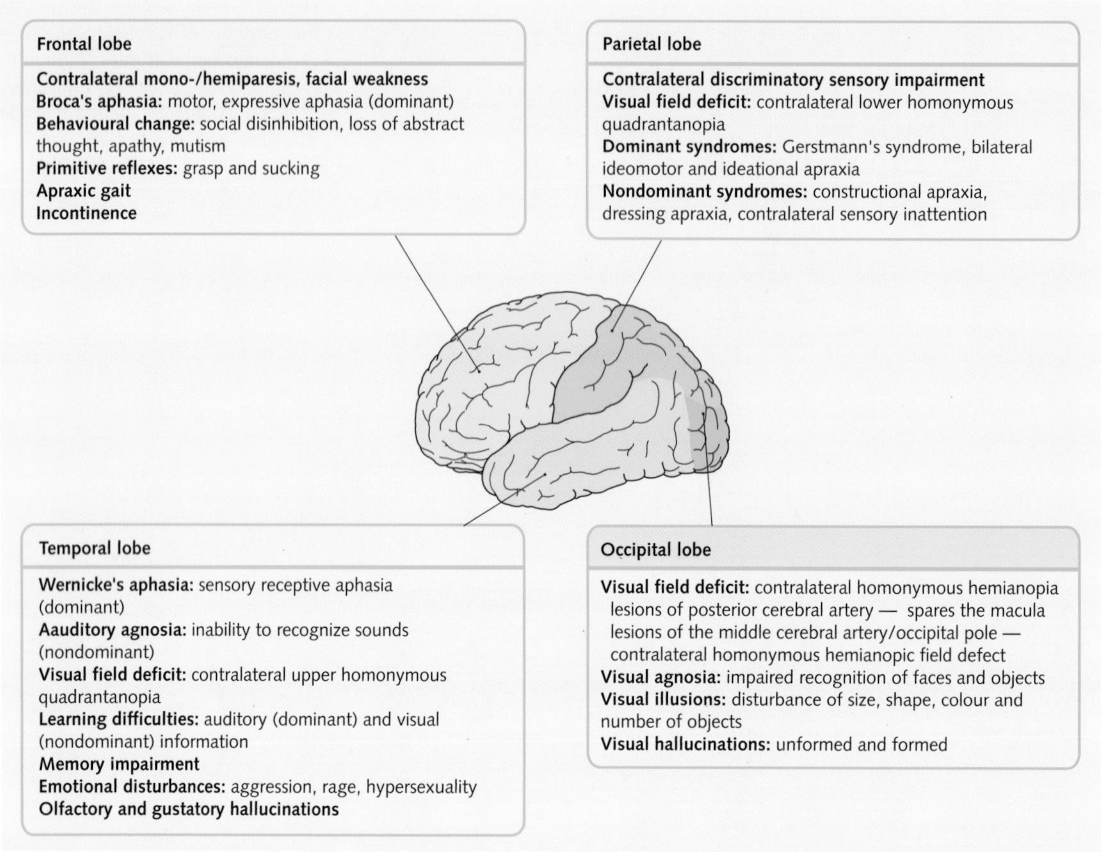

Frontal lobe
Contralateral mono-/hemiparesis, facial weakness
Broca's aphasia: motor, expressive aphasia (dominant)
Behavioural change: social disinhibition, loss of abstract thought, apathy, mutism
Primitive reflexes: grasp and sucking
Apraxic gait
Incontinence
Parietal lobe
Contralateral discriminatory sensory impairment
Visual field deficit: contralateral lower homonymous quadrantanopia
Dominant syndromes: Gerstmann's syndrome, bilateral ideomotor and ideational apraxia
Nondominant syndromes: constructional apraxia, dressing apraxia, contralateral sensory inattention
Temporal lobe
Wernicke's aphasia: sensory receptive aphasia (dominant)
Aauditory agnosia: inability to recognize sounds (nondominant)
Visual field deficit: contralateral upper homonymous quadrantanopia
Learning difficulties: auditory (dominant) and visual (nondominant) information
Memory impairment
Emotional disturbances: aggression, rage, hypersexuality
Olfactory and gustatory hallucinations
Occipital lobe
Visual field deficit: contralateral homonymous hemianopia
lesions of posterior cerebral artery — spares the macula
lesions of the middle cerebral artery/occipital pole — contralateral homonymous hemianopic field defect
Visual agnosia: impaired recognition of faces and objects
Visual illusions: disturbance of size, shape, colour and number of objects
Visual hallucinations: unformed and formed

Fig. 6.3 Damage to a focal area of the brain and the corresponding symptoms.

Posterior
Fasciculus gracilis
Fasciculus cuneatus
Dorsal or posterior column (proprioception and vibration)
Posterior horn
Corticospinal (motor)
White matter
Spinocerebellar tract
Grey matter
Anterior horn
Spinothalamic tract (pain and temperature)
Anterior

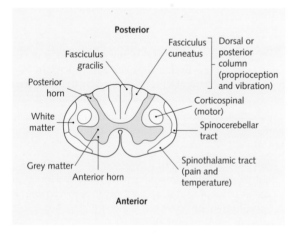

Fig. 6.4 Cross-section of the spinal cord showing the principal spinal tracts.

Drug-induced dyskinesias

Antipsychotic drugs can cause a range of dyskinesias (abnormal movements):

- Acute dystonic reaction:
  - Acute dystonia (sustained involuntary muscular contractions leading to repetitive or abnormal postures) within hours of neuroleptic drug, particularly metoclopramide
  - Spasm of mouth and jaw, may affect eyes and limbs
  - Treatment: benztropine, procyclidine
- Akathisia:
  - Inner sense of restlessness
  - Patients move about endlessly
  - Often caused by drugs for parkinsonism and by antipsychotics
  - Treatment: may improve on drug withdrawal
- Tardive dyskinesia:
  - Abnormal mouth and tongue movements months or years after antipsychotic drug treatment
  - Difficult to treat
  - Withdrawing drug may help, may worsen
  - Tetrabenazine may help
- Neuroleptic malignant syndrome:
  - Potentially fatal reaction to neuroleptic therapy
  - Characterised by high fever, rigidity, autonomic disturbances, fluctuating consciousness
  - Treatment: drug withdrawal, bromocriptine and/or dantrolene.

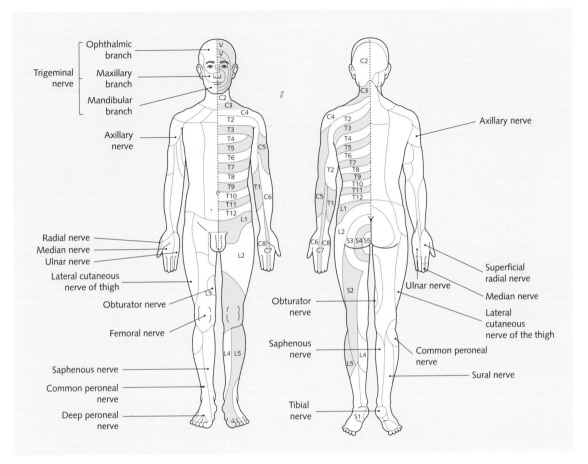

Fig. 6.5 The dermatomes.

Investigations

Abbreviated Mental Test Score

A screening questionnaire to assess for confusion (<7/10). One mark is given per question:

1. What is your age?
2. What year where you born?
3. What is the time (to nearest hour)?
4. What year is it?
5. Do you know where we are?
6. Can you identify two people either by name or job, e.g. doctor or nurse
7. Ask the patient to remember an address and later ask them to recall it, e.g. 42 West Street
8. Who is the current monarch?
9. What year did World War 2 start?
10. Can you count backwards from 20 to 1?

Blood tests

- CRP or ESR: ↑ in infection and inflammation
- Other specific tests for infections or inflammation

Electroencephalography (EEG)

Records the brain's electrical activity using electrodes taped to the scalp; used particularly in the investigation of epilepsy. Also used in intensive care setting to investigate and prognosticate in context of coma. Important patterns on EEG:

- Spike and wave: suggests epilepsy (may be normal between seizures)
- Periodic complexes: Creutzfeldt–Jakob disease (CJD), Alzheimer's disease
- Slowing of background rhythm: encephalopathy

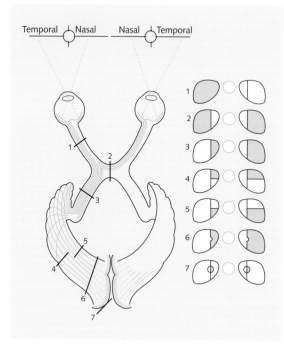

Lesion	Effect on vision
1. Optic nerve lesion	Monocular loss
2. Chiasmal lesion	Bitemporal hemianopia
3. Optic tract lesion	Homonymous hemianopia
4. Temporal lesion	Superior homonymous quadrantanopia
5. Parietal lesion	Inferior homonymous quadrantanopia
6. Optic radiation or cortex	Homonymous quadrantanopia (macular sparing)
7. Occipital pole lesion	Homonymous hemianopia

Fig. 6.6 Visual loss and the corresponding damage to the visual pathway.

Visual evoked responses

Measures the response of the optic nerve to stimulation of the eye:

- Used in the diagnosis of multiple sclerosis.

Electromyography

Records the electrical activity of muscle using electrodes inserted into the muscle:

- Used to investigate myopathies including myositis and muscular dystrophies.

Nerve conduction studies

Measures velocity and amplitude of electrical activity in nerves following direct stimulation:

- Used to investigate radiculopathies and peripheral neuropathies including carpal tunnel syndrome and radiculopathies.

Lumbar puncture

Investigates cerebrospinal fluid (CSF) with a number of diagnostic tests:

- Opening pressure (normal 10–20 cmH$_2$O): raised in idiopathic (or benign) intracranial hypertension
- Microbiology: microscopy, cell count and culture
- Virology: potential viral meningitis
- Biochemistry: glucose (compare with blood levels), protein
- Xanthochromia: yellow colouration of CSF is seen in subarachnoid haemorrhage
- Oligoclonal bands: bands of immunoglobulins increased in multiple sclerosis.

Can also be used therapeutically to remove CSF in idiopathic intracranial hypertension and normal pressure hydrocephalus.

CT

X-rays used to generate a 3D view of the brain:

- Useful for early diagnosis of haemorrhage and mass effect.

MRI

Uses magnetic field and pulses of radiowave energy so involves no ionising radiation, a potential problem with CT:

- Provides more detailed images of brain than CT
- Useful for investigating strokes, tumours and multiple sclerosis.

See also

- Endocrinology (Ch. 9): pituitary adenomas.
- Common presenting complaints (Ch. 14): headache, confusion, vertigo and dizziness, blackouts, coma, gait disorders, loss of vision.
- Clinical examinations (Ch. 15): peripheral motor and sensory neurological examination.

CEREBROVASCULAR DISEASE

STROKE: GENERAL FEATURES

Outline

General features:
- Sudden-onset focal neurological deficit due to a vascular lesion

- May be an ischaemic stroke or an intracerebral haemorrhage (see each below)
- Symptoms are usually 'negative' (loss of function).

Pathogenesis/aetiology

- Vascular lesion may include infarction, haemorrhage or embolism

- Causes are different depending on type.

Who

- ♀ < ♂
- Commonest neurological problem in the UK

- 2nd commonest cause of death in the developed world.

Clinical features

- Sudden onset
- Symptoms maximal at onset
- Loss of function
- Focal symptoms: dependent on site

Symptoms consistent with a stroke:
- Motor: unilateral weakness (face, arm or leg)
- Sensory loss: unilateral

- Aphasia (language disorder due to brain damage)
- Visuospatial neglect
- Visual symptoms: hemi- or quadrantanopia
- Other symptoms: diplopia, ataxia, vertigo, dysarthria, dysphagia
- Symptoms and signs are usually contralateral to the lesion unless cerebellar in origin or from cranial nerve lesions.

Investigations

Bloods tests

- FBC
- U&E

- fasting glucose
- fasting lipids

Imaging

- Imaging of brain:
  - Needed urgently particularly if thrombolysis is considered. Differentiates between ischaemic and haemorrhagic stroke
  - **CT**
  - **MRI** in some cases.

- Imaging of vessels:
  - Carotid Doppler US
  - CT angiogram of brain and neck vessels.

Other tests

- Cardiac investigations:
  - ECG

- Echocardiogram in some cases

Treatment

- Treatment particular to ischaemia or haemorrhage

General management:
- Admission to dedicated stroke unit: multidisciplinary input and rehabilitation

- Assess swallow: consider feeding via nasogastric tube
- Investigate and treat cause
- Hypertension: correct 2 weeks after event unless over 185 systolic (it often is!).

Prognosis and complications

Complications

Short term:
- Stroke recurrence
- Confusion
- Seizures (5%)
- Aspiration pneumonia
- Urinary tract infections
- Pressure sores

- Hyponatraemia
- DVT
- Pulmonary embolism

Long term:
- Dementia (30%)
- Depression (50%).

ISCHAEMIC STROKE

Outline

- Loss of blood supply to an area of brain
- 80% of strokes are ischaemic

- See also 'Stroke: general features'

Pathogenesis/aetiology

Causes

Cardiovascular causes:
- Large vessel atherosclerosis (50%):
- AF
- Mitral stenosis
- Prosthetic heart valves
- Bacterial endocarditis
- MI

- Haematological causes:
  - Sickle cell disease
  - Polycythaemia
  - Thrombophilias
  - Thombocythaemia
- Rarer causes:
  - Vasculitis: lupus, polyarteritis nodosa
  - Drug abuse
  - Infections: syphilis, HIV.

Who

Risks factors:
- Modifiable:
  - AF
  - Hypertension
  - ↑ Cholesterol
  - Smoking
  - Diabetes mellitus

- Oestrogens: oral contraceptive pill, hormone replacement therapy
  - Excess alcohol
- Non-modifiable:
  - ↑ Age
  - ♂
  - Family history
  - Heart disease.

A typical patient

A 65-year-old smoker presents to A&E with right sided arm weakness and aphasia which started 2 h ago.

Clinical features

- As for 'Stroke: general features'.

Investigations

- As for 'Stroke: general features'.

Treatment

- General management: As for 'Stroke: general features'
- Aspirin: 300 mg for 2 weeks, then 75 mg clopidogrel daily (scan first)
- Thrombolysis with IV tissue plasminogen activator (t-PA): give at dedicated centres within 3 h of onset.

- Contraindications to thrombolysis:
  - Head trauma <3 months
  - GI bleeding <3 weeks
  - Major surgery <15 days
  - Systolic BP >185 mmHg – treat BP, then can have thrombolysis
  - INR >1.5: reverse first
  - Recent stroke

Surgical management

- Carotid endarterectomy: if stenosis >70% on symptomatic side

- For hydrocephalus or brain swelling

Prevention before or after an event has occurred

To prevent stroke:
- Control modifiable risk factors
- Anticoagulation: for those with AF and prosthetic heart valves.

To prevent further episodes once a first stroke has occured:
- Manage risk factors:
  - Stop smoking
    - BP: ACE inhibitor, diuretics. Target <140/90

  - Diabetic control
  - Hyperlipidaemia: statins
  - Stop oestrogens
- Antithrombotic treatment:
  - 75 mg clopidogrel, as above
  - warfarin for AF (start 2 weeks after stroke)

Prognosis and complications

Prognosis

- One month mortality: 25%
- Full recovery in 40%: improvement greatest in first 6 months
- 10% risk of recurrence in 1 year

Poor prognostic factors:
- ↑ age
- Large area affected
- Loss of consciousness
- Severe motor impairment
- Persistent urinary incontinence
- Persistent neglect.

Complications

- As for 'Stroke: general features'
- Large infarcts: swelling and ↑ intracranial pressure (ICP)
- Haemorrhagic transformation of ischaemic area
- Obstructive hydrocephalus and brainstem compression: can be due to malignant middle cerebral artery

syndrome (cerebral swelling due to infarct, often young patients).

INTRACEREBRAL HAEMORRHAGE

Outline

- Stroke caused by bleeding directly into brain tissue
- 20% of strokes are caused by intracerebral bleeds.

- See also 'Stroke: general features'

Pathogenesis/aetiology

Causes

- Hypertension
- Amyloid angiopathy
- Rupture of an intracranial microaneurysm
- Vascular malformations, e.g. arteriovenous malformation
- Aneurysm

- Illicit drug abuse: cocaine
- Brain tumours
- Bleeding disorders, e.g. warfarin, congenital coagulation disorder
- Trauma.

Who

Risk factors:
- Hypertension

- Alcohol excess.

Clinical features

- Similar presentation to ischaemic stroke
- Headache
- Vomiting

- Loss of consciousness
- Seizures: more common
- May show progressive focal deficit.

Investigations

- As for 'Stroke: general features'

Treatment

- Not for thrombolysis
- If due to over-anticoagulation: reverse warfarin

General management:
- As for 'Stroke: general features'.

Prognosis and complications

Prognosis

- One month mortality: ∼30%
Poor prognostic factors:
- Large haemorrhage
- ↓ Glasgow Coma Scale
- ↑ age

- Hydrocephalus
- Intraventricular bleeding.

TRANSIENT ISCHAEMIC ATTACK

Outline

- Focal neurological deficit due to a vascular lesion that lasts less than 24 h
- Usually only lasts a few minutes

- Complete neurological recovery
- ↑ risk of further TIA or stroke within 1 month, therefore urgent treatment and follow-up.

Pathogenesis/aetiology

Causes

- As for ischaemic stroke.

Who

- Incidence: 0.05% per year

Risk factors:
- As for stroke.

A typical patient

65-year-old man presents to his GP one day after developing right-sided weakness and disturbed speech for 15 min. His symptoms have completely resolved and he wants to drive home.

Clinical features

- Sudden onset
- Symptoms maximal at onset
- Loss of function
- Focal symptoms – depends on the site of the lesion:
Carotid territory:
- Amaurosis fugax: painless fleeting loss of vision to one eye
- Contralateral weakness/numbness
- Dysphasia (language disorder, e.g. in speech or comprehension)
- Hemianopia (loss of half of visual field in one or both eyes) usually affects both eyes

Vertebrobasilar territory:
- Ataxia (↓ coordination)
- Vertigo
- Diplopia (double vision)
- Dysphagia (unable to swallow)
- Dysarthria (motor speech disorder)
- Bilateral visual loss
- Hemianopia
- Contralateral limb weakness
- Ipsilateral cranial nerve palsy.

Investigations

Blood tests

- FBC
- U&E

- Fasting glucose
- Fasting lipids including cholesterol

Imaging

Imaging of brain:
- MRI
- CT

Imaging of vessels:
- Carotid Doppler US
- CT Angiogram

Other tests

Cardiac investigations:
- ECG
- Echocardiogram in some cases.

Treatment

- Urgent referral to stroke clinic: seen within 1 week, 24 h if high risk

Risk factor modification:
- Smoking cessation
- ↓ salt and alcohol intake
- Control BP
- Screen for diabetes and hypercholesterolaemia

Drug treatment:
- Aspirin 300 mg immediately and continue for 2 weeks; then clopidogrel 75 mg daily for life
- Consider warfarin if in AF (only after imaging)
- Simvastatin

Other interventions:
- Consider carotid endarterectomy (surgical procedure to remove the clot) if >70% stenosis
- Avoid driving for 1 month after TIA or stroke.

Prognosis and complications

Prognosis

- Risk of stroke after TIA is highest in first month: 15% risk at 30 days

ABCD2 Prognostic score predicts the risk of early stroke following a TIA. High risk if score ≥4:
- **A**ge ≥60: 1 point
- **B**P ≥140/90: 1 point
- **C**linical features: unilateral weakness: 2 points or change in speech: 1 point
- **D**uration ≥60 min 2 points, 10–59 min 1 point
- **D**iabetes: 1 point.

SUBARACHNOID HAEMORRHAGE

Outline

- Bleeding into the subarachnoid space of the brain
- Often catastrophic
- Can be multiple (15%).

Pathogenesis/aetiology

Causes

- Rupture of saccular (berry) aneurysm (80%): found in junctions of the cerebral arteries. Associated with:
  - polycystic kidneys
  - coarctation of the aorta
- arteriovenous malformations (5%)
- trauma
- coagulopathies.

Who

- Typical age: mean age onset 50 years
- Incidence 0.015% per year

Risk factors:
- +ve family history
- Smoking (3–10× ↑ risk)
- Bleeding disorders
- Hypertension.

A typical patient

A 50-year-old woman attends the emergency department describing a sudden-onset severe headache, typically occipital.

Clinical features

- Sudden onset
- May be on exertion
- Mild: patient conscious but drowsy
- Severe: unconscious or dead.

Symptoms

SAH:
- **S**ick: vomiting after headache
- **A**bsent: loss of consciousness or coma
- **H**eadache 'like being hit on the head'. Usually occipital, the pain may radiate to the neck and legs
- Headaches preceding the current event (sentinel bleed).

Signs

- Meningism (symptoms due to irritation of the meninges by blood): neck stiffness, photophobia, Kernig's sign (pain on passive knee extension with hips flexed)
- 3rd (cranial) nerve palsy: suggests aneurysm of the internal carotid or posterior communicating artery
- Hemiparesis and aphasia: suggests aneurysm of the middle cerebral artery
- Fundoscopy reveals subhyaloid venous haemorrhages.

Investigations

Imaging

- CT brain: detects 90% if within 24 h of event

Other tests

- Lumbar puncture: >12 h after event if clinically appropriate and no evidence of raised intracranial pressure. Typical findings:
  - Uniform blood staining
- Xanthochromia: straw/yellow CSF due to haemolysed RBCs. Present from 12 h to several days after subarachnoid haemorrhage
- ECG: non-specific ST changes may be seen.

Treatment

- Neurosurgical referral
- Bed rest
- Hydration: IV fluids to avoid vasospasm.

Medical

- Control severe hypertension
- Nimodipine to prevent cerebral vasospasm (calcium channel blocker acting preferentially on cerebral arteries)
- Analgesia

Interventional

- Early intervention to prevent further haemorrhage
- Surgical: opening the skull and clipping of vessels
- Endovascular: angiography with endovascular coils which reduce the aneurysm by forming blood clots within them.

Prognosis and complications

Prognosis

- 50% mortality before reaching hospital
- Of those surviving there is a high incidence of rebleed
- Rebleed rate highest in first 2 weeks
- 30% die within 3 months
- 30% of survivors are dependent on carers.

Complications

- Hydrocephalus
- Seizures
- SIADH
- Intracerebral haematoma
- Arrhythmias.

ACUTE SUBDURAL HAEMATOMA

Outline

- Bleeding in the subdural space between the dura and arachnoid layers
- Rupture of a vein running from cortex to sagittal sinus.

Pathogenesis/aetiology

Causes

- Usually from head injury
- Two forms:
  - Severe brain injury causing parenchymal laceration: patients present in coma, no lucid interval
- Tearing of bridging veins across extradural space: 1° brain damage less severe, may have a lucid interval
- 50% associated with skull fracture.

Who

- Typical age: may occur at any age

Risk factors:
- Anticoagulant therapy.

Clinical features

- Loss of consciousness
- May have a lucid interval followed by rapid deterioration depending on mode of injury.

Investigations

Imaging

- CT/MRI demonstrates clot and/or midline shift (Fig. 6.7).

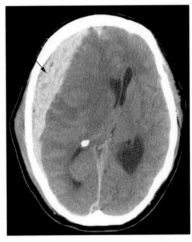

Fig. 6.7   CT showing a subdural haemorrhage (arrowed).

Treatment

- Surgical evacuation via burr holes (small holes made in the skull) or craniotomy.

Prognosis and complications

Prognosis

- 50% mortality
- Poor prognosis if severe injury and delay in diagnosis.

CHRONIC SUBDURAL HAEMATOMA

Outline

- Collection of blood in the subdural space hours or weeks after a brain injury.

Pathogenesis/aetiology

- Head injury
- Injury often mild, may not be remembered by some patients
- Elderly are at ↑ risk from cerebral atrophy tightening the veins making them vulnerable to sheering forces.

Who

- ♀ < ♂

Risk factors:
- Anticoagulation therapy
- Patients who fall: epilepsy, alcohol abuse.

Clinical features

- May have an insidious onset
- May be difficult to diagnose
- Confusion
- Drowsiness
- Headache
- Personality change
- Fluctuating levels of consciousness
- Focal neurological signs, e.g. hemiparesis.

Investigations

Imaging

- CT: subdural haematoma may be difficult to find, particularly if bilateral.

- May resolve spontaneously, monitor with CT

Surgical referral:
- To consider evacuation via burr holes or craniotomy.

- Better prognosis if diagnosed and treated early.

EXTRADURAL (EPIDURAL) HAEMATOMA

- Bleeding into the extradural space
- The extradural space lies between the skull and dura mater

- Usually due to bleeding from the middle meningeal artery or its branches as a result of head injury.

- May arise after mild head injury

- Skull fracture in 90%.

- Extremes of age suffer greater complications.

Head injury followed by:
- Brief unconsciousness with lucid recovery, then further deterioration in consciousness

- Headache
- Focal symptoms and signs
- Do not wait for focal signs or changes in consciousness.

- CT: lens-shaped/convex haematoma (Fig. 6.8).

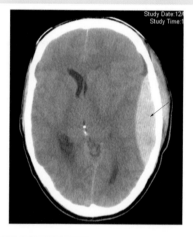

Fig. 6.8 CT showing typical convex appearance of an extradural haemorrhage (arrowed).

- Stabilise
- Urgent neurosurgical referral

- Clot evacuation via burr holes.

- Good prognosis if diagnosed and treated early

- 10% mortality.

DEMENTIA

GENERAL FEATURES

Outline

- Progressive disturbance of multiple higher cortical functions including memory, orientation and language without loss of consciousness

- Usually associated with a decline in social behaviour
- A symptom not a diagnosis.

Pathogenesis/aetiology

Causes

Neurodegenerative
- Alzheimer's (60%)
- Vascular dementia (20%)
- Dementia with Lewy bodies (15%)
- Frontotemporal dementia
- Progressive supranuclear palsy
- Corticobasal degeneration

Toxic
- Alcohol-related

Nutrition
- Thiamine, vitamin B_{12} deficiency

Metabolic
- Thyroid disease
- Renal disease

Prion disease
- CJD

Infective disorders
- HIV dementia
- Neurosyphilis

Inflammatory causes
- Multiple sclerosis

Structural
- Normal pressure hydrocephalus
- Frontal lobe tumour

Who

- Prevalence ↑ with age:
  - 10% of >65 years

- 20% of >80 years
- Rare below 55 years

Clinical features

- Affects higher cortical functions:
  - Memory
  - Orientation
  - Word finding difficulty
  - Personality
  - Judgement
  - Ability to cope with routine

Other symptoms
- Depression (note that depression in the elderly may mimic dementia)
- Paranoia
- Self neglect

Independent history from relatives is essential

Investigations

- Mini mental state examination

Depending on history, consider:

Blood tests

- FBC, ESR, U&Es, calcium, LFTs, TFTs, folate, vitamin B_{12}.

Urine

- Dipstick.

Imaging

- MRI
- CT

- EEG: if suspecting CJD

Other tests

- Lumbar puncture with CSF sample
- Genetic testing: Huntington's disease, CJD

- Brain biopsy: occasionally indicated, if rapidly progressive or vasculitis suspected.
- Syphilis serology

Treatment

- Treat reversible causes, e.g. hypothyroidism, vitamin B$_{12}$ deficiency
- Treatment is usually supportive:
  - Multidisciplinary team involvement: social services, geriatrician, carers' support
  - Long-term residential care

- Adaptation of the home
- Optimise correctable deficits, e.g. hearing aids, eyesight
- Psychological intervention
- Monitor for and treat depression
- Neuropsychiatric referral if appropriate.

Prognosis and complications

Prognosis

- Dementia is usually permanent and progressive

- Metabolic, nutritional and infectious causes may be reversible and therefore should not be missed.

ALZHEIMER'S DISEASE

Outline

- Dementia characterised by the presence of β-amyloid plaques and neurofibrillary tangles in the brain
- Can only be diagnosed definitively on pathological examination

- Clinically characterised by episodic memory impairment and progressive cognitive decline
- Commonest form of dementia
- May overlap with vascular dementia
- See also 'Dementia: general features'

Pathogenesis/aetiology

Pathology

- Deposition of:
  - β-amyloid plaques between nerve cells
  - neurofibrillary tangles within nerve cells composed of tau protein

- Diffuse cortical and subcortical neuronal loss

Genetics

- ApoE genotype
- Mutated genes:
  - Amyloid β-protein precursor gene (chromosome 21)
  - Presenilin 1 (chromosome 14)
  - Presenilin 2 (chromosome 1)

- Linked with Down syndrome: probably due to excessive β-amyloid due to the extra chromosome 21.

Who

- Typical age: over 70
- Commonest form of dementia

Risks:
- ↑ age
- +ve family history (10%): autosomal dominant
- Genetic predisposition.

A typical patient

75-year-old woman is brought in by her family who have noticed increasing forgetfulness and that she keeps getting lost.

Clinical features

- Insidious onset
- Progressive decline
- Episodic memory impairment (usually first symptom)
Followed by:
- Impairment of:
  - language
  - motor activities
  - executive functioning
  - visual perception and orientation

- daily functioning
- Depression: common
Late stage:
- Complete loss of intellectual function
- Motor disability
- Incontinence
- Seizures
- Return of infantile reflexes.

Investigations

- Mini mental state examination
- Exclusion of reversible causes (see above).

Imaging

- CT or MRI: atrophy of medial temporal lobe structures, enlarged ventricles (may appear normal in early disease).

Treatment

- Supportive intervention for patient and carers
- Home or residential care
- Treat anxiety, depression, insomnia

Drugs:
- Acetylcholinesterase inhibitors: donepezil, rivastigmine, galantamine
- Approved by NICE for mild and moderate Alzheimer's.

Prognosis and complications

Prognosis

- Progressive decline
- Median survival: 8 years from onset.

VASCULAR DEMENTIA

Outline

- Dementia due to ischaemic damage. Usually widespread.
- See also 'Dementia: general features'.

Pathogenesis/aetiology

Causes

- Ischaemic damage, clinical picture depends on location which differs between individuals.

Who

- ♀ < ♂
- 20% of dementia patients

Risks:
- Vascular risk factors (see 'Ischaemic stroke').

Clinical features

- Variable
- Often cortical as well as subcortical changes with generalised slowness of thinking

- Evidence of upper motor neuron involvement on examination, e.g. up-going plantars.

Investigations

- Mini mental state examination
- Exclusion of reversible causes (see above)

- Evidence of arteriopathy: hypertension, stroke, focal neurology.

Treatment

- Management of vascular risk factors:
  - Stop smoking

- BP control
- Diabetes control.

Prognosis and complications

Prognosis

- Progressive decline
- Often overlap with Alzheimer's disease.

DEMENTIA WITH LEWY BODIES

Outline

- Dementia with eosinophilic inclusions (Lewy bodies) in cortical neurons
- Associated with Parkinson's disease
- Classified as dementia with Lewy bodies if develop parkinsonism more than one year after onset of dementia

- Classified as Parkinson's dementia if dementia develops more than one year after onset of Parkinson's.
- See also 'Dementia: general features'.

Pathogenesis

- Lewy bodies are neuronal cytoplasmic inclusions that contain:
  - α synuclein
  - Ubiquitin

- They are found in the substantia nigra, medial temporal lobe and neocortex
- Amyloid plaques (as seen in Alzheimer's disease) are also commonly present.

Who

- 15% of dementia patients.

Clinical features

Progressive cognitive decline particularly in:
- Fluctuating cognition
- Visual hallucinations
- Repeated falls

- Variation in alertness
- REM sleep disorder: usually present
- Parkinsonism.

Investigations

- Mini mental state examination
- Exclusion of reversible causes (see above)

- Diagnosis based on history.

Treatment

- Acetylcholinesterase inhibitors: for agitation and hallucinations.

NB: Drugs such as haloperidol and other antipsychotics cause severe sensitivity reactions and increased mortality and are contra-indicated in dementia with Lewy bodies.

Prognosis and complications

Prognosis

- Progressive decline

Complications

- Death due to complications of immobility, poor nutrition and swallowing difficulties.

FRONTOTEMPORAL DEMENTIA

Outline

- Progressive cognitive decline with associated behavioural disorder and atrophy of frontal and temporal lobes

- Often associated with motor neuron disease.
- See also 'Dementia: general features'.

Pathogenesis/aetiology

Subtypes

1. *Behavioural variant*: impulsive or apathetic, loss of empathy

2. *Language variant*:
   2a. Semantic dementia: fluent speech but empty of content
   2b. Progressive non-fluent aphasia: effortful speech, loss of fluency

Pathology

- Accumulation of tau or TDP43 inclusion bodies.

Who

- Typical age: onset usually before 65

- Family history often present.

Clinical features

- Depends on subtype
- Insidious onset
- Cognitive impairment: mainly loss of language and frontal executive function
- Behavioural problems occur early
- Relative preservation of memory.

Investigations

- Mini mental state examination
- Exclusion of reversible causes (see above)

Imaging

- CT or MRI: focal atrophy of frontal and/or temporal lobes.

Treatment

- Supportive care.

Prognosis and complications

Prognosis

- Progressive decline.

PRION DISEASES

Outline

- Degenerative brain diseases caused by prions
- Prions are infectious proteins that cause abnormal folding of host proteins
- Prions can cause neurodegenerative disease by collecting extracellularly within the CNS to form plaques and lead to 'holes' or 'spongy tissue' within the brain

Types:
- CJD
- Gerstmann–Straussler–Scheinker syndrome.
- See also 'Dementia: general features'.

Pathogenesis/aetiology

Pathogenesis of CJD

- Prions convert PrPc (normal protein) to PrPsc (prion protein)
- PrPsc is protease resistant and causes spongiform changes, gliosis and neuronal loss in the brain. Amyloid plaques seen in some forms

Different forms of CJD:
- *Sporadic*
- *Familial*: autosomal dominant
- *Variant*: from eating contaminated meat
- *Iatrogenic*: transmission by neurosurgical instruments, human cadavers, e.g. corneal grafts and pituitary hormones.

Who

CJD

- Sporadic:
  - Mean age: 65
  - Incidence: 0.0001%
  - 85% of CJD cases
- Familial:
  - Autosomal dominant
- Variant:
  - Mean age: 27
  - 200 deaths in total, many in the UK.

Clinical features

CJD

- MAD:
  - **M**yoclonus (involuntary muscle jerks)
  - **A**taxia (↓ coordination) here due to cerebellar dysfunction
- **D**ementia: rapidly progressive over months
- Behavioural change
- Peripheral paraesthesia.

CJD

- Mini mental state examination
- Exclude reversible causes
- EEG: characteristic periodic complexes
- CSF: for 14-3-3 and S100 proteins

sCJD:
- MRI: cortical ribboning and ↑ signal in caudate and putamen

vCJD:
- MRI: Posterior thalamic change
- Tonsillar biopsy.

CJD

- No proven treatment.

Prognosis of CJD

- Uniformly fatal within approx 1 year.

HUNTINGTON'S DISEASE

- A rare inherited progressive disease characterised by choreiform movements (dance-like, rapid, jerky involuntary movements), behavioural and cognitive changes.

- See also 'Dementia: general features'.

Causes

- Autosomal dominant disease with anticipation (presents earlier in later generations)
- CAG trinucleotide repeat expansion in the Huntingtin gene on chromosome 4

- The larger the number of CAG repeats, the earlier the onset.

Pathogenesis

- Exact pathogenesis unknown
- Accumulation of Huntingtin protein in neuron nuclei

- Atrophy of the striatum: caudate nucleus and putamen.

- Typical age: onset usually between 30 and 50 years
- Younger onset associated with paternal transmission

- Incidence 0.004–0.007%.

Movement disorders:
- Chorea
- Akinesia (impaired muscular movement)
- Rigidity
- Dystonia (involuntary, sustained muscular contractions leading to abnormal postures or repetitive movements)
- Abnormal eye movements

Other changes:
- Personality change followed by dementia
- Psychiatric problems: particularly lack of empathy and insight.

- Genetic testing.

Treatment

- No specific treatment
- Symptomatic treatment:

- Tetrabenazine, reserpine (antipsychotics) for abnormal movements
- Genetic counselling.

Prognosis and complications

Prognosis

- Condition is relentless, with death within 15 years of 1st symptoms

- Poorer prognosis in younger patients.

EPILEPSY

GENERAL FEATURES

Outline

An epileptic seizure is a clinical event caused by the excessive discharge of neurons in the brain:
- Epilepsy is the tendency to have recurrent seizures (only 30–60% of first fits are followed by a second)

- Seizures may result in motor, sensory or behavioural symptoms or changes in consciousness.

Classification

Focal seizures:
- Onset within one hemisphere
- Seizure symptoms are related to location

Focal seizures with retention of awareness:
- Previously simple partial seizures
- No change in consciousness

Focal seizures with loss of awareness:
- Previously called complex partial seizures
- Consciousness impaired

Secondary generalised:
- Starts as focal seizure that spreads to both hemispheres;

Generalised seizures:
- Rapidly engaging bilateral networks, usually with no warning
- Loss of consciousness at onset

- Types include:
  - Tonic clonic
  - Absence
  - Myoclonic: may be part of benign seizure condition or part of progressive myoclonic epilepsies which are rare and severe
  - Atonic (rare)

Status epilepticus
- Seizure or series of seizures lasting more than 30 min without regaining consciousness
- Risk of permanent brain damage and mortality related to duration of status

Juvenile myoclonic epilepsy:
- Syndrome of myoclonic jerks, generalised clonic–tonic seizures and sometimes absence seizures.

Pathogenesis/aetiology

Causes of epilepsy

- Idiopathic (75%)
- Trauma: including birth trauma
- Tumours
- Vascular: stroke, arterial-venous malformations
- Infection: bacterial meningitis
- Alcohol
- Recreational drugs

- Multiple sclerosis
- Metabolic:
  - Hypocalcaemia
  - Hyponatraemia
  - Hypoglycaemia

Elements of a seizure

- *Prodrome*: change in mood or behaviour hours or days before seizure
- *Aura*: technically the onset of the seizure; includes abdominal sensations and feelings of déjà vu

- *Ictal event*: the seizure
- *Postictal*: after the seizure; patient is usually drowsy and confused

Driving and epilepsy

- Patient is responsible for informing the licensing authority (DVLA)

- Must be seizure-free for 1 year or have only experienced sleep seizures for 3 years with DVLA approval.

Neurology

- Typical age: peaks in those <20 and >60 years
- Prevalence: 0.7%.

A typical patient

A 20-year-old man presents to A&E. His friends describe that he fell to the ground, with all his limbs shaking and his eyes rolled back, lasting less than one minute. He is now very sleepy.

Clinical features

Focal seizures:
- Focal seizures with awareness:
  - Sudden onset and cessation
  - Symptoms depend on location:
    - Temporal lobe (60%):
  - Aura: epigastric sensations, olfactory hallucinations, déjà vu, jamais vu (feeling of unfamiliarity)
  - Automatisms: picking at clothes
    - Frontal lobe seizures (30%):
  - Forced head and eye turning
  - Loud cries
  - Bizarre limb movements, e.g. Jacksonian march, starts from thumb and involves hand, legs
  - Todd's paresis: post-ictal transient focal weakness
    - Occipital (rare):
  - Visual hallucinations
- Focal seizures with loss of awareness:
  - Often show 'automatisms'
  - Amnesia postseizure
- 2° generalised:
  - Tonic–clonic convulsions and loss of consciousness

Generalised seizures:
- Tonic clonic:
  - Tonic phase: rigidity, apnoea, tongue biting, cyanosis, falls
  - Clonic phase: violent convulsive movements of all limbs, incontinence
  - Postictal confusion, fatigue, headache, muscle pain
- Absence seizures:
  - Onset in childhood, usually resolve by adulthood
  - Brief loss of consciousness, blank stare, eyes flutter or roll
  - Rapid recovery
  - Often mistaken for day dreaming
  - May have multiple attacks/day
  - Associated with 3/s spike and wave discharges on EEG

Myoclonic seizures:
- Abrupt, brief, involuntary movement
- Immediate recovery
- Consciousness usually preserved

Atonic seizures:
- 'Drop attacks': loss of tone, fall to ground, no convulsions

Status epilepticus:
- Continuous seizure activity.

Investigations

Diagnosis is usually clinical. History should include:
- witness description
- birth trauma
- head injuries

- drug history including alcohol
- for regular attacks: frequency, prodromal symptoms, onset, duration, accompanying features

Consider other causes of collapse.

Blood tests

- FBC, U&Es, calcium, LFTs, glucose
- Drug screen

Imaging

- MRI brain for underlying cause.
- EEG:
  - Up to 5% of normal population may have an abnormal EEG

- 30% of patients with epilepsy have a normal EEG on first recording

Treatment

General priorities:
- Determine seizure type and cause
- Safety: avoid dangerous sports, unsupervised baths or swimming

- Avoid factors increasing risk: excess alcohol, lack of sleep, stress, fever, certain medications (flashing lights affects: <5%)
- Driving advice.

Medical

- Usually started after two seizures
- Aim for one drug
- Focal seizures: first line: carbamazepine, lamotrigine
- Generalised seizures: first line: valproate then lamotrigine

Side effects of major antiepileptics:
- Sodium valproate
- Nausea, weight gain, teratogenicity, hepatotoxicity
- Lamotrigine
- Rash, Stevens–Johnson syndrome, headache, vomiting
- Carbamazepine

Surgical

- May help where drugs have failed

Management of status epilepticus

- **A medical emergency**

General treatment:
- ABC approach: resuscitate, maintain airway, O_2 (100%), fluids
- Monitor

Medical:
- IV lorazepam or IV diazepam
- If continuing: add IV phenytoin

- Rash, Stevens–Johnson syndrome, aplastic anaemia, leucopoenia, headache
- Phenytoin
- Rash, hirsutism, weight gain, acne, cerebellar syndrome, gum hypertrophy, osteomalacia

Drug interactions:
- Hepatic enzyme inducers: carbamazepine, phenytoin. ↓ effectiveness of drugs metabolised by the liver e.g. the pill
- Hepatic enzyme inhibitors: sodium valproate:↑ effectiveness of other drugs, e.g. warfarin, lamotrigine, hypoglycaemics.

- Most benefit for patients with clear lesion, particularly hippocampal sclerosis: up to 60% seizure-free

- If continuing: consider IV phenobarbitone
- Thiamine and glucose IV if suspect malnutrition or alcohol abuse

If seizures persist >30 min:
- Transfer to ITU for intubation
- Continuous EEG
- IV propofol or thiopental
- Consider non-epileptic seizures.

Prognosis

- 50% will be seizure-free off medication
- 30% develop chronic epilepsy with difficult to treat seizures

Complications

- Sudden unexpected death in epilepsy (SUDEP)
- Accidents: drowning, including in bath, burns while cooking
- Psychiatric: social morbidity, e.g. unemployment
- Fetal malformations in pregnant women

- Status epilepticus: 10–15% mortality
- ↑ risk of death due to complications.

Pregnancy and epilepsy:
- Enlist specialist help
- All anti-epilepsy drugs ↑ risk of fetal malformations. Valproate associated with highest risk
- Aim for monotherapy at lowest possible dose
- Give folate 5 mg for conception and pregnancy
- Oral vitamin K during last month of pregnancy and vitamin K for newborn if mother taking enzyme inducing drugs.

MOVEMENT DISORDERS

PARKINSONISM

Outline

- Parkinsonism: a movement disorder characterised by bradykinesia and at least one of rest tremor, rigidity and postural instability
- Parkinson's disease: a neurodegenerative disease caused by disruption of dopaminergic neurotransmission in the basal ganglia

Parkinson plus conditions:
- Conditions with parkinsonian characteristics and additional features:
  - Progressive supranuclear palsy:
    - Initially abnormal vertical saccades, later all eye movements involved

- Symmetrical parkinsonian symptoms
- Poor response to L-dopa
- Multiple system atrophy:
  - Combination of parkinsonism, cerebellar and autonomic symptoms:
    - Parkinsonism: tremor may be absent and poor response to L-dopa
    - Cerebellar dysfunction
    - Autonomic: corticobasal degeneration parkinsonian features and higher cortical dysfunction, particularly apraxia and cortical sensory loss.

Pathogenesis/aetiology

Causes of parkinsonism

- Parkinson's disease (idiopathic parkinsonism)
- Inherited: Wilson's disease (copper deposition in the basal ganglia)
- Vascular: basal ganglia infarcts

- Drugs: dopamine antagonists (e.g. neuroleptics, antiemetics)
- Toxins: carbon monoxide
- Repeated minor head trauma (e.g. boxing, football)

Pathology in Parkinson disease

1. Loss of the pigmented neurons which produce dopamine in the substantia nigra:
   - The degeneration of dopaminergic neurons also reduces the normal inhibitory effect of acetylcholine, the increase of which leads to some of the parkinsonism symptoms

2. There are also intracellular eosinophilic inclusions called Lewy bodies in the midbrain.

Who

Parkinson's disease:
- Typical age at onset: 50–70 years
- ♀ < ♂

- Incidence: 0.5% in those >65 years
- Commonest of all movement disorders.

A typical patient

70-year-old man presents with a tremor of his right hand and increasing stiffness and slowness over several months.

Clinical features

TRAP: tremor, rigidity, akinesia/bradykinesia, posture change:
- Tremor:
  - 4–6 Hz tremor of the upper and lower limbs and sometimes the jaw. 'Pill rolling' of thumb moving rhythmically over fingers. Present at rest, worse when anxious/tired
- Rigidity:
  - ↑ Tone: limbs resist passive movement:
    - *Lead pipe* rigidity: ↑ rigid tone throughout movement
    - *Cogwheel rigidity*: combined with tremor so resistance is jerky
- Akinesia/bradykinesia:
  - Slow movement
  - Monotonous speech,
  - Expressionless face
  - Micrographia (small writing)

- Postural changes:
  - Stoop, shuffling forward, festinant gait (small accelerating steps)
  - Poor balance, reduced arm swing, difficulty turning, more likely to fall

Other features:
- Dementia (20%): late feature
- Depression (50%)
- Insomnia: REM sleep disturbance
- Bladder disturbance
- Muscle pains
- Constipation
- Drooling

Features suggestive of Parkinson's disease in a parkinsonism patient
- Unilateral onset
- Asymmetrical symptoms
- Weight loss
- Dysphagia
- Typical rest tremor
- Gradual progression
- Good response to levodopa.

Investigations

- Clinical diagnosis
- Lying and standing BP to detect autonomic failure.

Imaging

Brain imaging: to exclude other conditions.

Treatment

- Treatment is symptomatic
- Aim to restore dopamine and reduce acetylcholine

Conservative

- Multidisciplinary care: physiotherapy, speech therapy, occupational therapy, respite care.

Medical

Levodopa (L-dopa):
- Crosses the blood–brain barrier and converts to dopamine to replenish depleted dopamine
- Good for bradykinesia and rigidity
- Given with carbidopa or benserazide: extracerebral dopa decarboxylase inhibitors (which do not cross the blood–brain barrier) to prevent L-dopa breaking down peripherally to dopamine to cause side effects.
- Problems: diminishing response with long-term use, on–off syndrome (rapid fluctuations between being symptomatic and symptom control), dyskinesia, dystonia
- Side effects: orthostatic hypotension, confusion, nausea, nephrotoxicity
Adjuncts:
- Dopamine agonists, e.g. bromocriptine, ropinirole, pergolide, for tremor/rigidity. Monotherapy or with

L-dopa. Side effects: impulse control disorder eg excessive gambling. Also nausea, confusion, dyskinesia.
- Monoamine oxidase inhibitors, e.g. selegiline: inhibit breakdown of dopamine. May prolong action of L-dopa.
- Catechol-O-methyltransferase (COMT) inhibitors, e.g. entacapone: inhibit peripheral metabolism of L-dopa extending its action. Side effects: dykinesia, nausea, orange urine
- Anticholinergics (orphenadrine, benzhexol, procyclidine) improve tremor, stiffness, drooling, urinary urgency. Side effects: dry mouth, blurred vision, urinary retention, confusion
- Amantadine: for bradykinesia/rigidity
- Apomorphine: dopamine agonist.

Surgical

- For advanced disease, particularly if dyskinesias
- Deep brain stimulation: for motor fluctuations.

Prognosis and complications

Prognosis

Parkinson's disease:
- Progresses over 10–15 years
- 10–20% are unresponsive to treatment

- Overall survival is only slightly reduced
Progressive supranuclear palsy:
- Median survival <6 years.

DYSKINESIAS

TREMOR

Outline

- Rhythmic, regular movement
- May be most pronounced:
  - at rest
  - during maintained posture

- whilst executing a movement: intention or kinetic tremor. Intention tremors are more pronounced as movement nears completion.

Pathogenesis/aetiology

Causes

Rest tremor:
- Characteristic of parkinsonism
Postural:
- Benign essential tremor

- Also caused by: anxiety, drugs (β agonists, alcohol), thyrotoxicosis
Intention tremor:
- Characteristic of cerebellar disease.

Who

Benign tremor:
- 50% of patients have an autosomal dominant family history.

Clinical features

Benign tremor:
- Predominantly affects the upper limbs
- Symmetrical

- May involve head, face and voice
- Symptoms may improve with alcohol.

Investigations

Benign tremor:
- Clinical diagnosis.

Treatment

Benign tremor:
- Some respond to propranolol.

Prognosis and complications

Prognosis

Benign tremor:
- Slowly progressive

- Mostly a social disability.

DYSTONIA

Outline

- Involuntary sustained muscle contractions resulting in abnormal postures

- Can be 1° (idiopathic) or 2° (to another cause).

Pathogenesis/aetiology

Types of 1° dystonia:
- Generalised dystonia:
  - One example is torsion dystonia
  - Autosomal dominant disease associated with deletion in DYT1 on chromosome 9
- Focal dystonia:
  - Of a specific muscle or muscle group, e.g. writer's cramp

Causes of 2° dystonia:
- Cerebral palsy
- Infection: after encephalitis
- Post-anoxia
- Drug-related, e.g. neuroleptics, L-dopa
- Inherited degenerative diseases, e.g. Wilson's disease, lipid storage diseases.

Who

- Depends on cause

- Primary generalised torsion dystonia may run in families.

Clinical features

Generalised torsion dystonia:
- Onset in childhood
- Affects lower limbs and then spreads upwards

Focal dystonia:
- Blepharospasm: involuntary eye closure
- Oromandibular dystonia: recurrent spasms of the mouth, tongue and jaw
- Spasmodic torticollis (dystonia of the neck)
- Dystonic writer's cramp.

Investigations

- Clinical diagnosis.

Treatment

Generalised:
- Anticholinergic agents: trihexyphenidyl
- Levodopa extremely effective in dopa-responsive dystonia

Focal:
- Local injection of botulinum toxin.

Prognosis and complications

Prognosis

- Depends on cause:
  - Focal dystonias improve with botulinum injections

- Dopa responsive dystonia extremely responsive to treatment with L-dopa.

CHOREA

Outline

- Non-rhythmic, jerky, random movements that are purposeless and involuntary
- Appears dance-like

- Any part of the body can be affected: facial grimace, raised shoulders, flexion/extension of fingers
- Often occurs with athetosis (twisting and writhing movements).

Pathogenesis/aetiology

Causes

- Huntington's chorea
- Sydenham's chorea: postinfectious, associated with rheumatic fever (St Vitus' dance)
- Wilson's disease

- Drugs: phenytoin, antipsychotics, oral contraceptive pill, alcohol
- SLE
- Polycythemia rubra vera
- Thyrotoxicosis.

Who

- Can occur at all ages.

Clinical features

Ballismus:
- Violent, large amplitude, flinging movements
- Predominantly proximal muscles

- Often unilateral (hemiballismus): associated with lesions of the contralateral subthalamic nucleus
- A continuum of chorea.

Investigations

- Clinical diagnosis

- Investigate for underlying cause.

Treatment

- Tetrabenazine

- Treatment depends on the underlying disease.

Prognosis and complications

Prognosis

- Depends on cause

Complications

- Muscle aches or trauma from involuntary movements

- Swallowing difficulties leading to aspiration pneumonia and death.

MYOCLONUS

Outline

- Sudden, jerky shock-like movements
- May be due to abnormal electrical discharges of the cerebral cortex, brainstem or spinal cord

- May be rhythmic or irregular.

Pathogenesis/aetiology

Causes

- Epileptic myoclonus
- Degenerative disease:
  - Alzheimer's, CJD
- Progressive myoclonic ataxias:
  - Rare disorders causing ataxia and myoclonus, often with epilepsy

- Metabolic myoclonus:
  - Uraemia, hypocalcaemia, hyponatraemia
- 2° to cerebral anoxia
- Post-infectious myoclonus
- Idiopathic

Who

- One of the most common dyskinesias.

Clinical features

They occur:
- spontaneously
- in response to movement: action myoclonus
- in response to visual, auditory or somatosensory stimulation: reflex myoclonus, startle myoclonus.

Investigations

- Clinical diagnosis.

Treatment

- Some forms respond to sodium valproate or clonazepam
- Treat underlying cause.

Prognosis and complications

Depends on underlying cause

TICS

Outline

- Sudden, brief, involuntary movement that can be suppressed
- Suppression results in mounting tension with subsequent rebound
- May be vocalisations such as sniffs or grunts or more complex movements such as scratching the nose.

Pathogenesis/aetiology

Simple tics:
- Childhood tics
- Chronic simple tic

Complex tics:
- Gilles de la Tourette syndrome

Other causes:
- Drugs.

Who

Gilles de la Tourette syndrome:
- Typical age: onset before 18 years
- Prevalence: 0.05%

Associations:
- Obsessive compulsive disorder
- Attention deficit hyperactivity disorder.

Clinical features

Gilles de la Tourette syndrome:
- Multiple tics include vocalisations
- Coprolalia (obscene tics with swearing and inappropriate language) is relatively uncommon (15%)

- Tics commonly involve the face, arms and neck
- Fluctuation in severity
- Tics can change in character within the same patient.

Investigations

- Clinical diagnosis.

Treatment

- Pimozide, sulpiride (antipsychotics)
- Side effects of drugs may be worse than the actual tics

- Psychological support.

Prognosis and complications

Prognosis

Gilles de la Tourette syndrome:
- Usually lifelong symptoms

- Symptoms may improve with age.

CEREBELLAR DISEASE

Outline

- Disease of the cerebellum.

Pathogenesis/aetiology

Causes

- Multiple sclerosis
- Alcohol
- Space occupying lesion of cerebellum

- Drugs, e.g. anticonvulsants
- Endocrine, e.g. hypothyroidism
- Hereditary, e.g. Friedreich's ataxia.

Who

- Depends on cause.

Clinical features

DANISH:
- D: dysdiadochokinesis (impairment of rapid alternating movements)
- A: ataxia, broad-based gait

- N: nystagmus
- I: intention tremor
- S: slurred speech
- H: hypotonia.

Investigations

Imaging

- Brain imaging.

Other tests

- Thyroid function

- Genetic testing if appropriate.

Treatment

Depends on cause.

Prognosis and complications

Depends on cause.

INCREASED INTRACRANIAL PRESSURE AND HEADACHES

GENERAL FEATURES

Outline

- ↑ pressure in the cranium

- See also 'Headache' in Common presenting complaints (Ch. 14).

Pathogenesis/aetiology

Causes

- Head injury
- Space occupying lesion
  - Tumour
  - Abscess
- Hydrocephalus

- Benign (or idiopathic) intracranial hypertension
- Venous sinus thrombosis
- Infection, e.g. abscess, tuberculoma
- Haematoma
- Aneurysm.

Who

- Depends on cause.

Clinical features

Presentation of ↑ ICP:
- *Headache*: worse on waking, and with coughing, straining or lying down
- *Vomiting*: often without nausea, worse in the morning

- *Visual disturbance*: transient loss of vision, blurred vision due to papilloedema, diplopia (double vision) due to 3rd or 6th nerve palsy
- *Focal neurological signs*: sensation, movement, speech
- ↓ *consciousness*: sign of severity

Investigations

- Fundoscopy: papilloedema (swelling of the optic disc due to ↑ ICP).

Blood tests

- FBC, CRP, ESR

Imaging

- Brain imaging essential

Other tests

- Consider lumbar puncture once a mass has been ruled out.

Treatment

- Remove or treat underlying cause
- Dexamethasone for vasogenic oedema associated with tumours (not effective for cytotoxic oedema associated with head injury)

- Mannitol: osmotic diuretic, occasionally used in life-threatening situations
- Hyperventilation: may be protective by reducing CO_2 in the ITU environment.

Prognosis and complications

- Depends on cause.

BRAIN TUMOURS

Outline

Classification

Benign:
- Meningioma (15%):
  - Originates from the meninges
- Acoustic neuroma (schwannoma) (5%):
  - Originates from the Schwann cells on the 8th cranial nerve in the cerebellopontine angle
- Haemangioblastoma:
  - From CNS blood vessels
- Pituitary adenoma:
  - See endocrinology section

Malignant:
- Primary: glioma:
  - Commonest 1° brain tumour
  - Arises from glial cells
  - 4 grades with prognosis from good to poor:
    - *Grade 1*: paediatric only
    - *Grade 2*: low grade: slow growing
    - *Grade 3*: high grade: fast growing
    - *Grade 4*: glioblastoma multiforme, most malignant
- Secondary metastatic:
  - From lung, breast, kidney, malignant melanoma
  - Commoner than primary disease.
See also above: 'Increased intracranial pressure and headaches: general features'.

Pathogenesis/aetiology

Pathogenesis

- Primary brain tumours spread by direct extension
- Benign tumours may have a poor prognosis as they have a limited area to grow
- The increased pressure in the brain can lead to herniation of the cerebellar tonsils through the foramen magnum

Types of tumour by age:
- *In children*: mostly in the posterior fossa, e.g. medulloblastoma or ependyoma, commonest solid tumours of childhood
- *In adults*: gliomas or metastases.

Who

- Typical age: 20% in <15 years

- 10% of all cancers.

Clinical features

- Presentation depends on location of tumour and rate of growth:
  - *Epilepsy*: usually first symptom, particularly for low-grade glioma
  - *Symptoms of focal neurological deficits*: hemiparesis, dysphasia, visual field defects
  - *Symptoms of ↑ ICP*: headache, vomiting, drowsiness.

Gliomas:
- Low grade:
  - Generally present with epilepsy
- High grade:
  - Generally present with signs and symptoms of ↑ ICP

Acoustic neuroma:
- Hearing impairment, vertigo and facial weakness

Investigations

Blood tests

- FBC
- ESR.

Imaging

- CXR
- MRI of brain

Other tests

- Endocrine tests: if pituitary tumour suspected
- Tumour biopsy.

Treatment

Surveillance:
- Serial MRI scans for low-grade glioma (with symptomatic treatment) and small meningiomas

Drugs:
- Anticonvulsants if seizures present
- Steroids for ↑ ICP and oedema

Chemotherapy:
- Particularly for oligodendrogliomas
- First line for:
  - Lymphoma
  - Germ cell tumours

Radiotherapy:
- Good for:
  - Gliomas
  - Acoustic neuromas
  - Benign pituitary adenomas
  - Where recurrence is likely

Surgery:
- Neurosurgical referral
- Excision if benign and in non-eloquent region
- If malignant: consider palliative surgery for symptoms of raised ICP.

Prognosis and complications

Prognosis

Malignant tumours:
- High grade: 1 year survival <50%

Gliomas:
- Grade 1: good prognosis
- Grade 2: almost all transform into high-grade gliomas

- Grade 3: poor prognosis (do not metastasise)
- Grade 4: worst prognosis

Benign tumours:
- May be removed and cured.

CEREBRAL ABSCESS

Outline

- Site of abscess depends on mode of spread.
- See also above: 'Increased intracranial pressure and headaches: general features'.

Pathogenesis/aetiology

Causes

- Infection: bacteria, fungi or Toxoplasma
- Local spread, e.g. from ear or sinus
- Haematological spread: associated with multiple abscesses.

Who

Commoner in:
- immunocompromised
- IV drug abusers

- cyanotic heart disease patients
- pulmonary arteriovenous malformation
- following direct skull trauma.

Clinical features

- Symptoms and signs of raised ICP
- Pyrexia
- Drowsiness
- Seizures.

Investigations

Blood tests

- ↑ CRP, WBC, blood cultures.

Imaging

- CT or MRI of head: abscess (usually) surrounded by oedema

Other tests

- Lumbar puncture should not be done.

Treatment

- Drainage: if large abscess
- Prolonged antimicrobial therapy
- Serial imaging CT or MRI to assess progress.

Prognosis and complications

Complications

- Seizures.

BENIGN INTRACRANIAL HYPERTENSION

Outline

- Increased pressure in the brain with no known cause
- Also known as idiopathic intracranial hypertension
- Should not be thought of as benign, as if left untreated can cause progressive visual loss and optic atrophy.
- See also above: 'Increased intracranial pressure and headaches: general features'.

Pathogenesis/aetiology

Cause

- Unknown

Associations:
- Endocrine causes
- Oral contraceptive pill
- Drugs: tetracycline, vitamin A excess

Who

- Typical age: young
- ♀ > ♂

Risk factors:
- Obesity.

A typical patient

30-year-old woman presents with headaches in the morning which worsen when she lies down. She has noted blurred vision.

Clinical features

- Symptoms and signs of raised ICP but no mass lesion
- Headache
- Papilloedema
- Blurred vision
- Diplopia: secondary to 6th nerve palsy.

Investigations

Imaging

- Urgent CT: if papilloedema, to rule out mass lesions or venous sinus thrombosis.

Other tests

- Assess visual fields and size of blind spot
- Fundoscopy: papilloedema
- Lumbar puncture: ↑ opening pressure.

Treatment

- Stop causative agents
- Weight loss if obese: can be as effective as drugs
- Monitor visual fields
- ↓ pressure with lumbar punctures.

Medical

- Acetazolamide.

Surgical

- Lumboperitoneal shunt (shunt from CSF in the lumbar spine to the abdominal cavity)
- Or optic nerve fenestration.

Prognosis and complications

Prognosis

- Progressive visual loss and optic atrophy in 10%.
- See also above: 'Increased intracranial pressure and headaches: general features'.

HYDROCEPHALUS

Outline

- Excessive CSF in the ventricles of the brain.

Types

Obstructive or non-communicating hydrocephalus:
- Obstruction of outflow of CSF by: aqueduct stenosis, cerebral tumour or congenital malformation (e.g. Arnold Chiari malformation)

Communicating hydrocephalus:
- ↑ production of CSF or failure of its reabsorption into the cerebral sinuses due to scarring of arachnoid granulations, e.g. after meningitis

Normal pressure hydrocephalus:
- In the elderly or middle aged
- Chronic communicating hydrocephalus of unknown cause with initially high CSF pressure and enlarged ventricles, with pressure normalising over time.

Pathogenesis/aetiology

Pathogenesis

- Normally CSF is produced in the choroid plexus in the ventricles of the brain
- CSF flows through the foramina of Magendie and Luschka around the spinal cord and over the surface of the brain
- It is reabsorbed via the arachnoid granulations into the intracranial venous sinuses
- Hydrocephalus is caused by a blockage in the flow of CSF, increased production or failure of its reabsorption.

Who

- Typical age: bimodal distribution. Children affected by congenital malformations, adults more affected by normal pressure hydrocephalus at >60 years
- 1♀:1♂.

Clinical features

Children:
- ↑ head circumference, bulging fontanelles
- Subtle cognitive decline in older child
- Symptoms and signs of ↑ ICP

Adults:
- Headache
- Vomiting
- Visual symptoms
- Symptoms and signs ↑ ICP

Normal pressure hydrocephalus:
- Triad of symptoms – DIG:
  - D: dementia
  - I: urinary frequency then incontinence
  - G: gait disturbance: shuffling steps, falls.

Investigations

Imaging

- CT/MRI: including looking at the size of the ventricles.

Other tests

- Lumbar puncture good for normal pressure hydrocephalus and drainage of CSF once space-occupying lesion ruled out.

Treatment

- Treat underlying cause
- Drain CSF by shunt insertion:
  - Ventriculo-peritoneal (shunt from the brain ventricle to the abdominal cavity)
- Ventriculo-atrial shunts (shunt from the brain ventricle to the right atrium in the heart).

Prognosis and complications

Complications of CSF shunts

- Blockage
- Infection
- Subdural collection.

MIGRAINE

Outline

- Recurrent severe headaches with associated features often following visual auras
- Features include: nausea, vomiting, phonophobia, photophobia
- Duration 4–72 h

Frequency:
- Varies
- ~1.5 attacks per month
- Can develop chronic migraines: >15 days in a month (rare).

Pathogenesis/aetiology

Pathogenesis

- Not fully understood
- May involve changes in cerebral blood flow
- Serotonin, nitric oxide and noradrenaline may play a role

Triggers:
- Hunger
- Stress
- Relief of stress, e.g. holiday
- Sleep deprivation
- Changes to normal routine
- Hormonal link, e.g. during menstruation or with oral contraceptives
- Often none found.

Who

- Typical age: <40 years
- 2♀:1♂
- Prevalence: 10%

Associations:
- Family history.

Who

A typical patient

A 28-year-old woman with headaches once every 2 weeks which are unilateral, throbbing and associated with nausea. When she gets these headaches she lies down in a dark room.

Clinical features

Visual aura (15%):
- ~30 min before headache
- Flashing lights
- Scotoma (↓ vision in an area of the visual field)
- Fortification spectra: zig-zags resembling battlements gradually move across visual field
- Visual field loss

Headache:
- Can last hours or days
- Usually unilateral
- Throbbing or pulsating
- Mechanosensitivity: pain worse on head movement
- Allodynia: all stimuli produce pain
- Patients prefer to lie down in a dark and quiet room
- With nausea, vomiting and photophobia.

Investigations

- History.

Imaging

- Brain imaging if features suggestive of space occupying lesion.

Treatment

- Avoid triggers

Prophylaxis – only if more than 3 attacks per month:
- β-blockers: propranolol
- Tricyclics: amitriptyline
- Anti-epileptics (second line): valproate, gabapentin, topiramate

Symptomatic treatment:
- Analgesia: aspirin, paracetamol, ibuprofen
- Antiemetics: metoclopramide, domperidone
- 5 HT agonists: sumatriptan (also vasoconstrict). Contraindicated in heart disease, peripheral vascular disease.

Prognosis and complications

Prognosis

- Not life threatening.

Complications

- Analgesia headache from overuse of medication
- Chronic migraine

- ↑ risk of cerebrovascular disease with oral contraceptive pill use.

INFECTION OF THE BRAIN AND MENINGES

MENINGITIS

Outline

- Inflammation of the meninges
- Bacterial meningitis is a medical emergency
- This section primarily covers bacterial meningitis

- Occurs particularly in:
  - areas of overcrowding, poverty, malnutrition, e.g. students and military
  - after head injury
  - the immunocompromised.

Pathogenesis/aetiology

Causes

Bacteria:
- *Neisseria meningitidis* (meningococcus): several sero groups: A, B, C, Y and W135. Serotype B commonest in UK
- *Streptococcus pneumoniae* (pneumococcus): all ages particularly very young and old
- *Listeria monocytogenes*
- *Haemophilius influenzae*: predominantly in children <6 years: now rare due to success of vaccine

Viruses:
- Normally self limiting, mildest form:
- Echoviruses
- Coxsackie A and B
- HSV1 and HSV2
- Mumps

Mycobacteria:
- *M. tuberculosis*

Specific groups affected

Neonates BEL:
- Group B streptococci
- *Escherichia coli*: and other coliforms
- *Listeria monocytogenes*

Immunocompromised:
- *Listeria*
- *Cryptococcus*
- TB meningitis.

Who

- Typical ages: <4 years and 15–19 years
- Incidence: 2000/year in the UK
- Most cases are sporadic, but there may be outbreaks
- Peaks winter/spring.

Clinical features

- Fever
- Headache
- Meningism: neck stiffness, photophobia and Kernig's sign (pain on passive knee extension with flexed hips)
- Seizures
- Confusion
- Non-blanching rash: only in 2/3 of those with meningococcal disease

Raised intracranial pressure:
- Confusion
- ↓ conscious level
- Papilloedema
- Focal neurological signs, e.g. 6th nerve palsy
- In the young and the elderly, signs may be more subtle:
  - Infants: apathy, floppy, irritability, not feeding
  - Elderly: confusion and fever.

Investigations

Blood tests

- FBC
- U&Es
- CRP
- Glucose
- Blood culture.

Imaging

- CT: only if focal neurology, new seizures, or papilloedema

Other tests

Lumbar puncture:
- CSF changes (Table 6.2).
- Gram stain and culture
- CSF PCR
- Rapid bacterial antigen tests.

Table 6.2 Lumber puncture findings in meningitis

	CSF	Cells/mm^3	Protein (g/L)	Glucose
Normal	Clear	0–3	0.2–0.4	>2/3 plasma level
Viral	Clear	5–500 mononuclear cells (lymphocytes)	0.4–0.8	Normal (occasionally low)
Bacterial	Turbid	5–2000 polymorphs (neutrophils)	0.5–5	Low
TB	Turbid or fibrinous	5–1000 mononuclear cells (lymphocytes)	0.5–5	Very low

Treatment

Outside hospital:
- Prompt diagnosis and treatment saves lives
- Benzylpenicillin IM

In hospital:
- At once:
  - O_2
  - Fluid resuscitation
  - <55 years cefotaxime or ceftriaxone
  - >55 years cefotaxime and ampicillin to cover listeria
  - Dexamethasone reduces neurological sequelae: give before or with antibiotics, ideally within first 72 h.
- Organisms isolated:
  - Seek microbiological advice and alter medications based on culture sensitivities

- A notifiable disease
- Contact prophylaxis:
  - 'Kissing' and household contacts only
  - For meningococcal and haemophilus exposure: rifampicin or ciprofloxacin
- Prevention:
  - Routine universal vaccination against:
    - *Haemophilis influenzae* type B
    - *Neisseria meningitidis* serogroup C. Also A/C/Y/W135 for travel to high risk areas
    - *Streptococcus pneumoniae*: 7 serotypes.

Prognosis and complications

Prognosis

- 5% mortality.

Complications

Early:
- Hydrocephalus: may require shunt
- Focal infarcts

Late:
- 16% of survivors suffer long-term problems: epilepsy, deafness, learning difficulties

ENCEPHALITIS

Outline

- Inflammation of the brain parenchyma

- Usually caused by a virus.

Pathogenesis/aetiology

Causes

- Viruses: most common is HSV
- Also: arbovirus, enterovirus, varicella zoster virus, EBV, mumps, measles

- In immunocompromised: CMV, *Gondii Toxoplasma*
- Post-infectious: subacute sclerosing panencephalitis following measles.

Who

- Commonest cause in the UK is HSV1 (apart from in neonates).

Clinical features

HSV encephalitis:
- Prodromal illness
- Fever
- Behavioural changes
- Headache

- ↓ consciousness
- Seizures
- Focal neurological signs: particularly temporal and frontal lobes: olfactory hallucinations.

Investigations

Imaging

- CT/MRI of brain: changes in temporal lobes.

Other tests

Lumbar puncture:
- CSF analysis: ↑ protein, ↑ cells
- CSF PCR for viral DNA.

EEG:
- Diffuse slow-wave activity particularly with temporal localisation.

Treatment

HSV encephalitis:
- IV aciclovir: very effective if given promptly. Commence if HSV suspected

- Dexamethasone if mass effect.

Prognosis and complications

Prognosis

- Poor prognosis if treatment is delayed.

DISEASE OF THE BRAIN AND SPINAL CORD

MULTIPLE SCLEROSIS (MS)

Outline

- Chronic inflammatory demyelinating disorder affecting the CNS
- The episodes of demyelination must be separated in time and space

- Main sites affected are the cervical spinal cord, optic nerves, periventricular white matter and the brainstem and its cerebellar connections
- A relapse is a clinically evident attack of demyelination.

Classification

- Relapsing and remitting: lesions occur in different parts of the CNS at different times often with incomplete recovery. Makes up 70% of cases initially. Most convert to secondary progressive MS about 10 years from disease onset

- Secondary progressive: symptoms are more continuous and gradually worsen. Relapses are less frequent and with less recovery
- Primary progressive: continuously worsening symptoms with cumulative disability. Occurs in ~20% of patients.

Pathogenesis/aetiology

Causes

- Aetiology unknown

- Possibly autoimmune and genetic susceptibility

Pathology

- Autoimmune reaction against white matter of brain and spinal cord leads to inflammation, plaques of demyelination and axonal loss
- The demyelination delays or prevents conduction

- Local breakdown of the blood–brain barrier due to inflammation and immune response
- Partial remyelination may lead to improvement in symptoms between relapses.

Who

- Typical age: mean onset 25 years
- 3♀:1♂
- Incidence 120/100 000

- Commonest demyelinating disease
- Commoner in temperate climates.

A typical patient

A 22-year-old woman presents with painful visual loss in her right eye; 18 months later she develops paraesthesia in her legs.

Clinical features

- Symptoms evolve over days with total or partial resolution in weeks

Visual:
- Optic neuritis: optic nerve inflammation causing partial/total visual loss. Usually unilateral

- Symptoms: pain, blurred vision, loss of colour vision
- Signs: ↓ visual acuity, visual field defects, relative afferent pupillary defect. Fundoscopy: pale or pink swollen optic disc.

Clinical features

- Diplopia: from plaques involving 3rd, 4th, 6th cranial nerves or in the medial longitudinal bundle
- Internuclear ophthalmoplegia: disorder of conjugate lateral gaze. Affected eye has impaired adduction causing diplopia in extreme abduction. Compensatory nystagmus can be seen in the contralateral eye (Fig. 6.9)

Sensory:
- Paraesthesia
- Pain, e.g. trigeminal neuralgia
- Lhermitte phenomenon: electric shock sensation in limbs on neck flexion from spinal cord lesions

Motor:
- Limb weakness with ↑ tone
- Hyperreflexia

Cerebellar signs:
- Ataxia, nystagmus, intention tremor, dysarthria (motor speech disorder)

Psychiatric symptoms:
- Transient mood changes (70%)
- Intellectual impairments (50–60%): impaired memory and attention
- Depression: reactive, suicide risk
- Euphoria and lability 10–20%

Other manifestations:
- Bladder disturbance (50–75%): urgency, frequency, incontinence

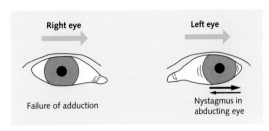

Fig. 6.9 Right internuclear ophthalmoplegia: failure of adduction of the right eye on adduction with nystagmus of the left eye in abduction.

- Sexual dysfunction
- Seizures
- Uhthoff phenomenon: symptoms worsen when hot, e.g. after a bath
- Fatigue: a prominent symptom

Final stages:
- Neurological deficits accumulate:
  - Dementia, ataxia, tetraparesis

Investigations

- Diagnosis is largely clinical, supported by MRI findings and other investigations to exclude other causes.

Blood tests

- FBC, ESR, U&Es, TFTs, B$_{12}$, folate

Imaging

- MRI: investigation of choice, 90% sensitivity

McDonald criteria:
- Combines clinical and MRI findings to diagnose MS.

Other tests

Electrophysiological tests:
- Visual evoked potentials: conduction delay along the visual pathways
- Somatosensory evoked potentials
- Brainstem auditory-evoked potentials (BAEPs)

Lumbar puncture:
- CSF: useful if diagnostic uncertainty.
- ↑ protein
- ↑ WBC
- Oligoclonal bands: ↑ in CSF > serum. Found in 95%.

Treatment

Management of an acute relapse:
- Steroids: ↓ duration of relapse but no effect on overall disability or disease course

Symptomatic treatment::
- Involve multidisciplinary team, ophthalmologists, urologists
- Bladder (urgency incontinence): intermittent self catheterisation, oxybutynin (anticholinergic)
- Neuropathic pain: carbamazepine for trigeminal neuralgia, amitriptyline, gabapentin

- Back pain: physiotherapy, transcutaneous electrical nerve stimulation (TENS), NSAIDs
- Spasticity: physio, baclofen
- Fatigue: graded exercise, pulsed steroids, amantadine, modafinil

Disease-modifying treatment (for relapsing remitting MS only):
- Interferons:
  - Interferon-β1a: avonex, rebif
  - Interferon-β1b: betaferon

Treatment

- 30% reduction in relapse rate, possible effect on progression
- Indications: must be ambulant with at least 2 significant relapses within last 2 years, or one disabling relapse in past year with new lesions on MRI
- Side effects: injection site reaction, flu like symptoms, myalgia, headache. Rarely bone marrow suppression and hepatotoxicity
- Glatiramer acetate:
  - Mimics myelin basic protein

- Indications: as for interferon
- Side effects: injection site reactions, anxiety and palpitations

Other treatments (in severe relapsing remitting disease):
- Natalizumab (mononclonal antibody): risk of developing multifocal leucoencephalopathy (1:1000): monitor with yearly MRI
- Mitoxantrone (doxorubicin analogue): chemotherapeutic agent. Has risk of cardiac toxicity and leukaemia.

Prognosis and complications

Prognosis

- Life expectancy is ↓ by 10–15 years
- 20 years after onset of symptoms:
  - 35% still working
  - 50% use walking aids

Better prognosis:
- Earlier age of onset
- Sensory symptoms or optic neuritis at onset
- Good remission after first exacerbation

Complications

- Spasticity
- Recurrent UTIs

- Bronchopneumonia.

MOTOR NEURON DISEASE

Outline

- Group of neurological disorders characterised by progressive degeneration of motor neurons in brain and spinal cord
- Rapid, progressive course leading to death within years
- Both upper motor neuron (UMN) and lower motor neuron (LMN) signs due to anterior horn cell involvement

Distinguishing motor neuron disease from other neurological diseases
- In motor neuron disease:
  - Usually there is no sphincter disturbances or loss of sensation
  - External eye movements are unaffected.

Pathogenesis/aetiology

Causes

- Aetiology unknown

- Mutations in *SOD1* gene encoding copper–zinc superoxide dismutase found in some patients. Other mutations include FUS and C90rf72

Who

- Typical age of onset 50–70 years
- 1♀:1.5♂
- Incidence: 6/100 000

- 5–10% have a family history suggestive of autosomal dominant inheritance

A typical patient

A 50-year-old man has noted weakness of his right arm over the last few months.

Clinical features

Four clinical types (BAPP):

1. **B**ulbar palsy:
   - Affects upper (pseudobulbar) and lower (bulbar) motor neurons of cranial nerves 9, 10 and 12, causing dysarthria and dysphagia
   - Progressive over 6–12 months
   - Risk of aspiration
2. **A**myotrophic lateral sclerosis:
   - Affects the lateral corticospinal tracts and the anterior horn cells
   - Combined LMN wasting and UMN hyperreflexia and spasticity, often in the same limb
   - Commonest form (~50%)
3. **P**rogressive muscular atrophy:
   - Anterior horn cell lesion
   - Pure LMN involvement with weakness, wasting and hand and arm fasciculation
   - Initially distal muscles, later spreads proximally
4. **P**rimary lateral sclerosis:
   - Primarily UMN involvement
   - Progressive tetraparesis
   - Rare

Can be a combination of all patterns
- Psychiatric symptoms:
  - Emotional lability, sleep disturbance, fatigue, depression
  - Mild to severe cognitive deficits.

Investigations

- Important to exclude any other cause of symptoms.

Blood tests

- ↑ Creatinine kinase

Imaging

- MRI: spinal imaging to exclude cord or root compression.

Other tests

- Electrophysiology:
  - EMG: spontaneous fibrillations and fasciculations.

Treatment

- Multidisciplinary approach: neurologist, physiotherapist, occupational therapist, speech and language therapist, palliative care

Symptomatic treatment:
- Joint pains: NSAIDs
- Constipation: laxatives
- Dysphagia: softened food diet, nasogastric tube, gastrostomy, e.g. percutaneous endoscopic gastrostomy insertion
- Respiratory failure: non-invasive ventilatory support

Disease-modifying treatment:
- Antiglutamate drugs, e.g. riluzole.
- Prolongs life by 3 months.

Prognosis and complications

Prognosis

- Mean survival from onset: 3–5 years
- Bulbar palsy has the worst prognosis, progressive muscular atrophy has the best prognosis

Complications

- Respiratory failure: main cause of death
- Aspiration pneumonia
- Venous thromboembolism due to immobility.

MYELOPATHY

GENERAL FEATURES

Outline

- Myelopathy is disease of the spinal cord
- In the adult, the spinal cord ends at the lower border of L1
- Nerve pathways are anatomically close, so sensory, motor and autonomic symptoms may be concurrent

Causes of spinal cord disease

- Compression: disc prolapse, syringomyelia
- Inflammation: MS
- Tumours: neurofibroma, meningioma
- Trauma: e.g. total resection, hemisection (Brown-Séquard syndrome).
- Infection: e.g. TB, syphilis

- Vascular: e.g. anterior spinal artery occlusion which mainly affects the anterior cord due to anatomy of the spinal artery. Causes paraplegia, loss of pain and temperature sensation, with sparing of joint position sense
- Hereditary: hereditary spastic paraparesis.

Who

- Depends on cause.

Clinical features

Motor:
- Bilateral UMN weakness and sensory loss
- Distribution of weakness depends on the level of the lesion
- LMN signs may also be present if nerve roots are involved
- Any cord lesion above C4 causes respiratory paralysis: 'C3, 4, 5 keeps the diaphragm alive' via the phrenic nerve

Sensory:
- Sensory loss below level of lesion
- But beware: level of sensory loss may not accurately reflect the level of the lesion (spinal imaging should be higher than the highest symptoms)

Autonomic:
- Bladder involvement
- Urinary urgency and frequency
- Sexual dysfunction.

Investigations

Blood tests

- FBC, vitamin B_{12}.

Imaging

- MRI of spine.

Treatment

- Depends on cause.

Prognosis and complications

Prognosis

- Depends on cause.

SPINAL CORD COMPRESSION

Outline

- Compression of the spinal cord
- May develop quickly or slowly depending on the cause

- This is an emergency: failure to relieve spinal cord compression can lead to irreversible paraplegia (lower limb weakness) and incontinence
- Needs urgent investigation and referral.

Pathogenesis/aetiology

Causes

- *Degenerative*: chronic degenerative disc disease
- *Tumours*: of the spinal cord, or metastatic deposits
- *Infection*: TB (Pott's disease), abscess
- *Haematoma*

- *Intervertebral disc herniation*: a tear in the outer annulus fibrosus of the intervertebral disc causes the nucleus pulposus to be herniated, compressing the spinal cord or nerve roots
- *Trauma*.

Who

- Depends on cause.

Motor:
- Limb weakness
- UMN signs: spasticity, brisk reflexes, extensor plantar response
- LMN signs may be present if acute, or if roots are involved

Sensory:
- Sensory loss below the level of the lesion

Other symptoms:
- Back pain
- Bladder sphincter involvement: hesitancy, frequency, painless retention
- Constipation.

- FBC, vitamin B$_{12}$.

- CXR
- Spinal X-rays
- MRI of spine (Fig. 6.10).

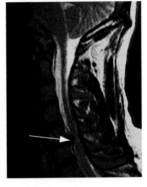

Fig. 6.10 MRI of spine showing cord compression (arrow).

- Urgent referral to neurosurgery
- Treat underlying cause

- Tumours: urgent radiotherapy and/or steroids
- Surgical decompression of the spinal cord.

- Depends on cause.

CAUDA EQUINA SYNDROME

- Dysfunction of the sacral and lumbar nerve roots in the lumbar vertebral canal causing bladder, bowel, sexual dysfunction and perianal numbness
- **This is an emergency**
- Always ask about the relevant symptoms

The cauda equine:
- Nerve roots coming down from the conus medullaris
- It starts below the termination of the spinal cord at the level of L1/L2 and consists of nerve roots L1–5 and S1–5.

- Disc prolapse is commonest cause
  - Particularly at L4/5 and L5/S1
- Tumours: primary or metastatic

- Trauma
- Infection: abscess, TB.

- 1♀:1♂.

Motor:
- LMN weakness of lower limbs
- Loss of ankle reflexes
- Can be bilateral or unilateral.

Sensory:
- Sensory changes in saddle distribution or perianal area

Autonomic:

- Urinary symptoms: poor stream, retention
- Bowel incontinence
- Constipation
- Loss of anal tone
- Impairment of sexual function

Other symptoms:
- Back pain.

Clinical examination

- Neurological examination

- PR examination to check for anal tone.

Imaging

Urgent:
- MRI.

- Requires urgent treatment
- Neurosurgical referral

- Surgical decompression.

Prognosis

- May be reversible if prompt treatment and not progressed to cause urinary retention

- If with urinary retention: prognosis is bad.

Complications

- Permanent bowel and genitourinary dysfunction

- Permanent leg weakness.

SYRINGOMYELIA

Outline

- A longitudinal cyst (syrinx) forms in the spinal cord
- Usually in the cervical region
- Fibres that cross from one side of the cord to the other are primarily affected leading to symptoms in a 'cape like distribution' over the upper trunk and limbs

Syringobulbia:
- Cavitation within the brainstem (rather than the spinal cord)
- The central area affects the trigeminal nuclei, sympathetic trunk, cranial nerves 9, 10, 11 and 12 and the vestibular system causing bilateral lower cranial nerve palsies and Horner syndrome.

Pathogenesis/aetiology

Causes

- Arnold–Chiari malformation: congenital abnormality with herniation of the cerebellar tonsils through the foramen magnum leading to blockage of CSF flow, allowing a syrinx to form. Commonest cause

- Infection
- Trauma.

Pathogenesis

- The cavity interrupts spinothalamic fibres that cross within the cord
- As it enlarges it extends into the anterior and posterior horn cells

- Further enlargement can affect the lateral and dorsal columns.

Who

- Incidence: 8/100 000

- Mean age at onset: 30.

Clinical features

Sensory:
- Loss of pain and temperature sensation in a cape distribution

Motor:
- LMN signs in upper limbs at the level of the syrinx as the anterior horn cells are damaged: wasting and weakness of the small muscles of the hands, ↓ reflexes
- UMN signs in lower limbs, below the level of the syrinx: spastic paraparesis, ↑ reflexes, due to corticospinal tract involvement

Horner syndrome:
- From sympathetic nerve damage

Syringobulbia:
- 5th cranial nerve: facial pain or sensory loss
- 8th cranial nerve: hearing loss and nystagmus
- 9th,10th,12th cranial nerves: tongue wasting and bilateral weakness.

Investigations

Imaging

- MRI of cervical spine.

Treatment

- Surgical decompression.

Prognosis and complications

Prognosis

- Symptoms can be static for years but worsen with increases in venous pressure.

BROWN-SÉQUARD SYNDROME

Outline

- Damage to one half of spinal cord
- See figure 15.8 for an illustration

Pathogenesis/aetiology

Causes

- Trauma
- Tumours
- Inflammation.

Who

- Rare.

Clinical features

- Ipsilateral loss of vibration and position sense (posterior columns)
- Contralateral loss of pain and temperature sense (spinothalamic)
- Ipsilateral motor activity loss.

Investigations

Imaging

- MRI of spine.

Treatment

- Cervical spine immobilisation
- High-dose steroids: for inflammation
- Treat cause
- Seek neurosurgical/orthopaedic advice.

Prognosis and complications

Prognosis

- Depends on cause

Complications

- Complications of spinal injury

SUBACUTE COMBINED DEGENERATION OF THE SPINAL CORD

Outline

- Deficiency of vitamin B_{12} leads to damage to corticospinal tracts, dorsal columns and peripheral nerves
- Both UMN and LMN signs.

Pathogenesis/aetiology

Causes

- Nutritional deficiency (vegans)
- Pernicious anaemia
- Terminal ileum disease
- Total gastrectomy
- Parasitic infection
- Copper deficiency can also present in this way.

Pathogenesis

- Myelin degeneration in the posterolateral columns.

Who

- Commoner in those >60 years
- Prevalence of vitamin B_{12} deficiency in Europe: 1.6–10%.

Clinical features

Use mneumonic SCD (like subacute combined degeneration)
S: sensory and motor peripheral neuropathy:
- Loss of light touch and weakness
- Absent ankle jerks
C: corticospinal tract damage:
- Spastic paraparesis
- Weakness

- Extensor plantars
D: dorsal column damage:
- Loss of vibration and proprioception sense
- Sensory ataxia
Others:
- Optic atrophy
- Dementia.

Investigations

Blood tests

- FBC: ↑ MCV with macrocytes
- Vitamin B_{12} levels
- Other vitamin levels for associated deficiencies

- Schilling test to measure vitamin B_{12} absorption
- Intrinsic factor antibodies and anti-parietal cell antibodies

Other tests

Nerve conduction studies:
- Axonal sensorimotor polyneuropathy (in up to 80%).

Treatment

- Vitamin B_{12} therapy indefinitely.

Prognosis and complications

Prognosis

- Symptoms usually improve after a few months of treatment, unless severe damage has occurred.

RADICULOPATHY AND PLEXOPATHIES

RADICULOPATHY

Outline

- Radiculopathies are lesions of the nerve root
- Leads to pain in a dermatomal distribution with numbness and tingling and weakness of affected muscles with loss of appropriate reflexes
- A description rather than a diagnosis

Polyradiculopathy:
- More than one nerve root is affected.

Pathogenesis/aetiology

Causes

- Degenerative changes
- Disc prolapse: commonest cause

- Trauma
- Tumours.

Pathogenesis

- The dorsal root contains sensory fibres, the ventral root contains motor fibres
- These fibres join to become the spinal nerve at the intervertebral foramen

- Nerve roots can be compressed or irritated producing signs relating to that root.

Who

- Depends on cause.

Clinical features

Commonly affected roots:
- C5: neck and shoulder pain, deltoid and biceps weakness, loss of biceps and supinator jerk
- C6: neck and lateral forearm pain, bicep weakness, loss of biceps and supinator jerk
- C7: neck, lateral arm pain, triceps and finger extensor weakness, loss of triceps jerk

- L4: front of thigh pain, quadriceps weakness, loss of knee jerk
- L5: lateral lower leg pain, weak extensor hallucis longus
- S1: back of thigh and sole of foot pain, weak plantar flexors, loss of ankle jerk.

Investigations

Blood tests

- FBC
- ESR
- Glucose

- Serum electrophoresis
- Calcium
- Phosphate.

Imaging

- MRI of spine.

Treatment

- Treat underlying cause
- Supportive measures: physiotherapy, emotional support
- Symptomatic treatment of neuropathic pain

- May resolve spontaneously
- Surgery may be required.

Prognosis and complications

Prognosis

- Depends on cause.

PLEXOPATHIES

Outline

- Lesion of the nerve plexus (network of nerves)
- Leads to weakness, wasting and areflexia.

Some brachial plexopathies:
- Neuralgic amyotrophy:
  - Acute inflammation of the brachial plexus
  - Unknown cause, may be viral
- Erb's palsy (C5–6):
  - Upper brachial plexus lesion
- Usually caused by injury during difficult delivery
- Klumpke syndrome (C8-T1):
  - Lower brachial plexus lesion
  - Usually traction injury caused by excess abduction of arm, usually during delivery at birth
- Thoracic outlet compression (C8-T1):
  - Compression of lower cord of brachial plexus.

Pathogenesis/aetiology

Causes

- Compression: cervical rib
- Tumours: lung (e.g. Pancoast tumour) or breast
- Radiotherapy
- Trauma: during birth, accidents.

Who

- Depends on cause.

Clinical features

- Weakness, wasting, areflexia
- ± associated Horner syndrome: depending on the cause and location of the compression
- Neuralgic amyotrophy:
  - Onset: severe pain shoulder, neck, arm for 2–3 weeks.
  - Then weak shoulder abduction and lateral rotation. Winging of scapular and ↓ reflexes
  - Recovery over 6–18 months
- Erb's palsy (C5–6):
  - Loss of biceps jerk, wasting and weakness of shoulder abduction
- Arm hangs medially rotated, with forearm pronated ('waiter's tip position'). Loss of sensation down lateral aspect of arm
- Klumpke syndrome (C8-T1):
  - Paralysis of the hand muscles
  - Claw hand and sensory loss along medial aspect of arm
- Thoracic outlet compression (C8-T1):
  - Pain and sensory loss of medial forearm with wasting and weakness of hand muscles
  - May have associated vascular symptoms, e.g. Raynaud's.

Investigations

Blood tests

FBC, immunoglobulins: to help identify immunological causes or tumours

Neurophysiology studies

- EMG
- Nerve conduction studies.

Imaging

- MRI of suspected site of involvement.

Treatment

- Treat underlying cause
- Immunoglobulin therapy if immune mediated cause
- Supportive measures: physiotherapy, emotional support
- Symptomatic treatment of neuropathic pain
- May resolve spontaneously
- Surgery may be required.

Prognosis and complications

Prognosis

- Depends on cause.

NEUROPATHY

PERIPHERAL NERVE DISEASE

Outline

- Diseases affecting the nerves
- Peripheral nerve damage
- Can affect motor, sensory, autonomic nerves or a combination.
- May affect one nerve (mononeuropathy) or many (polyneuropathy)

Mononeuropathy:
- Damage to individual nerves
- Often through trauma and entrapment, e.g. carpal tunnel syndrome (see below)

Mononeuritis multiplex:
- Separate involvement of 2/more nerves
- Usually associated with a systemic disease such as: PLANT WARDS
  - Polyarteritis nodosa
  - Leprosy
  - HIV (AIDS)
  - Neurofibromatosis
  - Tumour
  - Wegner's

- Amyloidosis
- Rheumatoid arthritis
- Diabetes mellitus
- Sarcoid

Polyneuropathy:
Mainly sensory polyneuropathy:
- Caused by:
  - Diabetes mellitus
  - Hypothyroidism
  - Amyloidosis
  - Drugs, e.g. isoniazid
  - Alcohol
  - Infections

Mainly motor polyneuropathy:
- Caused by:
  - Guillain–Barré
  - Porphyria
  - Lead
  - Hereditary neuropathies.
- Damage to many nerves

Pathogenesis/aetiology

Classification of peripheral nerve disease by cause

- Connective tissue disease:
  - Rheumatoid arthritis, lupus (SLE)
- Inflammatory:
  - Guillain–Barré (see below)
  - Chronic inflammatory demyelinating poly-neuropathy (CIDP) (see below)
  - Sarcoid
  - Vasculitis
- Toxins:
  - Drugs (isoniazid, amiodarone)
  - Alcohol
  - Lead
- Nutritional deficiencies:
  - Vitamin B_1, B_6 or B_{12}
- Associated with systemic disease:
  - Diabetes mellitus
  - Renal failure
  - Porphyria

- Amyloidosis
- Malignancy
- Infection:
  - HIV
- Hereditary neuropathies:
  - Hereditary motor sensory neuropathies or Charcot–Marie–Tooth disease:
    - Type 1:
      - Demyelinating, autosomal dominant most common.
      - Distal wasting of lower limbs (resemble inverted champagne bottles). Progresses to upper limbs. Pes cavus and clawing of the toes and hands. ↓ reflexes and loss of sensation
    - Type 2:
      - Axonal.

Who

- Common

- Depends on cause.

Clinical features

Symptoms and signs

- Sensory:
  - Numbness
  - Paraesthesia (tingling)
  - Burning sensations
  - Pain
- Motor:
  - Weakness
  - Wasting
  - Fasciculations
- Autonomic:
  - Postural hypotension (dizziness or fainting on standing: measure lying and standing BP)

- Erectile dysfunction
- ↓ sweating
- Diarrhoea or constipation
- Urinary retention
- Arrhythmias
- Autonomic changes common in diabetes amyloid disease and Guillain-Barré
- Other signs:
  - Loss of reflexes
  - Skin changes: loss of hair, dry skin
  - Skeletal changes: pes cavus, clawing of toes
  - High stepping gait
  - Foot drop.

Distribution

- *Mononeuropathy*: peripheral nerve distribution
- *Polyneuropathy*: glove and stocking distribution (extremities) most common pattern

- *Spinal root damage*: dermatomal distribution.

Investigations

Blood tests

- FBC
- CRP/ESR
- U&Es
- LFTs
- Glucose

- TFTs
- Vitamin B_{12}
- Folate
- Serum protein electrophoresis
- Auto-antibodies.

Urine

- Glucose

- Bence Jones proteins

Other tests

Further investigations depending on initial findings and symptoms:
- CXR: sarcoid or lung cancer
- Autonomic function tests
- Nerve conduction studies

- EMG
- Lumbar puncture for CSF analysis
- Nerve biopsy: only if other tests do not reveal a cause and vasculitis is suspected
- Genetic tests if hereditary cause suspected.

Treatment

- Treat underlying cause if possible
- Multi-disciplinary team involvement:
  - Physiotherapy
  - Occupational therapy: home adaptations

- Foot care
- Genetic counselling for inherited diseases.

Medical

- Steroids: for inflammation, autoimmune disease or vasculitic causes

- Gabapentin and amitriptyline for neuropathic pain.

Surgical

- Entrapment mononeuropathies: surgical decompression if possible.

Prognosis and complications

Complications

- Long-standing neuropathy may lead to joint deformities (Charcot joints) and neuropathic ulceration.

CARPAL TUNNEL SYNDROME

Outline

- Compression of the median nerve under the flexor retinaculum of the wrist

- An entrapment neuropathy.

Pathogenesis/aetiology

Causes

- Idiopathic
Associated with:
- Connective tissue disease: rheumatoid arthritis

- Endocrine changes: hypothyroid, acromegaly, diabetes, menopause, pregnancy, obesity.

Who

- Typical age: 40–50 years
- ♀ > ♂

- Commonest entrapment mononeuropathy.

A typical patient

A 54-year-old woman has noted pain and tingling in her left hand, particularly at night.

Clinical features

Sensory:
- *Paraesthesia*: tingling, pain, worse at night. May be relieved by hanging the hand down
- *Sensory loss*: in distribution of median nerve (often not precise)

Motor:
- *Weakness*: of abductor pollicis brevis (poor thumb abduction)
- *Wasting*: of thenar eminence (late feature).

Investigations

Clinical tests:
Tinel's sign (TAP):
- Percussion over median nerve, leads to paraesthesia
Phalen's test (Phlex):
- Hold wrist fully flexed for 2 min: may provoke sensory symptoms

Nerve conduction studies:
- ↓ sensory action potentials
- Look for cause
- Nerve conduction studies if not improving.

Treatment

- Splints
- Steroid injection

- Surgical decompression.

Prognosis and complications

Prognosis

- Depends on cause
- Usually resolves after pregnancy

- Good response to surgery.

ULNAR NERVE PALSY

Outline

- Paralysis of the ulnar nerve

- From damage anywhere along the nerve

Pathogenesis/aetiology

Causes

- Compression in the cubital tunnel at the elbow: commonest cause
- Compression at the wrist

- Diabetes
- Hereditary compression neuropathy.

- Any age.

Clinical features

- Symptoms depend on lesion site
- Tingling of little and ring finger and ulnar side of hand
- Weakness of small muscles of hand, sparing muscles supplied by the median nerve (LOAF: lumbricals 1 and 2, opponens pollicis, abductor pollicis brevis and flexor pollicis brevis)

- If at elbow: also weakness of long finger flexors to 4th and 5th fingers.

Investigations

- Look for cause

- Nerve conduction studies if not improving.

Treatment

- Rest
- Pressure avoidance

- Splinting if not resolving.

Surgical

- Decompression and transposition of nerve at elbow if needed.

Prognosis and complications

Prognosis

Depends on cause and extent of nerve damage.

COMMON PERONEAL NERVE PALSY

Outline

- Paralysis of the common peroneal nerve

- From damage anywhere along the nerve.

Pathogenesis/aetiology

Causes

- Compression at lateral knee as nerve winds around fibula: commonest cause, particularly in leg crossers
- Prolonged kneeling
- Lesion at fibula head

- Diabetes
- Vasculitis
- Hereditary compression neuropathy.

Who

- Any age.

Clinical features

- Weakness of ankle dorsiflexion causes a foot drop
- Also weakness foot eversion

- Sensory loss is variable: may involve lateral foot or just 1st dorsal webspace.

Investigations

- Look for cause

- Nerve conduction studies if not improving.

Treatment

- Depends on cause and extent of nerve damage.

Prognosis and complications

Compression usually recovers spontaneously within 12 weeks.

GUILLAIN–BARRÉ SYNDROME

Outline

- An acute inflammatory demyelinating polyneuropathy affecting mainly motor but also sensory and autonomic nerves
- Progresses within hours or days, reaching a peak within 4 weeks

- If it progresses after 8 weeks becomes defined as chronic inflammatory demyelinating polyneuropathy (see below).

Pathogenesis/aetiology

Pathogenesis

- Inflammatory demyelination of the peripheral nervous nerves, possibly due to an abnormal autoimmune response
- 2/3 of patients have a known infection in the weeks prior to onset of symptoms, particularly:

- *Campylobacter jejuni*
- CMV
- EBV
- *Mycoplasma pneumoniae*.

Who

- Incidence: 2/100 000/year.

Clinical features

Sensory (usually first symptoms):
- Pain and numbness in feet and hands

Motor:
- Symmetrical distal weakness, ascends to involve arms
- Cranial nerve involvement (50%): diplopia, drooling, dysphagia

- Severe cases: respiratory and bulbar muscle weakness

Autonomic (in 2/3 patients):
- Tachycardia or bradycardia, heart block, asystole, arrhythmia
- Unstable BP
- Urinary retention.

Investigations

Blood tests

- FBC
- U&Es

- Antiganglioside antibodies (25%)

Other tests

Special tests:
- EMG and nerve conduction studies: demyelinating disease, therefore a ↓ in conduction velocity

- ECG: for arrhythmias
- Lumbar puncture for CSF analysis: ↑ protein, normal white cell count.

Treatment

- **Medical emergency**
- Admit, observe
- Cardiac monitoring for arrhythmias
- Monitor FVC for respiratory depression and consider ventilation if respiratory weakness: if respiratory involvement, involve ITU early
- Intravenous immunoglobulin

- Plasma exchange if continued deterioration
- Steroids are not helpful

Prevent complications:
- Heparin for DVT and pulmonary embolism prophylaxis
- Careful nursing to prevent pressure ulcers
- Speech and language and physiotherapy involvement.

Prognosis and complications

Prognosis

- 80% make good recovery but may take months
- 10% have permanent disability or relapsing remitting disease
- 5–10% mortality

Worse prognosis:
- Older age
- Rapid onset
- Ventilator support
- Diarrhoea/*C. jejuni* preceding.

Prognosis and complications

Complications

- Pulmonary embolism
- Aspiration pneumonia
- Pressure ulcers.

CHRONIC INFLAMMATORY DEMYELINATING POLYNEUROPATHY

Outline

- A chronic inflammatory motor and sensory neuropathy characterised by demyelination and progression beyond 8 weeks from onset.

Pathogenesis/aetiology

Pathogenesis

- The cause is unknown but may be autoimmune.

Who

- Typical age: middle aged and the elderly
- $♀ < ♂$.

Clinical features

- Similar signs and symptoms as Guillain–Barré syndrome, but presents over a longer time

Sensory:
- Loss of proprioception
- Sensory loss in a glove and stocking distribution

Motor:
- Absent reflexes
- Bilateral symmetrical proximal and distal limb weakness
- Rarely bulbar or respiratory muscle weakness.

Investigations

- +ve Romberg test.

Blood tests

- FBC, ESR, U&Es

Other tests

Special tests:
- Nerve conduction studies: ↓ conduction velocity and conduction block
- CSF analysis: ↑ protein
- Nerve biopsy may be appropriate.

Treatment

Main treatments:
- Intravenous immunoglobulin
- Steroids
- Plasma exchange

Other treatments include:
- Azathioprine
- Cyclophosphamide
- Ciclosporin.

Prognosis and complications

Prognosis

- Lifelong disease: spontaneous remission rare except in younger patients
- 90% patients improve with the three main treatments.

CRANIAL NERVE LESIONS

(1) OLFACTORY NERVE LESIONS

Outline

- Damage to the olfactory nerve which is important for the sense of smell.

Pathogenesis/aetiology

Causes

- Head injury
- Nasal or sinus disease
- Tumours

- Genetic: Kallmann syndrome (hypothalamic hypogonadism).

Who

- Rare.

Clinical features

- Hyposmia, anosmia

- Altered taste.

Investigations

Clinical examination

- Any change in taste or smell?

Imaging

- Brain imaging if appropriate.

Treatment

- Treat underlying cause.

Prognosis and complications

Prognosis

- Anosmia secondary to head injury is often permanent.

(2) OPTIC NERVE LESIONS: PAPILLOEDEMA

Outline

- Swelling of the optic disc due to raised intracranial pressure (ICP).

Pathogenesis/aetiology

Causes

Raised ICP:
- Space occupying lesion: tumour, abscess
- Cerebral oedema
- Infection
- Hydrocephalus
- Idiopathic intracranial hypertension

Medical causes:
- Accelerated hypertension
- Polycythaemia rubra vera.

Who

- Rare

- 1♀:1♂.

Clinical features

Visual signs and symptoms:
- Usually no initial change in acuity
- ↑ ICP causes visual obscuration: loss of vision for a few seconds particularly on coughing or bending forwards
- Visual field defects: enlarged blind spot, constricted visual fields

On fundoscopy:
- Blurring of the disc margins
- Loss of venous pulsation
- Usually bilateral.

Investigations

Clinical examination

- Visual acuity and fields, colour vision testing, fundoscopy (Fig. 6.11).

Imaging

- MRI of brain to look for space occupying lesion.

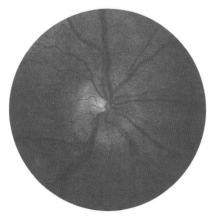

Fig. 6.11 Papilloedema apparent on fundoscopy.

Treatment

- Treat underlying cause.

Prognosis and complications

Prognosis

- Depends on cause.

(2) OPTIC NERVE LESIONS: OPTIC NEURITIS

Outline

- Inflammation of the optic nerve
- Leads to optic atrophy.

Pathogenesis/aetiology

Causes

- Multiple sclerosis (MS): presenting feature in 25% of MS
- Infections: viruses: measles, mumps, EBV.

Who

- Young adults: 15–40 years.

Clinical features

- Acute monocular visual loss
- Eye pain: particularly on movement
- Central scotoma
- Impaired colour vision

- Disc may be swollen (papillitis) or normal (retrobulbar neuritis)
- Relative afferent pupil defect: tested by the swinging light test: the affected pupil dilates when a light swings from the unaffected to the affected eye.

Investigations

Clinical examination

- Visual acuity and fields, colour vision testing, fundoscopy
- Visual evoked potentials

Imaging

- MRI of brain.

Treatment

- Steroids: may lead to earlier recovery of vision
- Refer to neurologist for consideration of disease-modifying drugs if suspicion of MS.

Prognosis and complications

Prognosis

- Vision usually returns within 6–8 weeks
- Some patients remain with severe visual loss
- 70% of patients with optic neuritis go on to develop MS (higher risk if abnormal MRI).

(2) OPTIC NERVE LESIONS: OPTIC ATROPHY

Outline

- Prolonged damage to the optic nerve produces a pale disc on fundoscopy.

Pathogenesis/aetiology

Causes

- Optic nerve compression: meningioma, glioma
- ↑ ICP
- Postoptic neuritis
- Nutritional: thiamine and vitamin B_{12} deficiency
- Drugs: ethambutol, isoniazid
- Toxins: alcohol, tobacco
- Inherited: Leber's hereditary optic atrophy.

Who

- 1♀:1♂
- Seen at any age.

Clinical features

- Impaired visual acuity
- Central scotoma
- Pallor of the disc on fundoscopy
- Relative afferent pupil defect (see above).

Investigations

Clinical examination

- Visual acuity and fields, colour vision testing, fundoscopy (Fig. 6.12)
- Vitamin B_{12} levels.

Imaging

- MRI of brain.

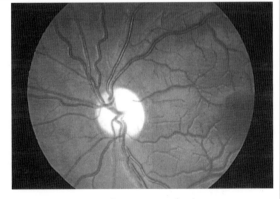

Fig. 6.12   Optic atrophy as seen on fundoscopy.

Treatment

- Treat underlying cause.

Prognosis and complications

Prognosis

- Depends on cause

Complications

- Visual impairment
- Blindness.

(3) OCULOMOTOR NERVE LESIONS

Outline

- Lesion of the oculomotor nerve which innervates most of the eye muscles, allowing the eye to move.

Pathogenesis/aetiology

Causes

- Diabetes mellitus
- Vasculitis
- Tumour
- Vascular infarct
- Cavernous sinus pathology: often associated with lesions of cranial nerves 4, 5 and 6 as these nerves all pass through the cavernous sinus together
- Trauma.

Who

- Depends on cause.

Clinical features

- Weakness of oculomotor muscles: inferior oblique, medial, superior and inferior rectus palsy so eye is turned down and out
- Ptosis: eyelid covers eye
- Pupil enlarged.

Investigations

Clinical examination

- Eye movements, direct and consensual pupillary light and accommodation reflex.

Blood tests

- Fasting glucose
- ESR.

Imaging

- MRI of brain.

Treatment

- Depends on cause.

Prognosis and complications

Prognosis

- Depends on cause.

(4) TROCHLEAR NERVE LESIONS

Outline

- Lesion of the trochlear nerve which innervates the superior oblique muscle of the eye.

Pathogenesis/aetiology

Causes

- Head trauma
- Ischaemic vasculopathy
- Cavernous sinus pathology.

Who

- 1♀:1♂.

- Superior oblique palsy: diplopia maximal on downward gaze while eye in adducted position with vertical or diagonal separation of images.

Clinical examination

- Eye movements, pupillary eye and accommodation reflexes.

- Prisms
- Botulinum toxin

- May need surgical correction.

Prognosis

- Depends on cause.

(5) TRIGEMINAL NERVE LESIONS

- Lesion of the trigeminal nerve which is important for facial sensation and chewing
- The trigeminal nerve has three major branches (thus its name): ophthalmic, maxillary and mandibular. The mandibular branch has a motor supply to the pterygoids and muscle of mastication

Trigeminal neuralgia:
- Unilateral facial pain within the distribution of the trigeminal nerve
- Most commonly affects the mandibular division
- Neuralgia: severe burning or stabbing pain following the course of a nerve.

Causes of trigeminal neuralgia

- Idiopathic
- Blood vessel close to nerve

- Rarely: space occupying lesion, e.g. MS, aneurysm.

- ♀ > ♂

- Age: >50

Trigeminal neuralgia

- Intense, sharp stabbing pain, electric shock like, lasting seconds
- Usually unilateral
- Tic douloureux: face screws up in pain
- Between pain, no abnormal signs

Triggers:
- Washing
- Shaving
- Eating
- Talking.

Clinical examination

- Trigeminal nerve: light touch in the three branches of the nerve, corneal reflex, test muscles of mastication by clenching the teeth and opening and closing the mouth, jaw jerk

Imaging

- MRI with views of the course of the trigeminal nerve to look for a compressive lesion.

Trigeminal neuralgia

- Carbamazepine: most effective
- Phenytoin
- Baclofen

- Surgical decompression if drugs fail.

Prognosis and complications

Prognosis of trigeminal neuralgia

- 2/3 patients: symptoms controlled with drugs.

(6) ABDUCENS NERVE LESIONS

Outline

- Lesion of the abducens nerve which innervates the lateral rectus muscle which abducts the eye

- The 6th nerve has a long intracranial course and is therefore vulnerable to damage by trauma or masses.

Pathogenesis/aetiology

Causes

- Diabetes
- Vascular damage
- Tumours
- Trauma

- Multiple sclerosis
- Brainstem infarct
- Cavernous sinus pathology.

Who

- All ages.

Clinical features

- Lateral rectus weakness: failure of abduction of the affected eye (unable to move the eye outwards) leading to diplopia with horizontal separation of images that is maximal on looking towards the affected side.

Investigations

Clinical examination

Eye movements, pupillary light and accommodation reflexes.

Imaging

- MRI.

Treatment

- Depends on cause
- Prisms

- May need surgical correction.

Prognosis and complications

Prognosis

- Depends on cause.

(7) FACIAL NERVE LESIONS

Outline

Bells palsy:
- Acute LMN facial nerve palsy of unknown cause producing weakness of the entire half of the face

- An upper motor lesion such as a stroke causes unilateral weakness of only the lower half of the face, with forehead sparing, as the upper facial muscles are supplied by the motor cortex of both sides.

Pathogenesis/aetiology

Causes

- Idiopathic: Bell's palsy
Brainstem lesions:
- Stroke, tumour
Infection:
- Viral: varicella zoster virus (Ramsey Hunt syndrome), HSV

*bilateral causes

- Lyme disease*
- Meningitis
Systemic disease:
- Diabetes mellitus
- Sarcoidosis*
- Guillain-Barré syndrome.*

Who

- Incidence: 15–40/100 00/year
- Highest incidence aged 30–50 years

- Risk increases with pregnancy and diabetes.

Clinical features

- Abrupt onset, within 24–48 h
- Unilateral facial weakness: eyebrow droop, drooping of side of the mouth
- Pain behind the ear, may precede weakness
- Hyperacusis

- ↓ taste in some patients
- Often have subjective sensory loss on affected side of face
- Herpetic vesicles may be visible in the external auditory canal if due to HSV.

Investigations

Clinical examination

- Test muscles of expression (lift eyebrows, close eyes tight, blow out cheeks, whistle, show teeth).

Blood tests

- FBC, ESR, fasting glucose.

Other tests

- EMG
- MRI if atypical or involvement of other cranial nerves

- ENT examination.

Treatment

- Recovery may be spontaneous
- Prednisolone: if within 3 days of onset increases chance of complete recovery
- Antivirals, e.g. aciclovir if possibility of HSV infection (but may not affect outcome)

- Eye care if incomplete eye closure, to prevent drying and ulceration of the cornea
- Plastic surgery occasionally used to restore symmetry if no recovery.

Prognosis and complications

Prognosis

- 80% recover within 2 months

- 15% have nerve degeneration and permanent weakness.

Complications

- Corneal exposure and ulceration due to poor lid closure

- Aberrant reinnervation may cause 'jaw winking' (winking of affected eye with jaw movement) due to periocular fibres regenerating to supply the mouth.

(8) VESTIBULOCOCHLEAR NERVE LESIONS

Outline

- Lesion of the vestibulocohlear nerve which is important for hearing and balance
- The nerve has two divisions: vestibular and cochlear:
  - *Vestibular nerve*: lesions lead to vertigo and loss of balance
  - *Cochlear nerve*: lesions lead to sensorineural deafness and tinnitus

Acoustic neuromas:
- These are benign tumours of the eighth cranial nerve. They are commonly found in the cerebellopontine angle
- The proximity to other nerves means that a lesion in this area also affects the 5th, 7th and sometimes 6th cranial nerves resulting in a mixed picture of: deafness, tinnitus and vertigo with loss of facial sensation and weakness.

Pathogenesis/aetiology

Causes

- Lesions: tumours (neuroma), multiple sclerosis
- Trauma
- Infection: basal meningitis
- Drugs: alcohol, gentamicin

Deafness can be:
- *conductive*: due to a problem in the mechanical conduction of sound to the inner ear, or
- *sensorineural*: due to a problem with the processing of sound either at the level of the inner ear, the vestibulocochlear nerve or in the brain.

Who

- Depends on cause.

Clinical features

- *Vertigo*: sensation of rotation or swaying, associated with nausea and nystagmus (eye oscillations).
- *Sensorineural deafness*

- *Tinnitus*: abnormal hissing or whistling sound internally heard when there is no external source of the sound.

Investigations

Rinne test and Weber test can distinguish normal hearing, conductive and sensorineural deafness (Table 6.3).
- Rinne test:
  - Compare loudness of tuning fork held to ear and mastoid process

- Weber test:
  - Tuning fork held against forehead
- Hallpike manoeuvre:
  - Rapid movement of patient from sitting to lying with head flexed forwards and tilted to one side will trigger vertigo and nystagmus.

Imaging

- MRI of brain.

Table 6.3   Tests to distinguish normal hearing, conductive and sensorineural deafness

	Rinne test	**Weber test**
Normal	Air conduction loudest	Equally loud in both ears
Conductive deafness	Bone conduction heard louder than air conduction	Sound heard better in deaf ear
Sensorineural deafness	Air conduction heard louder than bone conduction	Sound heard better in intact ear

Investigations

- Depends on cause
- Neuro-otological referral for caloric testing

- ENT referral if appropriate.

Prognosis and complications

Prognosis

- Depends on cause.

(8) VESTIBULOCOCHLEAR NERVE LESIONS: MENIERE'S DISEASE

Outline

- Disorder of the inner ear affecting hearing and balance and leading to a triad of tinnitus, deafness and vertigo.

Pathogenesis/aetiology

- Not caused by eighth nerve damage but by end-organ disease
- May be caused by excess fluid due to failure of endolymph reabsorption.

Who

- Age 30–50
- Incidence $\sim$100/100 000/year.

Clinical features

- Episodic vertigo: severe, often associated with nausea and vomiting
- Fluctuating deafness
- Tinnitus
- Recurrent attacks lasting minutes–hours.

Investigations

Clinical examination

Rinne test and Weber test:
- Hearing tests

Imaging

- MRI (usually normal) to exclude space occupying lesion.

Treatment

During attack:
- Bed rest
- Antiemetics
- Prochlorperazine
General treatment:

- Salt restriction
- Diuretics
- Betahistine – short-term use only
- Vestibular exercises

Surgical

- Destruction of labyrinth/vestibular nerve.

Prognosis and complications

Prognosis

- Deafness gradually progresses and may become permanent
- 80% of patients respond to treatment.

(9, 10) GLOSSOPHARYNGEAL AND VAGUS NERVE LESIONS: BULBAR AND PSEUDOBULBAR PALSY

Outline

- A collection of symptoms rather than a diagnosis
- Bulbar palsy:
  - LMN lesion to cranial nerves 9, 10, 11, 12 resulting in weakness of the tongue, muscles of chewing, swallowing, and facial muscles
- Pseudobulbar palsy:
  - UMN lesion of cranial nerves 9, 10, 11, 12
  - Due to corticobulbar lesions.

Causes

Bulbar palsy:
- Guillain–Barré syndrome
- Motor neuron disease
- Syringobulbia
- Tumours

Pseudobulbar palsy:
- Stroke
- MS
- Motor neuron disease
- Tumour

Note that motor neuron disease can cause both a bulbar and a pseudobulbar palsy.

- Pseudobulbar palsy is commoner than bulbar palsy.

Symptoms and signs in bulbar and pseudobulbar palsy are shown in Table 6.4.

Table 6.4 Symptoms and signs in bulbar and pseudobulbar palsy

Bulbar palsy	Pseudobulbar palsy
Nasal speech: quiet and hoarse	Slow monotonous speech, sometimes explosive
Absent jaw jerk	Brisk jaw jerk
Reduced or absent gag reflex	Brisk gag reflex
Nasal regurgitation of food, dysphagia	Dysphagia
Wasted tongue	Small, spastic tongue
LMN signs: flaccid, fasciculating tongue	Associated UMN signs in limbs
	Emotional lability

Clinical examination

- 9th nerve: gag reflex
- 10th nerve: ask patient to say 'ahh', look for uvula deviation.

Imaging

- MRI of brain.

- Depends on cause.

Prognosis

- Depends on cause.

(11) ACCESSORY NERVE LESIONS

Outline

- Lesion of the accessory nerve which has two parts: the spinal accessory nerve innervates the sternocleidomastoid and trapezius muscles and the cranial accessory nerve has some overlap with the vagus nerve.

Pathogenesis/aetiology

Causes

- Stroke
- Tumour
- Trauma
- Jugular foramen syndrome.

Who

- Very rare.

Clinical features

Very rare to find isolated lesion:
- Spinal accessory nerve lesion causes weakness of sternomastoid and trapezius.

Investigations

Prognosis

Clinical examination

- Look for trapezius and sternocleidomastoid wasting, ask patient to shrug shoulders and move their head against resistance

Other tests

- Nerve conduction studies.

Treatment

- Depends on cause.

Prognosis and complications

- Depends on cause.

(12) HYPOGLOSSAL NERVE LESIONS

Outline

- Lesion of the hypoglossal nerve which innervates the tongue

UMN:
- Unilateral produces little effect

- Bilateral produces a pseudobulbar palsy: dysarthria and dysphagia

LMN:
- Ipsilateral atrophy, fasciculations, weakness causing deviation towards the affected side.

Pathogenesis/aetiology

Causes

UMN:
- Cerebrovascular disease
- Motor neuron disease

LMN:
- Space occupying lesion of skull base, e.g. tumour.

- Isolated lower cranial nerve palsies are rare.

- Weakness of tongue movement
- Stiff movement if UMN lesion
- Atrophy and fasciculations if LMN lesion.

Clinical examination

Examine the tongue inside the mouth and ask patient to move it side to side:
- Test strength by asking patient to push tongue against inside of cheek against resistance

Imaging

- Look for space occupying lesion

Other tests

- EMG if fasciculations.

- Depends on cause.

Prognosis

- Depends on cause.

NEUROMUSCULAR JUNCTION DISORDERS

MYASTHENIA GRAVIS

Outline

- An acquired autoimmune disorder characterised by fatiguability and weakness of muscles due to autoantibodies against the neuromuscular junction

Two presentations:
- Younger women:
  - Acute illness associated with autoimmune disease and HLA-B8 and HLA-DR3
- Older men:
  - Disease associated with thymic and eye disease.

NB: There is cross over between these groups.

Pathogenesis/aetiology

Cause

- Aetiology unknown
- B and T cells implicated.

Pathogenesis

- In normal muscle contraction, nerve stimulation causes acetylcholine (Ach) to be released into the neuromuscular junction
- Ach binds to receptors causing the muscle to contract
- In myasthenia gravis, IgG autoantibodies bind to nicotinic Ach receptors at the neuromuscular junction
- This↓ the number of receptors available for acetylcholine binding, causing ↓ contraction and weakness.

Who

Associations:
- Autoimmune disease
- Thymic hyperplasia (70%): thymoma in 10% of patients
- Hyperthyroidism
- Rheumatoid arthritis
- Lupus (SLE).

Clinical features

- Muscular fatigue: worse at end of day and after exercise
- Weakness is episodic and variable
Muscles (listed in order affected):
- *Ocular muscles* (65%): ptosis, diplopia
- *Bulbar*: dysphagia, dysarthria, dysphonia: voice deteriorates when counting

- *Facial muscles*: myasthenic snarl on smiling
- *Neck*: head drops as extension weaker than flexion
- *Limb girdles*: weakness, mainly proximal muscles
- *Respiratory muscles*: respiratory weakness.

Investigations

Imaging

- CT chest for thymoma.
Tensilon test:
- IV edrophonium (short acting anticholinesterase): improves muscle weakness

- Only conduct test in hospital with resuscitation facilities available.

Other tests

- Ach receptor antibody (90%)

- Neurophysiology: ↓ response to repetitive nerve stimulation

Treatment

- Anticholinesterases, e.g. pyridostigmine, neostigmine. They prolong the activity of Ach by inhibiting acetylcholinesterase which breaks it down. Side effects: nausea, vomiting, diarrhoea, abdominal pain
- Immunosuppression: prednisolone, azathioprine

- Plasmapheresis: can be used in acute exacerbations
- Thymectomy: may induce remission in 50% 7–10 years later. Indicated for patients with thymoma but also improves symptoms in patients without thymoma or thymic hyperplasia.

Prognosis and complications

Prognosis

- With thymoma: 5 year survival is 70%.

Complications

- Respiratory muscle weakness can cause death

- Some drugs worsen myasthenia gravis including: β-blockers, aminoglycosides, erythromycin, ciprofloxacin, quinine, verapamil, phenytoin and lithium.

LAMBERT–EATON MYASTHENIC SYNDROME

Outline

An autoimmune disorder where autoantibodies bind to the calcium channels of the neuromuscular junction preventing release of acetycholine, which is vital for muscular contraction. Table 6.5 compares it with myasthenia gravis.

Table 6.5 Comparison of Lambert–Eaton myasthenic syndrome and myasthenia gravis

Myasthenia gravis	Lambert–Eaton
Autoantibodies to Ach receptors	Autoantibodies to calcium channels
Weakness ↑ with exercise	Weakness ↓ on exercise
Eye signs first	Limb weakness and gait problems before eye signs
No autonomic involvement	Autonomic involvement
Normal reflexes	Hyporeflexia
Responds to edrophonium	Weaker response to edrophonium

- Voltage gated calcium channel autoantibodies are present.

Causes

- Autoimmune
- Paraneoplastic manifestation of small cell lung cancer (or other cancers).

Who

- Rare
- Middle aged and older people
- Young people can also be affected

- 1♀:5♂
- Paraneoplastic in ∼60% of patients.

Clinical features

- Proximal muscle weakness with ↑ strength after exercise
- May also have ocular and bulbar weakness (with dysarthria)
- Autonomic symptoms: dry mouth, postural dizziness, urinary symptoms

- Reflexes are depressed, but strong contraction against resistance will increase reflexes
- Absent reflexes are restored by exercise.

Investigations

- Anti-P/Q voltage gated calcium channel antibodies (85%)
- EMG: ↑ response to repetitive stimulation

- Poor response to edrophonium test (see Myasthenia gravis, above)

Imaging

- CXR: to investigate lung malignancy.

Treatment

- Management of underlying malignancy
- 3′4-diaminopyridine: increases acetylcholine release

- IV immunoglobulin
- Steroids.

Prognosis and complications

Prognosis

- May remit if underlying malignancy is treated.

Complications

- Can precede cancer by many years: regular CXR should be performed if malignancy is not initially found.

MYOPATHIES

GENERAL FEATURES

Outline

- Muscle diseases

- Features suggestive of muscular, rather than nerve disease:
  - Tend to affect proximal muscles first (apart from myotonic dystrophy) symmetrically affected
  - Reflexes are preserved until late in the disease.

Pathogenesis/aetiology

Inherited:
- Muscular dystrophies (see below)
Acquired:
- Inflammatory: poly/dermatomyositis

- Metabolic: thyrotoxicosis, hypothyroidism, Cushing's disease
- Drugs: steroids, alcohol, statins.

Who

- Depends on cause.

Clinical features

- Muscular weakness
- Wasting
- Myalgia, muscular cramps, stiffness
- Waddling gait.

Investigations

- Creatine kinase
- EMG
- Muscle biopsy.

Treatment

- Depends on cause.

Prognosis and complications

Prognosis

- Depends on cause.

MUSCULAR DYSTROPHY

Outline

- Group of inherited disorders of progressive degeneration and weakness of skeletal muscles
- Muscle is replaced with fat and connective tissue giving a bulky appearance in Duchenne and Becker muscular dystrophies.

Pathogenesis/aetiology

Duchenne muscular dystrophy:
- X linked recessive
- Caused by mutation of the gene for dystrophin (a muscle protein) on short arm of chromosome X
- Usually in boys
- Progressive

Becker muscular dystrophy:
- Due to mutation in same gene, but less severe

Facioscapulohumeral muscular dystrophy:
- Autosomal dominant
- More benign.

Who

Duchenne muscular dystrophy:
- Commonest muscular dystrophy
- 25/100 000 male births

- Mostly in males

Facioscapulohumeral:
- Adolescent onset.

Clinical features

Duchenne muscular dystrophy:
- Muscle weakness, muscle wasting, calf pseudohypertrophy
- Children present with difficulty walking and clumsiness

- Gower's sign: patient uses their hands to climb up their legs to stand from lying down

Facioscapulohumeral:
- Weakness and wasting of face and shoulders
- Winging of scapulae.

Investigations

- Creatine kinase
- EMG
- Muscle biopsy
- Genetic testing.

Treatment

- Supportive treatment
- Genetic counselling.

Prognosis

Duchenne muscular dystrophy:
- Progressive
- Usually in wheelchair by teens
- Death by age 20 due to chest infection or cardiomyopathy

Becker muscular dystrophy:

- Onset in early teens
- Wheelchair required by age 20–30

Facioscapulohumeral muscular dystrophy:
- Slightly ↓ lifespan.

MYOTONIC DYSTROPHY

Outline

- An inherited multi-system disease characterised by myotonia which is a failure of muscle relaxation after contraction.

Pathogenesis/aetiology

Causes

- Autosomal dominant disease
- Caused by an expanded trinucleotide repeat in a gene on chromosome 19

- Shows anticipation (earlier and more severe presentation in subsequent generations)

Who

- Typical age of presentation: 20–50 years

- ♀ < ♂.

Clinical features

Muscles:
- Myotonia: unable to release grip, distal muscles mostly affected
- Facial weakness: bilateral ptosis, haggard appearance
- Sternomastoids, and temporalis weakness and wasting
- Cardiomyopathy: ECG abnormalities, arrhythmias, heart block

Endocrine associations:
- Diabetes mellitus
- Pituitary dysfunction

- Testicular or ovarian atrophy
- Gynaecomastia
- Frontal balding

Others:
- Cataracts
- Mitral valve prolapse
- Smooth muscle involvement causing constipation, dysphagia
- Mild intellectual impairment.

Investigations

- EMG
- Search for associated features

- Genetic testing if appropriate.

Treatment

- Treat associated disorders.

Prognosis and complications

Complications

- Respiratory muscle involvement causing pneumonia and daytime sleepiness

- Cardiac complications: heart block and arrhythmias.

Renal system 7

Faculty Contributor: Laurie Sharman

Kidneys

The kidneys are found on either side of the spine at levels T12–L3. Their function is:

- regulation of fluid volume and electrolyte balance
- regulation of acid–base balance
- regulation of BP
- regulation of calcium, phosphorus and bone metabolism
- endocrine processes: production of erythropoietin (the hormone stimulating erythopoiesis, red blood cell production), activation of vitamin D, production of renin
- removal of waste or toxic substances.

The nephron

The functional unit of the kidney, with around a million per kidney. Each consists of the Bowman's capsule, convoluted tubules, loop of Henle and collecting ducts.

Four layers make up the filtering apparatus of the glomerulus; each of these can be affected in renal disease with effects on filtration:

- basement membrane
- blood vessel lining (endothelial cells)
- podocytes (epithelial cells)
- mesangium (smooth muscle like cells with phagocytes).

Different hormones and medications target different parts of the nephron (Fig. 7.1).

Glomerular filtration rate

Kidney function can be measured using the glomerular filtration rate (GFR): the amount of filtrate formed every minute (usually 100–130 mL). GFR tends to be kept constant through renal homeostasis:

- Renal pathology may lead to ↓ GFR if ultrafiltration is reduced.
- Estimated GFR is calculated using creatinine clearance as daily creatinine production is constant and is freely filtered through the kidneys with little reabsorption.
- Creatinine can give an underestimation of renal impairment so a number of more sophisticated formulae can be used, e.g. the modification of diet in renal disease (MDRD) equation, which considers age, sex, race and serum creatinine levels.

Symptomology

Symptoms related to the lower urinary tract:

- Infection:
  - Frequency
  - Urgency
  - Dysuria
  - Haematuria
- Obstruction:
  - Hesitancy
  - Poor stream
  - Postmicturition dribbling
  - Incomplete voiding.

Dialysis

- Method to filter waste products from the blood in patients with renal failure
- Complications include: cardiovascular disease (MI and Stroke) and sepsis

Haemodialysis

- Removal of waste products from the blood as it passes through an external filter machine
- In the acute setting: performed via central venous access.
- In the chronic setting: repeated 3 times a week via a surgically created arterial-venous fistula often in the anterior cubital fossa. In exams look out for the fistula 'hum' on auscultation

Peritoneal dialysis

- For chronic renal failure patients to remove waste products through the peritoneum of the abdomen acting as a filter. Requires a peritoneal catheter inserted surgically but patients can be managed at home.

Investigations

Blood tests

- Hb: ↓ from ↓ erythropoietin production in renal disease

Fig. 7.1 The nephron and site of action of hormones and diuretics.

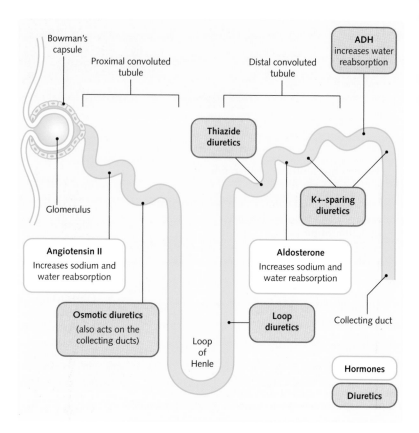

- U&Es:
  - Imbalance of ions in renal disease as the kidney helps to regulate ion homeostasis
  - Creatinine: used to calculate estimated GFR
  - Urea: ↑ in high protein diet, catabolism, GI bleeds (a source of protein in the gut), renal impairment.

Urine

- Dipstick: see table 7.1 for abnormalities seen.
- If positive result, may send for microscopy and culture.

Microscopy

Red blood cells: dipstick-positive haematuria must be sent for microscopy to determine presence of RBCs

White blood cells: >5 white blood cells per high power field suggests infection

Bacteria: UTI definition is $>10^5$/mL of urine

Casts: produced by the kidney and detection in the urine can indicate different pathology dependent on the type of cast. RBC casts indicate a glomerular cause of haematuria.

Radiography

Plain film radiography of kidneys, ureter, bladder (KUB) may show radiopaque stones in the renal tract.

Ultrasound

Good initial imaging for size, renal cysts and masses.

Intravenous urogram

Intravenous urogram (IVU) comprises serial radiographic films taken before and after IV contrast:

- Good for assessing kidney size, filling defects (including renal stone disease) and haematuria
- The contrast can precipitate an allergic reaction and is nephrotoxic.

Renal angiography

CT with IV contrast to image the renal vasculature:

- Good for the diagnosis of renal artery stenosis and renal vascular disease (Fig. 7.2).

Cystoscopy

Direct visualisation of the bladder with a cystoscope:

- Used to detect malignancy.

Renal biopsy

Tissue sampling of the kidney:

- Good for diagnosing patients with nephrotic or nephritic syndromes.

Table 7.1　Abnormalities seen on urine dipstick

Abnormalities on urine dipstick	Causes
Proteins	Kidney disease (glomerulonephritis and nephrotic syndrome) Multiple myeloma Urinary tract infection (UTI) Physiological: exercise, pregnancy, menstrual period, post-coital
Blood	UTI Kidney stone Kidney disease (nephritic syndrome) Trauma Tumour Bleeding disorders
Leucocytes	Just UTI Prostatitis Epididymo-orchitis Urethritis TB Glomerulonephritis Drugs: corticosteroid, cyclophosphamide
Nitrites	UTI High red meat consumption
Ketones	Diabetic ketoacidosis Starvation Alcohol
Glucose	Diabetes Pregnancy

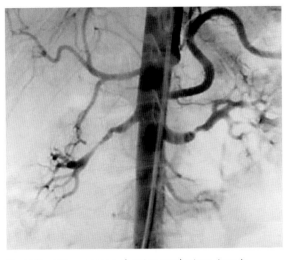

Fig. 7.2　MR angiogram showing renal artery stenosis.

See also

- Biochemistry (Ch. 12): sodium regulation
- Common presenting complaints (Ch. 14): enlarged kidney, haematuria, proteinuria, polyuria, oliguria, pruritus.

RENAL FAILURE

GENERAL FEATURES

Outline

A description rather than a diagnosis. Describes a reduction in glomerular filtration rate (GFR):
- GFR usually estimated from creatinine
- Creatinine ↑ >50% above baseline (normal level: 70–110 μmol/L)

Kidney failure can be acute or chronic, leads to impairment of:
- filtration: waste products such as creatinine and urea accumulate
- regulation of salt and water

- BP control
- erythropoietin production
- vitamin D formation
- acid–base balance

Questions to consider:
- Are there life-threatening complications?
- Is there acute or chronic failure?
- What degree of renal impairment is there?
- What is the cause?

Pathogenesis/aetiology

Distinguishing acute from chronic renal failure

Acute renal failure (ARF)
- Shorter duration of symptoms
- Symptom severity is worse
- Rapid reduction in urine output
- Usually reversible

Chronic renal failure (CRF)
- Longer duration of symptoms
- Usually irreversible
- Smaller kidneys
- Additional problems:
  - Anaemia
- Bone changes
- Long-standing hypertension
- Uraemic neuropathy
- End-stage renal failure

Who

See below.

Clinical features

- Uraemia:
  - Results from build up of nitrogenous waste normally excreted
  - Symptoms include nausea, vomiting, itching, lethargy, metabolic taste, bleeding, drowsiness, confusion, convulsions, death
  - Can lead to uraemic pericarditis and encephalopathy, which are life-threatening complications
- Poor regulation of salt and water:
  - Leads to oedema, breathlessness, hypertension.
- Symptoms:
  - Cardiopulmonary: breathlessness (anaemia), oedema, heart failure (fluid overload), pericarditis (from uraemia), arrhythmias (hyperkalaemia)
  - GI: nausea, anorexia, vomiting
  - CNS: fatigue, weakness (from anaemia), confusion, seizures, coma (from uraemia).

Investigations

- Blood tests
- Urine
- ECG:
  - Shows causes, e.g. long-standing hypertension or an MI
- Reveals complications, e.g. pericarditis, hyperkalaemia
- Imaging
- Biopsy: if no obvious cause.

Treatment

- Hyperkalaemia: calcium gluconate, insulin and dextrose (p. 503)
- Pulmonary oedema: O_2, diuretics, nitrates, opiates (p. 87)

Acute dialysis if

- Persistent hyperkalaemia
- Severe metabolic acidosis
- Persistent pulmonary oedema

- Uraemia: ↓ protein intake to ↓ nitrogenous waste
- Hypervolaemia: diuretics
- Acidosis: bicarbonate IV/orally
- Bleeding: fresh frozen plasma, platelets

- Uraemic pericarditis
- Uraemic encephalopathy.

Prognosis and complications

Complications

Life-threatening:
- Hyperkalaemia
- Pulmonary oedema
- Metabolic acidosis

- Hypertensive encephalopathy
- Uraemic encephalopathy
- Uraemic pericarditis.

ACUTE RENAL FAILURE/ACUTE KIDNEY INJURY

Outline

Reduction in GFR that occurs over hours, days or weeks and is usually reversible:
- **Medical emergency**
- Acute-on-chronic kidney failure is common.

Distinguishing prerenal from renal causes
- Prerenal: urine is concentrated as kidneys compensate for ↓ perfusion
- Renal: lose salt and water indiscriminately, as the problem is with the kidneys
- See Table 7.2

Table 7.2 Distinguishing prerenal from renal causes

	Prerenal	Renal
Urine sodium (mmol/L)	<20	>40
Urine osmolarity (mosmol/L)	>500	<350
Urine:plasma urea ratio	<20:1	<10:1

Pathogenesis/aetiology

Causes

Often multifactorial:
- Prerenal from ↓ blood flow to the kidneys:
  - Fluid loss, e.g. dehydration, burns, haemorrhage
  - ↓ Cardiac output, e.g. heart failure, MI
  - Shock
  - Renal artery obstruction, e.g. stenosis, thrombosis
  - Nephrotoxic drugs, commonly NSAIDs, ACE inhibitors, gentamicin, diuretics

- Renal from changes within the kidneys (40%):
  - Glomerular disease
  - Acute tubular necrosis
  - Ischaemia
  - Vasculitis
  - Pyelonephritis
- Postrenal from outflow obstruction:
  - Urinary tract obstruction, e.g. stones, prostatic hypertrophy
  - Renal vein thrombosis.

Who

- Any patient is at risk.

A typical patient

A 60-year-old patient, recently started on a diuretic, who has had some vomiting for 3 days and is dehydrated. On presentation, he is confused, oliguric and tachycardic. Blood tests reveal a high potassium.

Clinical features

- Often asymptomatic.

Symptoms

- Non-specific (listed under General features, above)
- Also usually oliguria, <400 mL/24 h, may be polyuria

- Acidosis: tachypnoea as a respiratory compensatory mechanism.

Investigations

Blood tests

- ↓ Hb
- ↓ Bicarbonate
- ↑ Urate
- ↑ Urea
- ↑ Potassium

- ↑ Phosphate
- ↑ Magnesium
- ↑ Creatinine >50% above baseline (altered GFR)
- ABG: metabolic acidosis with or without respiratory compensation.

Urine

- Dipstick
- Urinary urea <500 mmol/L (concentrated)

- Microscopy, culture and sensitivity

ECG

- Changes caused by ↑ potassium (wide QRS, peaked T waves, ↓ P waves)

Imaging

- CXR: pulmonary oedema in overload

- US of urinary tract to exclude obstruction.

Other tests

- Biopsy:
  - Commonest cause of acute renal failure seen in renal biopsy is renal vasculitis.

Treatment

As above for 'general features'. In addition:

Acute treatment: an emergency

- If in shock: ABC approach
- Treat pulmonary oedema and hyperkalaemia
- Monitor hourly: pulse, BP, central venous pressure and urinary output
- May need ITU input for inotropic support to maintain a BP for renal perfusion or for haemodialysis to treat life-threatening complications

- Monitor fluid balance and U&Es daily and correct (see Surgical chapter 13)
- Stop nephrotoxic drugs
- Adequate nutrition
- Establish cause and treat

Cause specific treatments:

- Bladder outflow obstruction: catheterise

- Sepsis: antibiotics, find source.

Prognosis and complications

Prognosis

- Depends on cause

- Renal function usually recovers within 2–6 weeks if cause removed.

Complications

- Sepsis: commonest cause of death

- Mortality risks as for General features, above.

CHRONIC RENAL FAILURE/CHRONIC KIDNEY DISEASE

Outline

Reduction in glomerular filtration rate (GFR) occurring over months or years that is progressive and usually irreversible:
- Commonly caused by diabetes, hypertension, glomerulonephritis.
- Long-term kidney failure gives rise to a number of complications
- Classified by GFR level (Table 7.3).
NB: Patients with CRF should be prescribed medication with care, as renal disease impairs excretion of certain drugs

Table 7.3 Classification based on GFR

Stage	GFR (mL/min)	Type of CRF
1	>90	GFR normal but evidence of kidney damage
2	60–90	Evidence of kidney damage with mild ↓ GFR
3A 3B	45–59 30–44	Moderate reduction in GFR
4	15–29	Severe reduction in GFR
5	<15	End-stage renal failure

Pathogenesis/aetiology

Causes

- Systematic causes:
  - Diabetes mellitus: commonest cause
  - Hypertension: common cause
  - Infection: HIV
  - Amyloidosis
  - Vascular disease: vasculitis
  - Malignancy: myeloma
  - Drugs: analgesics, HIV medication

- Renal specific causes:
  - Glomerular disease
  - Maldevelopment of kidney (particularly in children)
  - Inherited: autosomal dominant polycystic kidney (commonest genetic cause), Alport syndrome
  - Chronic renal ischaemia
  - Tubulo-interstitial disease: TB, multiple myeloma
- Urological causes:
  - Urinary tract obstruction: stones or prostatic hypertrophy.

Who

Incidence:
- 5% of population have an GFR of <60 mL/min (stage 3)

- 20% of those >70 years have a GFR of <60 mL/min (stage 3).

A typical patient

A 60-year-old woman with long-term diabetes and hypertension is lethargic. Her urine dipstick demonstrates protein and her GFR is 10 mL/min. On examination she has a large blood vessel that 'hums' on auscultation in her right anterior cubital fossa.

- May be asymptomatic until GFR <15 mL/min when dialysis may be needed.

Symptoms

As for General features, above. Other changes in CRF:
- General: malaise, anorexia
- Anaemia: more common in CRF because of reduction in erythropoietin, ↓ bone marrow activity, blood loss
- Bone changes: renal osteodystrophy (bone disease in CRF) includes:
  - Osteomalacia, osteosclerosis, osteoporosis from reduction in vitamin D synthesis
  - ↓ Calcium, leading to tetany (involuntary muscular contractions), cramps, spasms, 2° hyper-PTH
- Neurological: uraemic neuropathy including paraesthesia (numbness), carpal tunnel syndrome, autonomic dysfunction

- Cardiovascular disease: hypertension may lead to further vascular complications, uraemic pericarditis, heart failure
- Haematological: platelet abnormalities: bruising, bleeding
- Skin: pallor (anaemia), pruritus (uraemia), pigmentation (uraemia; causing a yellow/brown tinge to the skin.
- End-stage renal failure:
  - Volume overload
  - GI bleeds, platelet disorders, anaemia
  - Pericarditis, hypertension
  - Peripheral neuropathy
  - Abnormal immune function.

As for General features, above, plus:

Blood tests

- FBC: anaemia more common than in acute renal failure
- Haematinics: iron, ferritin, vitamin B_{12}, folate
- ↓ Calcium

- ↓ Vitamin D
- ↑ ALP
- Blood glucose: diabetes
- U&Es: ↑ potassium, urea, creatinine.

ECG

- Left ventricular hypertrophy (from hypertension), ischaemia.

Imaging

- CXR: left ventricular hypertrophy, fluid overload

- Bone scans.

Aim is to delay end-stage renal failure:
- Identify and treat cause
- As above for 'general features'
- In addition: may need long-term treatments

Additional CRF treatment:
- Anaemia: recombinant human erythropoietin
- Hypocalcaemia and hyperphosphataemia:
  - Vitamin D analogues, calcium supplements
  - Dietary restriction of phosphate
  - Phosphate-binding agents, e.g. calcium carbonate

- Hypertension: aggressive treatment in diabetic patients:
  - ACE inhibitors, caution if coexistent renal vascular disease
  - Angiotensin receptor antagonists
  - Diuretics
- Long-standing hyperkalaemia: diet restrictions
- Long-standing acidosis: sodium bicarbonate
- Dialysis: for severe symptomatic CRF
- Kidney transplant: consider transplantation if appropriate.

Prognosis

- Mortality: The majority of patients with chronic renal failure will die of renal failure or vascular complications.

- 50% of patients with CRF eventually need dialysis.

GLOMERULAR DISEASE: GLOMERULONEPHRITIS

GENERAL FEATURES

Outline

Damage to the glomerular filtering apparatus, leading to a reduction in the GFR and possibly renal failure. Damage can affect:
- any of the four layers of the glomerular structure

- part of the glomerulus (segmental) or the whole glomerulus (global)
- only some of the glomeruli (focal) or all the glomeruli (diffuse).

Classification

By presentation:
- Nephrotic: damage causes increased protein excretion
- Nephritic: damage causes blood in the urine (NB: haematuria does not equate to glomerulonephritis as there are other causes (see p. 624))

- Both: some diseases have both nephrotic and nephritic features, e.g. SLE

Pathogenesis/aetiology

Causes

- Primary:
  - Glomerular idiopathic disease
  - Hereditary: Alport syndrome, Fabry's disease

- Secondary:
  - From systemic disease: diabetes, SLE, amyloidosis, sarcoidosis, rheumatoid arthritis, bacterial endocarditis, HBV, HCV, myeloma.

Pathogenesis

Damage can be caused by:
1. Immune complex formation in situ: leading to inflammation:
   - Goodpasture's disease: against basement membrane
   - group A β-haemolytic streptococci
   - SLE
2. Immune complexes in the circulation being depositing in the glomeruli and leading to complement activation and inflammation:
   - group A β-haemolytic streptococci
   - HCV
   - lupus

3. Toxic-antibodies, causing damage without forming immune complexes
4. Cell-mediated injury: T-cell delayed type IV hypersensitivity reaction or cytotoxic T-cell reaction to target cells:
   - minimal change disease
   - focal segmental glomerulosclerosis
5. Activation of complement: bacteria stimulate complement; the by-products are deposited in the glomerulus: membranoproliferative glomerulonephritis.

Who

- 3rd commonest cause of end-stage renal disease.

Clinical features

- May be asymptomatic
- Nephrotic syndrome: proteinuria
- Nephritic syndrome: haematuria

- Hypertension
- Renal failure.

Blood tests

- FBC, U&E, LFTs, ESR, CRP
- Albumin
- Immunoglobins (for myeloma)
- Blood glucose (for diabetes)
- Antistreptolysin O titre: poststreptococcal glomerulonephritis
- HBV and HCV serology

Urine

- Dipstick: blood or protein
- Microscopy: renal casts

Imaging

- Renal US

Other tests

- Biopsy:
  - Renal sample for microscopy and immunofluorescence

- Autoantibodies:
  - ANCA
  - ANAs: lupus
  - Anti-double-stranded DNA (dsDNA): lupus
  - Anti-basement membrane: Goodpasture's disease
  - Rheumatoid factor.

- Bence Jones protein.

- CXR: Wegener's granulomatosis, Goodpasture's disease.

Nephrology referral, see below.

See below.

NEPHROTIC SYNDROME

Triad of:
- proteinuria: >3.5 g/24 h
- hypoalbuminaemia: <30 g/L
- oedema

A syndrome rather than a diagnosis and includes a range of disorders (see Nephrotic causes, below).

Other complications include:
- hyperlipidaemia
- infection
- hypercoagulability.

Causes

- Primary disease:
  - Minimal change nephropathy: commonest cause in children
  - Membranous nephropathy: commonest cause in adults

  - Focal segmental glomerulosclerosis
- Secondary causes:
  - Diabetic glomerulopathy, SLE, amyloid, hypertension, Henoch–Schönlein nephritis.

Pathogenesis/aetiology

Pathogenesis

- Proteinuria from glomerular damage, which affects filtration and allows protein to leak
- Hypoalbuminaemia from proteinuria and from ↑ catabolism of resorbed albumin in the proximal tubules
- Oedema from:
  - kidney resistance to atrial natriuretic peptide (normally would ↑ loss of water and salt from the kidneys)
  - low albumin in blood causes a low oncotic pressure, which activates the renin–angiotensin–aldosterone system and thus promotes reabsorption of water and salts

- Hypercoagulable state: loss of clotting inhibitors leads to DVTs, renal vein thrombosis
- Hyperlipidaemia from:
  - loss of apolipoproteins, which are important in lipid transport
  - ↑ albumin synthesis (to compensate for loss) requires cholesterol and triglyceride synthesis
- Infection: loss of immunoglobulins (proteinuria).

Who

- ♀ > ♂.

Clinical features

Symptoms

- Oedema: swollen ankles, genitals, ascites, face, arms, pleural effusions

- Xanthelasma: yellow plaques around eyelids from hyperlipidaemia.

Signs

- Hypertension.

Investigations

Blood tests

- Protein for proteinuria
- Serum albumin <30 g/L (can be normal because of hepatic synthesis as compensation)

- Lipids for hyperlipidaemia.

Urine

- Dipstick: proteinuria
- 24-h urinary protein

- Culture.

Imaging

To assess renal size.

Other tests

- Biopsy:
  - May be useful in some cases to confirm an underlying disease or to identify idiopathic disease. Not in children as very likely to be minimal change disease

Treatment

- Treat underlying cause:
- Bed rest
- Monitor U&E, BP, fluid balance, weight
- Oedema: fluid and salt restriction plus diuretics, e.g. furosemide

- Treat hypertension
- Proteinuria: ACE inhibitors, e.g. ramipril
- Hyperlipidaemia: statin, e.g. simvastatin
- Hypercoagulable state: anticoagulants.

Prognosis and complications

Prognosis

- Depends on histological type or 1° condition.

Complications

- CRF
- Hyperlipidaemia: atherosclerosis and cardiovascular disease
- Osteomalacia: loss of vitamin D
- Hypoalbuminaemia: muscle wasting, broken down to reuse albumin.

Renal vein thrombosis

- A possible complication
- Deterioration in renal function
- Loin pain
- Haematuria
- Enlarged kidney

NEPHRITIC SYNDROME

Outline

A syndrome, not a diagnosis: includes a range of disorders (see Nephritic causes, below). Combination of:
- haematuria
- proteinuria
- hypertension
- oedema
- oliguria
- uraemia

Rapid progressive glomerulonephritis:
- Nephritic disease following severe injury, renal failure can follow in weeks. May be caused by:
  - immune complex deposition
  - autoantibodies against neutrophil cytoplasmic antigens
  - autoantibodies against glomerular basement membrane.

Pathogenesis/aetiology

Causes

- Primary disease: IgA nephropathy (Berger's disease).
- Secondary disease:
  - Postinfectious streptococcal glomerulonephritis
  - SLE
  - Cryoglobulinaemia
- Goodpasture's disease
- Systemic vasculitis: Wegener's granulomatosis, Henoch–Schönlein pupura, microscopic polyarteritis
- Infection.

Who

- Depends on cause.

Clinical features

- Hypertension
- Oedema
- Oliguria or anuria
- Symptoms of uraemia
- Haematuria.

Investigations

Blood tests

- U&Es
- Creatinine clearance
- Serum albumin
- Blood glucose
- ANCA
- Infection screen.

Urine

- Dipstick: haematuria, proteinuria (proteinuria (<2 g/ 24 h; less than nephrotic syndrome)
- Culture
- Microscopy.

Imaging

- CXR

Other tests

- Renal biopsy.

Treatment

- Treat cause
- Treat hypertension with ACE inhibitors.
- DVT prophylaxis for prothrombotic state.

Prognosis and complications

Complications

- Renal failure
- Pulmonary oedema
- Hypertensive encephalopathy.

DISORDERS LEADING TO NEPHROTIC SYNDROME (SEE ABOVE)

MINIMAL CHANGE DISEASE

Outline

- Nephrotic syndrome with little change apparent on light microscopy.

Pathogenesis/aetiology

Causes

- Idiopathic (most common)
- Medication: NSAIDs
- Malignancy: lymphoma
- Food allergy.

Pathogenesis

- Thought to be caused by a disorder of T-cells leading to cytokine release that affects the podocytes of the glomerulus and, therefore, filtration.

Who

- Typical age: peaks at 2–3 years
- ♀ < ♂
- Commonest cause of nephrotic syndrome in children (90%) but also affects adults (20% of nephrotic cases).

Clinical features

- Symptoms of nephrotic syndrome (proteinuria, oedema, hypoalbuminaemia)
- May be haematuria.

Investigations

- Biopsy:
  - Light microscopy of renal biopsy shows minimal or no change but electron microscopy shows podocyte fusion.

Treatment

May resolve without treatment:
- Steroids
- Immunosuppressant therapy: cyclophosphamide, ciclosporin.

Prognosis

- Children:
  - 95% resolve with steroids; one third do not relapse; one third have regular relapses
- Adults:
  - 70% resolve with steroids; more likely to relapse.

Complications

- Renal failure in 1%.

FOCAL SEGMENTAL GLOMERULOSCLEROSIS

Outline

- Nephrotic syndrome where only some glomeruli are affected (focal) and only part of the glomerulus itself (segmental) is involved, leading to scarring of the kidney (glomerulosclerosis).

Pathogenesis/aetiology

Causes

- Primary disease: idiopathic
- Secondary disease:
  - IgA nephropathy
  - Alport syndrome
  - Obesity
- Heroin use
- HIV
- Ureteric reflux
- Vasculitis.

Pathogenesis

- Hypertension and hyperfiltration may be important.

Who

- 10% of nephrotic cases in children, 30% in adults.

Clinical features

- Symptoms of nephrotic syndrome
- Hypertension
- Impairment of renal function.

Investigations

- Biopsy:
  - Some glomeruli are partly sclerosed
- IgM and C3 may be found in mesangium and sclerotic areas under immunofluorescence.

Treatment

- Steroids: effective in 30%
- Immunosuppressant therapy: cyclophosphamide, ciclosporin
- Dialysis
- Renal transplant
- Treat underlying cause.

Prognosis and complications

Prognosis

- Majority develop end-stage renal failure within 10 years.

Complications

- Can recur after renal transplantation.

MEMBRANOUS GLOMERULONEPHRITIS

Outline

A slowly progressive nephrotic syndrome from inflammation of the glomerulus from immune complex deposition:
- Most immune complexes are formed in situ

- Affects the basement membrane but not the mesangium (membranoproliferative glomerulonephritis affects both).

Pathogenesis/aetiology

Causes

- Primary disease: idiopathic (85%)
- Secondary disease:
  - Infection: HBV, *Streptococcus viridans*, malaria, mumps, syphilis
  - Malignancy: melanoma, lymphoma, lung cancer

- Autoimmune: thyroid disease, SLE, rheumatoid arthritis
- Complement abnormalities
- Drugs: penicillamine, gold, heroin.

Pathogenesis

- Thickened glomerular capillary wall where immune complexes and complement are deposited on the basement membrane; complexes can form in situ following antigen trapping.

Who

- Typical age: 30–50 years
- ♀ < ♂

- Makes up 30–50% of nephrotic cases in adults and 2–5% in children.

Genetics

- HLA-DR3

- HLA-DR2 in Japanese.

Clinical features

- Symptoms of nephrotic syndrome (80%)
- Nephritic symptoms (35–50%)

- Hypertension.

Investigations

- Biopsy:
  - Thick basement membrane; silver stain shows many tiny spikes on the epithelial aspect of the basement membrane.

Treatment

- Steroids
- Immunosuppressant therapy: cyclophosphamide, ciclosporin, chlorambucil

- Dialysis and transplant for renal failure
- Treat underlying cause.

Prognosis and complications

Prognosis

- 30% remission, 25% partial remission, 25% slow progression, 20% end-stage renal failure

- Younger, female patients do best.

Complications

- Renal vein thrombosis.

ALPORT SYNDROME

Outline

- Genetic disease characterised by glomerulonephritis and deafness
- Ocular defects may also occur.

Pathogenesis/aetiology

Causes

- X linked (85%)
- Also autosomal inheritance
- Mutation of *COL4A*, encoding part of type IV collagen.

Pathogenesis

- Abnormal collagen IV of the basement membrane of the kidneys, inner ears and eyes
- Can lead to end-stage renal disease.

Who

- ♀ < ♂
- Prevalence 1:5000.

Clinical features

- Kidneys: haematuria
- Ears: sensorineural deafness
- Eyes:
  - Cataracts
  - Conical cornea
  - Lenticonus: bulging of the lens on examination.

Investigations

Urine

- Haematuria
- Proteinuria.

Imaging

- Initially normal, later small kidneys.

Other tests

- Biopsy:
  - Skin: structural abnormalities of collagen
  - Renal.

Treatment

- ACE inhibitor for proteinuria
- Dialysis and transplantation for renal failure.

Prognosis and complications

Prognosis

- Better in females.

IGA NEPHROPATHY/BERGER'S DISEASE

Outline

Nephritic syndrome from deposition of IgA antibody in the kidney leading to inflammation:
- Slowly progressive

- Henoch–Schönlein purpura also involves deposition of IgA and can be considered a systemic version of Berger's disease.

Pathogenesis/aetiology

Pathogenesis

- Mesangial deposits of IgA in the basement membrane; inflammatory response leads to glomerulosclerosis
- Unknown aetiology.

Who

- Typical age: older children and young adults
- ♀ > ♂

- Commonest form of glomerulonephritis world wide
- Associated with HLA-DR4.

Clinical features

Symptoms often begin 1–2 days after a respiratory tract infection:
- Haematuria

- Hypertension
- Symptoms and signs of nephritic syndrome.

Investigations

Blood tests

- ↑ IgA

Urine

- Proteinuria

- Haematuria.

Other tests

- Biopsy:
  - Renal mesangial proliferation with IgA and C3 deposits in mesangium.

Treatment

- Steroids
- Immunosuppressants: cyclophosphamide

- ACE inhibitors.

Prognosis and complications

Prognosis

- Worse in males

- Generally good.

Complications

- Renal failure in 25% after 30 years.

GOODPASTURE'S DISEASE

Outline

- Autoimmune disease causing lung haemorrhage and glomerulonephritis (nephritic syndrome): remember by **Good**pasture's: **g**loberulonephrits and **p**neumonitis).

Pathogenesis/aetiology

Pathogenesis

From autoantibodies (IgG) against Goodpasture antigens of the basement membrane of the glomerulus, and of the lung alveoli:
- Antigen is part of non-collagenous domain of α_1 or α_3 chain of collagen IV

- Trigger unknown though often follows a viral infection
- Classic type II hypersensitivity reaction.

Who

- ♀ < ♂
Associations:
- Autoimmune disease
- HLA-DR2 in 65%

A typical patient

A patient recovering from a viral infection begins to cough up blood. There are opacities on his CXR.

- Dry cough
- Dyspnoea
- Loss of appetite
- Nausea
- High BP
- Oedema
- Haemoptysis in 50% (from lung haemorrhage)
- Haematuria: from glomerulonephritis.

Investigations

Bloods tests

- FBC: iron-deficiency anaemia
- Basement membrane antibodies.

Imaging

- CXR shows infiltrates from pulmonary haemorrhage, usually in the lower zones.

Other tests

- Biopsy:
  - Renal or lung biopsy: diagnostic
- Renal biopsy: shows crescents with inflammatory cell infiltrate, linear staining on direct immunofluorescence.

Treatment

Medical

- Treat shock
- Plasma exchange: to remove antibodies
- Immunosuppressants: to ↓ immune response

Surgical

- Transplant only when in remission.

Prognosis and complications

Prognosis

- Poor, usually fatal if untreated
- Better prognosis if creatinine <500 mL/min or <50% crescents on biopsy.

POSTSTREPTOCOCCAL GLOMERULONEPHRITIS

Outline

Glomerular disease causing nephritic syndrome 1–3 weeks after infection with group A β-haemolytic streptococcal infection.

Pathogenesis/aetiology

Pathogenesis

- Immune complexes develop and deposit in the glomerulus (IgG) throughout the kidney
- Leads to inflammation and complement activation that can cause kidney damage.

Who

- Typical age: occurs in children/adolescents
- Rarer in developed countries.

Clinical features

- 1–2 weeks after a streptococcal skin or throat infection
- Symptoms and signs of nephritic syndrome.

Investigations

Blood tests

- ↑ Anti-streptolysin O titre (exotoxin from the bacteria)
- Anti-DNAseB
- Anti-hyaluronidase
- Complement: ↓ C3
- ↓ GFR.

(see below)

Investigations

Urine

- Dipstick: proteinuria, haematuria.

Other tests

- Biopsy:
  - Renal biopsy, rarely necessary, would show:
    - diffuse inflammation
    - granular IgG and C3 glomerular deposits.

Treatment

- Antibiotics for infection.

Prognosis and complications

Prognosis

- Children: excellent
- 60% adults recover.

Complications

- 40% of adults develop hypertension and renal failure.

TUBULAR DISEASE

RENAL TUBULAR ACIDOSIS

Outline

- Metabolic acidosis from a failure to correctly acidify the urine.

Classification

- *Type 1*: distal tubule failure to excrete hydrogen ions
- *Type 2*: proximal tubule failure to reabsorb bicarbonate; can be isolated or part of Fanconi syndrome (see below)
- *Type 3*: mixture of types 1 and 2
- *Type 4*: ↓ ammonium excretion in the distal tubules due to hypoaldosteronism; results in hyperkalaemia.

Pathogenesis/aetiology

Causes

Type 1:
- Idiopathic
- Autoimmune: SLE
- Genetic: Marfan syndrome

Type 2:
- Idiopathic
- Fanconi syndrome
- Wilson's disease
- Tubulointerstitial disease, e.g. myeloma

Type 4: hypoaldosteronism or aldosterone resistance.

Who

- All rare
- Type 4 > type 1 > type 2.

Clinical features

Symptoms and signs of metabolic acidosis

Type 1:
- Rickets or osteomalacia: from ↓ calcium as it is used to buffer hydrogen ions
- Renal calculi

- Symptoms and signs of hypokalaemia

Type 2: symptoms and signs of hypokalaemia

Type 4: symptoms and signs of hyperkalaemia.

Investigations

Type 1:
- Hypokalaemia
- Hyperchloraemia

- Metabolic acidosis
- Urine pH >5.5

Type 2:
- Hypokalaemia
- Hyperchloraemia
- Mild metabolic acidosis

Type 4:
- Hyperkalaemia
- Mild acidosis
- Plasma renin low
- ↓ Plasma aldosterone.

Type 1: sodium bicarbonate orally
Type 2: sodium bicarbonate orally
Type 4:
- Fludrocortisone (a mineralocorticoid to compensate for hypoaldosteronism)

- Diuretics: for hyporeninaemic hypoaldosteronism
- Calcium resonium if hyperkalaemia
- Treat cause.

- Depends on cause.

- Stones are a complication of type 1 disease: because of the hypercalciuria (stONEs for type ONE).

FANCONI SYNDROME

- Impaired proximal tubular function leading to ↓ reabsorption of glucose, amino acids, uric acid, potassium, sodium, phosphate and bicarbonate; as a result they are excreted into the urine

- Leads to renal tubular acidosis type 2.

- Idiopathic (may be inherited)
- Inherited:
  - Cystinosis, the accumulation of the amino acid cysteine
  - Wilson's disease

- Acquired: tubule damage from:
  - Heavy metal poisoning
  - Drugs
  - Renal disease.

- Commonest in children (6–9 months)

- Also occurs in adults.

- Polyuria: from osmotic diuresis
- Dehydration and thirst
- Vomiting
- Failure to thrive in children

- Symptoms and signs of hypokalaemia
- Low phosphate: hypophosphataemic rickets in children, osteomalacia in adults
- Low bicarbonate: renal tubular acidosis.

- Glucose
- Amino acids
- Uric acid

- Potassium, sodium
- Phosphate
- Bicarbonate.

Treatment

- Treat underlying cause
- Bone disease: vitamin D
- Correct fluid and electrolyte loss
- Genetic counselling where relevant.

Prognosis and complications

Prognosis

- Depends on cause
- Worse in inherited disease.

Complications

- CRF.

ACUTE TUBULAR NECROSIS

Outline

- Necrosis of the tubular cells of the kidney from ischaemia or toxins, which leads to a fall in GFR through haemodynamic changes, obstruction or back leak
- May get hyperkalaemia from failure to excrete potassium.

Pathogenesis/aetiology

Causes

- Ischaemic:
  - Trauma
  - Sepsis
  - Hypotension
  - Hypovolaemia: shock, dehydration, vomiting, diarrhoea
- Toxic:
  - Gentamicin, lead, gold
  - NSAIDs: prevent synthesis of prostaglandins, which protect the kidney from ischaemia by stimulating vasodilation.

Pathogenesis

- Ischaemia leads to hypoperfusion of renal cortex and necrosis
- Toxic substances cause tubular cells to detach and collect in the lumen of the tubules causing obstruction; regeneration of the tubules usually occurs.

Who

- Common cause of acute renal failure.

Clinical features

- Presents as acute renal failure: oliguria or polyuria.

Investigations

Blood tests

- ↑ Creatinine
- ↓ Sodium
- ↑ Potassium
- Metabolic acidosis.

Other tests

- Urinalysis
- Renal US: to exclude obstruction
- Renal biopsy.

Treatment

- Fluid and electrolyte correction
- Dialysis if needed.

Prognosis

- 50% mortality, depending on speed of treatment and cause

- Recovery of renal function in 1–3 weeks if 1° cause reversed.

Complications

- Hyperkalaemia can trigger cardiac arrhythmias.

TUBULOINTERSTITIAL NEPHRITIS

Outline

Inflammation of the kidneys affecting the tubules and interstitium surrounding the tubules:

- Normally occurs 2–40 days after ingestion of toxin
- Leads to fibrosis and tubular loss.

Classification

- Acute: usually from a hypersensitivity reaction (T-cell response) to drugs (commonest cause), infection or immune disorder

- Chronic: usually from an underlying disorder or large amounts of analgesics.

Pathogenesis/aetiology

Causes

- Acute:
  - Analgesia: NSAIDs
  - Antibiotics: penicillin, gentamicin, rifampicin, sulphonamides,
  - Diuretics: furosemide, thiazide
  - Heavy metals: mercury, lead, gold
  - Others: allopurinol, phenytoin
  - Infection: staphylococci, streptococci
  - Immune disorders: SLE

- Chronic:
  - Underlying disorder: pyelonephritis, diabetes mellitus, sickle cell
  - Large consumption of analgesics: chronic NSAID use inhibits synthesis of prostaglandins, which are important for vasodilation; leads to ischaemia and necrosis.

Who

- Primary tubulointerstitial disease: accounts for 10–15% of renal disease worldwide.

Clinical features

- Acute:
  - Fever
  - Skin rash
  - Eosinophilia, eosinophiluria
  - Haematuria
  - Proteinuria
  - Acute renal failure

- Chronic:
  - Polyuria
  - Proteinuria
  - Nocturia
  - Uraemia
  - Ureteric colic
  - CRF.

Investigations

Blood tests

↑ Urea and creatinine.

Urine

- Proteinuria
- Haematuria

- RBC casts.

Other tests

- Special tests:
  - Intravenous urogram (IVU): cortical scarring

- Renal biopsy.

Treatment

- Manage renal failure
- Supportive

- If cause is medication, stop the drug and use appropriate alternative
- Dialysis and transplant for end-stage renal disease.

Prognosis and complications

Prognosis

- Good.

Complications

- Chronic disease can lead to transitional cell carcinoma.

CONGENITAL KIDNEY DISEASE

ADULT POLYCYSTIC KIDNEY DISEASE

Outline

- An inherited disease where multiple cysts develop in both kidneys in adults, replacing normal tissue and leading to renal failure.

Pathogenesis/aetiology

Causes

- Autosomal dominant disease
- 50% results from new mutations

- Three genes involved that alter tubular epithelium growth:
  - *PKD1* on chromosome 16 (85% of cases)
  - *PKD2* on chromosome 4 (10% of cases)
  - *PKD3*, unmapped.

Pathogenesis

- Cysts can develop anywhere in the kidney
- Cysts increase in size slowly over years, leading to renal enlargement and destruction of normal kidney function

- Cysts can also develop in the pancreas, ovary, liver, lungs, spleen (remember POLLS)
- Hypertension develops, which leads to many of the complications.

Who

- Typical age: 30–50 years

- Prevalence 1:1000 (commonest inherited renal disease).

Clinical features

Symptoms

- Renal:
  - Initially asymptomatic
  - Hypertension
  - Large, palpable kidneys
  - Abdominal and back pain from renal enlargement
  - Haematuria
  - Urinary tract infections
  - Kidney stones
  - Symptoms and signs of CRF

- General:
  - Berry aneurysm in 10–20% of patients resulting from weak arteries and ↑ BP: risk of subarachnoid haemorrhage
  - Mitral valve prolapse
  - Hepatomegaly (liver cysts).

Imaging

US or CT:
- Large irregular kidneys
- Multiple cysts in kidneys

- Enlarged kidneys bilaterally
- Subarachnoid haemorrhage.

Treatment

- Monitor and control BP
- Monitor U&Es
- Treat urinary infections

- Dialysis or transplantation for CRF
- Genetic counselling and screening.

Prognosis and complications

Prognosis

- Cysts will enlarge and eventually dialysis or transplant may be needed.

Complications

- Polycythaemia
- Renal failure in 50% (accounts for 8–10% of CRF)

- Renal cell carcinoma (rare)
- Subarachnoid haemorrhage.

INFANTILE POLYCYSTIC KIDNEY DISEASE

Outline

- An inherited disease in infants where multiple cysts develop throughout both kidneys, replacing normal tissue

- Leads to chronic hepatic fibrosis, portal hypertension and early death.

Pathogenesis/aetiology

- Autosomal recessive disease, with a mutation affecting chromosome 6.

Who

- Rare: 1: 40 000.

Clinical features

- Palpable mass of enlarged kidneys (>12 times normal size)

- Signs of liver disease
- Stillbirth.

Investigations

Imaging

- US.

Treatment

- Manage respiratory failure, hypertension, respiratory problems.

Prognosis and complications

Prognosis

- More severe than adult disease, with most dying within 2 months

- Death is from renal or respiratory failure in neonates.

LOWER URINARY TRACT DISORDERS

RENAL CALCULI

Outline

Normally soluble material crystallises and forms stones in the collecting ducts:

- Stones are deposited in the urinary tract and can move and impact, commonly at the pelviureteric or vesicoureteric junctions, which can lead to obstruction and severe pain
- Calcium stones (calcium phosphate or oxalate) most common (80%), radiopaque

- Also from uric acid, struvite (magnesium aluminium phosphate, mostly from infection) and cysteine
- Staghorn calculus is where the stone takes the shape of the pelvis and branches into the calyces like a stag's antlers:
  - Common in stones induced by infection
  - Most commonly in struvite stones.

Pathogenesis/aetiology

Causes

A high concentration of solutes supersaturates urine and crystallises due to:

- Increase in urinary solutes:
  - ↑ Calcium: dietary, ↑ vitamin D, hyperparathyroidism
  - ↑ Urea or uric acid: gout and urinary infections
  - ↑ Oxalate: dietary (chocolate, tea), ↑ absorption (from small bowel disease)
  - ↑ Cysteine: cysteinuria (autosomal recessive condition)

- ↑ Struvite: from infection
- Abnormal tubular function
- Acid–base imbalance: alkaline urine favours calcium phosphate precipitation, acidic urine favours the precipitation of urate
- Decrease in urinary fluid: dehydration, which is common in warm climates
- Certain drugs: loop diuretics, antacids, steroids.

Who

- Typical age: 30–40 years
- 1♀:2♂

- Common: prevalence 2%.

A typical patient

A 40-year-old man presents to A&E with severe pain that radiates from the loin to the groin. The pain occurs in waves and causes him to writhe. Urine dip shows evidence of haematuria.

Clinical features

- Mostly asymptomatic
- Renal colic: severe loin to groin pain that occurs in waves because of peristalsis and dilatation proximal to obstruction
- Haematuria (90%): if no blood on dipstick unlikely to be a renal stone

- Nausea and vomiting
- May present with symptoms of infection
- May present with urinary obstructive symptoms if there is a urethral stone.

Blood tests

U&Es: calcium, urea, bicarbonate.

Urine

- Dipstick: haematuria
- pH
- Chemical analysis of stone passed
- Culture.

Imaging

- Plain KUB: 90% of calculi are radiopaque (as most contain calcium; Fig. 7.3)
  NB: 90% of gallstones are translucent
- CT kidneys, ureters, bladder to assess size of stone, site and amount of obstruction. Most common investigation
- intravenous urogram: demonstrates site and amount of obstruction.

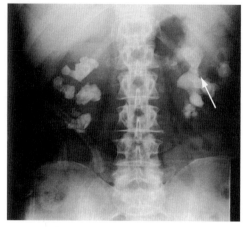

Fig. 7.3 Plain KUB showing staghorn calculus in the renal pelvis (arrow).

- Analgesic: NSAIDs (particularly diclofenac) or opiates
- Fluids
- Intervene if persistent pain, infection or obstruction
- Calculi <5 mm diameter will mostly pass spontaneously: discharge with pain relief
- Larger stone can lead to obstruction or infection:
  - Refer to urologist
  - Antibiotics if infection
- Stone removal:
  - Smaller stones: extracorporeal shock wave lithotripsy (ESWL) to break up the stone so it can pass
  - Larger stones: percutaneous nephrolithotomy (a needle is inserted through the skin to remove the stone) or open surgery
- Prevention of recurrence:
  - ↑ Fluid
  - ↓ Dietary sources.

Prognosis

- Good: either by passing the stone naturally or with intervention
- Recurrence rate is 50% within 5 years.

Complications

- Infection proximal to an obstructive stone: urosepsis, pyelonephritis
- Urinary fistula
- Abscess formation.

URINARY RETENTION

Outline

- Inability to urinate as a result of obstruction or ↓ detrusor power, which can lead to renal failure from rise in back pressure
- **An emergency if anuric**

- Obstruction can be partial or complete:
  - An emergency if complete
  - Often reversible
  - Can occur suddenly or gradually, depending on cause.

Detrusor muscle
Found in the bladder, this muscle contracts on parasympathetic nerve stimulation leading to release of urine. Sympathetic nervous stimulation stimulates detrusor relaxation, preventing loss of urine.

Pathogenesis/aetiology

Causes

Obstruction:
- Luminal:
  - Stones
  - Thrombosis
  - Tumour
- Mural:
  - Stricture
  - Neuromuscular dysfunction

- Extramural:
  - Abdominal or pelvic tumour
  - Pregnancy
  - Prostate: hypertrophy (commonest cause in men), cancer, faecal impaction
  - Phimosis
Detrusor failure:
- Rectal and orthopaedic surgery
- Diabetes mellitus
- CNS disease
- Anticholinergic drugs.

Pathogenesis

- Complete obstruction results in dilatation above the obstruction; can lead to hydronephrosis dilatation, distension of the renal pelvis and renal failure.

Who

- Common: ♀ < ♂ in the elderly.

Clinical features

Symptoms

- Hesitancy
- Poor stream
- Intermittent flow, postmicturition dribbling
- Incomplete emptying
- Anuria
- Overflow incontinence
- Irritative:
  - Frequency
  - Urgency
  - Nocturia

- Discomfort: intense desire to urinate if has occurred suddenly
- Location-specific symptoms and signs of obstruction:
  - Upper tract: loin pain, tenderness, enlarged kidney, anuria or polyuria (in partial obstruction from impaired renal function)
  - Lower tract: oliguria, suprapubic pain, palpable distended bladder, dull on percussion, leading to overflow incontinence and infection; may feel an enlarged prostate on rectal examination.

- Rectal examination
- Neurological examination.

Blood tests

- U&Es: impaired
- Prostate-specific antigen (PSA) to rule out prostate cancer.

Urine

Midstream specimen:
- Dipstick
- Microscopy, culture and sensitivity.

Imaging

- US
- Intravenous urogram (Fig. 7.4)
- CT.

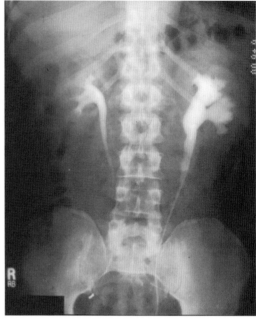

Fig. 7.4   Intravenous urogram showing dilated collecting system.

General

- Treat underlying cause
- Monitor weight, fluid balance, electrolytes

- Catheterise: if lower tract problem (flush if already catheterised)

Medical

- Alpha blockers for decreased detrusor power to relax the sphincters: alfuzosin, tamsulosin

Surgical/interventional radiology

- *Nephrostomy:* To relieve hydronephrosis. Urine drained directly from the skin into a bag from an artificial opening created between the kidneys and the skin surface

- Surgical intervention as appropriate for benign prostatic hyperplasia, strictures or stones

Prognosis

- Depends on cause. Worse prognosis if: complete obstruction, for long periods of time.

Complications

- Hydronephrosis: distention and dilation of renal pelvis
- UTI from stasis
- Bladder calculi

- Renal failure
- Bladder rupture: very rare.

URINARY INCONTINENCE

GENERAL FEATURES

Outline

- Demonstrable involuntary loss of urine.

Classification

- *Stress incontinence*: involuntary leakage of urine because of incompetent sphincter or loss of pelvic floor support (see below)
- *Urgency incontinence*: involuntary leakage of urine from urinary urgency (see below)
- *Mixed incontinence*: mixture of urgency and stress incontinence
- *Overflow incontinence*: leakage of a small volume of urine from an overfull bladder. Renal damage may develop if high intravesicular pressures persist. Mostly results from outflow obstruction but occasionally to detrusor failure

- *Functional incontinence*: incontinence caused by a coexistent physiological cause
- *Total incontinence*: continuous, passive loss of urine with no control; causes:
  - Congenital
  - Vesicovaginal fistulae
  - Paraplegia.

Pathogenesis/aetiology

Causes

- Depends on type
- Stress incontinence: see below
- Urgency incontinence: see below
- Functional incontinence: restricted mobility, difficulty in getting to the toilet on time

- Overflow incontinence: enlarged prostate (main cause in men)
- Drugs: diuretics, calcium channel blockers, α-adrenoreceptor antagonists (relaxes urethral sphincter), NSAIDs (fluid retention), acetylcholinergics.

Pathogenesis

- Parasympathetic nerve stimulation controls detrusor muscle contraction in the bladder, leading to release of urine.
- Sympathetic nervous stimulation stimulates detrusor relaxation and sphincter contraction, which prevents loss of urine.

- Anything interfering with the higher brain control, nervous coordination or muscular control can cause incontinence.

Who

- ♀ > ♂; occurs in 25% women
- Occurs in men later in life

- More likely if in institutional care
- 4% of elderly are also faecally incontinent.

Clinical features

- Involuntary loss of urine
- Frequency
- Hesitancy
- Urgency
- Poor stream: outflow obstruction or bladder problem

- Postmicturition dribbling
- Feeling of incomplete emptying
- Continual urine loss: suggests a fistula
- Faecal incontinence.

Investigations

Clinical examination

- Abdominal palpation: large bladder due to retention
- Neurological examination of legs

- Rectal examination to exclude faecal loading
- Frequency volume chart.

Urine

- Culture: exclude infection

- Cystometry and urine flow rate: reserved for specialist assessment.

Treatment

- Depends on cause.

General

- Fluid intake advice: ↓ caffeine, ↓ alcohol, appropriate daily fluid intake

- Toileting regimen: maintain bladder volume below that which triggers emptying.

Specific treatment

- Stress incontinence: see below
- Urgency incontinence: see below
- Functional incontinence: maximise toilet access

- Overflow incontinence: catheterisation can identify if this is the problem and treat cause.

Prognosis and complications

Complications

- Renal failure from back flow problems. Only an issue in the face of spinal cord injury and very occasionally in men with nocturnal enuresis.

STRESS INCONTINENCE

Outline

Involuntary leakage of urine as a result of:
- an incompetent sphincter or loss of pelvic floor support

- the rise in intra-abdominal pressure following exertion.

Pathogenesis/aetiology

Causes

- Pelvic floor weakness (33%): particularly in multiparous women

- Sphincter damage: possibly after surgery
- Prolapse of urogenital prolapse and bladder.

Who

Increased prevalence with ↑ age and with obesity:
- Common in pregnancy, after birth, postmenopausal women

- In men after prostatectomy.

Clinical features

- Loss of small volume of urine on coughing, laughing, posture change

- Sense of prolapse.

Investigations

Clinical examination

- Examine for prolapse

- Cough test: cough when standing up with a full bladder.

Treatment

Conservative

- Pelvic floor exercises
- ↓ Weight
- Ring pessary: plastic ring inserted into the vagina to support pelvic organs (for prolapse, not for SUI).

- Intravaginal electrical stimulation: stimulates the pelvic floor muscles to make them stronger.

Medical

- Duloxetine: (side effect nausea)

- Oestrogen creams if postmenopausal (for vaginal Sx associated with urogenital atrophy, not for incontinence).

Surgical

- Tension-free vaginal tape inserted under the urethra to support it
- Colposuspension: sutures each side of vagina to lift the bladder and urethra

- Injectable bulking substance such as collagen injected around the urethra.

Prognosis and complications

Prognosis

- Pelvic floor exercises can cure in 70% in the short term (>4 months therapy needed) but longer-term relapse is high

- Midurethral tapes: 80–90% effective for up to 10 years.

URGENCY INCONTINENCE

Outline

Involuntary leakage of urine preceded by urinary urgency:
- Socially disabling

- Worse than stress incontinence: one third are incontinent ('wet'), two thirds of patients only experience the symptoms of urgency

Pathogenesis/aetiology

Causes

Detrusor instability:
- Primary: exact pathogenesis unknown; other urological causes (infection, stones, tumour) need to be excluded before the diagnosis is made
- Secondary to local causes: infection, stones

- Secondary to brain damage: e.g. spinal cord injury, brainstem damage leading to malcoordination, multiple sclerosis, head injury, dementia, Parkinson's disease, stroke, multiple system atrophy.

Who

- ♀ > ♂, except in very late life

- Increasingly common with increased age.

Clinical features

- Often associated with troublesome frequency and nocturia.

Investigations

Neurological examination

- Spinal cord and CNS.

Treatment

Conservative

- Bladder retraining
- ↓ Caffeine, ↓ night fluid

- Regular voiding before actually needing to go.

Medical

- Anti-acetylcholinergics, e.g. oxybutynin, tolterodine
- Intravaginal oestrogens (see above)

- Antibiotics for infection.

Treatment

Surgical

- Intradetrusor botulinum injections: blocks acetylcholine at the neuromuscular junction
- Sacral nerve stimulation

- 'Clam' ileocystoplasty: bowel sutured into the bladder to interrupt unstable bladder contractions.

Prognosis and complications

Prognosis

- Condition waxes and wanes

- Patients may do well with behavioural techniques only but older people are more likely to need medication.

INFECTION

URINARY TRACT INFECTION

Outline

Defined as $>10^5$ colony-forming units (cfu)/mL of pure growth microorganism cultured from the urine:
- 10^2 cfu/mL can be symptomatic.

Classification

- Urethra: urethritis
- Bladder: cystitis
- Prostate: prostatitis
- Kidney, pyelonephritis: bacteria usually start in the urethra and ascend to the kidneys; can be acute or chronic (from long-standing or recurrent infection)

- Uncomplicated: normal tract and function
- Complicated: abnormal tract or function
- Sterile pyuria:
  - Urine with pus; causes:
    - kidney stones
    - partially treated UTI
    - TB of the urinary tract
    - malignancy.

Pathogenesis/aetiology

Infection often from patient's own bowel flora or skin organisms, which normally enter transurethrally: sexual intercourse and catheterisation facilitate this
- *Escherichia coli*: commonest (60–90%)
- Staphylococci

- Enterobacteriaceae
- Enterococci
- *Proteus* spp. (10%): associated with stone formation
- *Klebsiella* sp.

Predisposing factors

- Increased chance of bacterial invasion:
  - Females more than males: they have a short urethra close to the anus
  - Sexual intercourse
  - Bladder catheterisation

- Increased chance of infection:
  - Diabetes mellitus
  - Pregnancy: common complication (6%), if left untreated 20% develop acute pyelonephritis
  - Obstruction
  - Stones
  - Poor bladder emptying
  - An abnormal urinary tract.

Who

- Very common
- ♀ > ♂.

Epidemiology

- Females have a 35% lifetime risk
- Rarer in males and children, so needs investigating.

A typical patient

A pregnant woman presents to her GP with dysuria, and ↑ urinary frequency. Urine dip is positive for leukocyte esterase and nitrites.

Clinical features

Symptoms of infection:
- Frequency
- Urgency
- Dysuria
- Nocturia
- Haematuria
- Suprapubic pain and tenderness
- Fever.

- Cystitis:
  - Haematuria, suprapubic pain, dysuria, nocturia
- Prostatitis:
  - Backache, tender prostate on rectal examination
- Pyelonephritis:
  - Loin pain, fever, rigors, vomiting, tenderness, oliguria, weight loss, smelly urine, ↑ frequency, systemic symptoms

Symptoms in the elderly:
- Often atypical
- Confusion/delirium: always investigate in an elderly person presenting with acute onset confusion
- Incontinence
- Falls.

Investigations

Blood tests

- FBC: ↑ WBC
- ↑ CRP
- U&Es: renal function.

Urine

- Dipstick test:
  - **Leukocyte esterase**
  - **Nitrites**
  - Proteinuria
  - Haematuria
- Microscopy, culture and sensitivity.

Imaging

Indicated for single UTI in men and children and repeated infections in women
- KUB
- US

- CT kidneys, ureters, bladder
- Micturating cystogram: for vesicoureteric reflux, bladder and urethral tract abnormalities.

Treatment

- Oral antibiotics: trimethoprim, nitrofurantoin for 3–5 days, if abnormal tract for 5–10 days
- Cystitis: trimethoprim, ciprofloxacin
- Prostatitis: ciprofloxacin

- Modify antibiotic according to culture results
- High fluid uptake
- Follow up microscopy and culture to ensure treatment is complete

Acute pyelonephritis
Admit for IV fluids and antibiotics: cefuroxime, IV then oral (7 days).

Prevention
Women with recurrent infection:
- Prophylactic antibiotics 6–12 months
- ↑ Fluid intake

- Double voiding
- Void after intercourse.

Prognosis and complications

Prognosis

- If uncomplicated, good prognosis with rapid investigation and treatment.

Complications

- More common in those with complicated infections: renal papillary necrosis, renal abscess

- Pyelonephritis can lead to: urosepsis, pyonephrosis (pus around the kidney) and death.

URINARY TRACT CANCER

RENAL CELL CARCINOMA

Outline

- Cancer of the kidneys (also called hypernephroma and Grawitz tumour).

- Tumours are solitary, multiple or bilateral.

Pathogenesis/aetiology

Pathogenesis

- Cancer arises from the kidney lining
- Rounded, well demarcated mass
- Commoner in the upper pole

- Usually clear cell type: name comes from the cellular accumulation of fat and glycogen, which is lost in the histological preparation, resulting in clear cells.

Who

- Commonest renal tumour in adults
- Typical age: >50 years
- 1♀:2♂

Risk factors:
- Smoking
- Haemodialysis
- Genetic: von Hippel–Lindau syndrome (rare autosomal dominant disease).

Clinical features

- Haematuria
- Loin pain
- Flank mass
- Anaemia
- Left-sided varicocoele (rare) (enlargement of scrotal vein from obstruction of the renal vein)

- Symptoms of cancer: malaise, weight loss.
- Paraneoplastic syndromes:
  - Hypercalcaemia
  - Polycythaemia: from ↑ erythropoietin production, leads to hypertension.

Investigations

Bloods tests

- FBC: polycythaemia
- U&Es: ↑ Calcium
- ALP: ↑ if bone metastases.

Urine

- Dipstick: haematuria

Imaging

- US
- CT/MRI: for staging (Fig. 7.5).
- CXR: cannon-ball metastases are multiple, well-circumscribed nodules in the lungs seen on CXR; classically from renal cell carcinoma
- Bone scan: metastases

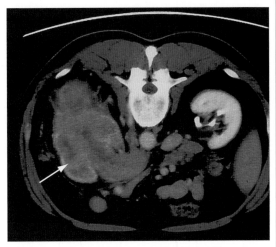

Fig. 7.5 CT showing renal carcinoma (arrowed).

Treatment

- Interferon-alpha, interleukin (IL)-2

- Resistant to chemotherapy and radiotherapy.

Surgical

Main treatment:
- Radical nephrectomy (removal of the kidney)

- Partial nephrectomy if small.

Prognosis and complications

Prognosis

- Metastases may regress after 1° tumour is removed
- 5-year survival: 40% (worse if metastases).

- 25% have metastases at presentation: to bone, liver, lung.

Complications

- Invasion of inferior vena cava.

WILMS' TUMOUR

Outline

- Cancer of the kidney, found mostly in children (also called nephroblastoma)
- An embryonic tumour from the primitive renal tubules and mesenchymal cells

- Aggressive and fast growing
- 10% bilateral.

Pathogenesis/aetiology

Associations and risks

- Chromosomal abnormality: deletion of short arm of 11

- Associated with Beckwith–Wiedemann syndrome.

Pathology

- Large, white, solid, firm masses

- Necrosis and haemorrhage.

- Typically in children <5 years
- Rare in adults
- Main abdominal malignancy in children
- Incidence 1:200 000.

Clinical features

- Large abdominal mass
- Haematuria
- Abdominal pain (rare)
- Hypertension (rare).

Investigations

Urine

- Dipstick for haematuria.

Imaging

- US
- IVU
- CT/MRI.

Treatment

- Radical nephrectomy
- Radiotherapy
- Chemotherapy postoperation.

Prognosis and complications

Prognosis

- 5-year survival ~85%.

BLADDER CANCER

Outline

Most often develops in the posterior and lateral walls of the bladder. Types:
- Transitional cell carcinomas: 98%
- Squamous cell carcinoma
- Adenocarcinomas.

Staging

- Tis: in situ in innermost layer of bladder lining
- Ta: just in the innermost layer of the bladder lining
- T1: extending into connective tissue beneath the bladder lining
- T2: extending through connective tissue into muscle
- T3: extending through muscle into fat
- T4: spread outside the bladder.

Pathogenesis/aetiology

Increased risk from:

- Smoking
- Chronic inflammation: schistosomiasis associated with squamous cell carcinoma
- Alanine dye contact (via industrial work)
- Drug exposure: cyclophosphamide.

Who

- 1♀:3♂
- Incidence: 15 000/year.

Clinical features

- Present early as protrudes into lumen
- Painless haematuria
- Symptoms of obstruction
- Symptoms of irritation: frequency, urgency, dysuria
- Recurrent UTIs (15%).

Investigations

Urine

- Cytology

Cystoscopy

- Direct visualisation
- Biopsy

Imaging

- Intravenous urogram (IVU): demonstrates filling defects
- CT/MRI: for spread and staging

Treatment

- Depends on staging:
  - Tis/Ta/T1: diathermy (heating) via cystoscopy
  - T2/T3: radical cystectomy (removal of all/part of the bladder) plus postoperative or neoadjuvant chemotherapy
- T4: palliative radiotherapy or chemotherapy; catheterisation can ↓ pain
- Follow-up frequency depends if high or low risk.

Prognosis and complications

Prognosis

- Tis/Ta/T1: 80% of patients, 5-year survival: 95%
- Fixed tumours and metastases: median survival: 1 year.

Complications

- Cystectomy can lead to sexual and urinary malfunction
- Metastases.

PROSTATE

BENIGN PROSTATIC HYPERPLASIA

Outline

- Enlargement of the male prostate; not premalignant.

Pathogenesis/aetiology

Cause

- Aetiology not well understood but may be related to changes in hormone balance with age (androgens fall) or periurethral gland sensitivity to oestrogen.

Pathogenesis

Hyperplasia (↑ cell number) of gland and hypertrophy (↑ cell size) of fibromuscular stroma:
- Mainly involves central periurethral area, causing urinary tract obstruction early as there is compression on the prostatic urethra and periurethral glands
- Prostate becomes nodular in appearance.

Who

- Typically more frequent with increasing age
- Common in men >70 years (75%).

Risk factors:
- Age
- Hormonal status.

- Symptoms of urinary obstruction:
  - Hesitancy
  - Poor stream
  - Postmicturition dribbling
  - Incomplete voiding
  - Urinary retention

- Symptoms of bladder irritation:
  - Frequency
  - Nocturia
  - Urgency
- Other symptoms and signs: enlarged prostate felt on rectal examination.

Blood tests

- FBC
- U&Es

- Prostate-specific antigen (PSA): if >4 more likely cancer rather than benign prostatic hyperplasia.

Imaging

- Kidney/ureter/bladder
- IVU

- US for bladder volume, and upper tract dilatation

Other tests

- Urodynamic studies

- Cytoscopy.

- Mild: watchful waiting

- Catheterisation for retention.

Medical

- α_1-Adrenoreceptor blockers: tamulosin, prazosin; these relax prostate and bladder smooth muscle to relieve flow (side effect, postural hypotension)

- $5\alpha_1$-Reductase inhibitors (e.g. finasteride) prevent conversion of testosterone to dihydrotestosterone, which is thought to cause prostatic hypertrophy (side effect ↓ libido).

Surgical

Transurethral resection of prostate (TURP):
- Removal of sections of the prostate through the urethra:
  - Early complications: infection, bleeding, clot retention
  - Late complications: haemorrhage, retrograde ejaculation (semen redirected to the bladder), incontinence, urethral strictures, impotence (3–5%), recurrent prostatic pregrowth.

Other options:
- Transurethral incision of the prostate
- Prostatectomy (open or laser).

Prognosis

- No worsening in 65% of mild dysplasia.

Complications

If undetected can lead to:
- bilateral obstruction
- infection
- renal calculi

- CRF
- compensatory hypertrophy of the bladder because of the high pressures.

PROSTATE CANCER

Outline

- Prostatic intraepithelial neoplasia is preinvasive precursor
- Usually adenocarcinoma, and often found incidentally on postmortem.

Pathogenesis/aetiology

Pathogenesis

- Aetiology not well understood but may be related to changes in hormones with ↑ age: testosterone is a growth factor for prostate cancer
- Usually arises in the peripheral prostate where it is non-obstructive; consequently often presents late (benign prostatic hyperplasia is more often central; see above).

Gleason score

- Used to predict prognosis of prostate cancer based on microscopic appearance
- Determined by analysing two areas, grading them and adding the scores together to reach a total between 2 (best score) and 10 (worst score).

Who

- Typical age >60 years
- 8% of all cancers in men (2nd commonest male malignancy).

Risk factors:
- Family history
- ↑ Testosterone.

Clinical features

- Asymptomatic
- Symptoms of urinary obstruction:
  - Hesitancy
  - Poor stream
  - Postmicturition dribbling
  - Incomplete voiding
- Symptoms of bladder irritation:
  - Frequency
  - Nocturia
  - Urgency
- Irregular prostate on rectal examination
- Symptoms from metastases (particularly bone metastases): weight loss.

Investigations

Blood tests

- ↑ Prostate-specific antigen: used to measure response to therapy
- U&Es: ↑ calcium if metastases.

Imaging

- US: transrectal
- CT/MRI of abdomen and pelvis: for staging
- Bone scan.

Other tests

- Biopsy

Treatment

- Microscopic tumours: watch and wait
- High Gleason score: more aggressive treatment.

Radiotherapy and chemotherapy
- Radiotherapy including brachytherapy (radioactive seeds implanted in prostate)

- Good if the patient is unfit for surgery, or for palliation.

Hormone therapy

With testosterone antagonists:
- LH-releasing hormone agonists (goserelin)

- Antiandrogens (flutamide, cyproterone acetate).

Surgical

- Radical prostatectomy for T1 (tumour present, but not detectable clinically or with imaging) and T2 (tumour can be palpated but has not spread outside the prostate)

- Relieve obstructive symptoms: transurethral resection of prostate (see above)
- Orchidectomy: to ↓ testosterone (rarely).

Prognosis and complications

Prognosis

- Good prognosis (even with metastases) if responding to hormonal treatment

- 10% mortality within 6 months.

Complications

- Treatment can cause impotence and incontinence

- Metastases: often to bone.

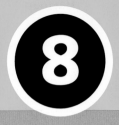
HAEMATOLOGY

Blood formation

Blood is composed of:

- White blood cells (WBCs): neutrophils, monocytes, basophils, eosinophils, lymphocytes
- Red blood cells (RBCs)
- platelets
- plasma.

The formation of blood cells is called haemopoiesis (Fig. 8.1). It occurs:

- in the embryo in the yolk sac
- in the fetus in the spleen and liver
- in adults in bone marrow.

Red blood cells (erythrocytes)

RBCs are formed by the process of erythropoiesis, which normally occurs in the bone marrow. The process is controlled by the hormone erythropoietin, which is synthesised in the kidney. RBCs contain:

- Hb, an iron-containing molecule that transports O_2:
  - fetal Hb (HbF) is mostly replaced by adult Hb in the first year after birth
  - in normal adults 97% of Hb is the HbA variant, composed of two alpha- and two beta-globin chains
  - other normal forms in adults, although in smaller quantities, include HbA_2 and HbA1c
  - abnormal variants include HbH and HbBarts (in alpha-thalassaemia) HbS (in sickle cell disease), HbAS (sickle trait)
- glycoproteins, attached to the surface of the cell, determine blood group:
  - the ABO blood group system is the most commonly used; it includes four groups: A, B, AB, O (Table 8.1)
  - minor blood groups include Rhesus (+ve or −ve), Duffy and Kidd.

Haemostasis

The clotting process is vital to prevent blood loss:

- Platelets, blood vessel endothelium and clotting factors are all required

- Haemostasis involves constriction of the blood vessel, formation of a temporary platelet plug and the cumulation of the blood clotting process into a fibrin mesh
- Coagulation cascade has two pathways that meet in the final common pathway, resulting in the formation of a fibrin mesh from fibrinogen by activation of thrombin:
  - *Intrinsic pathway*: contact activation pathway
  - *Extrinsic pathway*: tissue factor pathway
- Natural inhibitors of coagulation are protein C, antithrombin III, protein S.

Investigations

Blood tests

Full blood count (FBC)

- Hb:
  - Normal range 13.5–17.5 g/dL for men, 11.5–15.5 g/dL for women
  - Low in anaemia, high in polycythaemia
- Mean corpuscular volume (MCV): measures average RBC volume and is useful in identifying causes of anaemia:
  - Normal range 76–96 fL
  - Lower than normal, microcytosis
  - Higher, macrocytosis
- Mean cell Hb concentration (MCHC): Hb concentration in an average RBC:
  - Calculated by dividing Hb by the haematocrit
  - Raised in conditions such as hereditary spherocytosis
  - Decreased in microcytic anaemias
- Red blood cell distribution width (RDW): measure of the variability of the width of red blood cells in a sample
- Reticulocyte count: number of immature RBCs (reticulocytes), which have a reticulin framework of RNA that can be stained:
  - Increased in RBC haemolysis and in response to treatment for anaemia (more blood cells are being formed)
- Platelets:
  - Normal: 150×10^9 to 400×10^9/L
  - Thrombocythaemia: increased platelets, e.g. malignancy and infection

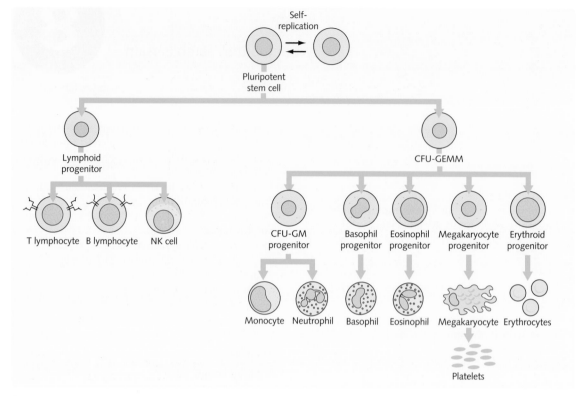

Fig. 8.1 Haemopoiesis. CFU–GEMM, multipotential myeloid stem cell; CFU–GM, granulocyte–macrophage colony-forming cell; NK, natural killer cell.

Table 8.1	ABO blood groups	
Phenotype/red cell antigens	**Genotype**	**Antibodies**
O	OO	Anti-A, anti-B
A	AO or AA	Anti-B
B	BO or BB	Anti-A
AB	AB	None

- Thrombocytopenia: decreased platelets, e.g. in marrow failure, idiopathic thrombocytopenic purpura (ITP), disseminated intravascular coagulation (DIC), hypersplenism and viral infection
- WBC: includes neutrophils, lymphocytes and eosinophils:
  - Normal 4×10^9 to 11×10^9/L
  - Causes of raised or low levels shown in Table 8.2
- Note that pancytopenia is the decrease in all types of blood cell:
  - Presents with infection (low WBCs), bleeding and bruising (low platelets), tiredness and shortness of breath (low RBCs)

- Caused by bone marrow failure, drugs, bone marrow infiltration, severe sepsis, paroxysmal noctural haemoglobinuria, or destruction of all blood cells peripherally, e.g. hypersplenism.

Haematinics
- Iron studies: total iron, serum total iron-binding capacity, iron-binding saturation, serum ferritin (iron-storage molecule)
- Folate
- Vitamin B_{12}.

Inflammatory markers
- Erythrocyte sedimentation rate (ESR):
  - Measure of rate of sedimentation of RBCs over an hour
  - Indicator of inflammation, infection or malignancy
- C-reactive protein (CRP): indicator of inflammation and infection

Markers of haemolysis
- Coombs' test (direct antiglobulin test) demonstrates the presence of antibodies or complement on the surface of RBCs:
  - Positive in haemolytic anaemias with an immune component
- LDH increased
- Haptoglobin decreased

Table 8.2 White cells and variation in normal values

Type of white cell and normal values	Causes of ↓	Causes of ↑
Total WBC • 4 to 10×10^9/L	=*Leucopenia* • Viral infections • Drugs: phenytoin, chemotherapy • Autoimmune: Felty's • Racial: African/Middle East	=*Leucocytosis* • Infection • Inflammation • Trauma • Malignancy

Neutrophils
• 2 to 7.5×10^9/L
• 40 to 75% of total WBC
	=*Neutropenia*
	• Congenital: Kostman
	• Acquired: Fanconi anaemia
	• Bone marrow failure or infiltration
	• Vitamin B_{12} or folate deficiency
	• Autoimmune disease
	• Immunodeficiency
	• Sequestration:
	  • hypersplenism
	  • Iatrogenic - chemotherapy and radiotherapy
		=*Neutrophilia*
		• Bacterial infection
		• Inflammation
		• Trauma
		• Steroids
		• Chronic myeloid leukaemia (CML)

Lymphocytes • 1.3 to 3.5×10^9/L • 20 to 40% of total WBC	=*Lymphopenia* • Bone marrow infiltration • SLE • HIV infection • Drugs: chemotherapy	=*Lymphocytosis* • Viral infection mainly • Chronic lymphocytic leukaemia (CLL)
Eosinophils • 0.04 to 0.44×10^9/L • 1 to 6% of total WBC		=*Eosinophilia* (HHHH) • Haematological malignancies (including Hodgkin's lymphoma) • Histamine (asthma, allergies) • HIV • Helminths

• Bilirubin - raised unconjugated
• Sphenocytosis
• Reticulocytosis
• Macrocytic anaemia

Blood film
• Blood as seen under the microscope (Fig. 8.2):
• Essential for investigating haematological disease or for identifying parasites
• Table 8.3 describes different types of abnormal cells seen on blood film and their interpretation.

Coagulation tests

Prothrombin time (PT): tests for any abnormalities in the extrinsic pathway of the coagulation cascade

International normalised ratio (INR): A ratio of the PT compared with a normal control sample is used to monitor warfarin therapy

Activated partial thromboplastin time (APTT): measures the intrinsic pathway of the coagulation cascade

Thrombin time: a measure of the final common pathway

Platelet function analyser 100 (PFA-100): time taken for blood to occlude in an artificial membrane. Measure of platelet function as long as $>100 \times 10^9$/L

D-dimers: a fibrin degradation product and a measure of fibrinolysis. It can indirectly help to eliminate unlikely venous thromboembolism.

Table 8.4 summarises the investigations for coagulopathy and their interpretation.

Bone marrow: aspirate and biopsy
• To investigate important haematological haemolytic malignancies (diagnosis, staging, monitoring) or infiltration of disease into the bone marrow
• Performed under local anaesthetic
• Aspiration: semi-liquid bone marrow for microscopy, PCR, chromosome analysis, cytogenetics and immunophenotyping
• Bone marrow biopsy (also called a trephine biopsy): solid piece of bone marrow for microscopy and special staining.

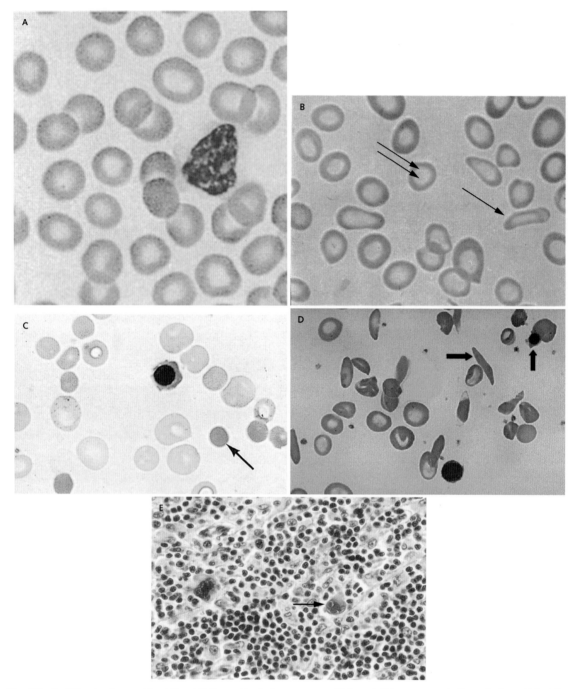

Fig. 8.2 Red blood cells on a blood film. (A) Normal typical appearance; (B) iron-deficiency anaemia (from Forbes 2003 with permission); (C) spherocytes (arrowed); (D) target cells and sickle cells (arrowed); (E) Reed–Sternberg cell.

Positron emission tomography

Nuclear medicine imaging where a radioactively labelled isotope is introduced to the body so that metabolically active tissues can be identified in a 3D image. It can be combined with CT and MRI.

- Useful for haematological malignancies but also for general staging and in neurology to measure brain activity.

Table 8.3 Cells seen on blood film

Cell seen under microscope	Description and examples of diseases
Abnormalities seen in red blood cells	
Microcytosis	Small cells, found in microcytic anaemia
Macrocystosis	Large cells, found in macrocytic anaemia
Hypochromia	Faint coloured red blood cells due to↓ Hb synthesis: found in iron deficiency anaemia
Target cells	Red blood cells with staining in the centre: found in iron deficiency anaemia, liver disease, thalassaemias and HbC
Pencil cells	Pencil shaped cells seen in iron deficiency anaemia
Howell Jolly bodies	DNA fragments seen in RBC, normally removed by spleen: seen in hyposplenism
Burr cells	Irregular spherical, rather than disc shaped red blood cells with spike-like projections, seen in uraemia
Heinz bodies	Precipitates of denatured Hb within the red blood cells, e.g. in glucose-6-phosphate dehydrogenase deficiency, thalassaemia
Reticulocytes	Younger, larger red blood cells: found in bleeding and haemolysis
Spherocytes	Small rounded red blood cells seen in hereditary spherocytosis and autoimmune haemolytic anaemia
Sickle cells	Sickle shaped cells seen in sickle cell disease
Tear drop cells (dacrocytes)	Tear dropped shaped red blood cells seen in myelofibrosis
Poikilocytes	The term for any abnormally shaped cell, e.g. spherocytes, dacrocytes, burr cells
Rouleaux formation	Stacking of red blood cells, seen in myeloma
Basophilic stippling	Small dots seen at the periphery of red blood cells from the accumulation of rRNA. Seen in sideroblastic anaemia, megaloblastic anaemia and in beta-thalassaemia
Other cells	
Auer rods	Crystals of coalesced granules seen in blast cells in acute promyelocytic leukaemia. They have a rod like appearance on microscopy
Reed Sternberg cell	Large bi or multi nucleate malignant B lymphocytes that are pathognomonic of classical Hodgkin's lymphoma
Blasts	Premature precursor cells: acute leukaemia

Table 8.4 Coagulation tests and their interpretation

Underlying cause	INR	APTT	Thrombin time	Platelets	D-dimer	PFA-100
Liver disease	↑	↑	↑	↓	↑	↑
Vitamin K deficiency	↑	(↑)	–	–	–	–
Haemophilia	–	↑	–	–	–	–
Von Willebrand's	–	↑	–	–	–	↑
Platelet disease	–	–	–	↓ or –	–	↑
DIC	↑	↑	↑	↓	↑	N/A
Heparin	(↑)–	↑	↑	–	–	–
Warfarin	↑	–(↑)	↑	–	–	–
TTP	–	–	–	↓	–	N/A

ONCOLOGY

Basic oncological terminology

Benign: a non-malignant tumour, one that cannot metastasize. The difference between benign and malignant tumours is shown in Table 8.5.

Malignant: tumour characterised by invasiveness, metastases and differentiation of cells.

Dysplasia: disordered cell development resulting in an alteration in their size, shape, or organisation

Metaplasia: reversible change from one type of differentiated tissue to another. May precede neoplasm

Neoplasm: the process of tumour growth

Carcinoma in situ: cancer that has not invaded the basement membrane (common in exam questions)

Invasive carcinoma: cancer that has invaded beyond the basement membrane

Cancer grade: this is the histological measure of how differentiated cancer cells are from those around then:

- Grade 1: low-grade tumour, well differentiated
- Grade 2: moderately differentiated
- Grade 3: high-grade tumour, undifferentiated.

Cancer stage: this is related to prognosis. Solid tumours can be staged according to the TNM system, tumour (T; size), node (N; involvement of regional lymph nodes), metastases (M):

T0: no tumour

Tis: carcinoma *in situ*

T1–T4: depends on size

N0: no lymph node involvement

N1–N3: depends on lymph node spread

M0: no distant metastases

M1: metastases.

Cancers can be classified according to the origin of the cell (Table 8.6):

Certain cancers produce 'markers' that can be measured. These are useful for diagnosis and for monitoring disease progression and treatment (Table 8.7).

Oncological emergencies

Some aspects of cancer must be dealt with urgently:

- Tumour lysis syndrome
- Febrile neutropenia
- Spinal cord compression
- Hypercalcaemia
- Superior vena caval obstruction.

Tumour lysis syndrome

A complication of chemotherapy that can be lethal. Chemotherapy can lead to the rapid death of tumour cells, leading to the release of their intracellular ions:

- Results in ↑ potassium, ↑ phosphate, ↑ urate, ↓ calcium, which can precipitate renal failure
- More common after the treatment of haematological malignances
- Prevention involves allopurinol and intravenous hydration before chemotherapy.

Febrile neutropenia

Temperature of >38 °C in a neutropenic patient (neutrophils $<1.0 \times 10^9$/L):

- Most commonly due to septicaemia, can be life threatening
- Treat according to local antibiotic protocol.

Spinal cord compression

The tumour compresses the cord or affects the blood supply of the cord (see spinal cord compression p. 248, Ch. 6):

- Image with urgent MRI and treat with IV dexamethasone
- Urgent radiotherapy or surgical decompression is necessary to preserve neurological function.

Hypercalcaemia

Results from bone metastases or tumour production of parathyroid hormone (PTH)-related peptide (a paraneoplastic hormone that acts like PTH, increasing osteoclast activity and, therefore, calcium) (see hypercalcaemia, p. 423):

- Treat with IV fluids and IV bisphosphonate.

Table 8.5 Differences between benign and malignant tumours

Characteristics of benign versus malignant tumours	
Benign	**Malignant**
Localized	Metastatic spread
No invasion	Invasion of normal structures
No metastases	Metastases
Relatively slow growth rate	Relatively rapid growth rate
Good differentiation	Poorly differentiated
Few mitoses	Many mitoses
Normal nuclear chromatin	Increased nuclear chromatin
Uniform size cells	Cells and nuclei vary in size
Exophytic growth	Endophytic growth
Compression of normal tissue	Invasion and destruction of normal tissue

Table 8.6 Classification of cancers according to cell origin

Type of cell	Type of cancer	
	Benign	Malignant
Epithelium		
Squamous cell	Squamous cell papilloma	Squamous cell carcinoma
Glandular mucosa	Adenoma	Adenocarcinoma
Transitional cell	Transitional cell papilloma	Transitional cell carcinoma
Neuroendocrine	Melanocytic naevus	Malignant melenoma
Mesenchymal (Connective tissue)		
Bone	Osteoid osteoma	Osteosarcoma
Cartilage	Chondroma/osteochondroma	Chondrosarcoma
Fibrous tissue	Fibroma	Fibrosarcoma
Bone marrow	Haemangioma	Angiosarcoma
Glia	Glioma	Glioma
Adipose	lipoma	Liposarcoma
Skeletal	Rhabdomyoma	Rhabdomyosarcoma
Smooth	Leiomyoma	Leiomyosarcoma
Haemopoietic	–	Leukaemia
Lymph	–	Lymphoma

Table 8.7 Tumours markers

Tumour marker	Type of cancer
Ca 125	Ovarian cancer
Ca 19–9	Pancreatic cancer
Carcinoembryonic antigen (CEA)	Colorectal cancer
Prostate-specific antigen (PSA)	Prostate cancer
Human chorionic gonadotrophin (hCG)	Testicular teratoma and seminoma
α-Fetoprotein	Hepatocellular carcinoma and testicular teratoma

Superior vena caval obstruction

Can be caused by malignant mediastinal tumours (commonly small cell carcinoma of the lung and NHL).

Obstruction impairs filling of the right side of the heart, causing venous engorgement and oedema of the head, neck, arms and upper thorax:

- Can lead to airway compromise
- Symptoms include breathlessness, blackouts, headaches

- Investigate with Pemberton's test: facial plethora and ecyanosis when the arms are lifted above the head for >60 s
- Treat with radiotherapy or a vena cava stent.

Cancer treatment

You should know:

- that cancer can be targeted with radiotherapy, chemotherapy or surgery
- palliative care (symptom control) is for untreatable or unresponsive cancer
- the terminology for cancer treatment.

Terminology for cancer treatment

Neoadjuvant: therapy given before the main treatment, e.g. neoadjuvant chemotherapy before surgery to shrink a tumour

Adjuvant: therapy given after the main therapy, e.g. chemotherapy or radiotherapy after surgery

Concomitant: different therapy modalities given simultaneously

Chemotherapy: aims to affect cancerous cells more than the cells of the body; cytotoxic drugs target rapidly dividing cells, often during DNA synthesis:

- Side effects include hair loss, vomiting, nausea, infertility, myelosuppression and secondary cancers

Immunotherapy: includes:

- tumour-specific monoclonal antibodies to target cancerous cells, e.g. rituximab
- vaccines to provide non-specific immunostimulation and to raise an adaptive immune response against cancer, e.g. BCG in bladder cancer
- cytokines to regulate the immune response to target the cancer
- recombinant colony-stimulating factors to reduce neutropenia after chemotherapy.

See also

- Endocrinology (Ch. 9): pituitary tumour, malignant thyroid, hypercalcaemia.
- Surgery (Ch. 13): malignant breast disease, GI malignancies, malignant melanoma, basal cell carcinoma, squamous cell carcinoma.

ANAEMIA

GENERAL FEATURES

Outline

- A reduction in the level of haemoglobin (Hb), the O_2 carrying pigment within the RBCs
- Due to:
  - ↓ Production of RBC
  - ↑ Destruction of RBC
  - Loss of RBC
- Defined by Hb level:
  - *Men*: <13.5 g/dL (norm: 13.5–17.5 g/dL)
- *Women*: <11.5 g/dL (norm: 11.5–15.5 g/dL)
- Not a diagnosis but result of an underlying problem
- Dependent on speed of onset, severity, age, oxyhaemoglobin dissociation
- Slow onset tolerated better than rapid onset

Sideroblastic anaemia:
- A rare disorder of Hb synthesis where iron cannot be incorporated into the protoporphyrin ring to form Hb.

Pathogenesis/aetiology

Causes

- Many causes that can be classified in many ways
- In the pages that follow the anaemias will be classified by cause into:
  - deficiency anaemias: ↓ production due to reduction in one element needed for RBC synthesis
  - haemolytic anaemias: ↑ RBC destruction
  - Acute blood loss
- A typical classification is by mean corpuscular volume (Table 8.8).

Table 8.8 Classification by mean corpuscular volume

Microcytic <80 fL	Normocytic 80–95	Macrocytic >95 fL
Stop Those Incy Little cells S: sideroblastic anaemia T: thalassaemia I: iron deficiency L: lead poisoning C: chronic disease	*Medium RBC* M: marrow failure or infiltration R: renal failure (lack of erythropoeitin) B: blood loss C: chronic disease	*FAT RBCs* F: folate deficiency A: alcohol T: thyroid: hypothyroid R: reticulocytosis (haemolysis) B: B_{12} deficiency C: cytotoxic drugs, cirrhosis (liver disease) s: smoking

Who

- Common
- ♀ > ♂
- 10% of women (due to menstruation).

Clinical features

Symptoms

- Lethargy
- Shortness of breath from ↓ O_2 carriage
- Weakness
- Light-headedness/dizziness
- Palpitations
- Angina.

Signs

- Pallor: visible at mucous membranes, skin creases if moderate to severe
- Jaundice: if anaemia is due to haemolysis
- Hyperdynamic circulation:
  - Tachycardia
  - Collapsing pulse
  - Systolic flow murmur
- Bone abnormalities: frontal bossing
- Hepatosplenomegaly
- Retinal haemorrhage (rapid onset).

Investigations

Blood tests

- FBC
- Reticulocyte (immature RBC) count: measure of production of blood cells
- U&Es
- LFTs

- ESR
- Haematinics: levels of iron, vitamin B_{12}, folate
- Blood film
- LDH.

Further tests

To investigate an underlying cause:
- e.g. endoscopy in iron deficiency anaemia and colonoscopy

- Bone marrow aspirate.

Treatment

- Treat underlying cause

- May need a blood transfusion.

Prognosis and complications

Prognosis

- Dependent on cause.

Complications

- Heart failure (acute)

- Iron overload (chronic effect with regular blood transfusions).

DEFICIENCY ANAEMIAS

IRON DEFICIENCY

Outline

- Deficiency of iron in the body
- Due to excessive chronic blood loss or insufficient absorption of iron

Iron in the body:
- Iron is an essential component of the haem component of Hb
- It is absorbed in the duodenum and jejunum
- 70% of iron is contained in circulating Hb and reused following RBC death:

- *Transferrin*: transports iron in the plasma and constitutes <0.2% of iron
- *Ferritin and haemosiderin*: stores of iron. Found in hepatocytes, skeletal muscle and reticuloendothelial system
- In iron deficient states the body compensates by:
  - using ferritin stores
  - releasing iron from macrophages

Pathogenesis/aetiology

Causes

Insufficient intake:
- Low dietary iron: purely breast fed child, lack of red meat, fish, lentils, chickpeas
- ↑ Requirements: growth, pregnancy, prematurity, infancy

Malabsorption:
- Coeliac disease
- Gastrectomy
- Achlorhydria (no production of gastric acid)

Loss:
- *Bleeding: may be a presenting sign of malignancy, e.g. GI or pulmonary. NICE guidelines for urgent referral for*

suspected bowel cancer include: any man or non-menstruating woman with unexplained iron-deficiency anaemia
- *Parasitic infection*
- *Inflammatory bowel disease*
- *GI ulcers*
- *Menorrhagia*

Plummer–Vinson syndrome:
- A syndrome of iron-deficiency anaemia together with dysphagia and the formation of oesophageal webs (thin membranes of oesophageal tissue that can cause dysphagia). Aetiology is unclear.

Who

- Typical age: commoner in young people
- Commonest cause of anaemia
- ♀ > ♂
- 10% of women are iron deficient due to menorrhagia
- Rarer in men and the elderly so always perform endoscopy to check for malignancy or bleeding in these groups

A typical patient

- A 26-year-old vegetarian presents to her GP because she is always tired. She has long, heavy periods. On examination she has pale conjunctiva and is slim.

Clinical features

Symptoms and signs of anaemia

- See 'General features' above
Signs of iron deficiency:
- Koilonychia: brittle spoon nails
- Angular cheilosis or angular stomatitis: sore areas at the corner of the mouth
- Atrophic glossitis: smooth tongue (due to loss of papillae) that may be tender
- Dysphagia: in Plummer–Vinson syndrome

Consider source of bleeding:
- Haematuria
- Haemoptysis
- Haematemesis
- Melaena
- Menorrhagia.

Investigations

Blood tests

- Microcytic anaemia: ↓ Hb, ↓ MCV
- ↓ Reticulocyte count: in relation to degree of anaemia
- ↓ Serum iron
- ↓ Serum ferritin: may be normal or high in an acute inflammatory response
- ↑ Total iron-binding capacity and transferrin <10%
- ↑ Platelet count

Blood film (Fig. 8.2B):
- Microcytic hypochromic RBCs
- Target cells
- Pencil cells
- Poikilocytosis: varied shape RBC

Other tests

Bone marrow aspiration:
- Absence of iron from intracellular stores and erythroblasts when stained with Perl's Prussian blue stain
Investigate source of blood loss:
- Lower GI bleed: rectal examination, colonoscopy

- Upper GI bleed: OGD, duodenal biopsy, tissue transglutaminase antibodies
- Investigate causes of menorrhagia
- Haematuria: cystoscopy
- Haemoptysis: CXR.

Treatment

Iron replacement:
- Oral: ferrous sulphate, or ferrous gluconate
- Parenteral: intravenous or intramuscular iron, for:
  - malabsorption
  - high iron requirements, i.e., ongoing GI loss
  - oral replacement fails
- Required for >3 months to replenish stores and correct anaemia

- Side effect: abdominal pain, dark/black stool, nausea, change in bowel habit (IV also causes anaphylactic shock)
Other:
- Treat underlying cause:
  - Blood transfusion

Prognosis and complications

Prognosis

- With iron replacement therapy expect a rise in Hb of 2 g/dL every 3 weeks.

Complications

- Lower IQ in children (improves with correction of iron levels).

VITAMIN B$_{12}$ DEFICIENCY

Outline

- Deficiency of vitamin B$_{12}$ in the body
- Due to insufficient intake or poor absorption

Vitamin B$_{12}$:
- Daily requirement: 2.4 mcg
- Found in meat, milk and eggs
- Absorbed in the terminal ileum
- Intrinsic factor produced by gastric parietal cells (in the stomach) is required for the absorption of vitamin B$_{12}$
- Vitamin B$_{12}$ is stored in the liver (enough for 2–4 years supply)
- Transported to the bone marrow by transcobalamin

- B$_{12}$ deficiency results in the formation of RBC megaloblasts, which are then destroyed (as they are abnormal) resulting in haemolytic jaundice

Vitamin B$_{12}$ function:
- Involved in the synthesis of nucleic acids and DNA
- Required in the maintenance of myelin
- Required to convert serum folate to an active intracellular form (via methylation of homocystine to methionine). Therefore, vitamin B$_{12}$ deficiency and folate deficiency often coexist
- Acts as a coenzyme for the production of succinyl A.

Pathogenesis/aetiology

Causes

Insufficient intake:
- Dietary deficiency, e.g. vegans
- Increased requirement: some bacteria consume B$_{12}$

Malabsorption:
- Any disease affecting the terminal ileum, e.g. Crohn's disease; Zollinger–Ellison syndrome
- Lack of intrinsic factor
- Partial gastroectomy
- Pernicious anaemia:
  - Immune mediated atrophy of gastric mucosa and parietal cells

- No intrinsic factor is produced and vitamin B$_{12}$ cannot be absorbed
- Mostly occurs in middle aged or elderly women
- An autoimmune disorder that occurs with other autoimmune disorders
- Occurs more often in people with premature grey hair and blue eyes, and those with blood group A
- Overgrowth by vitamin B12-consuming bacteria or fish-tapeworms

Drugs:
- Metformin.

Who

Pernicious anaemia:
- Typical age: more in the elderly

- 1: 1000

A typical patient

A 50-year-old woman with fair hair and blue eyes presents with a 1 month history of paraesthesia of her digits with occasional clumsiness and lethargy for 6 months. She has also lost 2 kg over that time. On examination she has coarse facies and pallor with mild jaundice and glossitis.

Clinical features

- Develops insidiously

Signs

- Angular cheilosis
- Glossitis
- Lemon yellow tint

Neurological complications (not seen in folate deficiency):
- Subacute combined degeneration of cord (see neurology chapter 6): weakness, ataxia, paraplegia

- Pancytopenia and megaloblastosis.

- Peripheral neuropathy: symmetrical, paraesthesia of fingers and toes. Affects the lower limbs more than the upper limbs and dorsal columns
- Optic atrophy (rare)
- Dementia
- Paraesthesia an early sign

Investigations

Blood tests

- ↓ Serum B$_{12}$
- ↓ RBC folate but ↑ serum folate
- Intrinsic factor antibodies in 50% with pernicious anaemia.
- ↓ Reticulocytes

Blood film:
- Macrocytic anaemia: ↓ Hb, ↑ MCV and ovalocytes
- Megaloblasts
- Neutrophils: hypersegmented nuclei

Investigations

- Megathrombocytes
- Poikilocytosis: oval cells

- Pancytopenia: ↓ Hb, ↓ WBC, ↓ platelets

Schilling test

- To assess if symptoms are from B_{12} or intrinsic factor deficiency
- *Part I*: B_{12} given by intramuscular injection to saturate levels. Radioactively labelled B_{12} then given orally
- Metabolite levels: serum homocysteine and methylmalonic acid rise as B_{12} falls

- 24 h urine collected: normal individuals have >10% of the oral dose contained in the urine. If <10% there is a problem with B_{12} absorption
- *Part II*: as in Part 1, but intrinsic factor added orally
- If there is an ↑ in the % contained in the urine it suggests an intrinsic factor deficiency rather than B_{12} deficiency

Other tests

- Endoscopy or barium meal: if suspecting underlying intestinal disease, including carcinoma

Bone marrow aspirate:
- Megaloblasts: (see Folic acid deficiency section below)
- Bone marrow biopsy: confirmatory.

Treatment

- Stores replenished with intramuscular hydroxocobalamin (B_{12})

- Maintain every 3 months for life
- Avoid blood transfusions: risk of cardiac failure.

Prognosis and complications

Prognosis

Following treatment:
- Symptomatic improvement within 24 h
- Hb rise 2–3 g/dL every 2 weeks
- White cell and platelets normal by 7–10 weeks

- Bone marrow normal after 48 h
- Peripheral neuropathy improves in 3–6 months but cord signs will not, so treat as soon as possible.

Complications

- Gastric carcinoma
- Sterility
- ↓ Osteoblast activity
- Cardiovascular disease

- Epithelial abnormalities, hyperpigmentation
- Weight loss
- Neurological disease: subacute, combined degeneration of the spinal cord; paraesthesias.

FOLATE DEFICIENCY

Outline

- Insufficient intake or poor absorption
Folic acid:
- Daily requirement: 100–200 µg/day
- Found in liver, yeast and green vegetables like broccoli or spinach

- Absorbed from the small bowel
- Important in the synthesis of nucleic acid and DNA
- The metabolic role of folic acid is interdependent with vitamin B_{12}: both are required by rapidly dividing cells
- A deficiency of one can lead to deficiency of the other.

Pathogenesis/aetiology

Causes

Insufficient intake:
- Dietary: commonest cause
Increased requirements:
- Pregnancy, lactation
- Haemolytic anaemia
- Malignant disorders: ↑ use
- Dialysis: ↑ excretion

- Psoriasis
Malabsorption:
- Crohn's disease, coeliac disease, tropical sprue
Other:
- Sulfasalazine, pyrimethamine, methotrexate, trimethoprim, anticonvulsants

Who

A typical patient

A lady with known long-term coeliac disease presents with tiredness and shortness of breath. Blood film shows macrocytic anaemia and megaloblasts.

Clinical features

- Symptoms and signs as for anaemia: see 'General features' above
- Develops faster than B_{12} deficiency, usually in patients with malnutrition and other vitamin deficiencies

- No neuropathy unless concurrent B_{12} deficiency.

Investigations

Blood tests

- ↓ RBC folate
- ↑ Bilirubin and ↑ LDH: from ↑ destruction of abnormal RBCs

Blood film:

- Macrocytic anaemia: ↓ Hb, ↑ MCV
- Megaloblasts
- Neutrophils: hypersegmented nuclei
- Poikilocytosis: oval cells

Other tests

- Jejunal biopsy: for coeliac disease if history does not suggest dietary deficiency.

Bone marrow aspirate:

- Megaloblasts: these are large RBCs with delayed maturation of the nucleus due to inhibition of DNA

synthesis. The commonest causes are Vitamin B_{12} and folate deficiency.
- Bone marrow biopsy: confirmatory

Treatment

- Oral folic acid 5 mg daily for four months (longer if cause is malabsorption)
- Pregnant women: should take folic acid to prevent neural tube defects in the fetus: 400 µg daily

- **Ensure adequate vitamin B_{12} levels before giving folate: otherwise, subacute combined degeneration of the cord and neuropathy may develop**
- Avoid blood transfusions, unless given very slowly with diuretic cover.

Prognosis and complications

Prognosis

- See Vitamin B_{12} Prognosis section above

Complications

- Neural tube defects in fetus of pregnant women
- Sterility
- Cardiovascular disease

- ↑ Homocysteine, occlusive vascular disease and osteopenia.

HAEMOLYTIC ANAEMIAS

GENERAL FEATURES

Outline

- Abnormal destruction of RBCs

- RBC lifespan reduced to <120 days.

Classification

Extravascular destruction:

- Destruction is within the reticuloendothelial system: spleen, marrow, liver, phagocytes
- Destroyed RBCs are removed by macrophages (mostly in the spleen)

Intravascular destruction:

- Destruction occurs within the blood vessels: oxidised Hb appears in the plasma.

Pathogenesis/aetiology

Most of the following are expanded in the tables immediately following:

- Congenital causes:
  - Metabolic defects:
    - Glucose-6-phosphate dehydrogenase deficiency
    - Pyruvate kinase deficiency

- Membrane defects:
  - Hereditary spherocytosis
- Haemoglobin defects:
  - Thalassaemia
  - Sickle cell anaemia

Pathogenesis/aetiology

- Acquired causes:
  - Immune:
    - Autoimmune haemolytic anaemia
    - Drug induced
  - Non immune:
    - *Hypersplenism*: pooling of blood leads to panyctopenia and haemolysis
- *RBC fragmentation syndromes*: from heart valves, DIC, malignant hypertension
- *Paroxysmal nocturnal haemoglobinuria*
- *Renal/liver disease*
- *Drugs*: dapsone, phenacetin
- *Infection*: toxins, burns.

Who

- Family history
- 5% of all anaemia.

Clinical features

Signs

- Pallor
- Jaundice
- Urine turns dark on standing due to urobilinogen
- Splenomegaly
- Pigment gallstones.

Investigations

Blood tests

- Evidence of ↑ RBC breakdown:
  - Hyperbilirubinaemia (unconjugated): bilirubin is a breakdown product of haem in RBCs
  - ↑ Urobilinogen (break down product of bilirubin)
  - ↓ Haptoglobulin (released from RBCs)
  - Abnormal RBC morphology
- *Evidence of ↑ RBC production*:
  - ↑ Reticulocytes
  - ↑ Marrow activity
  - ↑ LDH

Blood film changes:
- Normocytosis, macrocytosis (due to reticulocytosis), microcytosis (in paroxysmal nocturnal haemoglobinuria)
- ↑ Reticulocytes
- Spherocytes
- Eliptocytes
- Fragments of RBCs
- Schistocytes
- Target cells

Treatment

- Depends on cause.

Prognosis and complications

Prognosis

- Depends on cause.

GLUCOSE-6-PHOSPHATE DEHYDROGENASE DEFICIENCY

Outline

- An inherited deficiency of glucose-6-phosphate dehydrogenase leads to precipitation of RBCs under certain conditions, causing haemolytic anaemia
- Due to acute intravascular haemolysis.

Pathogenesis/aetiology

Causes

- X-linked recessive disorder
- Some react to a chemical within broad beans (favism).

Pathogenesis

- Glucose-6-phosphate dehydrogenase maintains glutathione in a reduced state
- Glutathione protects against oxidant injury in RBCs
- RBCs deficient in the enzyme and exposed to oxidative stress causes Hb to oxidise and form precipitates called Heinz bodies
- The Heinz bodies adhere to the RBC membrane causing intravascular lysis and removal by the spleen.

- Commonest RBC enzyme defect
- Mostly in ♂ (X-linked recessive)
- 200 million people world wide particularly in:
  - Mediterranean
- West Africa
- Asia
- Similar geographic distribution to malaria

An 18-year-old Greek youth who recently started some anti-malarials for a holiday abroad develops jaundice and lethargy.

- Usually well between episodes
- Recurrent jaundice and dark urine which resolves spontaneously
- Features of anaemia
- May present as neonatal jaundice.

Between episodes:
- ↓ Glucose-6-phosphate dehydrogenase levels on assay

Acute episode:
- Reticulocytosis
- Features of haemolysis: ↑ unconjugated bilirubin, ↓ haptoglobin and ↑ urinary urobilinogen

Blood film:
- Heinz bodies (Hb precipitated in RBC)
- Bite cells with portions removed from the circumference from phagocytosis in the spleen of Heinz bodies at the cell edge
- Fragments

See 'General features' of haemolytic anaemia above.

- Avoid precipitants, e.g. beans, drugs
- Treat any underlying infection
- Monitor Hb if unwell
- Fluid resuscitation to maintain good urinary output
- Packed RBC transfusion if severe
- In neonates: consider phototherapy and exchange transfusion if severe anaemia.

- Often self limiting as new RBCs are made rapidly in response to haemolysis.

- Anaemia
- Kernicterus: brain damage in neonates from raised levels of bilirubin
- Shock.

PYRUVATE KINASE DEFICIENCY

- An inherited disorder where a deficiency of the pyruvate kinase enzyme leads to ↓ survival of RBCs causing haemolytic anaemia.

- An autosomal recessive disorder.

- Pyruvate kinase in an important enzyme in production of ATP
- Without ATP, RBCs, are unable to control ion pumps leading to ↑ intracellular sodium, and therefore entry of water into cells causing lysis.

Who

- 1♀:1♂
- Common in:
  - N. Europe

- Japan
- United States.

Clinical features

- Splenomegaly
- Relatively mild symptoms: jaundice and gallstones are commonest

- Frontal bossing (prominent forehead): rare.
- Most patients are asymptomatic but are susceptible to ↑ oxidant stress, e.g. drugs (e.g. anti-malarials), infection

Investigations

Blood tests

- Hb 4–10 g/dL
- ↓ Pyruvate kinase levels on assay

Blood film:
- Poikilocytes
See Haemolytic anaemia above.

Treatment

- Splenectomy
- Folic acid

- Packed RBC transfusion if severe.

Prognosis and complications

Complications

- Gallstones
- Aplastic crisis (↓ reticulocytes)

- Hypersplenism.

HEREDITARY SPHEROCYTOSIS

Outline

- An inherited disorder where a defect in the RBC membrane causes the cells to have a spherocytic shape that is more rigid than normal making them vulnerable to destruction and therefore leads to haemolytic anaemia.

Pathogenesis/aetiology

Causes

- Autosomal dominant with variable expression.

Pathogenesis

- Defects in proteins of the RBC membrane (including spectrin and ankyrin) cause the RBCs to become more spherical with increasing permeability

- There is ↑ osmotic fragility of RBCs
- RBCs become trapped in the spleen where they are haemolysed.

Who

- Incidence: 1/5000

- Common in N. Europeans.

Clinical features

- Anaemia
- Jaundice: fluctuates

- Gallstones
- Splenomegaly.

Blood tests

- Coombs' test (direct antiglobulin test) negative (see Autoimmune haemolytic anaemia)
- ↑ Osmotic fragility
- Raised mean cell haemoglobin concentration

Blood film:
- Spherocytes (Fig. 8.2C)
- Reticulocytosis (↑ reticulocytes)
See 'General features' of Haemolytic anaemia above.

Treatment

- No treatment if mild or young
- Folic acid supplementation

- Splenectomy: if severe
- Screening of family members.

Prognosis and complications

Complications

- Gallstones
- Aplastic crisis due to parvovirus B19 infection

- Megaloblastic anaemia due to ↑ folate utilisation.

THALASSAEMIA

Outline

- An inherited disorder where an abnormal globin gene leads to reduced globin synthesis and therefore abnormal Hb synthesis and anaemia

- The number and type of gene affected affects the phenotypic outcome.

Classification

Alpha (α) thalassaemia:
- Reduced α chain formation
- *One abnormal gene*: silent carrier
- *Two abnormal genes*: α thalassaemia trait
- *Three abnormal genes*: HbH disease
- *Four abnormal genes*: hydrops fetalis. HbBarts replaces HbA Normally incompatible with life

Beta (β) thalassaemia:
- Reduced β chain formation
- *One abnormal gene*: β thalassaemia minor (heterozygote), asymptomatic carriers. May have mild anaemia
- *Two abnormal genes*: β thalassaemia major (homozygote)
- Thalassaemia intermedia: an intermediate condition, with moderate anaemia.

Pathogenesis/aetiology

Causes

- Autosomal recessive inheritance.

Pathogenesis

- Haemoglobin is composed of two α and two β globin chains
- These are coded for by four α globin genes (two on each chromosome 16) and two β globin genes (one on each chromosome 11)
- Mutations in these genes leads to reduced or absent synthesis of one or more of the globin subunits of Hb
- This results in excess of the other chain
- The unmatched unstable Hb precipitates leading to:

1. damage to the RBC membranes causing precipitation of globin chains and haemolysis
2. ineffective erythropoiesis leading to extramedullary haemopoiesis (formation of blood outside of the bone marrow)
- Whilst severe disease can cause major problems the milder forms do provide an advantage in infection from malaria

Who

α thalassaemia:
- ↑ Incidence in:
  - Mediterranean
  - Middle East
  - Africa
  - SE Asia

β thalassaemia:
- ↑ Incidence in:
  - Mediterranean
  - Middle East
  - China
  - India.

Clinical features

α thalassaemia:
- Silent carrier: asymptomatic
- Alpha-thalassaemia trait:
  - Normally asymptomatic
- HbH disease:
  - Haemolytic anaemia
  - Splenomegaly
  - Bone changes
- Hydrops fetalis:
  - Stillborn/early death
  - Hepatosplenomegaly
  - Oedema
  - Extramedullary haemopoiesis

β thalassaemia:
- β thalassaemia minor:
  - Normally asymptomatic
- β thalassaemia intermedia:
  - Extremeduallary haemopoiesis

- Hepatosplenomegaly
- Skeletal deformity
- Gallstones
- Leg ulcers
- β thalassaemia major:
  - Failure to thrive from 3–6 months (as the body switches from synthesising HbF to HbA)
  - Severe anaemia
  - Hepatosplenomegaly
  - Jaundice
  - Skeletal deformity including frontal bossing from bone marrow hyperplasia
  - Haemosiderosis
  - Recurrent infections
  - Heart failure
  - Growth failure, and delayed puberty
  - Diabetes
  - Gallstones.

Investigations

Blood tests

For all types:
- Iron studies: normal ferritin
- Anaemia
- Hypochromia with microcytosis (apart from silent carriers in α thalassaemia) and ↑ RBC

HbH disease:
- Reticulocytosis
- Target cells

Hydrops fetalis:
- Reticulocytosis
- Target cells

β thalassaemia intermedia:
- Target cells

β thalassaemia major:
- Target cells
- Basophilic stippling
- Nucleated RBC
- Reticulocytosis

Other tests

- Hb electrophoresis:
  - HbH disease: HbH
  - Hydrops fetalis: ↑ HbBart
  - β thalassaemia major: ↑ HbF, ↑ HbA2, ↓ or absent HbA
  - β thalassaemia minor: ↑ HbF, ↑ HbA2
- Alpha/beta chain synthesis studies of DNA analyses
- PCR assay to distinguish α- and β-thals gene mutation

Treatment

α thalassaemia:
- HbH disease:
  - Folate supplements
  - Blood transfusions if necessary with iron chelation therapy
  - Splenectomy if increasing transfusion requirements (will need infection prophylaxis)

β thalassaemia:
- β thalassaemia minor: no treatment
- β thalassaemia intermedia: may need occasional transfusions
- β thalassaemia major:

- Transfusion every 4 weeks to maintain Hb >10 g/dL. Important in childhood to ensure normal growth
- Folate supplements
- Iron chelators, e.g. desferrioxamine s.c. (to ↓ risk of iron overload) given with ascorbic acid (vitamin C) to ↑ iron excretion
- Splenectomy if increasing transfusion requirements (will need infection prophylaxis)
- Bone marrow transplant in patients <16 years with normal liver function. Can be curative

Prevention:
- Genetic screening.

Prognosis and complications

Prognosis

α thalassaemia:
- HbH disease: variable survival
- Hydrops fetalis: stillborn or death soon after birth

β thalassaemia:
- Major: death in childhood without treatment. Bone marrow transplant may be curative
- Intermedia: good survival even without treatment, rarely requires blood transfusion.

Prognosis and complications

Complications

- Skull bossing and fractures: due to bone expansion causing a thin cortex
- Splenomegaly
- Iron overload from multiple transfusions: causes toxicity of heart, liver, pituitary, parathyroid, thyroid, pancreas
- Transfusion transmitted infections.

SICKLE CELL DISEASE

Outline

- An inherited condition where a mutation of the gene for beta globin results in the formation of HbS instead of HbA, which causes the Hb to form an abnormal 'sickle' shape.

Classification

- Homozygote: sickle cell anaemia (HbSS): 80–90% HbS
- Heterozygote: sickle cell trait (HbAS): <50% HbS. No disability, although vasoocclusive events can occur in hypoxic conditions. Confers protection from malaria
- Double heterozygote (HbSC) for HbS and HbC characterised by moderate clinical severity, with increased risk of thrombosis

Lifetime progression:
- Symptoms only from 3rd month onwards (delay as fetal form, HbF is present, which is protective)
- Childhood: hand-foot infarction, impaired growth and delayed puberty
- Pregnancy: ↑ mother and fetal morbidity and mortality
- Old age: renal failure.

Pathogenesis/aetiology

- Inheritance: autosomal recessive.

Pathogenesis

- Caused by a single base mutation in the β globin gene on chromosome 11 where valine replaces glutamic acid resulting in sickle B (HbS)
- HbS polymerises in hypoxic conditions (infection, hypoxia, hypothermia, acidosis) causing cells to become insoluble and rigid
- The erythrocyte shape becomes distorted and changes from a biconcave disc to a 'sickle' shape
- 'Sickling' leads to two main features: vasoocculsion and haemolyis
- Patients often present with a 'crisis' (see below).

Who

- Afro-Caribbeans
- Middle East.

A typical patient

A 17-year-old Afro-Caribbean male student presents with painful limbs and back and a fever. He has had a 3 week history of preceding coryzal symptoms and a cold. He has slight jaundice and is dehydrated.

Clinical features

- Results in haemolysis with an Hb of 6–8 g/dL with intermittent crises and complications

Vaso-occlusion effects:
- Painful crises:
  - Bone pain:
    - Adults: ribs, spine, pelvis
    - Children: hands and feet
  - Chest syndrome in 30%: commonest cause of death in adults with sickle cell from infection, fat embolism and pulmonary sequestration. Presents with chest pain, cough, dyspnoea
- Cerebral infarction: strokes (particularly in children), fits and hemiplegia
- Retinal ischaemia: visual loss
- Priapism: persistent and painful erection from sequestration of sickle cells in corpora cavernosa. Needs decompression, can cause impotence

- Bone necrosis/osteomyelitis
- Splenic atrophy: they become susceptible to infection

Haemolytic effects:
- Anaemia (less symptoms than would be expected as HbS has less affinity for O_2 than regular Hb)
- Gallstones
- Jaundice
- Splenomegaly
- Heart failure and cardiomyogaly: from hyperdynamic circulation

Late symptoms and signs:
- Chronic ill health
- Leg ulcers
- Long-term lung complications
- Renal failure
- Liver dysfunction: due to sequestration.

Clinical features

Sickle cell crises:
1. *Vaso-occlusive crises:*
   - Sickled cells are trapped in the microcirculation
   - Precipitated by dehydration, hypoxia, infection, acidosis and cold
   - Microinfarcts occur in the bone, lung, spleen, brain and spinal cord
2. *Haemolytic crises:*
   - Haemolysis of fragile sickled RBC in the spleen after 10–12 days rather than 120, leading to ↓ Hb
   - In chronic disease Hb is ↓ , but can drop further due to infection, drugs, and with coexistent glucose-6-phosphate dehydrogenase deficiency

Other crises:
- *Aplastic crisis:*
  - Bone marrow aplasia often triggered by parvovirus B19 which infects RBC precursors
  - Self limiting but transfusion may be required
- *Visceral sequestration:*
  - Sickled RBCs pool in the liver and spleen causing pain, anaemia, hepatosplenomegaly, shock and death. Leads to splenic atrophy with ↑ infection risk
  - Need exchange transfusion.

IN A CRISIS

Investigations

Blood tests

- FBC: ↓ Hb, ↑ Reticulocytes (20–30%)
- U&Es: ↑ Cr in renal failure
- ↑ Bilirubin

- ↑ LDH
- ABG: hypoxia, acidosis.

Infection screen

- Cultures: blood, sputum, urine

- CXR: new infiltrate on X-ray in chest syndrome

For diagnosis

- Blood film:
  - Target cells
  - Sickle cells (Fig. 8.2D)

- Electrophoresis:
  - To confirm diagnosis
  - Distinguishes HbSS and HbAS

Prenatal diagnosis

- Maternal blood sampling for fetal DNA then PCR
- Chorionic villus sampling

- Fetal blood sampling (mid-2nd trimester).

Treatment

Crisis:
- Treatment is only symptomatic:
  - Analgesia
  - O_2 +/− respiratory support
  - Hydration with IV fluids
  - Warm support
  - Antibiotic therapy if infection present
  - Blood transfusion
  - Exchange transfusion if recurrent crisis or significant organ damage
  - Venous thromboembolism prophylaxis: LMWH and compression stockings
Prevention of crises and infection:
- Long-term folic acid: to maintain ↑ Hb production

- Immunisation against pneumococcus and *H. Influenza* (encapsulated organisms)
- Long-term prophylactic penicillin V
- Avoid precipitating factors: cold, dehydration, violent exercise, hypoxia, infection
- Before surgery or pregnancy: exchange transfusion or RBC transfusion
- Genetic counselling
Long term:
1. Bone marrow transplant: only if <16 years
2. Regular blood transfusions sometimes indicated, e.g. organ damage or risk of stroke: aim to keep HbS <30%
3. Hydoxycarbamide if >1 chest crisis in 2 years or >3 painful crisis in 1 year
4. Splenectomy for hypersplenism.

Prognosis and complications

Prognosis

- 5% mortality in first 10 years of life
- Average lifespan: 40–50 years

- Spleen normally infarcted by age 6.

Prognosis and complications

Complications

- Cerebrovascular accident
- Infection (hyposplenism: encapsulated organisms), particularly *Salmonella* for bone and joint infections
- Infarctions
- Cholelithiasis
- Social/schooling absentism

- Glaucoma
- Nephrotic syndrome
- Limb ulceration
- Iron overload from multiple transfusions: causes toxicity of heart, liver, pituitary, parathyroid, thyroid, pancreas
- Infertility.

AUTOIMMUNE HAEMOLYTIC ANAEMIA

Outline

Immunological destruction of RBCs by autoantibodies:

- Leads to haemolysis

- Classified into warm or cold types depending on the optimal temperature for antibody binding.

Pathogenesis/aetiology

Pathogenesis

- Table 8.9 gives the differences between warm and cold types.

Table 8.9 Differences between warm and cold types

Warm	Cold
Reacts at 37 °C	Reacts at < 4 °C (antibody comes off RBC at warmer temperatures)
IgG antibody	IgM antibody: complement
1° cause: idiopathic. If associated with idiopathic thrombocytopenic purpura = Evans's syndrome	1° cause: idiopathic
2° causes: – Autoimmune disorders (50%), e.g. SLE – Lymphoma, CLL – Drugs: e.g. methyldopa, penicillin, quinidine	2° causes: – Infections, e.g. glandular fever (anti-i), malaria, *M. pneumoniae* (anti-I) – Lymphoma – Paroxysmal cold haemoglobinuria: rare
Mainly extravascular haemolysis	Mainly intravascular haemolysis

Who

- Typical ages: all
- 1♀:1♂

Associations:

- Other autoimmune disorders (50%).

Clinical features

Symptoms of anaemia

Cold:

- Chronic anaemia worse when cold
- Occurs with Raynaud's, acrocyanosis (cyanotic discolouration of the fingers)

Warm:

- Splenomegaly.

Investigations

Blood tests

- Coombs' test detects antibodies on RBCs = direct antiglobin test
- *Warm*: IgG
- *Cold*: C3d complement

Blood film:

- Features of haemolysis:
  - *Warm*: spherocytes, microspherocytes
  - *Cold*: agglutination

- Reticulocytosis schistocytes and helmet cells - intravascular haemolysis
- Schistocytes and helmet cells - intravascular haemolysis

Investigate for 2° causes:

- *Warm*: ANA, anti-dsDNA, immunoglobulins, paraprotein
- *Cold*: mycoplasma serology, Donath–Landsteiner antibody (in paroxysmal cold haemoglobinuria)
- ↓ haptoglobin–intravascular.

Treatment

- Remove underlying cause

Warm type:
- Steroids
- Folic acid
- Immunosuppressant drugs, e.g. azathioprine, cyclophosphamide, vincistine, IVIG, rituximab
- Danazol
- Splenectomy

Cold type:
- Keep warm
- Chlorambucil, steroids, cyclophosphamide

Life-threatening anaemia:
- RBC transfusion (least incompatible blood).

Prognosis and complications

Prognosis

- Depends on underlying cause.

PAROXYSMAL NOCTURNAL HAEMOGLOBINURIA

Outline

- An acquired RBC membrane disorder making RBCs susceptible to haemolysis by the complement pathway
- Features of the clinical syndrome include:
  - haemolytic anaemia
  - venous thromboses (of the large vessels)
  - pancytopenia
  - aplastic anaemia
  - iron deficiency.

Pathogenesis/aetiology

Causes

- Mutation of the *pig*-A gene on the X chromosome which synthesises glycosylphosphatidylinositol, which is important for attachment of cell surface proteins
- Some of the surface proteins, such as CD55 and CD59, play a role in stopping the complement process, without them, complement continues leading to haemolysis.

Who

- Rare.

Clinical features

- Abdominal pain
- Dark urine in the morning (from Hb in the urine)
- Haemolysis
- Thrombosis, e.g. Budd–Chiari syndrome
- Anaemia
- Aplastic anaemia
- Iron deficiency.

Investigations

Blood tests

- Pancytopenia
- Flow cytometry to detect CD55 and CD59 on RBCs (absence is diagnostic)
- HAM test (RBC lysis at low pH).

Imaging

- For suspected venous thromboses.

Treatment

- Symptomatic treatment – RBC transfusion
- Iron therapy
- Folic acid
- Eculizumab (anti-complement 5)
- Stem cell transplant
- Steroids
- Anticoagulation.

Prognosis and complications

Prognosis

- May be stable
- Can develop into aplastic anaemia or leukaemia or myelodysplastic syndrome.

BLEEDING DISORDERS

GENERAL FEATURES

Outline

Bleeding disorders are caused by:
1. platelet disorders: from a ↓ in function, number thrombocytopenia or both

2. blood factor disorders
3. blood vessel defects
4. coagulation factor disorders.

1. PLATELET DISORDERS

PLATELET FUNCTION DISORDERS

Outline

- Bleeding impairment due to a problem with platelet function.

Pathogenesis/aetiology

Causes

- Disorders of adhesion:
  - Platelet-type Von Willebrand disease
  - Impaired adhesion to collagen
  - Bernard–Soulier syndrome: GP1b deficiency
- Storage pool disease: abnormality/deficiency of alpha dense granules: Wiskott-Aldrich syndrome
- Disorders of aggregation:
  - Glanzmann's thrombasthenia: glycoprotein (GP) IIb/IIIa deficiency
  - Essential athrombia

- Acquired disorders:
  - Drugs: aspirin, NSAIDs, alcohol
  - Uraemia, liver disease
  - Myeloproliferative and myelodysplastic disorders
  - Paraproteinaemia
- Cardiopulmonary bypass
  - Isolated platelet factor III deficiency

Who

- Relatively rare.

Clinical features

- Bleeding of mucosal lining
- Petechial rash and spontaneous shin purpura

- Prolonged bleeding after trauma and postpartum
- Lifelong bleeding (in Glanzmann's and Bernard–Soulier).

Investigations

Blood tests

- Platelet count normal
- Bleeding time: prolonged
- Platelet function analyser 100: prolonged

- Blood film: congenital platelet dysfunction, myelodysplastic picture
- Platelet aggregation studies.

Treatment

- Platelet transfusion
- Tranexamic acid (if bleeding)

- Avoid: aspirin, NSAIDs.

Prognosis and complications

Prognosis

- Dependent on underlying cause.

THROMBOCYTOPENIA

Outline

- Bleeding impairment due to a ↓ number of platelets ($<150 \times 10^9$/L)

- Can be due to an underproduction of platelets or excess destruction.

Underproduction:
- Bone marrow infiltration: malignancy, sarcoidosis
- ↓ megakaryotes: aplastic anaemia, excess alcohol, severe megaloblastic anaemia
- Drugs
- Infection

Excess destruction:
- Drugs: quinine, amiodarone, rifampicin, thiazide diuretics
- Heparin-induced thrombocytopenia
- DIC, bacterial sepsis
- Thrombotic thrombocytopenic purpura and haemolytic uraemic syndrome (see both below) and HELLP
- Platelet pooling in the spleen: myleofibrosis, splenomegaly
- HIV, hepatitis C
- Autoimmune:
  - ITP see below
  - Posttransfusion

- 1♀:1♂.

Platelets
- $20-50 \times 10^9$/L: bruising and petechiae following minor trauma
- $<20 \times 10^9$/L: mucosal bleeding

- Purpura
- Spontaneous haemorrhages
- Lymphadenopathy
- Splenomegaly (uncommon in ITP).

- Platelet count is low

- Platelet associated antibody

- Bone marrow examination if >60 years or unusual signs or symptoms: exclude paroxysmal nocturnal haemoglobinuria by the immunophenotyping,

myelodyplastic syndrome, malignancy, or bone marrow infiltration.
- Investigation for underlying causes.

- Treat underlying cause

Acute crisis:
- Platelet transfusion
- Cryoprecipitate (blood product from fresh frozen plasma).

- Bleeding

IMMUNE THROMBOCYTOPENIA (ITP)

- An autoimmune disorder with thrombocytopenia due to platelet destruction
- Often follows a viral infection particularly in children. 30% of children go on to have chronic ITP compared with almost all adult cases

- Can be idiopathic or associated with a secondary cause.

Primary:
- Idiopathic

Secondary:
- Associated with SLE, chronic lymphocytic leukaemia, HIV, HCV, *Helicobacter pylori* infection.

- An IgG autoantibody develops against a glycoprotein receptor on the platelet membrane

Acute ITP:
- 1♀:1♂
- 5/100 000
- Children only

Chronic ITP:
- ♀ > ♂
- 3–5/100 000
- 20–40 year olds.

- Easy bruising
- Purpura

- Mucosal bleeding: nose bleeds, menorrhagia (heavy periods)
- Prolonged bleeding from skin cuts.

Blood tests

- Platelet count is low
- Immature platelet fraction is high

Blood film:
- Giant platelets

Other tests

Bone marrow examination:
- Not always required

- Exclude all other causes for thrombocytopenia.

- Children normally do not require treatment
- *H. pylori* eradication if implicated
- Suppress immune response:
  - Prednisolone
  - IV Immunoglobulin (for crises)
  - Anti-D immunoglobulin (for crises)

- Rituximab
- Azathioprine
- Splenectomy (2nd line) with pneumococcal vaccine and lifelong penicillin
- Thrombopoietic stimulating agents.

Prognosis

- 15–25% lasting remission
- 2/3 respond to steroids

- Most have a relapsing–remitting course
- ITP patients: 80% enter remission after medication

Complications

- Bleeding

- Fatigue (side effect from medication)

THROMBOTIC THROMBOCYTOPENIC PURPURA

Outline

- A disorder with a pentad of abnormalities where there is thrombocytopenia due to platelet consumption in platelet-rich thrombi
- Abnormalities are caused by microvascular thrombi including renal failure and thrombocytopenic purpura

- Mechanical fragmentation of RBC during flow through partially occluded high shear small vessels
- Only 20–30% present with full pentad
- **A haematological emergency**

Causes

- Associated with:
  - Quinine, simvastatin, trimethoprim, oestrogen-containing drugs
  - HIV, pregnancy
  - Transplant
  - Malignancy

- Pancreatitis
- Idiopathic:
  - Abnormal ADAMTS13 (an enzyme that breaks down von Willebrand factor) in thrombotic thrombocytopenic purpura (normal in haemolytic uraemic syndrome).

- Rare
- Commoner in adults

- ♀ > ♂.

Clinical features

- Pentad of abnormalities:
  1. Micro-angiopathic haemolytic anaemia, jaundice
  2. Thrombocytopenia (usually 10-30 x 10^9/L)
  3. Neurological abnormalities, e.g. fits, decreased consciousness
  4. Renal disease – proteinuria and microhaematuria
  5. Fever.

Investigations

Blood tests

- FBC: ↓ Hb, ↓ platelets, ↑ reticulocytes
- Clotting profile: normal
- ↑ D-dimer and fibrinogen (helpful in distinguishing thrombotic thrombocytopenic purpura from DIC)
- Direct antigobulin test negative
- Baseline troponin
- ↑ LDH

- ↓ Haptoglobins
- U&Es: ↑ Cr
- ↑ bilirubin (haemolysis)

Blood film:
- Schistocyte (fragments of RBC).
- ADAMTS13 activity ↓ and antibody ↑

Urine

- Full virology screen

- Proteinuria

Other tests

CT:
- If suspected cardiovascular vascular accident.
  - Head (stroke)
  - Investigate for malignancy with CT around chest, abdomen and pelvic areas if suspicious

ECG
Echocardiogram

Treatment

- Plasma exchange with fresh frozen plasma (75–90% respond)
- Do not transfuse platelets

- Folic acid
- Methylprednisolone.

Prognosis and complications

Prognosis

- Untreated: 90% mortality
- Relapse rate: 13–36%

- If refractory, treat with rituximab.

Complications

- Stroke

- Myocardial infarction

HAEMOLYTIC URAEMIC SYNDROME (HUS)

Outline

- Intravascular haemolysis with fragmentation of RBCs
- Renal failure is the predominant symptom

- Normally follows an infection of **Escherichia coli 0157:H7**.

Pathogenesis/aetiology

Causes

- Associated postdiarrhoeal infection with:
  - Escherichia coli O157:H7

- *Shigella dysenteriae.*

Who

- Commoner in children.

Clinical features

- Renal failure is more severe than in thrombotic thrombocytopenic purpura (commonest cause of acute renal failure in children) and neurological manifestations are rarer

- May occur after symptoms of acute infection, particularly gastroenteritis with bloody diarrhoea.

Investigations

Investigations

Blood tests

- FBC: ↓ Hb, ↓ platelets, ↑ reticulocytes
- Clotting profile: normal
- U&Es: ↑ Cr
- Small vWF multimers
- ↑ Bilirubin (haemolysis)

Blood film:
- Schistocyte (RBCs from damage as they move past thrombi)
- Normal ADAMTS13 activity.

Urine

- Haematuria.

Other tests

Stool culture: may detect Escherichia coli.

Treatment

- Mainly supportive: including fluids, nutrition, antihypertensives

- Often requires haemodialysis
- Plasmapheresis if severe.

Prognosis and complications

Prognosis

- Mortality ~5%
- 5% have CRF

- Adults have a poorer prognosis than children.

2. BLOOD FACTOR DISORDERS

VON WILLEBRAND DISEASE

Outline

- Bleeding disorder due to inherited deficiency of von Willebrand factor (vWF) or dysfunction
- Acquired or inherited

vWF:
- A plasma protein that acts as cofactor for platelet adhesion to damaged subendothelium
- Acts as a stabliser for factor VIII, i.e. prevents degradation.

Pathogenesis/aetiology

Causes

- Gene on chromosome 12
- Type 1: autosomal dominant condition. Reduced vWF (quantitative)
- Type 2: autosomal dominant condition. Dysfunction of vWF (qualitative)

- Type 2C: autosomal recessive
- Type 3: most severe form. Autosomal dominant homozygous. Lack of vWF

Who

- Commonest inherited bleeding disorder
- 0.1% population

- Affects both sexes.

Clinical features

- Superficial bruising, menorrhagia and nosebleeds
Types 1 and 2:
- Mucosal bleeding: epistaxis, GI bleeds, bleeding gums
- Prolonged bleeding after surgery
- Menorrhagia, postpartum haemorrhage

- Deep haematomas uncommon
Type 3:
- Severe symptoms and signs: some as severe as haemophilia A–haemarthrosis.

Investigations

Blood tests

- VWF antigen: type 1 and normal type 2: ↓
- Decreased VIII: C
- APTT: prolonged
- PT: normal
- vWF RiCof activity decreased type 1
- Thrombin time: normal
- PFA-100: prolonged

- Ristocetin induced platelet aggregation: to distinguish types 1 and 2
- Hyperresponsive in type 2B
- Multimers:
  - Large multimers are decreased in type 1B and absent in type 2A

Treatment

Bleeding:
- Desmopressin (DDAVP) to ↑ natural levels (challenge 1st to ensure response). It stimulates release of factor VIII by endothelial cells
- Tranexamic acid (anti-fibrinolytic)
- vWF concentrates

Prevention:
- Avoid aspirin
- Preoperative desmopressin
- Can give desmopressin if responsive; if not, vWF concentrates
- In acquired vWD, bleeding is often very severe, therefore surgery should be avoided.

Prognosis and complications

Prognosis

- Deep haematomas: rare, only with type 3

- Normal life expectancy usual except with acquired vWD.

3. BLOOD VESSEL DEFECTS

GENERAL FEATURES

Outline

- Abnormalities in the blood vessels leading to bleeding disorders.

Pathogenesis/aetiology

Causes

Hereditary:
- Hereditary haemorrhagic telangiectasia
- Autosomal dominant disease with characteristic red spots
- CT disorder: Ehlers–Danlos, Marfan's syndrome

Acquired:
- Severe infection: meningococcal
- Drugs: steroids
- Allergic: Henoch–Schönlein purpura
- Scurvy, senile purpura
- Easy bruising syndrome.

Who

- Depends on cause.

Clinical features

Hereditary haemorrhagic telangiectasia:
- Epistaxis
- Recurrent GI bleeding
- Telangiectasia (localised collection of distended capillary vessels causing red spots which blanch on pressure)

General (not in hereditary haemorrhagic telangiectasia):
- Easy bruising
- Bleeding into the skin (rarely severe)
- Other symptoms depend on cause.

Investigations

- Laboratory investigations are normal

- Bleeding time: normal in vitro.

Treatment

- Tranexamic acid.

Prognosis and complications

Prognosis

- Depends on cause.

4. COAGULATION DISORDERS

HAEMOPHILIA A

Outline

- Coagulation disorder due to factor VIII deficiency.

Classification

- Mild: >5% of normal factor VIII levels
- Moderate: 1–5%
- Severe: if <1%
- Carriers have 50% normal level.

Pathogenesis/aetiology

- Inherited: **X-linked recessive**
- Family history of males affected on the maternal side of the family.

Pathogenesis

- Factor VIII is important in the intrinsic pathway of the coagulation cascade acting as a cofactor with factor IX to activate factor X.

Who

- Prevalence: 1/8000 ♂
- Affected women are asymptomatic carriers
- 30% have no family history (new mutations).

Clinical features

- Bleeding can be spontaneous or 2° to trauma

Mild:
- Post-traumatic bleeds and easy bruising

Severe:
- Spontaneous bleeding into muscles or joints
- Deep haematomas
- Arthropathy from bleeding into joints particularly of knees, elbows, ankles, wrists, shoulders and hips
- Intracranial bleeding
- Haematuria.

Investigations

Blood tests

- Factor VIII: antigen and activity ↓
- APTT: prolonged
- PT: normal
- Thrombin time: normal
- PFA-100: normal.

Other tests

- Antenatal diagnosis: fetal blood sampling or chorionic villus sampling
- Gene mutation analysis
- Von Willebrand assay to exclude type 3 von Willebrand's disease.

Treatment

- Managed in specialised haemophilia centres

For bleeds:
- IV recombinant factor VIII concentrate: for moderate/ severe bleeds
- IV desmopressin: for small bleeds. Stimulates release of factor VIII by endothelial cells

General management:
- Physio/hydrotherapy: with factor VIII cover. Minimises joint deformity and maintains mobility
- Analgesia
- Rest and elevation of haemarthrosis

Prevention:
- Avoid contact sports
- Good dental hygiene
- No NSAIDs or IM injections
- Prophylactic factor VIII: 3 × a week after one spontaneous joint bleed
- Genetic counselling.

Prognosis and complications

Prognosis

- With treatment: normal life expectancy.

Prognosis and complications

Complications

- Recurrent bleeding leading to permanent deformity or arthritis
- Haemophilic pseudo-tumours
- Development of inhibitors to factor VIII (30%): refractory to further replacement therapy
- HIV/Hep C infection if received blood products before 1986.

HAEMOPHILIA B

Outline

- Coagulation disorder due to inherited deficiency of plasma factor IX
- Also called Christmas disease.

Pathogenesis/aetiology

- Inherited: X-linked recessive.

Pathogenesis

- Factor IX is important in the intrinsic pathway of the coagulation cascade part of a process activating factor X with factor VIII cofactor.

Who

- Prevalence: 1/30 000 ♂
- Affected women are asymptomatic carriers.

Clinical features

- As for haemophilia A.

Investigations

Blood tests

- Factor IX low
- APTT: prolonged
- PT: normal
- Thrombin time: normal
- PFA-100: normal.

Treatment

- Recombinant factor IX concentrates
- Desmopressin not effective
- General management and prevention; otherwise, as for haemophilia A.

Prognosis and complications

Prognosis

- Normal life expectancy with treatment
- Development of inhibitors less common than in haemophilia A.

ACQUIRED COAGULATION DISEASES

Outline

These include:
- Vitamin K deficiency:
  - Vitamin K is required for the formation of factors II, VII, IX, X

Liver disease:
- Commonest cause of acquired coagulation disease
- Results in:
  - Thrombocytopenia and platelet abnormalities
  - ↓ Synthesis of clotting factors
  - ↓ Vitamin K absorption due to cholestasis.

Pathogenesis/aetiology

Causes of vitamin K deficiency:
- Malabsorption
- Malnutrition (including ICU patients)
- Newborns: poor vitamin K stores
- Liver disease: see hepatology chapter 5.

Who

- Commoner than inherited coagulation disorders
- Neonates.

- Bruising
- Haematuria
- GI bleeds
- Cerebral bleeds.

Blood tests

- APTT: prolonged
- PT: prolonged
- Thrombin time: normal (but severe disease causes ↓ fibrinogen, which causes a ↑ TT):
- PFA-100: normal.

- Phytomenadione (vitamin K) orally
- Vitamin K given to newborns prophylactically
- Correct underlying cause.

Complications

- Bleeding.

DISSEMINATED INTRAVASCULAR COAGULATION (DIC)

- Widespread, inappropriate intravascular deposition of fibrin from release of procoagulant substances into the blood or release of tissue factor leading to consumption of coagulation factors and platelets
- Consumption of coagulation factors leads to ↑ risk of bleeding
- Microthrombotic events from vessel occlusion by platelets (in 5–10%) leading to ischaemia and infarction.

Causes

Release of procoagulant substances into the blood:
- Malignancy: acute promyelocytic leukaemia, mucin-secreting adenocarcinoma, pancreatic cancer
- Haemolytic transfusion reaction–incompatible RBC
- Trauma
- Amniotic fluid embolism, placental abruption

- Liver disease
- Severe falciparum malaria
Endothelial tissue damage:
- Tissue damage: rhabdomyolysis, burns
- Infection: Gram − ve meningococcal septicaemia, virus
- Snake bites.

- Occurs in ∼1% of hospitalised patients.

- Mild to life-threatening
- Haemorrhage from any site
- Bruising
- Thrombotic events leading to: ischaemia or infarction in lungs, heart, brain, kidneys, liver, DVT, PE.

Blood tests

- APTT: prolonged
- PT: prolonged
- Thrombin time: prolonged
- ↓ Platelets
- Fibrinogen: ↓ (as widespread fibrin formation)
- D-dimers (product of fibrin degradation): ↑ due to increased break down of excess fibrin deposits
- Blood film: fragmented RBCs from haemolysis.

Treatment

- Treat underlying cause
- Supportive care: antibiotics, fluids, debridement
- Transfuse: platelets, fresh frozen plasma, cryoprecipitate, RBCs if bleeding

- Heparin or antiplatelet to slow activation of coagulatory factors if thrombotic problems are severe
- Antithrombin concentrates or activated protein C in severe sepsis or acute fatty liver of pregnancy.

Prognosis and complications

Prognosis

- Mortality 80% in acute DIC.

Complications

- Renal failure.

THROMBOTIC DISORDERS

- Thrombosis: blood clot within a vessel
- Emboli: fragments that break off a thrombus and block downstream vessels

- Thrombotic disorders can be arterial or venous, each of these are addressed in turn below:

ARTERIAL THROMBOSIS

Outline

- Formation of a thrombus in an artery
- Platelets play an important part

- Clot: platelet rich, RBC poor, pale, friable.

Pathogenesis/aetiology

Pathogenesis

- Usually from an atheroma (fatty deposits in the walls of vessels) formed in areas of turbulent blood flow, e.g. at the bifurcation of arteries
- Platelets adhere to damaged endothelium stimulating coagulation and leading to thrombosis and obstruction

- Emboli from this thrombus can break off and move down stream causing myocardial infarcts, strokes/TIAs and blockage of smaller vessels.

Who

Risk factors:
- Atherosclerosis:
  - Male
  - ↑ Age
  - Smoking
  - Hypertension
  - ↑ Cholesterol

- Diabetes mellitus
- Family history
- Antiphospholipid syndrome
- Hyperhomocysteinaemia
- Collagen vascular disease
- ↑ Factor VII
- ↑ Fibrinogen.

Clinical features

- MI/acute coronary syndrome
- Strokes/TIA

- Mesenteric arterial thrombosis causing ischaemic bowel.

Investigations

Clinical investigations

- BP.

Blood tests

- Lipid profile
- Fasting glucose
- Folate
- Homocysteine.
- Troponin
- Antibodies:
  - ANA

- Anti-dsDNA
- Anti-cardiolipin

For antiphospholipid syndrome:
- Anti-[beta]2glycoprotein 1
- Anticardiolipin antibodies
- Lupus anticoagulant

Investigations

Cardiac investigations

- ECG
- Echocardiogram

Imaging

- Carotid artery doppler US
- CT head: stroke.

Other tests

- Methylenetetrahydrofolate reductase (MTHFR) mutation analysis (leads to hyperhomocysteinaemia).

Treatment

Prevention: anti-platelet therapy:
- Aspirin: inhibits cyclooxygenase, ↓ thromboxane A$_2$ production
- Dipyridamole: inhibits platelet activation
- Clopidogrel: blocks platelet aggregation
- Abciximab, eptifibatide, tirofiban: block receptor for glycoprotein IIb/IIIa inhibiting the final pathway of platelet aggregation

Treatment:
- Thrombolytic therapy:
  - Streptokinase: forms complex with plasminogen to form plasmin (side effect: haemorrhage)
  - Tissue-type plasminogen activator (tPa)
  - Contraindications: recent major bleed, uncontrolled hypertension, recent surgery, bleeding disorders
- Surgery or angioplasty:
  - May be appropriate depending on location of thrombus or emboli.

Prognosis and complications

Prognosis

- Dependent on artery affected.

Complications

- Dependent on location of thrombus or emboli.

VENOUS THROMBOEMBOLISM (VTE)

Outline

- Thrombus in a vein
- Usually in deep veins of the legs causing a DVT
- The thrombus can dislodge and travel to the lungs leading to a pulmonary embolism
- Clot is dark red: rich in RBC, poor in platelets

Virchow's triad:
- Categories of risk factors for venous thrombus formation:

1. Abnormal blood flow, stasis: immobility, venous obstruction, ↑ viscosity
2. Vessel wall abnormalities: damage to vessel wall: trauma, thrombophlebitis (inflammation of a vein due to a clot), malignancy, vasculitis
3. Abnormal blood constituents: hypercoagulable states, e.g. protein C and protein S deficiency.

Pathogenesis/aetiology

Precipitating risks:
1. Stasis:
   - Hyperviscosity
   - Dehydration
   - Nephrotic syndrome
   - Pelvic obstruction
     - HONK
   - Postoperative (particularly orthopaedic)
   - Immobility
2. Vessel wall abnormalities:
   - Trauma
   - Vasculitis
   - Thrombophlebitis
   - Varicose veins

3. Hypercoagulable states:
Acquired:
- ↑ Oestrogen: puberty, hormone replacement therapy, contraceptive pill
- Pregnancy
- Obesity
- Malignancy
- ↑ Homocysteine
- ↑ Factors: VII, VIII, IX, XI
Hereditary:
- Abnormal fibrinogen
- Hereditary thrombophilias
- Paroxysmal nocturnal haemoglobinuria.

Pathogenesis

- RBCs and fibrin accumulate around venous valves forming thrombi

- The clot enlarges increasing the risk of embolisation (most commonly to the pulmonary vessels)
- Usually multiple risk factors involved.

Who

- Common, 1:1000/year in high-risk groups
- Commoner in older age

- 70% of patients with symptomatic PE will have asymptomatic DVT as well.

Clinical features

Clinical syndromes:
- Often asymptomatic (up to 75%)
- DVT (see Ch. 13)

- Pulmonary embolism (see Ch. 3)
- Budd–Chiari syndrome (hepatic vein occlusion)
- Acute abdomen: mesenteric vein thrombosis.

Investigations

Blood tests

- FBC (including platelets), clotting screen, D-dimers:
  - High negative predictive value for DVT
  - Investigate for paroxysmal nocturnal haemoglobinuria

- Investigate for risk factors and screen for malignancy if >40 years old
- Consider hereditary thrombophilia with relevant investigations (see below) if family history.

Imaging

- Depends on clinical syndrome: Doppler ultrasonography for DVT; CTPA for PE.

Treatment

Prevention:
- Mobilisation and hydration
- Risk stratification on admission to hospital
- Compression stockings: thigh length
- LMWH/inferior vena cava filter: filter used in high risk patients (often with a known DVT) who cannot receive anticoagulation to prevent pulmonary emboli

Mechanical interventions
- Graduated elastic stockings for post thrombotic syndrome
- Inferior vena cava filler if contraindication for medical coagulation

Pharmacological interventions:
- LMWH:
  - Continued until warfarin treatment is begun and the therapeutic target INR is attained.

- Unless due to malignancy when LMWH is continued instead of warfarin
- Vitamin K antagonist e.g. Warfarin
  - Target INR 2–3 (with regular monitoring)
  - Anticoagulated for 3–6 months if there is a definite trigger that has been eliminated and this is the 1st event
  - Ongoing treatment if there are persistent multiple risk factors or this is the second episode
- Factor Xa inhibitors, e.g. fondaparinux, rivaroxaban.

Thrombolysis
- For certain criteria in DVT and PE

Prognosis and complications

Prognosis

- Pulmonary embolus accounts for 5% of all hospital deaths

Complications

- Post-thrombotic syndrome: permanent pain, swelling, oedema, venous eczema from destruction of deep vein valves

- Recurrence of thrombosis
- Bleeding on anticoagulant therapy, drug interactions.

HEREDITARY THROMBOPHILIA

Outline

- Hereditary disease state causing increased risk of thromboses

- Usually predisposes to venous thromboses.

Causes

- Multifactorial interplay of environment and genetic predisposition
- Factor V Leiden (see below)
- Antithrombin deficiency: usually presents in early adulthood

- Protein C and S deficiency: these proteins inhibit factors V and VIII
- PG2O21OA mutation leads to ↑ prothrombin
- Antiphospholipid syndrome.

- Prothrombin gene mutation prevalence: ~2%.

Suspect if:
- Patient has unprovoked VTE under the age of 40 or arterial thrombotic disease under 30
- Thrombosis in unusual sites, e.g. cerebral vein

- Recurrent thromboses (unprovoked)
- Strong family history
- Recurrent miscarriages: antiphospholipid syndrome.

Blood tests

- Clotting profile
- Fibrinogen

- Protein C and protein S levels
- Antithrombin level and function.

Genetic testing

- DNA PCR:
  - Factor V Leiden

  - PG2021OA

Other tests

- Venous compression

- Ultrasound CTPA.

- Treat any thrombosis with anticoagulation ± thrombolysis

Prevention:
- Lifelong anticoagulation in antithrombin deficiency

- Precautions in surgery, pregnancy, puerperium, inhospital stay, travel
- Avoid oral contraceptive pill or hormone replacement therapy
- Modify risk factors for thrombotic disease.

- As above.

FACTOR V LEIDEN

- Commonest inheritable cause of thrombosis (but not the highest relative risk compared with other inherited defects).

- Inherited: autosomal dominant with incomplete dominance

- Gene on chromosome 1.

Pathogenesis

- Factor V is important in the coagulation cascade
- Normally deactivated by protein C
- In factor V Leiden, protein C is unable to deactivate abnormal factor V

- Results in overactivation of the clotting cascade and an increased tendency to form venous thromboses.

- Prevalence: 4% for heterozygotes
- 20–40% of patients with VTE have factor V Leiden

Risk factors:
- Heterozygotes: 5–8 × ↑ risk of VTE
- Homozygotes: 30–130 × ↑ risk.

Clinical features

- As above for hereditary thrombophilia.

Investigations

Genetic testing

- PCR.

Other tests

- Activated protein C resistance test.

Treatment

- Only treat if VTE occurs
- No evidence for 1° prophylactic anticoagulation
- If strong family history of VTEs:

- Screen
- Incidental finding of factor V Leiden: prophylactic LMWH during high-risk situations.

Prognosis and complications

Prognosis

- Absolute risk of venous thrombosis is multifactorial.

HAEMATOLOGICAL MALIGNANCIES

These include:
- Lymphomas

- Leukaemias
- Paraproteinaemias.

LYMPHOMAS

GENERAL FEATURES

Outline

- Malignant tumour of lymph nodes
- Proliferation of lymphocytes (B and T cells) forming solid lumps within lymphoid tissue

- <25% in bone marrow (compared with leukaemia).

Classification

- Based on morphology, immunophenotyping and genotype
- WHO classification system:
  - Hodgkin's lymphoma

- Non-Hodgkin's lymphoma (NHL):
  - B precursor
  - B mature
  - T precursor
  - T mature
  - Natural killer neoplasms.

Pathogenesis/aetiology

Ann Arbor staging system:
- Stage I: single node region
- Stage II: 2 or more node regions on same side of diaphragm
- Stage III: nodes both sides of diaphragm

- Stage IV: extralymphatic involvement: liver/bone marrow, bone, lung
- Suffix A: no B symptoms
- Suffix B: B symptoms
- Suffix E; single contiguous extranodal site
- Suffix X: bulking disease.

Who

- More common than leukaemia

- Young people.

Clinical features

- Lymphadenopathy (large lymph nodes):
  - Cervical
  - Axilla
  - Inguinal

- B symptoms:
  - Fever: >38 °C
  - Drenching night sweats
  - Weight loss: >10% in 6 months
  - Lack of energy

Investigations

- Fresh tissue not only fine-needle aspirations
- Each MDT must have a pathologist to review material for all new diagnoses and integrate all investigations

- Cytogenetic analysis by FISH
- Bone marrow biopsy for staging

Treatment

Standard chemotherapy regimes used in treatment:
- Hodgkin's lymphoma:
  - ABVD: adriamycin, bleomycin, vinblastine, dacarbazine
  - BEACOPP: bleomycin, etoposide, adriamycin, cyclophosphamide, vincristine, procarbazine, prednisolone

- NHL:
  - R-CHOP: rituximab, cyclophosphamide, doxorubicin (hydroxydaunorubicin), vincristine, prednisolone.
- CUF: Cyclophophamide, vincristine, prednisone
- Fludarabine
- Etoposide

Prognosis and complications

Prognosis

- Worse with B symptoms and resistant or relapsed disease

- Salvage therapy is most difficult following BEACOPP than ABVD

Complications

- Side effects of radiotherapy or chemotherapy
- 2° malignancies
- Pulmonary and cardiac toxicity

- Subfertility
- Relapse.

HODGKIN'S LYMPHOMA (HL)

Outline

- Pathognomonic of classical Hodgkin's lymphoma is the Reed–Sternberg cell: large bi- or multinucleate malignant B lymphocytes (Fig. 8.2e)
WHO classification:
- Classical Hodgkin's lymphoma:
  - Nodular sclerosing
  - Mixed cellularity
  - Lymphocyte rich

- Lymphocyte depleted
- Nodular lymphocyte-predominant Hodgkin's lymphoma:
  - No Reed–Sternberg cells (Fig. 8.2E)
  - 'Popcorn' nuclei
  - Rare B symptoms
  - 5% of Hodgkin's lymphoma.

Pathogenesis/aetiology

Causes

- Unknown

- Associated with EBV infection.

Pathogenesis

- Usually spreads to adjacent nodal groups (contiguous)
- Lymphadenopathy is supradiaphragmatic in 90%

- Liver, spleen, lung and bone marrow may be affected.

Who

- 1♀:2♂
Classic Hodgkin's lymphoma:
- 5/100 000
- 2nd commonest malignancy in 15–34-year-old adult males

- Caucasian groups
- ♀: peak at 30s then decreases
- ♂: peaks at 30 then remains constant

Clinical features

- Enlarged rubbery lymph nodes:
  - Particularly in the neck
  - Usually painless
  - May present with alcohol-related pain
- Pruritus
- Anaemia (30%)
- Cachexia
- Hepatosplenomegaly

Hasenclever index (a prognostic score for advanced Hodgkin's lymphoma):
- Each is associated with an additionally poor prognosis
- Hb <10.5 g/dL
- Albumin <40 g/L
- Stage 4
- Male
- WBC >15 × 10^9/L
- Lymphocyte <0.6
- Age >45 years.

Investigations

Blood tests

- FBC:
  - Normochromic normocytic anaemia
  - Lymphocytopenia
  - Neutrophilia
  - Eosinophilia
  - Thrombocytosis

- ↓ Albumin
- ↑ LDH (from ↑ cell turnover)
- ↑ ALP
- ↑ ESR.

Imaging

- CXR: pulmonary opacities and mediastinal lymphadenopathy

- CT, PET of the chest, abdomen and pelvis: for staging and restage after salvage.

Other tests

- Lymph node biopsy: for diagnosis or relapsed or primary resistant

- Bone marrow aspirate and biopsy: if infiltration is suspected (stage 3 or B symptoms present).

Treatment

Classic Hodgkin's lymphoma:
- Stage 1A–IIA and no adverse risk factors:
  - Radiotherapy with chemotherapy
- Stage IIB–IV and Hasenclever 4 or >4:
  - Chemotherapy
- Stage IIB–IV and Hasenclever score <4:
  - ABVD chemotherapy 6–8 cycles depending on response
- Older or unfit patients:

- Low-toxicity chemotherapy
- Radiotherapy
- Relapse:
  - Salvage chemotherapy
  - Stem cell autograft transplantation

Nodular lymphocyte-predominant Hodgkin's lymphoma:
- Stage 1A: radiotherapy
- Stage 2–4: treat as for classical Hodgkin's lymphoma.

Prognosis and complications

Prognosis

- 5 year survival: 75%
- Many cured only after second/third-line therapy
- Poor prognosis:
  - **Lymphocyte-depleted** Hodgkin's lymphoma

- **B symptoms**
- **High stage**
- **↑ age**
- **↑ ESR, ↑ LDH.**

Complications

- Predisposition to HSV
- Side effects of radiotherapy or chemotherapy

- Tumour lysis syndrome
- Relapse.

NON-HODGKIN'S LYMPHOMA

Outline

WHO classification:
1. Mature B-cells:
   a. Follicular:
      - Grades 1&2: indolent (slow growing), rarely require treatment

- Grade 3A & 3B: aggressive, treated as diffuse large B-cell lymphoma
   b. Marginal zone lymphomas:
      - Mucosa-associated lymphoid tissue, extranodal
      - Nodal marginal zone.

Outline

- Splenic marginal zone
- c. Diffuse large B-cell lymphoma: high grade and aggressive
- d. Mantle cell lymphoma: low grade and aggressive, high risk of relapse
- e. Burkitt's lymphoma: very aggressive
2. Mature T-cell, natural killer cell lymphoma/leukaemia
3. Precursor B-cell or T-cell leukaemia/lymphoma (lymphoblastic lymphoma) – common in boys

Pathogenesis/aetiology

Causes

Multifactorial:
- Genetic predisposition – none established
- Immunosuppression
- Viruses, e.g.
  - EBV causing Burkitt's lymphoma and B-cell NHL
- Human T-lymphotropic virus (HTLV-1) causing T-cell NHL
- HIV-Burkitt's and DLBL
- Radiation
- *H.pylori*-Mucosa-associated lymphoid tissue

Who

- Typical age: uncommon before 40
- ♀ < ♂ for NHL
- Incidence:
  - 12/100 000 per year
  - ↑ with age, NHL in 60–70 years
- 4% of all cancers
- More common than Hodgkin's lymphoma
- Commonest forms: diffuse large B-cell lymphoma and follicular lymphoma.

Clinical features

- Painless lymphadenopathy (75%)
- B symptoms: more common in high-grade lymphoma
Extranodal manifestations:
- Any organ may be affected
- Hepatosplenomegaly and bone marrow involvement more common than in Hodgkin's lymphoma
- Bone marrow infiltration:
  - Anaemia
    - Recurrent infections
    - Bleeding

Investigations

Blood tests

- FBC: ↓ Hb, ↓ platelets, ↑ WBC
- LFTs
- LDH
- β_2-Microglobulins
- Serum paraproteins and immunoglobulins
- HIV: in those with 1° CNS disease.

Imaging

- CXR: for mediastinal lymph nodes
- CT head, chest, abdomen and pelvis: for staging
- CT, PET: to confirm stage I

Other tests

- Lymph node biopsy (core or excision): for diagnosis.
- Bone marrow aspiration and biopsy
- Lumbar puncture with CSF analysis: to assess for CNS involvement
- Immunophenotyping
- Monospot test: for EBV.

Treatment

Follicular:
- Stage I/II: radiotherapy
- Stage II–III and asymptomatic: monitor
- Stage III–IV: R-CHOP. If old and unfit: chlorambucil
Diffuse large B-cell lymphoma:
- Stage I: R-CHOP and radiotherapy
- Radioimmunotherapy
- Stage II–IV: R-CHOP

Burkitt's:
- Chemotherapy
Mantle cell:
- Fit and <60 years: chemotherapy then stem cell transplant.

Treatment

- Unfit or >60 years: R-CHOP or rituximab cyclophosphamide, fundarabine

Marginal zone:
- Mucosa-associated lymphoid tissue:
  - *H. pylori* eradication (curative)
  - Chlorambucil (second line)
  - Rituximab (third line)

Relapse
- Retreat if had good response
- Myeloablative (destroys bone marrow cells) chemotherapy with autologous stem cell rescue or allogenic bone marrow transplant
- Novel chemotherapy combinations.
- Assess treatment success.

Prognosis and complications

Prognosis

International Prognostic Indicator (IPI) scores:
- Differs for each subtype of NHL
- For follicular NHL:
  - Functional ability
  - Age >60
  - Stage III/IV disease
  - ↑ LDH

- Spread to > 1 site beyond the lymph nodes
- Hb <12
- >4 nodal sites
- Overall 5 year survival rate:
  - 0–1 factor: 90%
  - 2 factors: 78%
  - 3–5 factors: 53%.

Complications

- Side effects of radiotherapy or chemotherapy: 2° malignancy, pulmonary and cardiac toxicity, subfertility

- Relapse

LEUKAEMIAS

GENERAL FEATURES

Outline

- ↑ Number of non-functional haemopoietic blood cells produced by the bone marrow
- Cells spill out into the blood and can infiltrate organs including the liver, spleen and lymph nodes

- Within the bone marrow the excess leukaemic cells suppress production of normal white cells, RBCs and platelets.

Classification

Stage of cell development:
- *Acute*: block in cell differentiation so immature blast cells accumulate. Aggressive and rapidly fatal if not treated. Cells accumulate in the bone marrow causing bone marrow failure
- *Chronic*: mature haemopoietic cells accumulate. Follows a less aggressive and slower course

Type of cell:
- *Erythroid*: red blood cells
- *Myeloid*: eosinophils, neutrophils, basophils and megakaryocytes
- *Lymphoid*: lymphocytes
- *Plasmacyatoid*: plasma cells

Types of leukaemia:
- Acute myeloid leukaemia (AML)
- Acute lymphoblastic leukaemia (ALL)
- Chronic myeloid leukaemia (CML)
- Chronic lymphocytic leukaemia (CLL).

Pathogenesis/aetiology

Cause

- Mostly unknown
- Genetics
- Environmental:

- Chemicals
- Drugs
- Radiation.

Pathogenesis

- Critical cellular pathways corrupted by accumulating genetic damage leading to autonomous proliferation of a stem cell clone

- CNS and testes tend to act as sanctuary sites for the cancer.

Who

- ALL commoner in children

- AML, CLL, CML more common in the elderly.

Clinical features

General:
- Due to bone marrow failure:
  - ↓ Functional WBC: ↑ susceptibility to infection, fever
  - ↓ Platelets: bruising and bleeding, purpura, petechiae
  - ↓ RBCs: anaemia, lethargy, pallor, dyspnoea
  - Hepatosplenomegaly: extramedullary haemopoiesis due to marrow failure
- Bone marrow infiltration
  - Bony pain
- Leucostasis (abnormal intravascular clumping of leucocytes) only common in CML with very high numbers of leukaemic cells:

- Confusion and drowsiness
- Blurred vision
- Fever
- SOB and cough

Specific:
- B cells (produced in the bone marrow):
  - Features depend on the site of lymphadenopathy: in the abdomen: effusions and ascites
- T cells (produced in the thymus):
  - Large mediastinal mass
  - Affects heart and great vessels: superior vena cava obstruction

Investigations

Blood tests

- FBC: ↑ WBC, lymphocytes in CLL and neutrophils and metamyelocytes in CML, monocytes in CMML ↓ RBC, ↓ platelets ↓ neutrophils
- U&Es

- ↑ Urate
- ↑ LDH
- Clotting abnormal in APML
- Blood film: blasts in acute leukaemia

Imaging

- CXR: mediastinal mass in T-cell ALL

Other tests

- Bone marrow trephine biopsy and special stains: diagnostic test
- Bone marrow aspirate for immunophenotyping, cytochemistry and morphollogy

- Lumbar puncture: to check for CNS infiltration
- Cytogenetics

Treatment

- Specialist management
- Chemotherapy:
  - Hickman line: for long-term venous access
  - Aims:
    - Induce complete remission
    - Consolidate complete remission
- ± stem cell transplant (for high risk patients)
- Monoclonal antibodies for targeted and less cytotoxic therapy
- Bone marrow transplant:
  - Autologous: patients own cells are stored and then returned at a later date – rare in leukaemia treatment

- Allogenic: genetically similar but not identical donor, a sibling or matched unrelated donor

Supportive care:
- Immediate treatment of neutropenic sepsis
- Blood and platelet transfusion as needed
- Prophylactic antiviral and antifungal medication
- Mouth washes
- Adequate hydration and allopurinol to reduce risk of tumour lysis syndrome during treatment
- Consider CMV negative blood products.

Prognosis and complications

Complications

- Side effects of radiotherapy or chemotherapy
- 2° malignancies
- Pulmonary and cardiac toxicity
- Subfertility

- Neutropenic sepsis
- Fungal infections
- Reactivation of CMV.

ACUTE MYELOID LEUKAEMIA (AML)

Outline

- Acute: block in differentiation
- Myeloid: eosinophils, neutrophils and basophils affected
- Immature blasts accumulate in the bone marrow causing bone marrow failure

- Blasts infiltrate the liver, spleen, skin and gums

Outline

Classification

Depends on affected cell:
- MI: undifferentiated myeloblastic
- M2: myeloblastic.
- M3: acute promyelocytic leukaemia (APML), associated with DIC

- M4: myelomonocytic: associated with skin and meningeal infiltration
- M5: monocytic: lymphadenopathy, meningeal and skin infiltration
- M6: erythroleukaemia: leukaemia
- M7: megakaryocytic.

Pathogenesis/aetiology

Causes

- Radiation
- Chemotherapy: alkylating agents, topoisomerase II inhibitors
- Predisposing diseases: myelodysplastic syndrome, rarely myeloproliferative disease
- Aplastic anaemia

- Congenital disorders, e.g. Down's syndrome, Fanconi anaemia, neurofibromatosis

Cytogenetics:
- t(15:17) in acute promyelocytic leukaemia
- KIT, CEBPA, TP53, RUNXI mutations

Who

- Incidence:
  - 2/10 000 children per year
  - 15/10 000 older adults per year

- 20% of all leukaemias
- More common in the elderly, especially as transformation from myelodysplastic syndromes.

Clinical features

- Symptoms and signs of bone marrow failure as above
- Infiltration:
  - Hepatomegaly
  - Splenomegaly
  - Lymphadenopathy
  - Bone pain

- Chloroma: a collection of leukaemic cells outside the bone marrow (only in M5)
- Skin infections
- DIC in type M3
- Hyperviscosity if very ↑ WBC
- CNS involvement rare in AML.

Investigations

Blood tests

- FBC:
  - Normochromic, normocytic anaemia
  - ↓ WBC and ↑ blasts
  - ↓ Platelets
  - Pancytopenia in APML
  - ↑ Urate, LDH and calcium

Blood film:
- Blasts: (Auer rods (crystals of coalesced granules with a rod-like appearance on microscopy (Fig. 8.3))
- >30% of blasts resemble promyelocytes in APML

Bone marrow:
- Hypercellular, ↑ blast cells

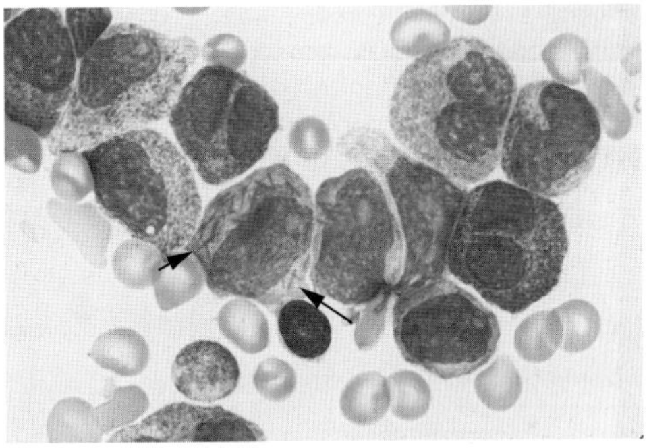

Fig. 8.3 Blast cells in AML with Auer rods in the cytoplasm (arrowed), which are typical of the disease.

Other tests

- Cytogenetic analysis: t(15:17), t(8:21).

- Molecular analysis

Treatment

- Supportive, particularly treating infections urgently
- Chemotherapy and immunotherapy, e.g. immunotoxin, gemtuzumab (anti-CD33)
- Stem cell transplant

APML:
- Emergency if deranged clotting (DIC):
  - All trans-retinoic acid
  - Chemotherapy
  - These can only be given once blast count has fallen.

Prognosis

- Rapidly progressive
- Mean survival: 2 months if untreated (usually due to sepsis)
- 3 year survival after chemotherapy: 20%

Poor prognosis:
- ↑ Age
- ↑ Blast cell count

ACUTE LYMPHOBLASTIC LEUKAEMIA (ALL)

Outline

- Acute: immature blasts
- Lymphoblastic: lymphoblasts

Classification

- Common B ALL 50%
- T-cell ALL 24%

- Other B-cell ALL 26%
- Can also be classified by microscopic appearance of blasts.

Pathogenesis/aetiology

Causes

Genetics:
- Translocations:
  - Philadelphia chromosome t(9,22): translocation between chromosomes 9 and 22 (combining the genes bcl and abr) which ↑ tyrosine kinase activity
  - t(4,11), t(8,14)

- Down's syndrome
- Ataxia telengiectasia

Environmental:
- Radiation exposure
- Transformation from CLL.

Who

- ♀ < ♂
- Commonest malignancy in childhood (23%)

- Peak incidence: aged 4 or >65 years
- T-cell ALL commonest in adolescent boys.

Clinical features

- Symptoms and signs of bone marrow failure as for 'General features above'
- Bleeding (30%)
- Infection (30%)
- Bone pain is a common presentation
- Short history as disease is aggressive
- Lymphadenopathy and splenomegaly (50%): not as pronounced as in CLL
- CNS involvement (60%)

T-cell ALL:
- Mediastinal mass
- Pleural effusion

Mature B-cell ALL:
- Leukaemic infiltration
- Retina, skin, tonsils.

Investigations

Blood tests

- FBC:
  - Normochromic normocytic anaemia
  - ↑ WBC
  - ↓ platelets

- ↓ Reticulocyte count
- ↑ Urate
- Coagulation usually normal
- Blood film: lymphoblasts

Imaging

- CXR: mediastinal mass in T-cell ALL.

Other tests

Bone marrow:
- Characteristic lymphoblasts in blood and bone marrow
- Lymphoblasts >20% of bone marrow cells (should be 5%).

Cytogenetics:
- Philadelphia chromosome.

Treatment

- Supportive care: hydration, prophylactic antibiotics, allopurinol
- Chemotherapy
- CNS prophylaxis: intrathecal (into the spinal canal) methotrexate
- Allogenic stem cell transplant if prognosis is poor.

Prognosis and complications

Prognosis

- 5 year survival:
  - Children 80%
  - Adults 30% if poor, 60% if good
- Poor indicators:
- Age <2 years or >9 years
- Male
- T-cell ALL
- Philadelphia chromosome
- WBC $>30 \times 10^9$/L
- Complications:
- Relapse sites are bone marrow, CNS, testes.

CHRONIC MYELOID LEUKAEMIA (CML)

Outline

- Chronic: mature cells accumulate
- Myeloid: eosinophils, neutrophils and basophils affected
- Considered a myeloproliferative disorder (see below)
- Can be divided into three phases:
  - A chronic phase lasting many years
- Then an accelerated phase: signals progression of the disease and that transformation to blast crisis is soon
- Followed by a blast phase or blast crisis where CML transforms to AML. Survival rates are lower.

Pathogenesis/aetiology

Causes

- Unknown
- Radiation
- Philadelphia chromosome t(9,22): >90% of patients with CML.
- The abnormally constitutively active tyrosine kinase (as a result of Philadelphia chromosome) causes autophosphorylation of downstream cell signalling pathways, making them resistant to apoptosis and leading to uncontrolled proliferation.

Who

- ♀ < ♂
- Incidence: 1/100 000 per year
- Peak incidence: 50–60 years
- 20% of all leukaemias.

Clinical features

- Insidious onset
- General symptoms:
- Fever
- Tiredness
- Weight loss
- Night sweats
- Gout (↑ urate)
- Marrow infiltration:
- Symptoms of bone marrow failure as for 'General features' if anaemia, thrombocytopenia and leucopenia
- Massive splenomegaly with abdominal pain
- Hepatomegaly 50%
- Lymphadenopathy uncommon.

Investigations

Blood tests

- ↑ Neutrophils and metamyelocytes, in accelerated phase – increase in basophils
- FBC: ↓ Hb, ↑ WBC, ↑ platelets
- ↑ Urate
- ↑ LDH
- ↑ Vitamin B$_{12}$
- Blood film:
- Leukoerythroblastic picture
- >20% blasts is blastic phase

Other tests

- Bone marrow:
- ↑ myeloid cells
- Hypercellular.
- Cytogenetics:
- Philadelphia chromosome.

Treatment

- Supportive care

Chronic and accelerated phase:
- Imatinib: a first-generation tyrosine kinase (TK) inhibitor for chronic and accelerated phase disease. Eliminates the mutant stem cell clone but must be taken lifelong. 10% do not respond
- Second-generation TK inhibitor: if no response or unable to tolerate imatinib

- Allogenic stem cell transplant: if above are unsuccessful

Chronic phase treatment:
- Interferon-alpha or hydroxycarbamide, to control cell counts and TK inhibitor

Blastic phase:
- Treat as for AML or ALL with the addition of imatinib.

Prognosis and complications

Prognosis

- With imatinib: 5 year complete haematological response: 98%.

Complications

- Leucostasis: treat with urgent plasmaphoresis

- 60% transform to AML, 30% to ALL.

CHRONIC LYMPHOCYTIC LEUKAEMIA (CLL)

Outline

- Definition: $\geq$5000 B-lymphocytes/μl peripheral bleed for $\geq$3 months
- Uncontrolled proliferation and accumulation of mature non-functional peripheral lymphocytes (95% are B-cell

CLL). Lymphoctyes proliferate in marrow, blood and lymphoid tissue
- T-cell CLL occurs rarely.

Pathogenesis/aetiology

Cause

- Unknown
- Familial predisposition (7x increased risk)
- Overexpression of Bcl2 gene

- Antigen stimulation within specific microenvironments and failure of apoptosis

Differential diagnosis

- Leukaemic phase of NHL
- Viral infection

- Prolymphocytic leukaemia

Progressive disease

Any of:
- Lymphocyte doubling time <1 year
- Decreasing platelets

- Decreasing Hb
- >50% increased organomegaly
- Constitutional symptoms.

Who

- Incidence increases in the elderly
- $\female < \male$
- Caucasians more common

- 25% of all leukaemia in adults
- 4.2 per 100 000/year

Clinical features

- Generalised lymphadenopathy (60%)
- Splenomegaly (30%)/organomegaly
- B symptoms
- ↑ Infection: from ↓ immunoglobulins

Stages:
- Stage A: <3 lymph nodes areas + Hb$\geq$10 g/dL, platelets $\geq$100 $\times$ 10^9/L
- Stage B: 3–5 lymph node areas + Hb$\geq$10 g/dL, platelets $\geq$100 $\times$ 10^9/L
- Stage C: Hb <10 g/dL, platelets <100 $\times$ 10^9/L.

Investigations

Blood tests

- FBC: ↓ Hb, ↑ WBC, ↓ platelets
- ↑ Urate
- ↑ LDH
- ↑ β_2-microglobins
- Coombs' test (direct antiglobulin test)
- Bilirubin: to exclude haemolytic anaemia
- ↓ γ-globulins

Blood film:
- Smudge cells: mature lymphocytes which are fragile (Fig. 8.4)

Other tests

Bone marrow:
- Aspirate and biopsy
- Increased mature lymphocytes (>30%).
- Cytogenetics.

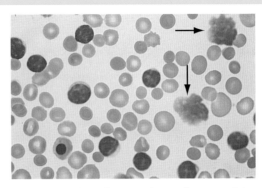

Fig. 8.4   Smudge cell (arrowed) typically seen in CLL.

Treatment

- Mostly supportive with monitoring

Chemotherapy:
- Stage A: watch and wait and monitor
- Stage B if symptomatic: chemotherapy
- Stage C or progressive disease: or B symptoms and chemotherapy

Chemotherapy:
- Old/unfit: chlorambucil or bendamustine
- Young/fit: fludarabine and cyclophosphamide and rituximab (anti-CD20)

Allogenic stem cell transplant:
- If young or poor prognosis (e.g. p53 mutation).

Prognosis and complications

Prognosis

- Worse prognosis:
  - Presenting with marrow failure

- T-cell CLL
- Death normally from infection.

Complications

- 10% transform to a high-grade lymphoma (Richter transformation). Very bad prognosis
- Associated with autoimmune haemolysis or ITP

- Complications of chemotherapy
- Immune suppression.

PARAPROTEINAEMIAS

GENERAL FEATURES

Outline

- Presence of monoclonal (produced from a single clone of plasma cells) immunoglobulins in the blood
- The paraproteins can be:
  - whole immunoglobulins

- part of the immunoglobulin:
  - heavy chains
  - light chains: when monoclonal light chains are filtered through the kidney they are known as Bence Jones. These can be measured and are commonly found in paraproteinaemias, particularly multiple myeloma.

Causes

- Myeloma
- Waldenström's macroglobinaemia
- Leukaemia and lymphoma
- 'Monoclonal gammopathy of undetermined significance' (MGUS). Defined as:
  - Paraprotein IgG <35 g/d or IgA < 20 g/L

- Urine light chains <1 g/24 h
- No immunoparesis (reduction in immunoglobin)
- Bone marrow plasma <10%
- No lytic bone lesions
- Normal Hb, calcium and renal function.

- Seen in older patients.

- Depends on cause.

- Identified by a single band on serum electrophoresis

- Classified by immune fixation (IgG, IgM, IgA, IgD, IgE and light chain).

Urine

- Bence Jones proteins.

- Depends on cause.

Complications

- MGUS requires regular follow-up as may later develop myeloma or lymphoma.

MULTIPLE MYELOMA

- Malignant proliferation of the plasma cells of the bone marrow
- Plasma cells are antibody (immunoglobulin) producing cells formed from B lymphocytes
- The malignant cells produce a monoclonal immunoglobulin (60% IgG, 30% IgA) and suppress normal immunoglobulin production

- In the majority of cases, immunoglobulin light chains are filtered at the glomerulus and can be found as Bence Jones proteins in the urine (see 'General features' above).

Causes

Most cases present de novo
- Genetics:
  - >50% have abnormalities of chromosomes. Useful for prognosis. Also linked with some genes

- Environmental:
  - Radiation
  - Inflammation and infection
- Monoclonal gammopathy of undetermined significance:
  - A significant percentage of patients develop myeloma.

Pathogenesis/aetiology

Pathogenesis of symptoms

- Recurrent bacterial infections:
- Due to ↓ in immunoglobulin

Skeletal abnormalities: 60%:

- Osteolytic lesions and pathological fractures: neoplastic cells produce osteoclastic activating factors which ↑ osteoclast activity, weakening bone.

Renal failure in 20–30% from several causes:

- 2° metabolic disturbances such as hypercalcaemia and hyperuricaemia affect the kidney

- Side effects of treatment are nephrotoxic, e.g. NSAIDs
- ↑ Risk of renal amyloidosis
- Light chain deposition in the glomerulus

Hyperviscosity syndrome:

- Due to polymerisation of a monoclonal antibody

Bone marrow infiltration:

- Pancytopenia.

Who

- Median age: >70
- ♀ < ♂
- Incidence: 5/100 000

- 1% of all malignancies
- Higher incidence in Afro-Caribbeans.

A typical patient

A 78-year-old female with back pain, anaemia and weight loss presents to her doctor. She is pale, with a tender spine but no evidence of cord compression. She is anaemic with a low total protein, renal impairment and a high calcium.

Clinical features

- Infections
- Bone pain and fractures
- Renal failure: presenting complaint in 20–30%
- Hyperviscosity symptoms: epistaxis, visual disturbances, headaches, confusion

- Hypercalcaemia: bones, stones, abdominal groans and psychic moans (see also Biochemistry chapter 12)
- Marrow failure: symptoms of pancytopenia
- Spinal cord compression

Investigations

Blood tests

- FBC: ↓ Hb
- U&E: ↑ Cr
- ↑ Calcium
- ↑ Urate
- ↓ Albumin
- ↑ β_2-microglobulin
- ↑ ESR and CRP
- Serum free light chains

Blood film:

- Rouleaux formation: RBC sticking together (Fig. 8.5)

Electrophoresis or immunofixation:

- Monoclonal paraprotein band
- May have immunoparesis (low levels of one or more immunoglobins).

Urine

- Bence Jones protein

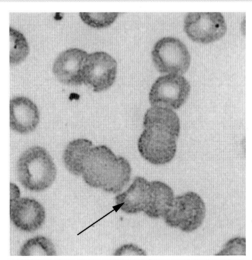

Fig. 8.5 Rouleaux formation of RBCs seen in myeloma.

Imaging

- X ray: 'punched out' lesions such as 'pepper pot' skull or osteolytic lesions (Fig. 8.6) = osteolytic lesions
- Skeletal survey
- There is a lack of osteoblastic (bone formation) reaction on bone scans
- CT to clarify the significance of ambiguous x-ray findings.

Other tests

Bone marrow aspirate and biopsy:
- Plasma cell infiltration >15%
- Gold standard.
- Quantification of the paraprotein
Cytogenetics:
- Chromosomal analysis.

Differential diagnosis

- MGUS
- AL amyloidosis
- Solitary plasmacytoma
- Bl-NHL
- CLL.

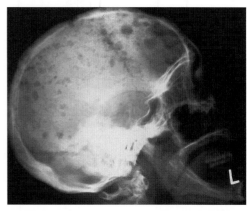

Fig. 8.6 Osteolytic lesions or 'pepper pot' skull seen in multiple myeloma.

- Incurable
Supportive:
- Analgesia: opiates and bisphosphonates
- Infection: antibiotics
- Blood product transfusions
- Hypercalcaemia and renal failure: hydration and bisphosphates
- Cord compression or fractures: emergency surgery or radiotherapy
- Hyperviscosity: plasmapheresis

Chemotherapy:
- Alkalating agents: melphalan, cyclophosphamide
- Younger patients: viscristine, adriamycin, dexamethasone
- Thalidomide
Radiation therapy:
- For bone pain
Others:
- Allogenic stem cell transplantation: may be curative, but has a high mortality so rarely done.

Prognosis

- Mean survival: 2–3 years
- Poor prognosis:
  - ↑ β_2-microglobulin levels

- ↓ Albumin
- Abnormalities of chromosome 13
- Deletions of p53, t(4:14), t(14:16).

Complications

- Death from renal failure or infection
- Spinal cord compression

- Amyloidosis of AL type in 10% (see below).

MYELOPROLIFERATIVE DISORDERS

GENERAL FEATURES

Outline

- A group of diseases of the bone marrow where there is clonal uncontrolled overproduction of one or more of the early cell lines: either erythroid, myeloid, megakaryocyte

- The precursors retain their ability to differentiate.

ESSENTIAL THROMBOCYTOSIS

Outline

- An increase in the number of platelets
- Platelets $>450 \times 10^9$/L sustained
- Platelets may be abnormal and have impaired function

- No other myeloid malignancy
- No reactive cause for ↑ platelet.

Pathogenesis/aetiology

Causes

Primary/essential thrombocythaemia:
- Myeloproliferative disorders

Secondary:
- Chronic bleeding

- Iron deficiency
- Trauma
- Inflammation: neoplasm, chronic infection.

Who

- Typical age: 50–60 year olds

- Rare in children.

Clinical features

- Asymptomatic
- Venous thromboembolism
- **Bleeding** (mainly of the GI system)
- Bruising
- Cerebrovascular symptoms

- Arterial thrombosis
- Systemic symptoms:
  - Weight loss
  - Pruritus
  - Sweats.

Investigations

Blood tests

- FBC: ↑ Platelets
- U&Es.
- Differentiate from secondary thrombocytosis due to:
  - Chronic bleeding

- Iron deficiency
- Inflammation
- Infection
- Malignancy.

Genetic studies

- JAK2 mutation
- MPL exon 10

- If JAK2 and MPL negative then test BRCA61 to exclude CML

Other tests

- Bone marrow examination.

Treatment

Primary:
- Busulfan, hydroxyurea, interferon-alpha.

Prognosis and complications

Complications

- Thromboses

- Progression to acute leukaemia or myelofibrosis

POLYCYTHAEMIA

Outline

- Disorder of a raised haematocrit (the proportion of blood volume taken up by RBCs)
- Absolute: ↑ in number of RBCs:
  - *Primary* (polycythaemia rubra vera): from a myeloproliferative disorder

- *Secondary*: ↑ erythropoietin production
- Relative/apparent: ↓ in total plasma volume with normal RBCs volume.

Pathogenesis/aetiology

Causes

Absolute: primary:
- Polycythaemia rubra vera: a malignant myeloproliferative disease of excessive proliferation of erythroid, myeloid and megakaryocytic progenitor cells. Due to a failure in apoptosis. Leads to hyperviscosity and thromboses

Absolute: secondary:
- Chronic hypoxia: heart or lung disease, high altitude
- Inappropriate erythropoietin production: renal/ liver disease

Relative:
- Stress
- Alcohol excess
- Smoking
- Dehydration
- Burns: plasma loss.

Who

Polycythaemia ruba vera

- Typical age: age 45–60 years
- Incidence: 1.5/100 000/year.

Clinical features

Polycythaemia ruba vera

- Aquagenic pruritus (in water)
- Erythema
- Facial plethora
- Tiredness
- Gout
- Arterial or venous occlusive event

- Raynaud's
- Angina
- Stroke/TIA
- Hyperviscosity symptoms: headaches, visual disturbances, tinnitus, dizziness
- Splenomegaly (60%).

Investigations

Polycythaemia rubra vera

Blood tests
- ↑ Hb
- ↑ Haematocrit
- ↑ Packed cell volume
- ↑ RBC
- ↑ WBC (↑ neutraphils in 60%)
- ↑ platelets (in 50%)

- **↓ or normal serum erythropoietin.**

Other tests
- US abdomen
- **Genetic studies: JAK2 mutation** in 95% of ruba vera
- Bone marrow aspirate: erythroid hyperplasia is a second line investigation

Secondary or relative causes

Must be excluded by:
- Careful history and examination
- ↑ **erythropoietin** (may be normal)
- **ABG**
- CXR

- α-fetoprotein
- Renal US.

Treatment

- Venesection to maintain haematocrit <0.45
- Aspirin
- Cytoreductive therapy: hydroxyurea, busulfan, chlorambucil, anagrelide, interferon

- if poor tolerance if venesection or symptomatic splenomegaly or disease progression or ↑ platelet
- Folic acid

Conservative measures:
- Reduce risk factors of arterial thromboembolism and VTE.

Prognosis and complications

- Rubra vera.

Prognosis of polycythaemia ruba vera

- Variable
- ~10–15 years survival with treatment.

Prognosis and complications

Complications of polycythaemia ruba vera

Transformation to:
- Leukaemia: 5%
- Myelofibrosis: 30%

- Thromboses
- Haemorrhage
- Iron deficiency.

MYELOFIBROSIS

Outline

- Disorder where there is massive fibrosis of the marrow due to hyperplasia of the megakaryocytes (precursor for platelets found in the bone marrow).

Pathogenesis/aetiology

Pathogenesis

- Hyperplasia of megakaryotes (therefore classified as myeloproliferative) which produce platelet derived growth factor
- This causes fibrosis of the marrow and bone marrow failure

- Haemopoiesis is redirected to the liver and spleen
- Cause of hyperplasia is unknown
- In 25% of cases there is a history of polycythaemia rubra vera.

Who

- Uncommon.

Clinical features

- Lethargy
- Night sweats
- Fever
- Weakness
- Weight loss
- Bone pain
- Hepatosplenomegaly: massive due to haemopoiesis

Marrow failure:
- Bruising and bleeding
- Symptoms of anaemia
- Infection.

Investigations

Blood tests

- ↓ Hb unexplained
- Blood film: dacrocytes, teardrop-shaped RBC leukoerythroblastosis (Fig. 8.7).

Other tests

- Bone marrow aspirate for diagnosis: often dry tap
- US abdomen
- JAK2 mutation or MPL mutation

Exclude relative and secondary polycythaemia:
- Serum erythropoietin, ABG, α-fetoprotein, CXR

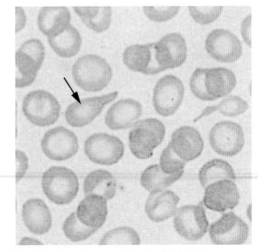

Fig. 8.7   Teardrop appearance of red RBCs in myelofibrosis.

Treatment

- Supportive: blood transfusion, folic acid, analgesics
- Hydroxyurea: reduces metabolic activity, WBC and platelets↑, anagrelide or interferon
- erythropoietin
- Hydroxycarbamide
- prednisolone
- Novel therapy: thalidomide
- Splenic irradiation or splenectomy
- Stem cell transplant

Prognosis and complications

Prognosis

- Median survival: 3 years.

Complications

- Transformation to AML: 10–20%.

DISORDERS OF THE BONE MARROW

BONE MARROW FAILURE

Outline

- A disorder of the haemopoietic stem cells of the marrow
- In adults, haemopoeisis (the formation of blood cells) occurs in the bone marrow
- Can be due to an inherited or acquired cause
- Bone marrow failure can affect one or all of the cell lines: RBCs, white blood cells and platelets

Pancytopenia:
- ↓ RBCs, white blood cells and platelets

Aplastic anaemia:
- Marrow hypoplasia (hypocellularity) leading to pancytopenia. The commonest cause of marrow failure. Can be due to congenital cause or acquired.

Pathogenesis/aetiology

Causes of bone marrow failure:

Congenital (15–20%)

- Fanconi's congenital aplastic anaemia: a rare autosomal recessive disorder characterised by short stature, aplastic anaemia and a predisposition to malignancy

NB: not the same as Fanconi syndrome.

Acquired

- Hypocellular marrow:
  - Idiopathic
  - Autoimmune
  - Drugs: NSAIDs, chloramphenicol, gold, phenylbutazine, chemotherapy
  - Radiotherapy
  - Paroxysmal nocturnal haemoglobinuria (see below)
  - Infection: hepatitis, HIV, parvovirus
- Infiltrated marrow:
  - Haemotological malignancies
  - Secondary cancers
- Differentiation defect:
  - Myelodysplasia.

Who

- Uncommon but serious
- 5/1000 000 each year
- Commonest cause is aplastic anaemia.

Clinical features

Reduced RBCs:
- Symptoms of anaemia

Reduced white blood cells:
- Infection

Reduced platelets:
- Thrombocytopenia
- Bleeding
- Bruising

Investigations

Blood tests

- FBC: pancytopenia, low or absent reticulocytes, normocytic anaemia
- Blood film.

Other tests

- Bone marrow examination: hypocellular marrow.

Treatment

- Treat cause
- Supportive:
  - Low WBC: antibiotics and antifungal
  - RBC transfusion
  - Platelet transfusions
  - If ferritin levels >1000 mg/L, give iron chelation

If severe:
- Bone marrow transplant (HLA matched sibling donor) if <40 years and severe or very severe
- Immunosuppressants: ciclosporin, high dose steroids
- Antithymocyte globulin (ATG).

Prognosis and complications

Prognosis

- Untreated: death within 6 months
- Prognosis worse if WBC is very low.

MYELODYSPLASIA

Outline

- Ineffective production in the bone marrow of all three myeloid lines (RBCs, neutrophils, platelets) due to a clonal defect in stem cells suppressing function of normal stem cells
- Progresses to AML.

Pathogenesis/aetiology

Causes

Primary:
- Often idiopathic

Secondary:
- Aggressive treatment for other previous cancers.

Who

- Typical age: usually >60 years old.

Clinical features

- Lethargy
- Fever
- Bruising
- Symptoms of anaemia
- Bleeding
- Infection: due to ineffective granulopoiesis
- Splenomegaly (10–20%).

Investigations

Blood tests

- Macrocytic anaemia
- ↑ MCV
- ↑ Monocytes

For diagnosis, requires:
- Bone marrow aspirate: shows ring sideroblasts, pelgeroid (hyposegmented) neutrophils, megakaryocytes with abnormal nuclei
- Bone marrow biopsy: hypercellularity.

Other tests

- Cytogenetics.

Treatment

- Supportive: RBC and platelet infusions, iron chelation therapy, erythropoietin ± granulocyte colony-stimulating factor to stimulate bone marrow production of granulocytes

- Chemotherapy
- Allogenic bone marrow transplantation depending on age, and if there is a matched donor.

Prognosis and complications

Prognosis

- Survival: 6 months to 6 years.

Complications

- Progression to AML: 30%
- Life-threatening bleed

- Neutropenic sepsis.

PARAPROTEIN DYSCRASIA

AMYLOIDOSIS

Outline

- Group of disorders where there is extracellular deposition of abnormally folded protein in organs
- These proteins are amyloids: insoluble fibrous protein aggregates
- Symptoms depend on the site of deposition

Classification of some systemic forms:
- *AL amyloidosis:*
  - Abnormal monoclonal immunoglobulins forming excess light chains, e.g. Bence Jones proteins in myeloma
  - Light chains deposit in the kidneys, heart, nerves, gut, and blood vessels

- Associated with chronic B lymphoproliferative disorders, e.g. myeloma, NHL
- *AA amyloidosis:*
  - Abnormal acute phase protein
  - Related to chronic inflammatory disorders and infection, e.g. rheumatoid arthritis, IBD, TB
- *Familial amyloidosis:*
  - Autosomal dominant
  - Most common form due to abnormal transthyretin
  - Causes sensory or autonomic neuropathy.

Pathogenesis/aetiology

Causes

- Acquired or inherited.

Pathogenesis

- Amyloids are extracellular proteins with a beta-pleated sheet crystalline structure
- There are many different forms depending on the precursor plasma protein:
  - Sustained, abnormally high concentration of proteins, e.g. β_2-microglobulin in renal failure

- Prolonged exposure to an amyloidogenic protein, e.g. beta protein in Alzheimer's disease
- Inherited or acquired variant protein, e.g. monoclonal immunoglobulin light chain (AL).

Who

- Typical age: >65 years old.

Clinical features

AL and AA:
- General: fatigue, weight loss, faints, oedema
- Kidney: glomerulonephritis, nephrotic syndrome, proteinuria
- Heart: angina, restrictive cardiomyopathy leading to dyspnoea
- Nerves: painful sensory neuropathy, autonomic neuropathy
- GI system: constipation, diarrhoea, hepatosplenomegaly

Specific to AL:
- Macroglossia
- Cardiac involvement more common than for other forms

Familial amyloidosis:
- Causes sensory or autonomic neuropathy
- Cardiomyopathy
- Mild renal disease.

Blood and urine tests

- FBC, U&Es, LFTs, albumin, coagulation, calcium
- Serum and urine free light chains

- Paraprotein studies and immunofixation.

Imaging

- Echocardiogram: speckled appearance
- Skeletal survey

- Serum amyloid P scintigraphy (nuclear medicine test forming 2D images).

Other tests

- ECG: for cardiomyopathy
- Biopsy of affected organ
  - best site often rectal biopsies

- Stained with Congo red: apple-green birefringence under polarised light

- Treat underlying disease: suppression of clonal disease with: melphalan, prednisolone, or vincristine, doxorubicin and dexamethasome
- Dialysis

- Organ transplantation
- AL responds to myeloma therapy
- Autologous stem cell transplant.

Prognosis

- 1–2 years
- Myeloma makes prognosis worse
- AL amyloidosis has a worse prognosis than AA form

- If cardiac failure at presentation, median overall survival: 6 months
- Very poor if autonomic or liver involvement.

Complications

- Restrictive cardiomyopathy causing:
  - Pulmonary hypertension

- Right ventricular hypertrophy and failure.

TRANSFUSION REACTIONS

GENERAL FEATURES

Outline

General hazards of transfusion:
- Acute:
  - Bacterial complications: septicaemia, shock (contamination ↓ by: citrate, cold storage, antibiotics)
  - Hypothermia: with rapid infusion of cold blood
  - Circulatory overload
- Chronic/delayed:
  - Iron overload
  - Infection: HBV, HCV, HIV, human T-lymphotropic virus, parvovirus, CMV, malaria, syphilis, vCJD prions

- Graft versus host transfusion reaction:
  - Donor lymphocytes recognise recipient as foreign and attack
  - Rash on palms and soles
  - Mostly in immunocompromised
- Serum sickness:
  - 7–12 days after injecting foreign antigen there is deposition of large immune complexes in arteries (vasculitis), kidneys (nephritis) and joints (arthritis).

ACUTE HAEMOLYTIC TRANSFUSION REACTIONS

Outline

- Immediate haemolysis of donated RBCs due to host antibody attacking foreign antigens on RBCs
- Most commonly due to ABO blood group incompatibility from blood given in error
- Reaction can occur in minutes (usually within 1 hour of starting transfusion)

- **Medical emergency**
- Can also get delayed haemolytic transfusion reactions, which are secondary immune responses of the host against donor RBC transfused in an immunised recipient.

Pathogenesis/aetiology

Pathogenesis

Intravascular haemolysis:
- Antibody response to donor RBCs: IgM
- Activates complement cascade and haemolysis

Extravascular haemolysis:
- Can be caused by anti-RhD, -E,-C, anti-K: mediated IgG preformed.

Who

- ~1 in 40 000 transfused units.

Clinical features

Intravascular: IgM mediated:
- Unconscious:
  - Hypotension
  - Uncontrollable bleeding: DIC
- Conscious:
  - Rigor
  - Chest tightness
  - Flank pain

- Tachycardia
- Oliguria and haemoglobinuria
- Facial flush
- Nausea and vomiting

Extravascular: IgG mediated:
- Jaundice
- Fever.

Investigations

- Return donor blood unit and take post-transfusion sample into EDTA tube (ethylenediaminetetraacetic acid) for analysis:
  - Repeat pre- and post-transfusion grouping and cross-match

- Coombs' test (direct antiglobulin test)
- Blood cultures
- FBC: for Hb level
- Urine for Hb
- Bilirubin.

Treatment

- Stop transfusion at once
- Fluid resuscitation and close observation
- Resuscitate and keep IV access patent
- IV colloid
- Fluid balance: ensure adequate urine output

- Establish recipient identity and their compatibility with the transfused unit
- IV hydrocortisone and IV chlorphenamine
- IV adrenaline if severe shock
- In acute renal failure: central venous access and dialysis.

Prognosis and complications

Complications

- Acute renal failure: due to Hb released by haemolysis

- DIC.

ALLERGIC REACTIONS

Outline

- Urticaria or anaphylaxis due to a blood transfusion.

Pathogenesis/aetiology

Causes

- Urticaria may be due to foreign protein reacting with recipient IgE

- Anaphylaxis: due to IgA from donor reacting with anti-IgA in recipient who is IgA deficient.

Who

- Uriticarial reactions are common.

Clinical features

Urticaria:

- Itchy rash from release of histamine by mast cells: swelling appears and resolves spontaneously within hours. Commonest effect, usually mild

Anaphylactic shock:

- Sudden hypertension, then hypotension, substernal pain, dyspnoea, wheeze.

Investigations

- Clinical diagnosis

- Check IgA status of patient.

Treatment

- ABC approach (see acutely unwell patient p. 2)

Severe urticaria:

- Slow transfusion rate
- Antihistamine

Anaphylaxis:

- Stop transfusion

- IM adrenaline
- IV hydrocortisone
- IV fluids

Prevention:

- IgA deficient patients: always transfuse IgA depleted blood.

Prognosis and complications

Prognosis

- Urticaria: most are not severe.

Complications

- Death if untreated anaphylaxis.

FEBRILE NON-HAEMOLYTIC TRANSFUSION REACTIONS

Outline

- Febrile reaction to a transfusion resulting from initial sensitisation and circulating leucocyte antibodies.

Pathogenesis/aetiology

Pathogenesis

- Initial sensitisation causes circulating low-level IgG anti-HLA

- Secondary exposure results in a massive antibody reduction against donor white cell HLA.

Who

- Common in those who have been pregnant or previously transfused

- Commonest reaction to donated blood.

Clinical features

- Fever
- Rigors

- 30–60 min after transfusion.

Investigations

- Test recipient blood for anti-HLA antibodies.

Treatment

Mild:

- Slow infusion
- Paracetamol
- Piriton

Severe:

- Stop transfusion
- Hydrocortisone
- Chlorphenamine
- Prevention: leucocyte depleted blood.

Prognosis and complications

Complications

- Can lead to transfusion-related lung injury (see below).

TRANSFUSION-RELATED ACUTE LUNG INJURY

Outline

- Reaction between recipient leucocytes and donor anti-leucocyte antibodies occurring within 1–2 weeks of transfusion leading to severe lung injury.

Pathogenesis/aetiology

Pathogenesis

- Acute respiratory distress from antibody reacting against HLA or HNA (human neutrophil antigen)
- Leads to complement activation, endothelial and epithelial injury and pulmonary vascular permeability.

Who

- Uncommon: 0.1–0.2% of transfusions
- More likely with fresh frozen plasma transfusion.

Clinical features

- Fever
- Chills
- Non-productive cough
- Dyspnoea
- ↓ O_2 saturations.

Investigations

- CXR: perihilar and lower lung shadowing.

Treatment

- Stop the infusion
- Supportive: in ITU or a high dependency unit
- Monitor O_2 saturations
- Maintain IV access
- Fluid resuscitation as required
- Careful fluid balance
- Prevention: leucocyte depleted blood.

Prognosis and complications

Prognosis

- Endotracheal intubation required in 70–75% of patients.

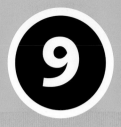
- Hormones are chemical messengers released from a gland in the body into the blood to act at distant sites by binding to receptors (either intracellular or extracellular)
- Most hormone systems are controlled by a feedback mechanism
- Organs of the endocrine system are interlinked leading to control of final hormone secretion (Fig. 9.1).

The main hormones, including their sites of action and roles, are summarised in Table 9.1.

The pituitary gland

Anterior pituitary

- Production of hormones by the anterior pituitary is regulated by hormones produced by the hypothalamus, which is connected to the pituitary gland
- The anterior pituitary makes and releases six hormones:
  - Growth hormone (GH): regulated by growth hormone-releasing hormone (GHRH)
  - Prolactin: inhibited by dopamine from the hypothalamus, stimulated by thyrotrophin-releasing hormone (TRH)
  - Adrenocorticotrophic hormone (ACTH): regulated by corticotrophin-releasing hormone (CRH)
  - Thyroid-stimulating hormone (TSH): regulated by TRH
  - Follicle-stimulating hormone (FSH): regulated by gonadotrophin-releasing hormone (GnRH)
  - luteinizing hormone (LH): regulated by GnRH.

Posterior pituitary

Releases hormones made in the hypothalamus:

- oxytocin
- antidiuretic hormone (ADH; vasopressin)

The adrenal gland

The adrenal glands are found just above the kidneys on both sides. They are made up of an external cortex and an inner medulla, both of which produce hormones:

- The external cortex has three layers each of which produces a different hormone:
  - Glomerulosa (outer zone): mineralocorticoids, e.g. aldosterone
  - Fasiculata (middle zone): glucocorticoids
  - Reticularis (inner zone): the sex hormones
- The internal medulla produces catecholamines, specifically adrenaline (epinephrine) and noradrenaline (norepinephrine), from chromaffin cells
- Sex hormones and glucocorticoid production is controlled by ACTH from the anterior pituitary; the amount of ACTH is, in turn, controlled by CRH released from the hypothalamus.

Figure 9.2 summarises the process of negative feedback in the hypothalamic–pituitary–adrenal axis.

Aldosterone production

The amount of aldosterone produced is controlled by the **renin–angiotensin–aldosterone** system:

- Pathway important for the control of BP and fluid balance
- Pathway involves several hormones: renin, angiotensin and aldosterone (Fig. 9.3)
- Renin is secreted by the kidneys in response to low BP and low levels of sodium:
  - Converts angiotensinogen (from the liver) into angiotensin I
- Angiotensin I is converted to angiotensin II by Angiotensin converting enzyme, ACE (produced in the lungs)
- Angiotensin II increases BP by
  - Vasoconstriction
  - Inhibits renin production by −ve feedback
  - Stimulates aldosterone production by the adrenal cortex
- Aldosterone increases BP by:
  - ↑ sodium reabsorption in the kidneys
  - ↑ potassium excretion.

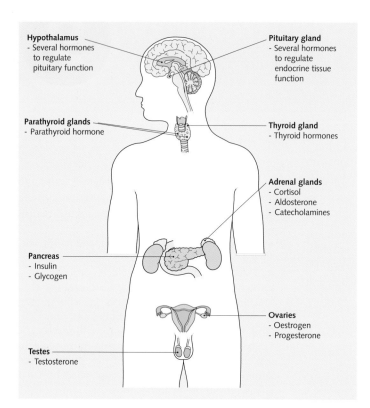

Fig. 9.1 The organs and hormones of the endocrine system.

The pancreas

The islets of Langerhans in the pancreas contain alpha, beta and delta cells, which produce specific hormones:

- Alpha cells release glucagon, which increases blood glucose levels by breaking glycogen down into glucose
- Beta cells release insulin, which reduces glucose blood levels by stimulating:
  - uptake of glucose into skeletal muscle/adipose tissue
  - synthesis of glycogen from glucose in liver
  - uptake of amino acids in tissue
  - action of insulin is opposed by glucagon (Fig. 9.4)
- Delta cells produce somatostatin, which inhibits release of GH and TSH and suppresses the release of some GI hormones; it also suppresses the release of glucagon and insulin.

The thyroid

The thyroid hormones are thyroid-stimulating hormone (TSH), thyroxine (T_4) and triiodothyronine (T_3):

- T_4 is relatively inactive and regarded as a prohormone for T_3
- T_3 and T_4 act on multiple tissues to:
  - ↑ basal metabolic rate
  - balance growth and development
  - modulate the action of other hormones.

Care should be taken when interpreting thyroid values during acute illness as the normal pattern of TSH and T_4 may be abnormal. This is called 'euthyroid sick syndrome'.

Calcium and vitamin D

Calcium in the body is necessary for:

- bone and teeth (99% of body calcium)
- nerve function
- muscle contraction
- blood clotting.

Normal levels of calcium are 2.12–2.65 mmol/L:

- Calcium in blood is either bound to albumin or freely ionised
- Levels of calcium are controlled by PTH, calcitonin and calcitriol (Table 9.2).

Vitamin D in its active form, 1,25-dihydroxycholecalciferol (calcitriol), increases plasma calcium and has widespread effects including on bone health. Vitamin D metabolism involves the skin, liver and kidneys (Fig. 9.5):

- In skin it can be made from cholesterol under the influence of UV light, which transforms 7-dehydrocholestrol into a form that is transferred and modified in the liver and then the kidneys to the active form calcitriol.

Table 9.1 Summary of the principle hormones including their site of action and role

Gland	Hormone produced	Role of hormone	Site of action	Too much produced	Too little produced
Hypothalamus	TRH GnRH CTRH GHRH	Release of hormones from the anterior pituitary TRH: release TSH GnRH: release FSH and LH CTRH: release ACTH GHRH: releases growth hormone (GH)	Anterior pituitary	Depends on hormone affected	Clinical picture of panhypopituitarism
Anterior pituitary	TSH	Stimulate T_4 and T_3 synthesis	Thyroid	Secondary hyperthyroidism	Secondary hypothyroidism
	ACTH	Stimulate release of cortisol and dehydroepiandrosterone (DHEA)	Adrenal	Cushing's disease	Adrenocortical insufficiency
	GH	Acts on most cells of the body: ↓ Glucose metabolism ↑ Lipolysis ↑ Protein synthesis ↑ Insulin-like growth factor production ↑ Differentiation of cartilage Growth promotion (indirectly: via insulin-like growth factor)	Cartilage Liver	Children: gigantism Adults: acromegaly	GH deficiency
	Prolactin	Lactation, breast development Contraction of uterine muscle,	Mammary glands Uterus	Hyperprolactinaemia	–
Posterior pituitary	ADH (vasopressin)	↑ Water reabsorption in the kidneys to concentrate the urine. High concentrations ↑ BP	Kidneys	SIADH	Diabetes insipidus Cranial: impaired ADH secretion Nephrogenic: renal resistance to action of ADH
Thyroid	Thyroxine (T_4) and triiodothyronine (T_3)	Acts on most cells of the body: ↑ Basal Metabolic Rate Balanced growth and development Modulates action of other hormones	Target cells on multiple tissues	Hyperthyroidism	Hypothyroidism
Para-follicular C cells	Calcitonin	↓ Release of calcium from bone Inhibits calcium absorption	Osteoclasts	Hypocalcaemia	Hypercalcaemia
Parathyroid	PTH	↑ Serum calcium ↓ Serum phosphate	Osteoclasts, renal tubules, intestine	Hyperparathyroidism	Hypoparathyroidism
Skin/liver/ kidney	Calcitriol	↑ Serum calcium Facilitates action of PTH	Osteoblasts Distal renal tubules	Hypercalcaemia	Children: rickets Adults: osteomalacia

Continued

Table 9.1 Summary of the principle hormones including their site of action and role—cont'd

Gland	Hormone produced	Role of hormone	Site of action	Too much produced	Too little produced
Adrenal cortex	From zona graunulosa: aldosterone	↑ Na reabsorption ↓ Potassium reabsorption/↓ H reabsorption ↑ BP and plasma volume ↑ sensitivity of muscle to vasoconstrictors	Distal tubule and collecting duct of kidney	Primary hyperaldosteronism	Congenital adrenal hyperplasia
	From zona fasiculata: cortisol	↑ Plasma glucose Bone catabolism Anti inflammatory (impair wound healing) ↑ renal blood flow	Widespread action Helps restore homeostasis after stress	Cushing's syndrome (↓ ACTH) Cushing's disease (↑ ACTH) Glucocorticoid resistance (cortisol doesn't work)	Addison's (↑ ACTH) Congenital adrenal hyperplasia
	From zona reticularis: DHEA	Prohormone for sex steroids, In men stimulates sperm maturation and secondary sexual characteristic development	Prohormone for sex steroids	Polycystic ovary syndrome in females	Hypogonadism Addison's disease
Adrenal medulla	Noradrenaline, adrenaline	Widespread action Act as part of the autonomic system	Part of autonomic system	Phaeochromocytoma	–
Pancreas	α-Glucagon	Glucose homeostasis: ↑ glucose levels	Various	Gluacogonoma	–
	β-Insulin	Glucose homeostasis: ↓ glucose levels	Various	Insulinoma	Diabetes mellitus
	λ-Somatostatin	Inhibit release of insulin and glucagon	Anterior pituitary, stomach, pancreas	–	–
Ovaries	Oestrogen	Secondary sexual characteristics, reproduction	Widespread	–	–
Testes	Testosterone	Secondary sexual characteristics, reproduction	Widespread	Virilism (in females)	–

(Thyrotropin-releasing hormone (TRH), gonadotrophin-releasing hormone (GnRH), corticotrophin-releasing hormone (CRH), growth hormone-releasing hormone (GHRH), adrenocorticotrophic hormone (ACTH), thyroid-stimulating hormone (TSH), luteinizing hormone (LH), follicle-stimulating hormone (FSH), syndrome of inappropriate ADH (SIADH))

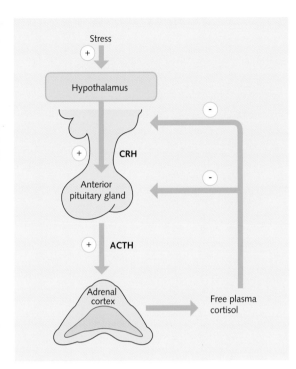

Fig. 9.2 The hypothalamic–pituitary–adrenal axis. CRH, corticotrophin-releasing hormone, ACTH, adrenocorticotrophic hormone.

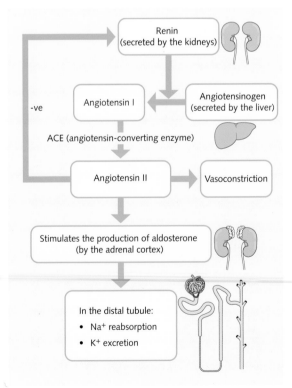

Fig. 9.3 The renin–angiotensin–aldosterone system.

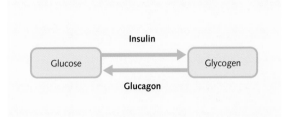

Fig. 9.4 Role of insulin and glucagon in storage of glucose.

Table 9.2	Hormones affecting levels of calcium		
Hormone	Source	Main function	Role
PTH	Parathyroid gland chief cells	↑ Calcium: ↓ Phosphate:	Releases calcium from bone (see below) ↑ Calcium absorption ↑ Levels of calcitriol
Calcitriol	Part of vitamin D metabolism (see below)	↑ Calcium	↑ Uptake of calcium from the intestine ↑ Reabsorption from the kidneys ↑ Bone reabsorption which releases calcium
Calcitonin	Thyroid gland C cells	↓ Calcium ↓ Phosphate	↓ Release of calcium from bone Inhibits calcium absorption

Body mass index

Body mass index (BMI) is a useful measure of whether a person is under- or overweight after accounting for their height: BMI = weight (kg)/height (m)^2 (Table 9.3).

See also

- Surgery (Ch. 13): endocrine tumours of the pancreas, gastrinoma.
- Common presenting complaints (Ch. 14): weight loss.

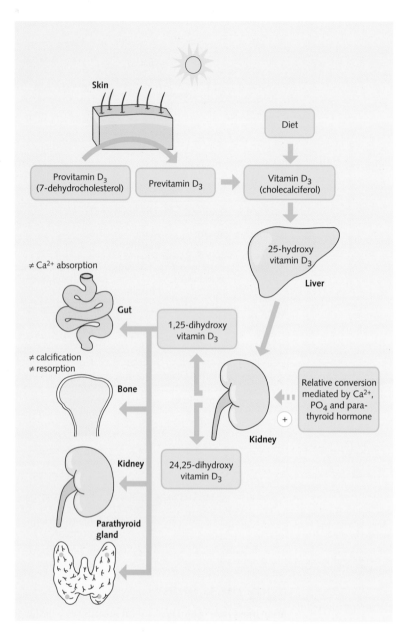

Fig. 9.5 Metabolism of vitamin D.

Table 9.3 Body mass index as a guide to healthy weight

	BMI	
	Non-Asian	**Asian**
Underweight	<18.5	<18.5
Normal (healthy weight)	18.5–24.9	18.5–22.9
Overweight	25–29.9	23–24.9
Obese	30–40	25–30
Morbidly obese	>40	>30

DISORDERS OF THE PITUITARY GLAND

PITUITARY TUMOUR

Outline

- A tumour in the pituitary gland
- Most commonly a benign adenoma
- Problematic due to:
  - functioning tumour: ↑ hormone production leading to hyperpituitarism
  - non-functioning tumour: ↓ in hormone production leading to hypopituitarism
  - tumour growth in a limited space

Commonest functioning tumours:
- ↑ Prolactin: prolactinoma: (35%)
- ↑ GH: acromegaly or gigantism (20%)
- ↑ Prolactin and GH: (7%)
- ↑ ACTH: Cushing's disease (7%)
- ↑ LH/FSH/TSH (1%)
- No obvious hormone, or more than one: (30%).

Pathogenesis/aetiology

Causes

- 10–20% of intracranial tumours
- Mostly benign adenomas
- Functioning tumours smaller than non-functioning tumours

Histological types (based on staining):
- *Chromophobes*: (the majority) poorly stained. ↑ in prolactin, ACTH, GH or non-secretory
- *Acidophils*: stains with eosin. Secrete GH or prolactin
- *Basophils*: stained with haemotoxylin. Secrete ACTH, LH, FSH, TSH.

Who

Typical age:
- 25–35 year olds: prolactin, ACTH secreting tumours
- 35–50 years: GH secreting
- 60 years: non-functioning tumours

Risk factors:
- Multiple endocrine neoplasia (MEN) see p. 422.

Clinical features

Signs and symptoms

Effects of hormone hypersecretion:
- Depends on hormone:
  - Prolactin excess: see below
  - GH excess: acromegaly or gigantism, depends on age
  - ACTH excess: Cushing's disease (see below p. 396)
  - Excess LH, FSH, TSH: rare
Effects of hormone suppression:
- Depends on hormone (see hypopituitarism):
  - ↓ *ADH*: diabetes insipidus

Pressure effects from tumour mass:
- Headache
- Visual field defects: usually bitemporal hemianopia from pressure on optic chiasm
- Seizures
- Hydrocephalus
- Cranial nerve palsy of III, IV, VI which run through the cavernus sinus
Effects from extension into the hypothalamus:
- Obesity: altered appetite and thirst from hypothalamic involvement
- Altered sleep
- Altered temperature regulation.

Investigations

Examination and hormone tests

- Visual field assessment
Hormone tests:
- Measure hormone levels: basal levels and tests of pituitary feedback
- Insulin tolerance tests: gold standard for the hypothalamic–pituitary–adrenal axis
- Short Synacthen test (see p. 401): for the adrenal axis
- Water deprivation test for diabetes insipidus (see below)

Imaging

- Pituitary CT/MRI assessment (Fig. 9.6).

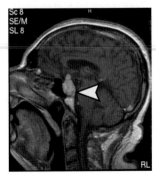

Fig. 9.6   MRI illustrating a pituitary adenoma (arrowhead).

Treatment

Medical

- Hormone replacement as needed.

Surgical

- Excision: trans-sphenoidal (usually) or transfrontal if large

Radiotherapy

- If surgical removal is not possible.

Prognosis and complications

Prognosis

- Metastases rare.

Complications

- Recurrence after surgery
- Fertility may be reduced after surgery due to ↓ in gonadotrophins.

HYPOPITUITARISM

Outline

- Decrease of some or all of the pituitary hormones
- Panhypopituitarism is deficiency of all the hormones
- Due to pituitary disease affecting hormone production directly, or from hypothalamic disease that affects hormone production of releasing hormones that stimulate production of anterior pituitary hormones

Hormones affected (in this order):
- GH
- FSH, LH
- Prolactin
- TSH
- ACTH.

Pathogenesis/aetiology

Causes

Hypothalamic disease:
- Mass: tumour, cyst, inflammation
- Infection: TB, meningitis
- Kallmann syndrome: gonadotrophin deficiency with anosmia (loss of smell), colour blindness, renal problems

Pituitary disease:
- Mass: non-functioning pituitary adenoma 70% of cases
- Idiopathic: surgery/radiation following tumour removal

- Pituitary apoplexy (haemorrhage of pituitary where there is an adenoma)
- Ischaemic necrosis, particularly Sheehan syndrome (pituitary infarction after postpartum haemorrhage)
- Congenital syndrome: rare

Other:
- infiltrative disease, e.g. sarcoidosis, amyloidosis.

Who

- No specific risk.

Clinical features

Signs and symptoms

Depends on deficiency: see also sections on individual hormones:
- ↓ GH:
  - May be silent in adults
  - Fatigue
  - Reduced muscle strength
  - Central adiposity
- ↓ Prolactin:
  - ↓ Lactation, hypogonadism
- ↓ TSH:
  - Fatigue, weakness, dry skin, cold sensitivity, weight gain

- ↓ Gonadotrophin:
  - Loss of libido
  - Infertility
  - Impotence
  - Dyspareunia (painful sex)
  - Regression of secondary sexual characteristics
  - Women: amenorrhoea, breast atrophy
- ↓ ACTH:
  - Fatigue, nausea and vomiting, anorexia, pallor, weakness, loss of pubic hair
- Pituitary tumour symptoms (where relevant):
  - Headache and visual field defects (bitemporal loss).

Investigations

Examination and hormone tests

- Visual field assessment

Hormone tests:

- Measure hormone levels: basal levels and tests of pituitary feedback

- Insulin tolerance tests: gold standard for the hypothalamic–pituitary–adrenal axis
- Short Synacthen test (see p. 401): for the adrenal axis.

Imaging

- CT/MRI assessment

Treatment

Treat cause:
- GH:
  - For growing children
- Gonadotrophin:
  - Androgens and oestrogens
  - LSH and FSH analogues for fertility
- TSH:
  - Thyroid hormones for life: give steroids before T_4 (T_4 can precipitate an adrenal crisis)

- ACTH:
  - Steroids for life
- Tumour:
  - Surgery/radiotherapy for tumour (see Pituitary tumour above).

Prognosis and complications

Prognosis

- Following diagnosis and hormone replacement: normal life expectancy.

HYPERPROLACTINAEMIA

Outline

- ↑ In prolactin

Normal prolactin production:
- Prolactin is important for lactation and uterine muscle contraction
- It is inhibited by dopamine from the hypothalamus: therefore any interruption to dopamine can lead to hyperprolactinaemia

- It is also stimulated by TRH which is part of the thyroid axis
- ↑ Prolactin inhibits GnRH, affecting development of sex hormones and leading to hypogonadism resulting in many of the symptoms.

Pathogenesis/aetiology

Causes

- Physiological: pregnancy, breast feeding, stress
- Prolactin secreting pituitary adenoma: prolactinoma (commonest cause)

- Interference of dopamine: hypothalamic or pituitary tumours, drugs (dopamine antagonists: metoclopramide, haloperidol, phenothiazine)
- Primary hypothyroidism (from high TRH)
- Drugs: oestrogens.

Who

- More easily diagnosed in women due to changes in their menstrual cycle.

A typical patient

A patient presents with irregular periods. The doctor notices visual field defects on examination.

Signs and symptoms

Women:
- Galactorrhoea (milk production from the breast in women who are not breast feeding)
- Irregular menstruation including late menarche, amenorrhea (no periods), oligorhoea (few periods)
- Impotence
- Infertility

Men:
- Infertility, erectile dysfunction, hypogonadism

Pituitary tumour symptoms (where relevant):
- Headache and visual field defects (bitemporal loss).

Examination and hormone tests

- Visual field assessment

Hormone levels:
- ↑ Serum prolactin level

- ↓ LH and FSH
- Thyroid function tests
- Pregnancy test

Imaging

- MRI/CT of pituitary and hypothalamus.

- Depends on cause

- Withdraw causative drugs.

Medical

- Dopamine agonists: inhibit prolactin
- Bromocriptine: lowers serum level and improves galactorrhoea

- Cabergoline: side effect: nausea, headache, nasal stuffiness.

Surgical

- For tumour removal

Radiotherapy

- For tumour

Prognosis

- Spontaneous normalisation in 30% over 15 years.

POSTERIOR PITUITARY: DIABETES INSIPIDUS

Outline

- Deficiency in ADH or the inability to use it leads to a disorder where the urine cannot be concentrated and the patient is always thirsty. Patients pass >3 L of dilute (<300 mOsm/kg) urine a day.

ADH:
- Produced in the posterior pituitary
- Its role is to regulate reabsorption of water in the kidneys
- It is 'anti-diuretic': it reduces diuresis (production of urine) when there is too little water in the blood and therefore concentrates the urine

- Acts at:
  1. V2 receptors in the kidney for water absorption: more released from the pituitary when the blood is concentrated
  2. V1 receptors in the arterioles causing vasoconstriction

Classification

- Cranial DI: impaired ADH secretion

- Nephrogenic DI: renal resistance to action of ADH

Pathogenesis/aetiology

Causes

Cranial:
- Head injury/surgery
- Pituitary tumour
- Haemorrhage
- Infection: meningitis.
- Inherited: autosomal dominant or part of DIDMOAD syndrome (diabetes insipidis, diabetes mellitus, optic atrophy, deafness)
- Status epilepticus

Nephrogenic:
- Hypokalaemia
- Hypercalcaemia
- Diabetes mellitus
- Chronic renal failure (CRF)
- Drugs: lithium, dimethylchlorotetracycline.

Who

Risk factors:
- Previous trans-sphenoidal surgery

A typical patient

A patient complains of polyuria and polydipsia. Blood tests reveal a high osmolarity with low urine osmolarity.

Clinical features

Signs and symptoms

- Polyuria
- Polydipsia
- Dilute urine

- Dehydration
- Serum osmolarity increased as water is excreted (normally:285–295 Osmol/kg).

Investigations

Blood tests

- U&Es: hypernatraemia (see Biochemistry p. 501)

- ↑ Plasma osmolarity.

Urine

- ↓ Osmolarity

Water deprivation test
- Test confirms DI and can distinguish between cranial/nephrotic cause.
- Water restricted for 8 h, then desmopressin is given
- Weight, blood and urine osmolality measured hourly for 16 h after
- If after desmopressin ↓ urine output and ↑ osmolarity: cause is cranial e.g. failure of ADH production
- If no change: cause is renal (Can not respond) (see Table 9.4)
- After a desmopression test:
  - **C**oncentrated urine **C**ranial cause
  - **N**o effect **N**ephrogenic

Imaging

- Hypothalamus and pituitary MRI.

Table 9.4   Water deprivation test with desmopressin

Urine osmolarity after fluid deprivation (mOsmol/kg)		Condition
Before desmopressin	After desmopressin	
<300 (dilute)	<300	Nephrogenic DI
<300	>300	Cranial DI
>800	>800	Polydipsia

Treatment

Nephrogenic:
- Treat cause
- Bendroflumethiazide, indomethacin or amiloride if it persists

Cranial:
- Find cause
- Desmopressin.

Prognosis and complications

Prognosis

- No affect on life expectancy if treated.

SYNDROME OF INAPPROPRIATE ADH SECRETION (SIADH)

Outline

ADH is secreted even when the blood is dilute and more urine should be produced. This leads to water retention and haemodilution. Features include:

- hyponatraemia
- excess of urinary sodium >20 mEq/L)

- inappropriately elevated urine osmolality (>200 mOsm/kg)
- ↓ serum osmolality.

See also hyponatraemia, Ch. 12, p. 502.

Pathogenesis/aetiology

Causes

- Endocrine disturbance: problem with hypothalamic–pituitary secretion, hypothyroidism, Addison's disease
- Ectopic production of ADH: e.g. small cell lung cancer, pneumonia, abscess, TB
- Neoplasia: lung, pancreas, ovary, lymphoma, thymoma

- CNS: tumour, trauma, infection, stroke, subarachnoid haemorrhage, multiple sclerosis, Guillain–Barré syndrome
- Infection
- Drugs: diuretics, NSAIDs, selective serotonin receptor inhibitors, tricyclic antidepressants, opiates, haloperidol, monoamine oxidase inhibitors, nicotine.

Who

- Typical age: commoner in older people. Rare in childhood

- Commonest cause of hyponatraemia in hospitalised adults.

A typical patient

A patient recovering from a subarachnoid haemorrhage develops nausea and confusion. Blood tests reveal low sodium.

Clinical features

Signs and symptoms

- Weakness
- Malaise
- Nausea
- Headache
- Confusion (due to low sodium)

- Irritability
- Fits
- Coma
- Death.

Investigations

Blood tests

- Check renal, adrenal and thyroid function to ensure they are normal.

- ↑ Serum sodium (often <125 mmol/L).

Urine

- Urine osmolarity much higher than plasma osmolarity
- Urine osmolality >500 mOsmol/kg

- Urine sodium >20 mmol/L.

Treatment

- Water restriction
- Dimethylcholotetracycline: inhibits ADH action on the kidney
- Hypertonic saline: prevents circulatory overload (expert advise only)

- Diuretic: furosemide (severe cases)
- Vaptans: New V2 receptor antagonists which promote free water loss.

Prognosis and complications

Complications

- Beware of central pontine myelinolysis (damage to myelin of nerve cells in the brainstem) with rapid sodium correction. Aim for 0.5–1 mmol/h correction.

GROWTH AXIS DISORDERS

GIGANTISM

Outline

- Increased GH secretion prepuberty causing excessive growth.

Pathogenesis/aetiology

Causes

- Hypersecretion from anterior pituitary
- 1% from ectopic GHRH secretion

- McCune–Albright syndrome, MEN1 and the Carney complex include gigantism as well-recognised features.

Who

- Rare disorder: about 0.6% of pituitary tumours in children.

Clinical features

Signs and symptoms

- ↑ Height
- Localised effects of tumour

- Hypopituitarism.

Investigations

- Oral glucose tolerance test: to demonstrate high levels of GH.

Imaging

- MRI: to detect pituitary adenoma

- CXR/AXR: for ectopic GH secreting tumours.

Treatment

Medical

- Somatostatin analogues, e.g. octreotide (inhibits GH)

- Dopamine agonists as adjuvants, e.g. bromocriptine.

Surgical

- Trans-sphenoidal surgery for pituitary tumours.

Prognosis and complications

Prognosis

- Mortality 2–3 × the general population.

Complications

- Diabetes mellitus (GH suppresses insulin)
- Blindness
- Delayed puberty

- Acromegaly
- Cardiovascular risk.

ACROMEGALY

Outline

- Increased growth hormone (GH) post puberty, after the epiphyseal plate cartilage has fused

- Causes ↑ growth in certain places such as the hands, feet and face.

Pathogenesis/aetiology

Causes

- Usually from functioning benign pituitary adenoma: 95% (see above)
- Carcinoma: rare

- Carcinoid tumours releasing GH: rare
- Excessive growth-hormone-releasing hormone (GHRH): 5%.

- Typical age: most present aged 30–50 years
- 1♀=1♂
- Incidence: 5/1000 000 per year.

A typical patient

A man presents to his GP as he has noticed his hands have got bigger. He has also noticed that he has coarse oily skin and recently been having headaches.

Signs and symptoms

Effects of ↑ GH:
- Neck: goitre
- Face: coarse facial features – prominent supraorbital ridge, large tongue, interdental separation, large nose, prognathism (protruding mandible) (Fig. 9.7)
- Axilla: acanthosis nigricans (brown-black pigmentation of the skin in areas of skin folding e.g. the axilla)
- Extremities:↑ hand and foot size
- CV system: heart failure, cardiomyopathy, hypertension
- Neuropathy: carpal tunnel syndrome
- Joints: arthritis, kyphosis
- Skin: coarse oily skin
- Endocrinology: diabetes 30%, impotence, sweaty
- Other: sleep apnoea

Effects from pituitary tumour (10%):
- Visual field deficits
- Cranial nerve palsies
- Headaches.

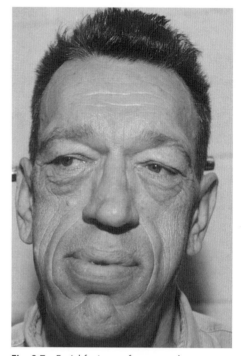

Fig. 9.7   Facial features of acromegaly.

Examination and hormone tests

- Look at old photos for comparison
- Visual field assessment
- Hormone tests:
  - Serum GH not diagnostic

- Oral glucose tolerance test is diagnostic: normally there is suppression of GH in response to glucose load. In acromegaly there is no suppression
- Serum insulin-like growth factor-1.

ECG

- For cardiac complications.

Imaging

- MRI of pituitary fossa

Medical

- Somatostatin analogue inhibits GH release: octreotide
- Dopamine agonists: bromocriptine

- GH receptor antagonist: pegvisomant.

Treatment

Surgical

For pituitary adenoma (see pituitary tumour above):
- Trans-sphenoidal: treatment of choice

- Transfrontal if large
- External irradiation following surgery or alone.

Prognosis and complications

Prognosis

- 90% cured
- Physical features are irreversible so diagnose quickly

- Untreated: mortality $2 \times$ the general population.

Complications

- Diabetes mellitus
- Large bowel tumours
- Cardiomyopathy

- Deaths from heart-related problems: heart failure and hypertension.

THYROID AXIS DISORDERS

HYPOTHYROIDISM

Outline

- ↓ Amounts of thyroid hormones (T_3 and T_4) resulting in typical symptoms such as lethargy, cold intolerance, weight gain and dry skin

- May lead to a goitre (enlarged thyroid gland).

Classification

1° hypothyroidism:
- Hypothyroidism from pathology in the thyroid gland: TSH is raised due to negative feedback

2° hypothyroidism:
- Hypothyroidism from pathology in the pituitary gland: TSH is low, and this is what causes low levels of T_4

Myxoedema:
- Infiltration of skin with mucopolysaccharides leading to dry waxy skin swelling in patients in a severely hypothyroid state

Myxoedema coma:
- A severe form of hypothyroidism:
  - where there is confusion and coma
  - where there is heart failure, hypothermia, hyponatraemia, hypoxia
  - that is a life-threatening condition
  - that occurs in the elderly
  - where there may be precipitating factors: cold, infection
  - that is uncommon.

Pathogenesis/aetiology

Causes

Hashimoto's disease:
- Autoimmune disease leading to hypothyroidism due to antibodies against the thyroid tissue
- Antibodies against:
  - thyroid peroxidase 95%
  - thyroglobulin 70%
  - TSH receptor
- Commonest cause of hypothyroidism
- Leads to goitre formation

Idiopathic atrophic hypothyroidism:
- Autoimmune, associated with thyroid microsomal antibodies
- Lymphoid infiltration leading to fibrosis and atrophy, with no goitre

Drug induced:
- Amiodarone, lithium, iodine

Iatrogenic:
- 40% following treatment for hyperthyroidism

Iodine deficiency:
- Particularly in mountainous areas (little seafood)
- Goitre common
- Commonest cause of hypothyroidism world-wide

Congenital defects:
- Routine screening of neonates
- Associated with cretinism (stunting of physical and mental growth from untreated congenital hypothyroidism)
- Commonest cause is Pendred syndrome (genetic disorder with hearing loss and goitre)

2° hypothyroidism:
- Pituitary failure, Sheehan syndrome (pituitary infarction after postpartum haemorrhage). Rare.

Who

- Typical age: ↑ with age
- ♀>♂
- Prevalence: up to 2%

Hashimoto's disease:
- Women
- Age 60–70 years
- Associated with HLA-B8, HLA-DR3, HLA-DR4, HLA-DQB1*03

Associations:
- Autoimmune diseases
- Down's syndrome
- Turner's syndrome
- Cystic fibrosis.

A typical patient

A patient presents to her GP as she feels tired all the time. On questioning, she admits to recent onset of weight gain, constipation, and dry skin and hair.

Clinical features

Signs and symptoms

General:
- Lethargy
- Cold intolerance
- Weight ↑, poor appetite
- Constipation
- Low, hoarse voice
- Bradycardia
- Confusion
- Goitre: depends on cause

Skin:
- Dry skin and hair
- Hair loss
- Little sweating
- Myxoedema

Psychological and neurological:
- Depression
- Dementia
- Peripheral neuropathy

- Cerebellar ataxia
- Carpal tunnel syndrome
- Deafness and cretinism
- Slow relaxing reflexes

Muscular:
- Myalgia

CV system:
- Bradycardia
- Angina
- Pericardial effusion
- Non-pitting oedema

Development:
- Poor growth
- Delayed puberty
- Mental retardation

Reproductive:
- Menorrhagia
- Infertility.

Investigations

Blood tests

- Normochromic macrocytic anaemia
- Thyroid hormones: ↓ T_4, ↓ T_3, ↓ or ↑ TSH

- Hashimoto's disease: autoantibodies against: thyroid peroxidase thyroglobulin.

ECG

- Sinus bradycardia.

Treatment

- Levothyroxine (T_4 tablets) daily for life
- Monitor thyroid levels

Myxoedema coma:
- ABC approach
- Supportive measures: O_2, fluid

- T_3 IV
- Hydrocortisone IV
- Dextrose IV: to prevent hypoglycaemia
- Surgery for large goitre with tracheal or oesophageal compression.

Prognosis and complications

Complications

- In Hashimoto's disease: follicle destruction leads to fibrosis

Complications of thyroid surgery:
- Haemorrhage
- Laryngeal nerve palsy and hoarseness: 1%
- Hypothyroidism

- Damage to parathyroid glands leading to hypoparathyroidism and low calcium in 2.5%
- Tracheal damage
- Thyroid storm: thyrotoxicosis causes acutely increased metabolism: life-threatening tachycardia, hypertension, fever.

HYPERTHYROIDISM/THYROTOXICOSIS

Outline

- ↑ Amounts of thyroid hormones resulting in typical symptoms such as heat intolerance, agitation and weight loss.

Types

1° hyperthyroidism:
- Pathology originating in the thyroid gland: TSH is low due to negative feedback

2° hyperthyroidism:
- Pathology that originates in the pituitary leading to raised levels of TSH that lead to high levels of thyroid hormones

Thyroid storm–thyroid crisis:
- A life-threatening episode of extreme hyperthyroidism
- Precipitated by illness, thyroid surgery
- Symptoms: fever, restlessness, nausea and vomiting, abdominal pain, sweating, tachycardia, hypotension, cardiac failure, delirium and then coma.

Pathogenesis/aetiology

Causes

1° hyperthyroidism:
- Graves' disease (see below)
- Toxic adenoma
- Toxic multinodular goitre
- De Quervain's (subacute) thyroiditis: transient inflammation of the thyroid due to a viral cause. Often starts with hyperthyroidism and then hypothyroidism
- Iatrogenic: from over treating hypothyroidism

2° hyperthyroidism:
- Pituitary adenoma
- Rare cause of hyperthyroidism.

Pathogenesis

- Symptoms due to ↑ metabolic activity from excess hormone

- Sympathetic over activity is the main cause of the cardiac problems.

Who

- Up to 5% of women
- 1/1000 ♂

- ♀>♂.

Clinical features

Signs and symptoms

General progression:
- Fatigue
- Heat intolerance
- Tremor
- Weight ↓ /appetite ↑
- Muscle wasting
- Diarrhoea
- Onycholysis (separation of nail from the nail bed)
- Goitre may be present

Skin:
- Thinning hair
- Palmar erythema
- Warm peripheries

Psychological and neurological:
- Emotional lability
- Psychosis
- Anxiety
- Restlessness
- Irritability

Muscular:
- Myopathy

CV system:
- AF
- Tachycardia
- Cardiac failure

Reproductive:
- Oligomenorrhoea.

Examination and hormone tests

- Test visual fields
- Thyroid Hormones: $\uparrow T_4$, $\uparrow T_3$, $\downarrow$ or $\uparrow$ TSH
- Serum antibodies for autoimmune disease

Imaging

- Thyroid scan if de Quervain's thyroiditis suspected

Thyroid storm

- Identify precipitant
- *Bloods*: FBC, blood glucose, urea and electrolytes
- *Imaging*: CXR, ECG.

Treatment

Medical

- Carbimazole. Methimazole: $\downarrow$ thyroid activity by blocking thyroglobulin synthesis (SE rashes, sore throat, fever)
- Propylthiouracil: inhibits thyroid peroxidase and blocks peripheral conversion of T_4 to T_3 (side effect hepatitis, nephritis, aplastic anaemia, leucopenia)
- Propranolol: B blocker for symptomatic relief

De Quervain's:
- Aspirin or NSAIDs
- Beta-blocker if needed
- Prednisolone if severe

Thyroid storm:
- Supportive:
  - ABC approach
  - O_2, IV fluids
  - Treat cause
- Antithyroid medication:
  - Propranolol
  - Carbimazole
  - Hydrocortisone (stops T_4 conversion to T_3)
  - Oral iodine solution.

Radiotherapy

- Ablation by radioactive iodine which accumulates in the gland and destroys it by local radiation

Surgical

- Thyroidectomy

Prognosis and complications

Prognosis

- Thyroid storm has a 50% mortality.

Complications

- Dermopathy (localised skin lesions) in severe cases
- Thyroid storm
- Complications of surgery if the thyroid glands are removed (see hypothyroidism).

GRAVES' DISEASE

Outline

- An autoimmune disease where autoantibodies stimulate the TSH receptor leading to $\uparrow$ production of TSH and therefore $\uparrow T_3$ and T_4
- Leads to a diffusely enlarged thyroid with pathognomonic features including exophthalmos
- Most common cause of hyperthyroidism.

Pathogenesis/aetiology

Pathogenesis

- IgG antibodies bind to TSH receptors stimulating TSH which leads to excess thyroid hormone production (Graves' disease caused by IgG class)
- There is infiltration of extraocular muscles and preobital CT by lymphocytes and macrophages probably because there is a TSH receptor-like protein in orbital preadipocytes.

Who

- Typical age: women aged 30–50 years
- ♀9:♂1
- 75% of all cases of hyperthyroidism

Genetics:
- 22% concordance in twins
- HLA-DR3
- HLA-DRB1*03
- HLA-DQA1*0501
- CTLA-4
- CD40
- PTPN22
- Protective gene: HLA-DRB1*0701.

Clinical features

Signs and symptoms

- Thyrotoxicosis as above

Pathognomonic features (only in Graves'):

- Ophthalmopathy (90%): limitation of eye movements, grittiness, ↑ tear production, proptosis (protrusion of the eye ball), diplopia, corneal ulceration
- Exophthalmos: protrusion of the eyeball due to endocrine cause (Fig. 9.8)
- Pretibial myxoedema (3%): rough patches over the tibia
- Thyroid acropachy (1%): digital clubbing in Graves' disease due to subperiosteal bone formation

Other features:

- Thyroid bruit
- Vitiligo: symmetrical white patches on skin, an autoimmune disease that occurs with other autoimmune diseases
- Diffusely enlarged thyroid
- Goitre in 90%.

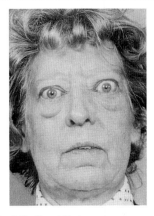

Fig. 9.8   Exophthalmos appearance.

Investigations

Blood tests

- ↓ TSH, ↑ T$_4$/T$_3$
- Serum microsomal and thyroglobulin antibodies:
  - Autoantibodies which stimulate TSH receptor present in >95%

- Autoantibodies against thyroid peroxidase and thyroglobulin in 75% of patients
- Measured by agglutination, ELISA or immunofluorescence.

Imaging

- Radioisotope thyroid scan: if cause is unknown.

Treatment

As for hyperthyroidism above.

Prognosis and complications

Prognosis

- Risk of long-term hypothyroidism with antithyroid medication.

Complications

- Mother can pass antibody to newborn which has disease until maternal antibody is catabolised.

THYROID LUMPS

Outline

- Lumps of the thyroid
- A goitre is an enlarged thyroid gland

Lumps can be:

- nodular or smooth

- toxic (hyperthyroid) or non-toxic
- single or multiple nodules: multinodular lumps tend to occur in thyroids subject to long-term stimulation.

Pathogenesis/aetiology

Causes of a goitre:

A GOITRE:

- **A**utoimmune: Hashimoto's/viral thyroiditis/Graves'
- **G**oitrogens, e.g. lithium
- **O**nset of puberty
- **I**odine deficiency, **i**nfection
- **T**hyrotoxicosis/**T**umour
- **R**eproduction (pregnancy)
- **E**nzyme deficiencies: ↓ thyroid hormone production leading to ↑ TSH and hyperplasia of thyroid follicles (commonest cause).

Causes of a single lump:

- Cyst
- Cancer (see below). Solitary nodules are more likely to be malignant (10%)
- Single nodule in multinodular goitre: 50%

Multinodular thyroid:

- Multinodular colloid goitre: commonest type. Usually non-toxic. Likely autoimmune.

Who

- ♀>♂

- Prevalence of goitre: 9%.

Clinical features

Signs and symptoms

- Neck lump
- Goitre (Fig. 9.9)
- Dysphagia: compress oesophagus
- Dyspnoea: compress trachea.

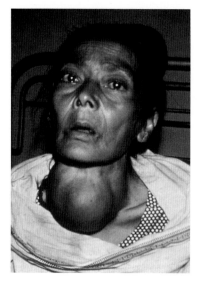

Fig. 9.9　Goitre.

Investigations

Clinical examination

- Thyroid examination.

Blood tests

- FBC, U&Es, ESR
- T_3/T_4, TSH

- Calcitonin: tumour marker
- Thyroid autoantibodies.

Imaging

- CXR: goitre or metastases
- US
- CT scan

- Radioisotope thyroid scan: appear as hot or cold nodules. Cancers are usually cold (low radioisotope uptake, non-functioning), but only 15% of cold spots are cancers.

Other tests

- Fine needle aspiration.

Treatment

- Mostly nothing is done
- Treat any hyper- or hypothyroidism.

Medical

- Iodine, if deficiency is the cause
- Antibiotics for bacterial infection

Surgical

- Cosmetic reasons
- Pressure effects: on trachea or oesophagus
- Symptoms of hyperthyroidism
- Malignancy.

Prognosis and complications

Complications

- Tracheal obstruction
- Complications of thyroid surgery (see hypothyroidism).

MALIGNANT THYROID

Outline

- Cancer of the thyroid

Benign:

- Follicular adenoma:
  - Normally cold nodules (low radioiodine uptake) but can be hot nodules

Malignant: mostly carcinoma:

- Papillary carcinoma (70–80% of thyroid malignancies):
  - From thyroid follicle epithelium
  - Asymptomatic thyroid enlargement
  - Common in women 20–30 years
- Medullary carcinoma (5%):
  - From calcitonin-producing C cells
  - Rare, familial with poor prognosis

- Associated with MEN2 syndrome
- Follicular carcinoma (20%):
  - From thyroid follicle epithelium
  - Solitary cold nodules
  - In 50–70 year olds
- Anaplastic carcinoma (rare):
  - Aggressive and locally invasive tumour in older patients
  - Normally incurable
- Lymphoma (2–5%):
  - Can arise within the thyroid
  - 1° or part of systemic disease.

Pathogenesis/aetiology

Causes

- Radiation exposure: particularly papillary carcinoma
- Oncogenes: (mutations of RET: codes for tyrosine kinase receptor) important in papillary and medullary carcinoma of the thyroid

- Families with MEN2 carry germline mutations of RET oncogene.

Who

- Uncommon but most common endocrine tumour
- 2–3% of all cancers.

Clinical features

Signs and symptoms

- Thyroid mass
- Malignant nodules normally painless
- Dysphagia or dyspnoea from mass effect

- Hoarseness: involvement of recurrent laryngeal nerve and vocal cord paralysis
- Weight loss
- Symptoms and signs of metastases.

Investigations

- As above
- Fine needle aspiration cytology distinguishes benign and malignant nodules

- Radioisotope thyroid scan: 10% of cold nodules are malignant.

Treatment

Surgical

- Lobectomy for local disease or thyroidectomy
- After removal: thyroid replacement which can also suppress residual tumours

- Recurrences: radioactive iodine ablation
- Node excision in papillary carcinoma and medullary carcinoma

Lymphoma

- Radiotherapy, chemotherapy.

Prognosis and complications

Prognosis

Papillary carcinoma:
- 90% survival

Medullary carcinoma:
- Poor prognosis

Follicular carcinoma:
- 10 year survival is 20%

Lymphoma:
- May respond

Complications

- Recurrence
- Complications of thyroid surgery (see hypothyroidism)
- Hypothyroidism

- Hypoparathyroidism
- Recurrent laryngeal nerve palsy.

ADRENAL AXIS DISORDERS

CUSHING'S SYNDROME

Outline

- Prolonged raised levels of cortisol
- Due to raised cortisol or raised level of adrenocorticotropic hormone (ACTH) causing a raised cortisol
- If the raised cortisol levels are specifically due to a raised ACTH from a pituitary tumour this is Cushing's disease (see below)
- Leads to chronic exposure to glucocorticoids

A useful mnemonic:
- **CUSHING**:
  - **C**entral obesity/**C**ervical fat pads/**C**ollagen fibre weakness/**C**omedones (acne)
  - **U**rinary free cortisol and glucose increase
  - **S**triae/**S**uppressed immunity
  - **H**ypercortisolism/**H**ypertension/**H**yperglycaemia/**H**irsutism
  - **I**mmunity suppressed
  - **N**eoplasms
  - **G**lucose ↑.

Pathogenesis/aetiology

Causes

Raised cortisol:
- Iatrogenic: administering steroids. Commonest cause
- Adrenal tumour, usually benign: 25%
- Pseudo-Cushing's: alcohol excess can mimic Cushing's syndrome

Raised ACTH:
- Ectopic ACTH: ACTH secreting tumour but not a pituitary tumour, e.g. lung, medullary carcinoma, thymoma
- Cushing's disease: (see below).

Who

- Typical age: 20–40 years

- ♀5:♂1.

A typical patient

A 30-year-old woman complains to her GP for weight gain, hirsutism and irregular periods.

Clinical features

Signs and symptoms

General:
- Plethoric face, central adiposity, dorso-cervical fat pad (buffalo hump) and proximal myopathy (Fig. 9.10)
- Hypertension
- Depression
- Impaired glucose tolerance

Skin:
- Hirsutism
- Tissue wasting
- Abdominal striae
- Bruising
- Acne
- Hyperpigmentation if ↑ ACTH as ACTH stimulates melanocytes

Musculoskeletal:
- Osteoporosis
- Fractures
- Limb muscle wasting

Immune system:
- Immune suppression

Reproductive changes:
- Menstrual irregularity/amenorrhoea
- Impotence

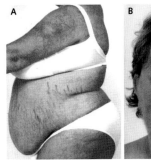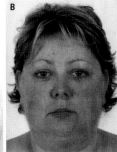

Fig. 9.10 Features of Cushing's syndrome and disease: (A) atraie, central adiposity; (B) cushingoid facies.

Investigations

Blood tests

- Polycythaemia

Hormone levels:
- ↑ Cortisol levels
- ACTH ↓ or ↑:
  - ↑ ACTH is the cause of the high cortisol
  - ↓ Cortisol is raised independently of ACTH leading to –ve feedback of ACTH
- Circadian rhythm studies: loss of normal fall of plasma cortisol at 24 h
- Evening serum and salivary cortisol level
- Dexamethasone–corticotropin-releasing hormone test
- Dexamethasone test

Dexamethasome suppression test (see table 9.5):
- Dexamethasone is a synthetic glucocorticoid that inhibits ACTH production by –ve feedback, thus reducing cortisol production
- First a low dose of dexamethasone is given then a high dose to distinguish between Cushing's disease and syndrome
- False-positive tests due to obedity, alcoholism and chronic renal failure

Urine

- ↑ Urinary free cortisol (24 hour collection) – used as a screening test

Imaging

- Establish cause using: CT, MRI.

Table 9.5 The dexamethasone suppression test

Dexamethasone		Condition
Low dose	High dose	
Cortisol ↓	Cortisol ↓	No pathology (Dexamethasone suppresses cortisol)
No change	Cortisol ↓	Cushing's disease: only causes suppression at high doses where levels are sufficient to suppress excess ACTH
No change	No change	Cushing's syndrome: levels of cortisol are high independent of ACTH

Treatment

- Depends on cause
- Iatrogenic: remove cause.

Medical

- Metyrapone (inhibits cortisol synthesis), aminoglutethimide
- Ketoconazole: blocks P450 dependent enzymes involved in the synthetic pathway of cortisol

Surgical

- First line for adrenal tumours or ectopic ACTH
- Removal of the adrenal gland/s. For adrenal adenomas, carcinomas. Hydrocortisone and fludrocortisone then given for life (if bilateral)

Prognosis and complications

Prognosis

- Surgical removal of tumour is curative
- Poor outcome for adrenal carcinomas. Survival <2 years
- Untreated: poor
- Treated: good prognosis.

Complications

- Osteoporosis
- Diabetes mellitus
- Cardiovascular compilations.

CUSHING'S DISEASE

Outline

- ↑ Cortisol levels specifically from inappropriate ACTH secretion from a pituitary tumour
- A type of Cushing's syndrome
- Cushing's disease: pituitary problem
- Cushing's syndrome: from some other cause.

Pathogenesis/aetiology

Causes

- From pituitary tumour.

Who

- Typical age: 30–50 years
- ♀ > ♂.

Clinical features

Signs and symptoms

- As above
- Hyperpigmentation of skin and mucous membranes from excess ACTH as ACTH stimulates melanocytes.

Investigations

Hormone levels:
- ↑ ACTH
- ↑ Cortisol
- Dexamethasone test (as above).

Imaging

- CT or MRI of the pituitary gland.

Treatment

- Metyrapone, ketoconazole if surgery cannot be performed.

Surgical

- Trans-sphenoidal removal: first line
- Rarely bilateral adrenalectomy if source can not be located but may lead to hyperpigmentation (nelson's syndrome) if ↑ ACTH continues.

Prognosis and complications

Prognosis

- Trans-sphenoidal surgery successful in 80%.

Complications

- As above.

PRIMARY HYPERALDOSTERONISM

Outline

- High aldosterone unrelated to the renin–angiotensin system
- Aldosterone increases sodium and water reabsorption and increases potassium excretion
- High aldosterone therefore causes hypernatraemia (antinatriuresis) and hypokalaemia (kaliuresis)
- Leads to fluid retention: hypervolaemia and hypertension.

Pathogenesis/aetiology

Causes

- Aldosterone-secreting adenoma: Conn's syndrome. Commonest cause 75%
- Adrenal carcinoma
- Bilateral hyperplasia of the adrenal cortex.

Who

- Rare

Clinical features

Signs and symptoms

- Often asymptomatic
- Hypertension
- Hypokalaemia symptoms: muscle weakness, polyuria and polydipsia, paraesthesia, abdominal distension, cramps
- Cardiac decompensation and complications of hypertension
- Metabolic alkalosis.

Investigations

Blood tests

- U&Es: sodium ↑, potassium ↓
- ↑ Aldosterone
- ↓ Plasma renin due to feedback mechanisms
- Adrenal venous sampling allowing selective assay of excess hormone.

ECG

- Changes due to low potassium.

Imaging

- CT/MRI: to differentiate adenoma from hyperplasia.

Treatment

Medical

- Aldosterone antagonist (spironolactone, eplerenone) for hypertension
- Calcium channel blockers: ↓ aldosterone levels.

Surgical

- Conn's: removal of the adenoma.

Prognosis

- Cured by removal of adenoma
- Poor in adrenal carcinoma.

Complications

- Those relating to chronic hypertension.

SECONDARY HYPERALDOSTERONISM

Outline

- High aldosterone from adrenal response to ↑ levels of renin.

Pathogenesis/aetiology

Causes

- Renal ischaemia: renal artery stenosis
- Chronic oedema (congestive cardiac failure, nephrotic syndrome, ascites)
- Hepatic failure
- Cardiac failure
- Hypertension
- Drugs: ACE inhibitors, NSAIDs.

Who

- Rare.

Clinical features

Signs and symptoms

- Often asymptomatic
- Hypertension
- Hypokalaemia symptoms: muscle weakness, polyuria and polydipsia, paraesthesia, cramps
- Cardiac decompensation
- Metabolic alkalosis.

Investigations

Blood tests

- U&Es: sodium ↑, potassium ↓
- ↑ Aldosterone
- ↑ Plasma renin (low in 1°) from decreased renal perfusion.

ECG

- Changes: associated with hypokalaemia.

Treatment

- Spironolactone (aldosterone antagonist) side effects: gynaecomastia, impotence, menorrhagia.

Prognosis and complications

Prognosis

- Varies depending upon underlying cause; good with early detection.

Complications

- See above.

CONGENITAL ADRENAL HYPERPLASIA

Outline

- Congenital adrenal hyperplasia (CAH) are a group of autosomal recessive congenital disorders which result in deficiency of one of the enzymes involved in the adrenal steroid synthesis pathway

- Leads to reduced glucocorticoid and mineralocorticoid synthesis
- A variety of disorders depending on which enzyme is deficient.

Classification

Salt wasting CAH:
- From 21-hydroxylase deficiency (95%): commonest CAH cause
- This enzyme is important in cortisol and aldosterone synthesis so neither is produced
- It is salt wasting as low mineralocortioid leads to salt loss, dangerous in neonates who may have salt losing crises

Salt sparing CAH:
- 11α-hydroxylase deficiency (3%)
- Cortisol is not produced but 11-deoxycorticosterone (DOC) replaces aldosterone as the mineralocorticoid so salt is not lost
- DOC does not respond to suppression of the renin–angiotensin system so more and more salt is retained. This leads to malignant, hypervolaemic hypertension.

Pathogenesis/aetiology

↓ Enzyme activity and their underlying genes:
- Several enzymes can be affected:
  - 21α-hydroxylase: cYP21A

- 11β-hydroxylase: cYP11B1
- 17α-hydroxylase: cYP17A
- Aldosterone synthetase: cYP11B2.

Pathogenesis

- As well as reduced synthesis of glucocorticoids and mineralocorticoids overall, low synthesis of cortisol and aldosterone leads to excess ACTH and other intermediate products (due to lack of negative feedback) leading to additional specific symptoms

For example, females present with pseudo-hermaphroditism as increased ACTH leads to increased dehydroepiandrosterone (DHEA), which leads to virilisation of external organs.

Who

- Typical age: children
- Commonest adrenal disorders of infancy

- Prevalence overall 1:16 000 population.

Clinical features

Signs and symptoms

- Depends on enzyme affected
- Virilism (secondary male sexual characteristics in females including ambiguous genitalia and hirsuitism) in the commonest forms
- Infertility

- Precocious/delayed puberty
- Primary amenorrhoea in females
- Vomiting and dehydration in early infancy
- 21-hydroxylase deficient males with salt wasting CAH present with failure to thrive.

Investigations

Blood tests

- ↑ ACTH from ↓ cortisol
- ↓ Aldosterone, ↑ potassium, ↑ renin in salt wasting forms
- In hypertensive forms:
  - ↓ Potassium, renin

21-hydroxylase deficiency:
- ↑ Serum 17-hydroxyprogesterone (usually >1000 ng/dL) in the presence of clinical features suggestive of the disease

Karyotype

- Essential.

Treatment

- Replacement therapy with cortisol or aldosterone

- Some need GnRH agonist induced delay in puberty.

Surgical

- Surgical treatment of ambiguous genitalia.

Prognosis

- Fatal if not treated or steroids inadequately replaced.

Complications

- Shortness of stature
- ↓ Fertility
- Testicular masses.

PRIMARY HYPOADRENALISM/ADDISON'S DISEASE

Outline

- Decrease in all three hormones of the adrenal cortex from acute destruction of the adrenal gland
- Also called Addison's disease
- Can be acute or chronic insufficiency

Classification of hypoadrenalism:

- 1° hypoadrenalism: direct destruction of the adrenal gland leading to ↓ synthesis of all adrenal steroids: Addison's disease
- 2° hypoadrenalism: hypothalamic–pituitary problem (see below)

Addisonian/adrenal crisis:

- An emergency from acute deficiency in adrenal hormones, mainly cortisol
- Patients develop hypovolaemic shock or hypoglycaemia
- Due to:
  - discontinuing long-term steroids without tapering the dose
  - acute stress in patients on long-term steroids
  - patients with chronic adrenal dysfunction
  - sepsis in adrenal gland
  - metastatic cancer.

Pathogenesis/aetiology

Causes

- Autoimmune (90%) 2♀:1♂
- Infection: TB, HIV
- Haemorrhage or infarction
- Malignancy: lymphoma, metastasis
- Infiltration: amyloidosis, haemochromatosis
- Inherited disorders
- Surgical removal
- Drugs: ketoconazole, busulfan, methadone

- Waterhouse–Friderichsen syndrome:
  - Haemorrhage into the adrenal glands from meningococcal septicaemia
  - Characterised by:
    1. Bacterial infection
    2. Hypertension leading to shock
    3. DIC with widespread purpura
    4. Fast-developing adrenocortical insufficiency with massive bilateral adrenal haemorrhage
  - Coma and death in 6 h.

Who

- Typical age: 20–40 years
- 4♀:1♂
- Uncommon

Associations:

- HLA-DR3/4, HLA-B8
- Other autoimmune diseases
- Autoantibodies to 21-hydroxylase, cytochrome P450 (and other autoantigens associated with adrenal cortical cells).

Clinical features

Signs and symptoms

From low cortisol:

- Hyperpigmentation: of skin and mucous membranes from excess ACTH as there is no − ve feedback from cortisol. ACTH stimulates melanocytes
- Reactive hypoglycaemia: lack of cortisol antagonism to insulin control

From low aldosteronism:

- Hyperkalaemia and hyponatraemia: lack of aldosterone causes renal loss of sodium
- Fluid loss
- Postural hypotension: from loss of water with the sodium

From low androgens:

- ↓ Growth of pubic hair in females

Non-specific features:

- Lethargy
- Depression
- Dizziness, confusion
- Vitiligo (associated with autoimmune diseases)
- Weight loss
- Abdominal pain
- Nausea/vomiting
- Constipation
- Arthralgia/myalgia.

Clinical features

Addisonian crisis:
- Fever
- Vomiting
- Abdominal pain
- Hypotension
- Tachycardia
- Hypovolaemic shock
- Collapse
- Coma.

Investigations

Blood tests

- FBC: eosinophilia, leucocytosis
- U&Es: sodium ↓, potassium ↑, urea ↑, glucose ↓
- Serum cortisol levels
- ACTH levels (high in Addison's disease)
- Renin and aldosterone
- Prolactin
- Adrenal antibodies: in 50%
- Screen for other autoimmune disease.

Synacthen test

- Synacthen is synthetic ACTH; the test demonstrates hypoadrenalism and distinguishes between 1° and 2° causes (Table 9.6)
- Short test: IV injection of Synacthen should cause normal rise of cortisol in 30 min. If not, shows hypoadrenalism
- Long test: IV injections for 3 days. Cortisol rises in 2° hypoadrenalism.

Imaging

- CXR, AXR to look for previous TB

Table 9.6 Synacthen test

ACTH dose		Condition
Short test	Long test	
Cortisol ↑	Cortisol ↑	No pathology
Cortisol not ↑	Cortisol ↑	2° hypoadrenalism
Cortisol not ↑	Cortisol not ↑	1° hypoadrenalism

Treatment

Acute treatment for adrenal crisis:
- ABC approach
- IV saline
- IV glucose if hypoglycaemic
- IV hydrocortisone
- Treat any underlying infection
- Identify cause

Maintenance therapy:
- Aldosterone replacement: fludrocortisone (side effect: risk of osteoporosis)
- Lifelong steroid replacement: hydrocortisone

Side effects of steroids:
- **BECLOMETHASONE**:
  - **B**uffalo hump
  - **E**asy bruising
  - **C**ataracts
  - **L**arger appetite
  - **O**besity
  - **M**oonface
  - **E**uphoria
  - **T**hin arms & legs
  - **H**ypertension/**H**yperglycaemia
  - **A**vascular necrosis of femoral head
  - **S**kin thinning
  - **O**steoporosis
  - **N**egative nitrogen balance
  - **E**motional liability.

Prognosis and complications

Prognosis

- Normal lifespan if treated.

Complications

- Renal sodium loss can cause circulatory collapse: needs urgent resuscitation.

SECONDARY HYPOADRENALISM

Outline

- A reduction in the hormones of the adrenal cortex from a problem with the hypothalamic–pituitary axis (inadequate ACTH production)

- Low cortisol and androgen, but normal aldosterone (stimulated by angiotensin II, not ACTH).

Pathogenesis/aetiology

Causes

- Iatrogenic: long-term steroid therapy leading to hypothalamic pituitary–adrenal suppression (commonest cause)

- Any disorder of hypothalamus or pituitary resulting in ↓ ACTH: metastases, infection, infarction, irradiation, haemorrhage, amyloidosis, sarcoidosis.

Who

- 4♀:1♂

- Incidence: 1/1 000 000.

Clinical features

Signs and symptoms

- Low cortisol and androgen effects as above
- Normal aldosterone, so no marked hyperkalaemia, or hyponatraemia

- No pigmentation as ACTH levels are low.

Investigations

- ACTH is low

- Synacthen test (see above).

Treatment

- Hydrocortisone.

Prognosis and complications

Prognosis

- If from longer-term steroid therapy, adrenals will recover as steroids are withdrawn.

PHAEOCHROMOCYTOMA

Outline

- Catecholamine (specifically adrenaline and mainly noradrenaline) producing tumour of chromaffin cells
- Leads to symptoms of sympathetic nervous system overactivity such as hypertension

- Phaeochromocytomas occur as part of MEN (see below) and other familial syndromes.

Pathogenesis/aetiology

Pathogenesis

- Originates from chromaffin cells, mainly of the adrenal medulla (∼90%) but can be extra-adrenal
- Tumours may compress the adrenocortical tissues
10% Rule:
- 10% bilateral
- 10% extramedullary

- 10% multiple
- 10% malignant
- 10% familial, e.g. MEN
- 10% in children
- 10% recur
- 10% present with strokes.

Who

- Typical age: 30–50 years olds and in childhood (∼10%)
- 2♂:1♀
- Rare 1:100 000

Associations:
- MEN2A, MEN2B
- Neurofibromatosis type 1
- Sturge–Weber syndrome
- Tuberous sclerosis.

Clinical features

Signs and symptoms

Phaeochros:
- **P**alpitations
- **H:** Headache/**hypertension**: can precipitate MI or stroke
- **A:** Anxiety
- **E:** excessive sweating
- **O:** l**O**ss weight

- **C**ardiomyopathy, myocarditis
- **H:** Hyperglycaemia
- **R**educed bladder control at night (nocturnal enuresis)
- F**O**ll**O**w up
- Signs may be episodic.

Investigations

Blood and urine tests

- Catcholamine levels in blood and urine (24-h collection)

- U&E, calcium, LFT

Other tests

- Fundoscopy: for hypertensive retinopathy

- Chromaffin reaction: dichromate fixative turns phaeochomocytoma brown.

Imaging

- CT/MRI

- Scintigraphy (two-dimensional nuclear imaging).

Treatment

Surgical

- Surgical excision: adrenalectomy

Medical

- Both alpha and beta blockade are required prior to surgery: alpha-blockers should be given first to prevent unopposed alpha-stimulation.

Prognosis and complications

Prognosis

- Normal life after surgery

- 90% are curable.

Complications

- Hypertension
- Diabetes mellitus

- Cardiomyopathy and congestive heart failure.

DIABETES AND ITS COMPLICATIONS

DIABETES MELLITUS

Outline

- Group of disorders of chronic hyperglycaemia from insulin deficiency, resistance or both

- The high levels of glucose lead to a number of vascular problems.

Classification

Type 1 (10%):
- Also called insulin-dependent diabetes (IDDM)
- From an total lack of insulin
- Due to an autoimmune attack on beta cells of the pancreas
- Islet cell autoantibodies to:
  - glutamic acid decarboxylase
  - anti-insulin B chain
  - anti-insulin receptor
  - IA-2 protein tyrosine phosphatase
- Insulin replacement is essential for treatment
- Associated with other autoimmune diseases

- Due to:
  - genetic predisposition: HLA-linked genes
  - environmental insults: viral infections, damage to altered beta cells, dietary
Type 2 (80–90%):
- Also called non-insulin-dependent diabetes (NIDDM)
- From a relative lack of insulin
- B cells cannot secrete insulin due to an altered response to hyperglycaemia
- There is also resistance to insulin by peripheral tissues
- Occurs in older people

Outline

- Due to:
  - environmental insult: obesity
  - genetic predisposition: multiple genetic defects

Other forms:
- Maturity-onset diabetes of the young: autosomal dominant, onset normally before 25. Strong family history
- Gestational diabetes (type 3): during pregnancy, resolves after delivery but can recur
- Genetic (type 4).

Pathogenesis/aetiology

Pathogenesis

- Uncontrolled hyperglycaemia causes complications
- Glucose is a reducing sugar that can react to change into a carboxyl group
- Leads to non-enzymic glycosylation of proteins
- Reacts irreversibly with proteins to form advanced glycosylation end-products (AGE) which affects protein function
- Causes both macro- and microvascular damage

Vascular damage:
- Macrovascular disease (larger vessels):
  - Cerebrovascular disease
  - Coronary artery disease (MI is the commonest cause of death in diabetes)
  - Peripheral vascular disease: accelerated atherosclerosis, gangrene, stroke, foot pain
- Microvascular disease (smaller vessels):
  - Diabetic eye disease: see below
  - Renal disease: see below
  - Neuropathy: mononeuritis, peripheral neuropathies, diabetic amyotrophy (painful weakness and wasting

of the quadriceps), autonomic neuropathies (including postural hypotension)

Skin disease:
- Lipoatrophy: fat necrosis at injection sites Recommended to vary the injection site
- Granuloma annulare: chronic benign condition where there is a ring of papules
- Acanthosis nigricans: pigmented roughened areas of thickened skin found in the axilla, neck or groin
- Necrobiosis lipoidica diabeticorum: shiny, yellow area on the shins
- Infections

Diabetic foot disease:
- 90% from neuropathy, also from peripheral vascular disease
- Infection
- Ulceration
- Can lead to amputation

Infection.

Who

- 2% of world population
- 3 million in the UK

Type 1:
- Typical age: younger, incidence peaks at puberty
- Usually thin
- Common in northern Europe
- Genetics:
  - HLA-DR3, 4 in >90%
  - Susceptibility: HLA-DQ8
  - Resistance: HLA-DR6
  - 50% twin concordance
  - Family history uncommon

Type 2:
- Typical age: >40 years
- Obese
- Often have had previous gestational diabetes
- Genetics: twins concordance 50%, family history common

2° causes:
- Pregnancy
- Cushing's
- Acromegaly
- Phaeochromocytoma
- Drugs: steroids, olanzapine
- Pancreatic conditions.

Clinical features

Signs and symptoms

- Lethargy
- Polydipsia
- Polyuria
- Vomiting
- Muscle weakness and wasting
- Weight loss: type 1
- Symptoms from complications: cerebrovascular disease, coronary artery disease, eye disease, diabetic foot disease, kidney disease, neuropathy, infection
- Impaired consciousness

Diabetic emergencies:
- May be the first presentation of diabetes
- Diabetic ketoacidosis (DKA): associated with type 1 disease (see below)
- Hyperosmolar non-ketotic acidosis (HONK): associated with type 2 disease (see below)
- Hypoglycaemia
- Lactic acidosis: metformin related.

Investigations

Diagnosed based on either a fasting blood glucose, random blood glucose or HbA1c level.
If symptomatic (e.g. polyuria, polydipsia, weight loss):
- single fasting plasma glucose >7

or

- single random plasma glucose >11.1

If asymptomatic: one of the following:
- a fasting glucose >7 on 2 separate occasions
- a random glucose >11.1 on 2 separate occasions
- HbA1c >6.5 on 2 separate occasions
- HbA1c and a raised fasting or random blood glucose

Glycated Hb:
- ↑ glucose reacts with N terminal amino acids of Hb β-chains leading to glycated Hb. The higher the glucose level, the higher the level of glycation
- Measure of glycaemic control over 8–12 weeks.

Autoantibodies:
- For type 1 diabetes. Can predict who will become diabetic

Insulin levels:
- Type 1: zero
- Type 2: normal or high

Each visit check:
- Home monitoring: blood sugar (Boehringer Mannheim test)
- HbA1c
- BMI
- Urinalysis: proteinuria
- BP
- Microalbuminuria

Annually:
- Pulses
- Feet
- Eyes
- Albumin/creatinine ratio
- Lipid profile
- TFTs.

Treatment

- Multidisciplinary team: diabetic nurse, consultant, dietician, mental health, podiatrist, ophthalmology
- Patient education and motivation
- Monitor regularly

Type 1:
- Insulin (side effects: weight gain, hypoglycaemia, lipohypertrophy). Several common regimes of insulin (Fig. 9.11)
- Slow acting insulin (usually given before bed): lantus, ultratard, glargine
- Fast acting insulin (usually given around meal times): novorapid, humalog, actrapid
- Insulin should never be stopped. If unwell: ↑ fluids, eat a little frequently, sip sugary drinks if vomiting and continue insulin

Type 2:
- Exercise/lifestyle/stop smoking
- Diet: low in fat, simple sugars, high in fibre and complex carbohydrates
- Treat hyperlipidaemia and BP to ↓ complications
- Regular checks
- Treatment is progressive, start with lifestyle change, then monotherapy, then two oral drugs, then insulin, then insulin with an oral drug
- Insulin given in persistent hyperglycaemia, pregnancy, recurrent illness or complications

Treatment protocol:
1. Lifestyle and metformin (if unsuitable for metformin consider sulfonylurea)
2. If HbA1c >6.5% add sulfonylureas (if unsuitable, consider gliptins or glitazones)
3. If HbA1c >7.5% add insulin (if unsuitable, consider sitagliptin or glitazone or exenatide/liraglutide)
4. If HbA1c remains >7.5% intensify insulin regimen and consider adding glitazone

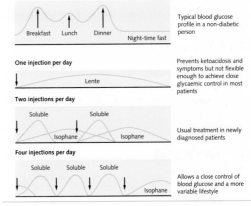

Fig. 9.11 Typical insulin regimens.

Medications:
- Metformin, a biguanide ↓ liver glucose production and sensitises target tissues to insulin. side effect: lactic acidosis
- Sulfonylureas e.g. glibenclamide, dolbutamine. Promote insulin secretion: side effects: appetite ↑, hypoglycaemia
- Glitazones e.g. pioglitazone. ↑ sensitivity to insulin and ↑ insulin secretion: side effect: hepatotoxicity
- Gliptins: DPP-4 inhibitors which prevent the breakdown of GLP-1 and allow continued insulin secretion. An alternative to insulin
- Exenatide/liraglutide: GLP-1 mimetics which increase insulin secretion. Result in weight loss.

Prognosis

- Life expectancy ↓ by 5–10 years.

Complications

- Type 1: diabetic ketoacidosis
- Type 2: hyperosmolar non-ketotic acidosis

- Long-term complications: cardiovascular (70%), kidney disease (10%), infection (6%) (see below).

DIABETIC EYE DISEASE

Outline

- Eye disease as a complication of diabetes
- Main problem is retinopathy which is caused by capillary damage within the eye leading to leakage and hypoxia of the vessels

- Eventually causes blindness
- Also cataracts, glaucoma, ocular palsies.

Pathogenesis/aetiology

Stages of retinopathy:

I. *Background*:
- Haemorrhages, dots and blots, hard exudates
- Action: review

II. *Preproliferative*:
- As above and soft exudates (cotton wool spots), venous beading and looping
- Action: ophthalmology referral

III. *Proliferative*:
- As above and new retinal vessel formation
- Action: urgent ophthalmology referral

IV. *Maculopathy*:
- As above and hard exudates, macula oedema
- Action: urgent ophthalmology referral, macular grid laser.

Who

- Commonest cause of blindness in people of working age

- 2% of young diabetics develop diabetic eye disease.

Clinical features

Signs and symptoms

- Cataracts
- Glaucoma

- Ocular palsies
- Blindness.

Investigations

- Fundoscopy

- Fluorescein angiogram of the eye.

Treatment

Prevention:
- Intensive glucose control in type 1 diabetes reduces incidence and progression
- BP control: slows the progression of diabetic retinopathy and reduces risk of vitreous haemorrhage

- Diabetic retinopathy screening: Annual UK screening for all diabetics over the age of 12

Laser therapy:
- Laser coagulation for microaneurysms and proliferative retinopathy.

Prognosis and complications

Prognosis

- 5% blind after about 30 years of diabetes

- Blindness is irreversible.

DIABETIC KIDNEY DISEASE:

Outline

- Kidney disease as a complication of diabetes
- Progresses from microalbuminuria and proteinuria to end-stage renal failure
- Responsible for 30–40% of end-stage renal failure

- United Kingdom Prospective Diabetes study: 10 years following diagnosis, prevalence of:
  - microalbuminuria, 25%
  - macroalbuminuria, 5%
  - end-stage renal failure, 0.8%
  - yearly rate of progression from macroalbuminaemia to renal failure was 2.3%.

Pathogenesis/aetiology

Pathogenesis

- Diabetes mellitus can damage kidney by:
  1. Glomerular disease: progresses from microalbuminaemia to macroalbuminuria to end-stage renal failure

  2. Ischaemic lesions of afferent and efferent arterioles
  3. Infection: UTIs, pyelonephritis.

Who

- 30% of type 1 diabetes
- 25–50% of type 2 diabetes

- More common in blacks than whites.

Clinical features

Signs and symptoms

- Features of renal disease.

Investigations

Blood tests

- U&Es for renal function

Urine

- Dipstick for protein

- ↑ Urine albumin:creatinine ratio: earliest evidence of diabetic glomerular disease is microalbuminuria (30–300 mg albumin over 24 h).

Treatment

Microalbuminuria:
- Control of BP is most important factor in ↓ progression
- Tight glycaemic control, ACE-I, angiotensin II inhibitors

Macroalbuminaemia:
- BP control, protein restriction

End-stage renal disease:
- Dialysis or renal transplant.

Prognosis and complications

Prognosis

- Glomerular disease affects 30% of diabetics diagnosed young.

Complications

- Renal papillary necrosis: rare complication of renal infection

- End-stage renal failure.

DIABETIC KETOACIDOSIS

Outline

- State of uncontrolled catabolism associated with insulin deficiency
- Patient is volume depleted, ketotic and acidotic

- Most commonly occurs in type 1 diabetic patients: typically with a history of poor control
- May be first presentation of diabetes
- **A medical emergency: life threatening**.

Pathogenesis/aetiology

Pathogenesis

- ↑ Glucose: lack of insulin leads to an ↑ in hepatic gluconeogenesis leading to high glucose levels which results in diuresis and dehydration
- ↑ Ketones: low insulin leads to fat catabolism. Lipolysis leads to formation of free fatty acids, which are broken by the liver to ketones leading to high anion gap metabolic acidosis. Stress hormones accelerate the processes. Ketones can be detected in the urine and in the breath (smell of nail remover) and lead to nausea and vomiting causing further dehydration

- The metabolic acidosis and dehydration lead to electrolyte imbalances

Precipitants:
- **6 I's:**
  - Insulin stopped/wrong dose
  - Initial presentation of diabetes
  - Infection
  - Intoxication – alcohol
  - Ischaemia
  - Infarction: MI.

Who

- ♀ > ♂

- Diabetic ketoacidosis accounts for 50% of diabetes-related admissions in young people and 1–2% of all primary diabetes-related admissions.

A typical patient

A 15-year-old girl presents to A&E with reduced consciousness. Blood sugars are 28 mmol/L. Her mum recalls that over the last few days she has been very thirsty. Her breath smells like nail remover.

Clinical features

Signs and symptoms

- 2–3 day history of gradual decline
- Polyuria
- Lethargy
- Anorexia
- Vomiting
- Abdominal pain: particularly in children

- Breathing: hyperventilation (Kussmaul's respiration), ketotic breath
- Dehydration: polydipsia, sunken eyes, dry mouth, hypotension
- Coma in 5%.

Investigations

Blood tests

- FBC: ↑ WBC in infection may be high in volume depletion
- U&Es:
  - Sodium ↓: may be high if dehydrated
  - Potassium ↑: patients are potassium depleted overall but levels may be normal or high as acidosis makes potassium move out of intracellular compartment. As acidosis is corrected potassium can fall very low
  - Urea/creatinine ↑: because of dehydration or catabolism
  - Bicarbonate levels
- Glucose elevation: often >20 mmol/L

- Blood gas:
  - pH <7.3
  - Bicarbonate low, metabolic acidosis
  - Pao_2 normal, $Paco_2$ low
- Later investigations: anti-insulin and anti-glutamic acid decarboxylase antibodies

Urine dip

- Ketones

- Glucose

ECG

- To monitor side effects of potassium changes.

Investigations

Other tests

Septic screen:
- Diabetic ketoacidosis may have been triggered by an infection: therefore do urine dip, consider CXR, blood or urine cultures particularly if pyrexial.

Treatment

Acute treatment

- **Emergency: ABC approach** (see acutely unwell chapter)
- O_2
For dehydration:
- Fluid IV: 0.9% saline: initially IL over 30–60 min, then continue, but at a reducing rate (if blood sugar drops to <10 mmol/L give 5% dextrose)
To correct lack of insulin:
- Insulin infusion IV: aim to normalise blood glucose slowly with a sliding scale
To correct ion imbalance:
- Potassium monitored and added to IV saline according to blood levels

- Consider bicarbonate only in severe acidosis
Monitoring:
- In a high dependency unit
- Check blood gas every 1–2 h initially (can use venous gas)
- Identify cause: treat any precipitating infection
If severe diabetic ketoacidosis, consider:
- Nasogastric tube if nauseated or unconscious (to prevent aspiration), urinary catheter if no urine passed, heparin in older or obese patients (risk of clotting)

The stable patient

- Once eating and drinking:
  - Stop insulin sliding scale and fluid and begin on sc insulin (ensure some overlap)
  - Continue to monitor glucose and electrolytes (initially hourly)

- If newly diagnosed diabetic: ensure contact with diabetic nurse and dietician before discharge and arrange follow-up.

Prognosis and complications

Prognosis

- Mortality 0.67% of all admissions with diabetic ketoacidosis

- Death if untreated.

Complications

- Cerebral oedema if treated too aggressively with fluids; therefore monitor headache and drowsiness during treatment (more common in children)

- Hypokalaemia
- Thromboembolism.

HYPEROSMOLAR NON-KETOTIC ACIDOSIS (HONK)

Outline

- Hyperosmolar non-ketotic state
- Life-threatening condition most commonly in type 2 diabetic patients where there is hyperglycaemia leading to severe dehydration and hyperosmolarity without significant ketoacidosis

- May be first presentation of diabetes
- **A medical emergency.**

Pathogenesis/aetiology

Pathogenesis

- A precipitating event leads to raised glucose. This leads to polyuria (osmotic diuresis), which in turn leads to dehydration and a further concentration of blood glucose

- The whole cycle then repeats causing intense hyperglycaemia, dehydration and reduced consciousness
- No significant ketosis.

Pathogenesis/aetiology

Precipitants

- Normally triggered by an illness
- Infection
- Glucose-rich fluids
- Infarction: MI, stroke
- Non-compliance with medication
- Drugs: beta-blockers, diuretics, alcohol, nutritional supplements, atypical antipsychotics, cocaine.

Who

- Typical age: more common in the elderly
- Type 2 diabetics
- In 30–40% of cases it is the first presentation of diabetes

A typical patient

- A patient presents to A&E with reduced consciousness. Blood sugars are recorded as 28 mmol/L

Clinical features

Signs and symptoms

- 7-day history of gradual decline
- Polyuria
- Thirst
- Confusion
- Lethargy/somnolence
- Visual changes
- Seizures
- Dehydration: polydipsia, sunken eyes, dry mouth, hypotension markedly increased skin turgor
- Symptoms of underlying precipitant
- Coma.

Investigations

Blood tests

- FBC
- U&Es
  - Sodium ↑: dehydration
  - Potassium ↑
  - Not acidodic
- ↑ Blood glucose
- ↑ Osmolarity

Other tests

Septic screen:
- May have been triggered by an infection: therefore do urine dip, consider CXR, blood or urine cultures, ECG.

Treatment

Acute treatment

- **Emergency: ABC approach** (see acutely unwell chapter)
- O$_2$

For dehydration:
- Fluid IV: 0.9% saline to slowly rehydrate over 48 h

To correct lack of insulin:
- Insulin IV, hyperosmolar non-ketotic acidosis more sensitive to insulin than diabetic ketoacidosis, so use a lower rate

To prevent thromboembolism:
- Treatment dose LMWH as risk of thrombosis from volume depletion and hyperglycaemia

Monitoring:
- In high dependency unit
- Monitor electrolytes and glucose after 1 h then every 2–4 h
- If severe: consider nasogastric tube and urinary catheter

The stable patient

- Once eating and drinking:
  - Stop insulin sliding scale and fluid and start SC insulin (best to have overlap between the two)
- Monitor glucose and electrolytes
- If new diagnosis: ensure contact with diabetic nurse and dietitian before discharge and arrange follow-up.

Prognosis and complications

Prognosis

- Mortality 20–30%.

Prognosis and complications

Complications

- Hypovolaemic shock
- Thromboembolism
- Confusion
- Coma: 10%.

HYPOGLYCAEMIA

Outline

- Plasma glucose <2.5 mmol/L (normal glucose range: 3.5–8.0 mmol)
- Hypoglycaemia leads to sympathetic activation
- Can also lead to ↓ availability of glucose for the brain

- **A medical emergency**
- Presume in all unconscious patients and those with rapid-onset confusion until proven otherwise.

Pathogenesis/aetiology

Causes

Diabetic patient:
- On insulin or oral hypoglycaemics
- Greatest risk: before meals, during the night
- Can be precipitated by poor glycaemic control, irregular eating, unusual exertion, excess alcohol

Non diabetic – **EXPLAIN**:
- **E**: exogenous drugs: insulin, alcohol, factitious/iatrogenic
- **P**: pituitary insufficiency
- **L**: liver disease
- **A**: Addison's disease
- **I**: insulinomas (see Surgery p. 638)
- **N**: non-pancreatic neoplasms

Pathogenesis

- Develops when hepatic glucose output < glucose uptake by peripheral tissues.

Who

- Commonest endocrine emergency.

Clinical features

Signs and symptoms

- Usually rapid onset

Glucose <3.5 mmol/L:
- Autonomic symptoms:
  - Sweating
  - Shaking
  - Anxiety
  - Tremor
  - Hunger
  - Palpitations
  - Tachycardia

Glucose <2.5 mmol/L:
- ↓ Cerebral glucose (neuroglycopenic):
  - Drowsy
  - Weakness
  - Irritability
  - Personality change/confusion
  - Change in vision: blurring
  - Seizures
  - Can mimic a stroke

Glucose <1.5 mmol:
- Coma
- Death.

Investigations

Blood tests

- Blood glucose: confirms diagnosis
- U&Es
- LFTs: liver disease can precipitate hypoglycaemia

- If no known history of diabetes: save serum to identify the cause
- Short Synacthen test if Addison's disease is suspected
- C-peptide: if exogenous source suspected.

Treatment

Patient is conscious:
- Sugary drinks
- Oral glucose
- Hypostop gel

Treatment

Patient is unconscious:
- 50% dextrose IV with saline flush (dextrose damages veins)

- IM glucagon: mobilises hepatic glycogen, useful when cannot obtain IV access
- If no prompt change: IV dexamethasone: to prevent cerebral oedema.

Prognosis and complications

Prognosis

- Fast recovery but recurrent or prolonged attacks lead to irreversible intellectual decline.

Complications

- Death.

REPRODUCTIVE SYSTEM DISORDERS

HYPOGONADISIM

Outline

- Defect in the function of the gonads: the ovaries and testes
- The gonads produce gametes and hormones: hypogonadism affects both these processes

- Can affect:
  - sexual development
  - fertility.

Pathogenesis/aetiology

Causes

Hypothalmic–pituitary disorder:
- Hypopituitarism
- Severe illness
- Malnourishment
- Hyperprolactinaemia: interferes with LH and FSH
- Kallmann syndrome (gondadotrophin deficiency with anosmia)

Gonadal disease:
- Congenital: Klinefelter's (in males: XXY), Turner's (XO) in females
- Acquired: trauma, radiation, infection (mumps, HIV), hepatic failure, renal failure, alcohol excess
Target tissues:
- Receptor deficiency.

Who

- Typical age: may occur at any age

- $♀ < ♂$.

Clinical features

Signs and symptoms

- Presentation: depends on age of onset
Males:
- Prepubertal onset:
  - Delayed puberty
  - Long limbs from continued growth of long bones
  - High pitched voice
  - Small penis, testes, scrotum
  - ↓ Muscle mass

- After puberty:
  - ↓ Public hair
  - Small prostate
  - ↓ Libido
Females:
- Amenorrhoea (no periods)
- Oligomenorrhoea (few periods)
- Breast/vaginal atrophy
- ↓ Public hair.

Investigations

Blood tests

- Measure LH, FSH, prolactin, oestrogen, testosterone

- Antiovarian antibody.

Imaging

- US of ovaries

- Pituitary MRI.

Investigations

Other tests

- Chromosome analysis
- Seminal fluids examination
- Ovarian biopsy.

Treatment

- Treat cause
- Androgen replacement
- LH, FSH, pulsatile GnRH if fertility is desired.

Prognosis and complications

Prognosis

- Replacement of sex steroids is main treatment but does not necessarily confer fertility or stimulate testicular growth in men.

Complications

- Osteoporosis
- Infertility without replacement hormones for those with hypothalamic or pituitary dysfunction.

POLYCYSTIC OVARY SYNDROME

Outline

- Multiple small cysts within the ovary from arrested follicular development
- Cysts cause excess androgen release from ovaries and adrenals
- Arrest of development due to ↓ secretion of LH.

Pathogenesis/aetiology

- Commonest cause of oligomenorrhoea and amenorrhea.

Who

- Common in females
- Starts shortly after menarche.

A typical patient

A 15-year-old girl goes to her GP as she has noticed hair growth under her chin. She also has irregular periods and a ↑ BMI.

Clinical features

Signs and symptoms

- Hirsutism (from ↑ androgen)
- Abnormal menstruation
- Infertility
- Insulin resistance: hypertension, hyperlipidaemia
- Acne
- Obesity.

Investigations

Hormone tests

- ↑ Testosterone
- LH ↑ /normal
- FSH normal
- ↑ LH:FSH.

Imaging

- Ovarian US: multiple cysts.

Treatment

- Symptomatic hair removal.

Medical

- Oral contraceptive pills (oestrogen with progesterone): control cycle and ↓ androgens
- Cyproterone acetate: anti-androgen, symptomatic relief
- Spironolactone: anti-androgen

- Clomifene: for fertility
- Metformin: biguanide (also used in diabetes), for fertility
- Finasteride: 5α-reductase inhibitor.

Prognosis and complications

Prognosis

- ↓ Fertility.

Complications

- ↑ Risk of endometrial cancer and type 2 diabetes.

OBESITY AND HYPERLIPIDAEMIAS

OBESITY

Outline

- Excess body fat with BMI >30 kg/m^2
  Metabolic syndrome:
- Obesity, BMI >30

And two of:
- ↑ Triglyceride: >1.7 mmol
- ↓ High density lipoprotein (HDL): <1.03
- ↑ BP: >130/85
- Fasting glucose: >5.6 mmol/L

Pathogenesis/aetiology

Causes

Endocrine causes:
- Cushing's
- Hypothyroidism
- Hypothalamic disease
- Hypogonadism

Others:
- ↑ Calorie intake
- ↓ Expenditure
- Genetics
- Psychological: appetite cueing, psychiatric disturbance.

Who

- Commoner in developed countries, becoming more common

- Metabolic syndrome associated with type 2 diabetes, polycystic ovaries, insulin resistance, cardiovascular disease.

Clinical features

Signs and symptoms

- ↑ Body weight, central fat distribution commoner in males
- Dyspnoea

- Lethargy
- Associated with depression.

Investigations

- Weight
- BMI

- Waist circumference.

Blood tests

- Lipids (hyperlipidaemia, see below)

- Fasting or random glucose or HbA1c.

Treatment

Conservative

- Weight reduction: reduce calories/increase exercise
- Group therapy.

Medical

- Orlistat: inhibits fat absorption
- sibutramine: promotes satiety sensation.

Surgical

If severe:
- Gastric banding or stapling
- Bypass surgery.

Prognosis and complications

Prognosis

- BMI > 40: ↓ life expectancy by 20 years in ♂, 5 years in ♀.

Complications

- Hypertension
- Heart disease
- Diabetes: type 2
- Obstructive sleep apnoea
- Gallstones
- Fatty liver
- Amenorrhoea
- Osteoarthritis of weight-bearing joints.

HYPERLIPIDAEMIA

Outline

- ↑ Lipid blood levels: cholesterol, triglycerides (TG) or lipoproteins
- A major risk factor for IHD
- Due to 1° familial hyperlipidaemias or a 2° cause
- Lipoproteins, composed of lipids, phospholipids, and apoproteins, transport lipid in the blood

Classification of lipoproteins:
- High density lipoprotein (HDL):
  - Transport cholesterol to the liver to be excreted
  - Protect against heart disease: ↓ cardiovascular (CV) risk
- Low density lipoprotein (LDL):
  - Transport cholesterol to the cells
  - Main contributor to atherosclerosis
  - Associated with CV risk
  - Synthesised from VLDL
- Intermediate density lipoprotein (IDL):
  - From peripheral breakdown of very low density lipoprotein (VLDL)
  - Return to liver to synthesise LDLs
- VLDL:
  - Transport triglycerides from the liver to the body for storage
- Chylomicrons:
  - Transport triglycerides from the gut to the body cells and the liver.

Pathogenesis/aetiology

Primary causes:
- Familial hyperlipideamias Fredrickson classification:
  - Type I: familial lipoprotein lipase deficiency: ↓ lipoprotein lipase causing ↑ chylomicrons (↑ TG)
  - Type IIa: familial hypercholesterolaemia: IDL receptor deficiency causing ↑ LDL (↑ cholesterol). Autosomal dominant
  - Type IIb: familial combined hyperlipidaemia: ↑ LDL and VLDL (↑ TG and ↑ cholesterol)
  - Type III: familial hyperlipoproteinaemia): ↑ IDL
  - Types IV and V: familial hypertriglyceridaemia: autosomal inheritance with ↑ VLDL or ↑ VLDL and chylomicrons. (↑ TG) increased risk of pancreatitis

Secondary causes:
- Alcohol: ↑ TG
- Diabetes
- Hypothyroidism
- Nephrotic syndrome
- Renal failure
- Hepatic dysfunction
- Drugs: oral contraceptives, beta-blockers, thiazides
- Diet and obesity
- Smoking: ↓ HDL, ↑ cholesterol.

Who

- Hypercholesterolaemia in >45% in the UK
- Familial hypercholesterolaemia: prevalence 1/500.

Clinical features

Signs and symptoms

- Mostly asymptomatic
- Obesity
- Corneal arcus: white opaque ring around the eye

- Xanthelasmata: yellow deposits around the eyelids
- Tendon xanthomata
- Pancreatitis (raised TG).

Investigations

Blood tests

- Fasting sample for total plasma cholesterol, triclyceride, HDL cholesterol

- Other tests to identify 2° causes: U&Es, LFTs, blood glucose

Other tests

- Electrophoresis of lipoproteins:
  - If specific 1° hyperlipidaemia suspected

- Genetic testing if family history of hyperlipidaemia.

Treatment

Lifestyle:
- Dietary therapy: fibre, fresh fruit and vegetables
- Exercise and weight loss

- Management of other CV risk factors: BP, smoking, alcohol.

Medical

NICE criteria for lipid modification:
- 2° prevention (patients with existing CV disease) – aim for:
  - Total cholesterol <4 mmol/L
  - LDL cholesterol <2 mmol/L
- 1° prevention (no vascular disease): treat if high risk (10 year risk of CV is >20%)
Statins (first-line therapy):
- Simvastatin, pravastatin
- Inhibitors of hydroxymethylglutaryl (HMG)-CoA reductase (role in cholesterol synthesis)

- Side effects: deranged liver function, muscle cramps, rhabdomyolysis, myositis, nausea and vomiting
Fibrates (second-line therapy):
- Nezafibrate
- ↓ triglycerides, ↓ LDL, ↑ HDL
- Side effect: myositis
Bile acid-binding resins:
- E.g. colestyramine and colestipol. Bind bile acids in the intestine to prevent their absorption

Screening

- Screen family members for familial hyperlipidaemias.

Prognosis and complications

Prognosis

- High levels of lipoprotein a predict an increase risk of vascular events
- In familial hyperlipidaemias children as young as 2 years old are at risk of early cardiac events

- Risk of IHD is higher if there are other risk factors for IHD including smoking and ↑ BP.

Complications

- Atherosclerosis
- IHD

- Early cardiac death if untreated.

CALCIUM DISORDERS

HYPERCALCAEMIA

Outline

- ↑ Calcium in the body: >2.65 mmol/L
- Causes salt and water loss leading to hypotension and renal failure

- 1° hyperparathyroidism and malignancy account for 80–90% of cases.
- A medical emergency if levels are >3.5 mmol/L

Pathogenesis/aetiology

Causes

- ↑ PTH: usually due to 1° hyperparathyroidism (see below)
- Malignancy: direct invasion of bone to release calcium and secretion of PTH-like peptide by the cancer
- ↑ calcium or vitamin D intake
- Specific disease: sarcoidosis, renal failure
- Drugs: lithium, thiazide diuretics, calcium and vitamin D supplements, theophyllines, retinoids

- Endocrine causes: **PATH**
  - **P**: phaeochromocytoma
  - **A**: Addison's
  - **T**: thyrotoxicosis
  - **H**: hyper-PTH
- Familial: familial benign hypocalciuric hypercalcaemia (rare defect in calcium sensing receptor).

Who

- Depends on cause.

Clinical features

Signs and symptoms

- Bones, stones, abdominal groans and psychic moans

Bones:
- Bone pain

Stones:
- Renal stones
- Renal failure
- Polyuria
- Polydipsia

Abdominal groans:
- Abdominal pain
- Vomiting
- Constipation
- Weight loss
- Peptic ulceration

Psychic moans:
- Depression
- Anorexia
- Weight loss
- Tiredness
- Weakness
- Confusion
- Mental changes

Also:
- Possible hypertension
- Arrhythmias/cardiac arrest.

Investigations

Blood tests

- FBC
- U&E: calcium, magnesium, albumin, creatinine, phosphate, ALP (phosphate and ALP may be high with low or normal albumin if malignancy is the cause)
- TSH: for thyroid cause

- Synacthen: for Addison's
- Level of PTH:
  - Hypercalcaemia and suppressed PTH: non-PTH cause
  - Hypercalcaemia and raised PTH: PTH cause.

ECG

- QT interval decrease.

Imaging

- If malignancy is suspected: bone scan and CXR

- If haematological malignancy suspected: blood film ± bone marrow aspirate.

Treatment

- IV fluids
- Bisphosphonates IV: pamidronate
- Diuretics: furosemide once rehydrated to induce calciuresis
- Monitor electrolytes

Treat underlying cause:
- Steroids if sarcoidosis or myeloma are the cause
- Surgery for 1° hyperparathyroidism or malignancy as indicated.

Prognosis and complications

Prognosis

- Depends on cause.

Complications

- Renal calculi (stones)
- Renal failure

- At levels >3.8 mmol/L: confusion, dehydration, clouding of consciousness, cardiac arrest.

HYPOCALCAEMIA

Outline

- Low calcium levels: <2.15 mmol/L.

Pathogenesis/aetiology

Causes

Decreased intake or transport:
- Low calcium diet and low vitamin D
- Malabsorption: coeliac disease
- Hypoalbuminaemia: chronic liver disease, malnutrition

Increased loss:
- CRF: commonest cause
- Phosphate therapy
- Blood transfusion

Hypoparathyroidism:
- Parathyroid gland removal
- Resistance to PTH: pseudohypo-PTH
- Congenital deficiency DiGeorge syndrome

Vitamin D deficiency:
- Osteomalacia, rickets

Drugs:
- Calcitonin, bisphosphonates

Others:
- Alkalosis, haemosiderosis, pancreatitis.

Who

- Rare, dependent upon cause.

A typical patient

A woman who has recently had her parathyroid glands removed presents with bone pain and numbness in her fingers.

Clinical features

Signs and symptoms

Neuropathy:
- Paraesthesia/numbness
- Tetany
- Papilloedema: swelling of optic disc
- Convulsion

Musculoskeletal:
- Muscle cramps
- Myopathy/bone pain

Psychiatric:
- Depression
- Behaviour disturbances

Others:
- Cataracts
- Laryngeal stridor

Chvostek's sign:
- Gentle tapping over facial nerve causes twitching of ipsilateral facial muscles from neuromuscular excitability

Trousseau's sign:
- Inflation of BP cuff above systolic pressure for 3 min induces spasm of fingers and wrist: carpopedal spasm.

Investigations

Blood tests

- U&Es: calcium, magnesium, ALP, vitamin D
- Serum and urine creatinine for renal disease

- PTH levels:
  - Hypocalcaemia and low PTH: hypoparathyroidism is the cause
  - Hypocalcaemia and raised PTH: non-PTH cause (except pseudohypoparathyroidism).

ECG

- ↑ QT interval, prolonged ST.

Imaging

- X-rays of metacarpals – short 4th metacarpals in pseudo-PTH.

Treatment

Mild:
- Oral calcium
- Monitor

Severe:
- Calcium gluconate IV
- Maintenance with alfacalcidol

For both:
- Treat cause
- Dietary supplementation.

Prognosis and complications

Prognosis

- Dependent upon underlying cause and duration of hypocalcaemia.

Complications

- Osteomalacia

- Rickets.

HYPERPARATHYROIDISM

Outline

- ↑ Levels of parathyroid hormone (PTH)
- Classified into primary, secondary and tertiary hyperparathyroidism depending on the cause

Effects of PTH:
- Overall effect:↑ calcium and ↓ phosphate in the plasma by:
  - ↑ Calcium absorption from the gut
  - ↑ Calcium and ↓ phosphate resorption in the kidney

- ↑ Osteoclast activity which are involved in bone resorption (break down) releasing Ca
- ↑ 1,25 dihydroxy vitamin D3 (calcitriol) production in the kidney which increases bone resorption, to ↑ calcium
- A medical emergency if calcium levels are >3.5 mmol/L

Pseudohyperparathyroidism:
- PTH-related protein is produced by some carcinomas from the kidney or lung.

Pathogenesis/aetiology

Causes

Primary:
- Levels of PTH ↑ due to hypersecretion
- From parathyroid adenoma, hyperplasia or carcinoma
- Associated with MEN syndromes

Secondary:
- PTH high in response to low calcium levels
- Calcium can be low/normal
- Due to chronic renal disease or vitamin D deficiency

Tertiary:
- Continued hyperparathyroidism after long-standing secondary PTH
- Often in renal disease (renal transplant)
- Plasma calcium and PTH are both high.

- Typical age of diagnosis: 50–55 years
- 3♀:1♂
- 21 cases per 100 000 person-years.

Clinical features

Signs and symptoms

- Mostly symptoms of hypercalcaemia (as above).

Investigations

Blood tests

- U&Es: calcium, phosphate, ALP (as a measure of osteoclast activity), PTH

Urine

- Calcium.

Imaging

- Radiographic evidence of bone resorption
- CXR, AXR, pelvic X-ray
- Isotope bone scan
- CT/MRI
- Parathyroid subtraction scans specifically investigating parathyroid pathology.

Treatment

- Treat cause
- Selective oestrogen receptor modulators (side effect RMs), e.g. raloxifene
- Bisphosphonates for those who are unsuitable for surgery

Primary hyperparathyroidism:
- Remove adenomas, remove PTH glands in hyperplasia

Secondary hyperparathyroidism:
- Restore calcium levels with vitamin D supplements, phosphate restriction

Tertiary hyperparathyroidism:
- Parathyroidectomy
- Monitor long term.

Prognosis and complications

Prognosis

- Good with treatment.

Complications

- 2–10% risk of recurrent or persistent disease.

HYPOPARATHYROIDISM

Outline

- ↓ Quantities of PTH

Pseudohypoparathyroidism:
- Condition where there is a failure of target cells to respond to PTH. May have characteristic facies.

Pathogenesis/aetiology

Causes

- Surgical removal during thyroidectomy: commonest cause
- Primary idiopathic hypoparathyroidism: autoimmune disorder associated with other autoimmune diseases
- Congenital: DiGeorge syndrome: parathyroid agenesis
- Severe hypermagnesaemia (magnesium inhibits PTH)
- Infiltration: infection, inflammation, malignancy
- Metal overdose: haemochromatosis, Wilson's disease, aluminium deposition in dialysis.

Who

- Uncommon: apart from transient surgical effects.

Signs and symptoms

- Mostly secondary to hypocalcaemia (as above).

Investigations

Blood tests

- Ca↓
- Phosphate↑

- Magnesium
- PTH low.

ECG

- Prolonged QT interval.

Treatment

- Restore calcium and vitamin D
- If tetany or severe presentation: IV calcium gluconate

- IV magnesium chloride if there is also low magnesium
- Long-term treatment: alfacalcidol or calcitriol.

Prognosis and complications

Prognosis

- Depends on cause.

POLYENDOCRINE DISORDERS

AUTOIMMUNE POLYENDOCRINE SYNDROMES

Outline

Autoimmune disease affecting more than one endocrine organ, although it can also affect other organs:
Type 1:
- Chronic mucocutaneous candidiasis (T-cell immune disorder leading to chronic infections of the mucosal surfaces). Usually first presentation
- Hypoparathyroidism
- Hypoadrenalism. Usually presents last
- May get other features including diabetes mellitus and hypogonadism

Type 2 (Schmidt syndrome):
- Autoimmune Addison's disease
- Autoimmune thyroid disease
- Diabetes mellitus type 1
- May get other features including hypogonadism.

Pathogenesis/aetiology

Type 1:
- Autosomal recessive
- Mutations in AIRE-1 (autoimmune regulator) on chromosome 21, a gene encoding a regulator of transcription

Type 2:
- Autosomal dominant with incomplete penetrance.

Who

- Rare
- Type 2 more common than type 1

Associations:
- Type 1 associated with HLA-A28
- Type 2 associated with HLA-A1, HLA-B8, HLA-DR3, HLA-DR4

Clinical features

Signs and symptoms

- Features of the specific endocrine abnormality
- All three manifestations do not need to be present to make a diagnosis

- May be associated with other autoimmune diseases: type 1 diabetes, hypogonadism, malabsorption, vitiligo, alopecia and pernicious anaemia.

- Investigation is guided by the identified endocrine abnormalities
- Serum endocrine autoantibody screen
- Individual hormone investigation.

- Treat each separate disease
- Monitor for possible new disease in a different gland.

- Based upon individual components of the syndrome.

MULTIPLE ENDOCRINE NEOPLASIA (MEN)

Tumours occur in several endocrine glands, at the same or different times:

- MEN1:
  - Benign adenomas of:
    - **PPPAT:**
      - **P**arathyroid: adenoma or hyperplasia
      - **P**ituitary (commonly prolactinoma, also GH secretion)
      - **P**ancreatic secreting tumours: usually gastrinomas or insulinomas
      - **A**drenal adenoma
      - **T**hyroid adenoma (follicular)
- MEN2:
  - 2A: **PAT:**
    - **P**arathyroid adenoma or hyperplasia
    - **A**drenal: phaeochromocytoma
    - **T**hyroid medullary carcinoma
  - 2B:
    - Like 2A but with intestinal and visceral ganglioneuromas and marfanoid appearance
    - No hyperparathyroidism.

- Autosomal dominant.

- MEN1: mutation in the tumour suppressor gene, menin on chromosome 11
- MEN2: mutation in Ret proto-oncogene on chromosome 10. Ret is a receptor tyrosine kinase important for nerves.

- Rare
- 0.02 cases per 1000.

Depends on tumour:

- MEN1:
  - Parathyroid adenoma: hypercalcaemia
  - Pituitary: prolactinoma, Cushing's disease, acromegaly (see above)
  - Pancreas: insulinoma, gastrinoma (see surgery chapter)
- MEN2:
  - Adrenal: phaeochromocytoma (see above)
  - Thyroid medullary carcinoma: diarrhoea, raised calcitonin, thyroid lump
  - Parathyroid: hypercalcaemia
- MEN2B:
  - Marfanoid appearance: tall, long limbs, arachnodactyly: long slender fingers and toes
  - Neuromas around the lips and the tongue.

Investigations

Urine and blood tests

- Type I: measure serum calcium
- Type II: pentagastrin-stimulated calcitonin test (diagnostic of thyroid medullary carcinoma), calcium infusion tests and serum calcitonin

- Urinary metanephrine (metabolite of adrenaline) measured for phaeochromocytoma.

Imaging

- For specific tumours.

Genetic testing

- Screen family members.

Treatment

- Excise tumours: hormone replacement as necessary
- Monitor

- Screen other family members.

Prognosis and complications

Prognosis

- Depends on tumour and tumour stage

- Gastrinomas (in type I) associated with a poor outlook.

Complications

- Tumour complications.

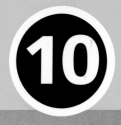
Useful bone terminology (Fig. 10.1)

Epiphysis: rounded end of long bone
Metaphysis: growing part of long bone between the diaphysis and epiphysis
Diaphysis: main/mid-section of shaft
Osteoclasts: involved in bone remodelling, resorbing bone
Osteoblasts: involved in bone remodelling, secreting extracellular matrix proteins and regulators responsible for bone formation
Cortical bone: dense compact outer layer of bone
Cancellous or tubular bone: spongy interior of bone responsible for its strength.

Seronegative vs. rheumatoid arthropathy

Seronegative arthopathies are a family of disorders, including **p**soriatic arthritis, **e**nteropathic arthritis, **a**nkylosing spondylitis and **r**eactive arthritis (remember by PEAR).
They are distinguished from rheumatoid arthritis by:

- lack of rheumatoid factor
- asymmetrical arthropathy
- association with HLA-B27
- clustering in families
- inflammation of enthesis (insertion of tendons/ligaments into bones) and joint ankylosis (stiffness)
- more limited joint involvement
- association with nail changes
- tending to involve major histocompatibility complex (MHC) class I.

Affected joints in rheumatological disease

The joint distribution affected in rheumatological disease can be useful for diagnosis (Fig. 10.2).

Antibodies in rheumatological disease

Many rheumatological diseases have associated antibodies (Table 10.1). In some cases, titre correlates with disease activity.

Investigations

Blood tests

- *FBC*: for anaemia caused by:
  - chronic rheumatological disease
  - side effects of rheumatological drugs (e.g. methotrexate/NSAIDs)
  - chronic bleeding
- *CRP and ESR*: ↑ in active inflammation
- *Serum uric acid*: ↑ in gout (not acute attacks)
- *Antistreptolysin O titre*: ↑ in rheumatic fever
- *Bone profile*: calcium, phosphate, ALP vary according to disease (Table 10.2).

Synovial aspirate

Aspirated from an inflamed joint. Can aid diagnosis:

- Clear, colourless: normal
- Turbid, yellow: septic and inflammation
- Clear, straw coloured: osteoarthritis
- Bloody: joint haemorrhage
- Send for microscopy for cell count, gram stain and polarised light microscopy for crystals.

Imaging

- Radiography useful for fractures, initial test for bone malignancies
- MRI is good for septic arthritis
- Isotope bone scan uses a tracer such as technetium injected into the bone, which localises to areas of high turnover due to inflammation or infection (Fig. 10.3). Examples of hot spots include:
  - bone metastases
  - fractures

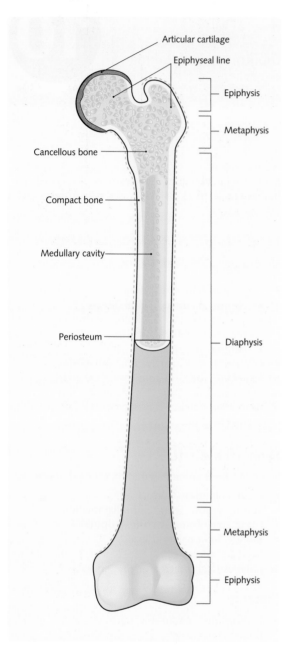

Fig. 10.1 The structure of long bones.

- osteomyelitis
- Paget's disease

NB: the bladder and kidneys often shows up as a hot spot as the tracer is excreted via the kidneys.

Dual energy X-ray absorptiometry (DEXA)

Low-dose X-ray radiation is used to measure bone mineral density, which is useful for assessing osteoporosis. The T scores compare the patient's bone mineral density values with those of young normal patient and the Z scores with an age-matched normal patient. The scores are calculated as the number of standard deviations below the normal peak values:

- normal bone: greater than -1
- osteopenia (mild): score between -1 and -2.5
- osteoporosis: less than -2.5.

Arthroscopy

Direct visualisation of a joint using an arthroscope or camera inserted into the joint. This approach may also be used therapeutically, e.g. to repair torn ligaments.

See also

- Common presenting complaints (Ch. 14): back pain.

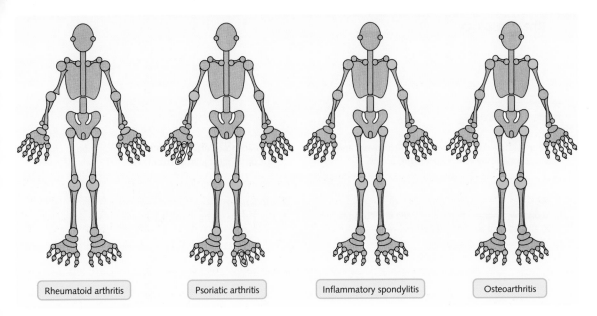

| Rheumatoid arthritis | Psoriatic arthritis | Inflammatory spondylitis | Osteoarthritis |

Fig. 10.2 Joints affected in different rheumatological diseases.

Table 10.1 Antibodies associated with rheumatological diseases

Disease	Autoantibody
Rheumatoid disease	Rheumatoid factor Anti–citrullinated peptide antibodies (anti-CCP)
SLE	Anti-dsDNA Antinuclear antibodies (ANA) Anti-ribonucleoprotein (RNP) such as anti-Ro (anti-SSA), anti-Sm (anti-SSB), anti-La Anti-cardiolipin
Sjögren's syndrome	Anti-Ro Anti-La ANA Rheumatoid factor
Anti-phospholipid syndrome	Anticardiolipin lupus anticoagulant antibodies Anti-beta-2-glycoprotein I
Polymyositis/ dermatomyositis	Anti-Jo1 ANA
Limited cutaneous scleroderma	Anti-centromere ANA
Diffuse cutaneous scleroderma	ANA Anti-Scl-70 Anti-RNA polymerase 1,2,3
Wegener's disease	(c-ANCA (proteinase 3))
Churg–Strauss	MPO-p-ANCA (myeloperoxidase)
Polyarteritis nodosa	p-ANCA (myeloperoxidase)
Mixed connective tissue disease	Anti-U1RNP

Table 10.2 Patterns of biochemical markers in bone disease

Bone disease	ALP	Calcium	Phosphate
Metastases	↑	↑ or −	↑ or −
Osteomalacia	↑	↓ or −	↓
Osteoporosis	−	−	−
Paget's disease	↑	−	−
1° hyperparathyroidism	↑	↑	↓
2° hyperparathyroidism	↑	−	↑
3° parathyroidism	↑	↑	↓

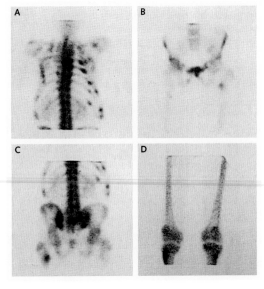

Fig. 10.3 Radioisotope bone scan showing multiple hot spots caused by small fractures in a vitamin D-deficient patient.

427

MECHANICAL DISORDERS

OSTEOARTHRITIS

Outline

- Degenerative disease of the joints, from wear and tear of articular cartilage which covers the bones
- Leads to cartilage loss and surrounding bone change
- Commonest joint problem.

Classification

1° (90%):
- Idiopathic: changes in prostaglandin and collagen III lead to altered load bearing properties
- No obvious predisposing cause
- Tends to occur in older people

2° (10%):
- Disease occurring in joints that are already damaged.

Pathogenesis/aetiology

Causes of 2° osteoarthritis:
- Previous rheumatoid/inflammatory arthritis
- Obesity
- Congenital deformity: developmental dysplasia of the hip and Perthes' disease
- Metabolic disorder

- Gout
- TB/septic arthritis
- Previously damaged joints through injury/trauma
- Certain occupations increase likelihood: pianist, typist, footballer, miners, removal men
- Sarcoid.

Pathogenesis

- The balance between cartilage synthesis and breakdown is disrupted from general wear, particularly in susceptible people
- Failure of the chondrocytes (cartilage cells that make and maintain the cartilage) to repair damaged cartilage
- Eburnation occurs: wearing of cartilage exposes bone. Leads to bone sclerosis (thickening and hardening) where bony surface becomes smooth, hard and white

- Underlying bone can remodel leading to formation of cysts
- Osteophytes form: bony projections at areas of cartilage destruction where new bone forms at the joint surface. Can catch nerves resulting in pain
- Overall results in cartilage fissures, disrupted collagen architecture, loss of prostaglandin.

Who

- Typical age: 50% of over 60s affected. More common in older people
- 3♀:1♂
- Less common in black Africans and Chinese
- Genetic factors may be important

Associations:
- Haemochromatosis
- Ochronosis (brown/black pigment in skin/cartilage)
- Family history: in certain types.

A typical patient

A 70-year-old retired builder with pain in the right knee. The pain is worse on walking, occurs every day and keeps him awake at night. He has varus deformity and fixed flexion in the right knee.

Clinical features

Pain:
- Stiffness
- Restricted range of movement
- Deformity
- Disability
- Tenderness

Timing of pain:
- Night-time pain suggests more severe osteoarthritis
- Hip and knee osteoarthritis give pain on weight bearing
- Relieved at rest, worse on movement
- Degenerative pain often gets worse during the day

Location:
- Non-symmetrical
- Joint instability

Common joints affected
Weight bearing:
- 1st carpometacarpal joint
- Cervical and lumbar spine
- Hip
- Knee (often varus deformity)
- Big toe metatarsophalangeal (MTP) joint

Non weight bearing:
- Distal and proximal interphalangeal joints (DIP and PIP)
- Heberden's nodes: bony swellings at DIP
- Bouchard's nodes: bony swellings at PIP, less common then Heberden's
- Thumb base

Investigations

Imaging

X-ray:
- Four features found on X-ray (Fig. 10.4). Remember by **O**steoarthritis **C**auses **N**arrow **S**paces
  - **O**steophytes
  - **C**ysts: dark shadowing on X-rays
  - **N**arrowing of joint space
  - **S**clerosis: white area just below the joint surface

MRI:
- If neurological sequelae, e.g. nerve root compression from spinal osteoarthritis

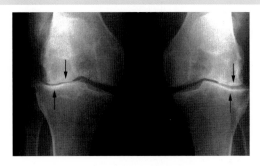

Fig. 10.4 Radiography of osteoarthritic knees showing features of osteoarthritis including loss of joint space (arrowed).

Other tests

Arthroscopy:
- Visualises early surface erosion of cartilage, sclerosis and eburnation

Treatment

Conservative

- Physiotherapy
- Weight reduction

- Walking aids (e.g. walking stick):
  - Hip: use on contralateral side
  - Knee: use on ipsilateral side
- Exercises.

Medical

- Analgesic ladder:
  - Paracetamol
  - NSAIDs
  - Weak opioids: codeine, tramadol (side effects – nausea, fatigue)

- Glucosamine and chondroitin to protect cartilage and slow progression but evidence of benefit is weak.

Surgical

- Often when pain is unbearable or with night pain:
  - Realignment osteotomy

- Arthoplasty: joint replacement.

Prognosis and complications

Prognosis

- Mild osteoarthritis: can be stable for years without getting worse

- Severe osteoarthritis: characterised by deformity in knees/hips, night pain. Needs surgical referral

Complications

- Remember by SAD:
  - Subluxation (partial dislocation)

- Ankylosis (joint stiffness)
- Deformities.

INFLAMMATORY CAUSES

RHEUMATOID ARTHRITIS

Outline

- Autoimmune, systemic, inflammatory disease affecting many tissues and organs but primarily affects the synovial lining of the joints leading to peripheral symmetrical inflammatory polyarthritis
- Summary – **SPIN PRAM**:
  - **S**ymmetrical
  - **P**eripheral
- **I**nflammatory
- **N**odules
- **P**annus
- **R**heumatoid factor
- **A**utoimmune
- **M**orning stiffness

Antibodies involved

1. Rheumatoid factor: an autoantibody (usually IgM) against the Fc portion of IgG. Note: 20% of patients are $-$ve and some healthy people are $+$ve
2. Anti-citrullinated protein antibody (ACPA): more specific for rheumatoid arthritis. Rarely $+$ve in those without the disease

- Positive results for rheumatoid factor and ACPA makes rheumatoid arthritis extremely likely
- Associated with many other antibodies, e.g. ANAs $<40\%$

Relevant syndromes

Felty syndrome:
- Triad of: rheumatoid arthritis, splenomegaly and neutropenia (look out for this in clinical examinations)
- 1% of patients with rheumatoid arthritis
- Destructive arthritis

- Vasculitis
- Associated with HLA-DR4

Caplan syndrome:
- Rheumatoid nodules and pulmonary fibrosis in patients with coal exposure, e.g. coal miners.

Pathogenesis/aetiology

Cause

- Exact cause unknown

- Autoimmune: T-cells, B-cells and cytokines are all involved and understanding this has led to development of new treatments.

Pathogenesis

- Synovium is permeated by inflammatory cells
- Inflammation thought to be caused by T-cell activation with pathogenesis mediated primarily by the cytokines TNF, IL-6, IL-1, IL-17. B-cells also involved. They produce rheumatoid factor and are involved in antigen-presentation
- Inflamed synovium proliferates, thickens and spreads from the joint lining to cover the cartilage surface and forms a 'pannus'
- Pannus: granulation tissue in the inflamed joint (contains T-cells and polymorphs)
- The thickened synovium causes cartilage, bone and tendon erosion by blocking blood supply to these areas and increased cytokinie production

- The underlying cartilage is eroded and the bone exposed

Other organs:
- Also affected. In severe form, there can be multi-organ dysfunction

Nodules:
- Form in 20% of patients: subcutaneous inflammatory granulomatous lesions that feel rubbery on touch. They form at pressure sites such as elbows and in extra-articular locations such as the pleura or pericardium
- Only occur in rheumatoid factor $+$ve patients.

Who

- Typical age: 30–40 years
- 3♀:1♂
- 2–3% of population

Associations:
- Smoking worsens symptoms
- Family history
- Genetics: associated with HLA-DR1 and HLA-DR4

A typical patient

A 32-year-old lady with swollen painful fingers and toes. She feels stiff in the mornings and has developed nodules over both elbows over the last three months.

Clinical features

American College of Rheumatology 2010 diagnostic criteria (>6/10 means a diagnosis of rheumatoid arthritis):

- A. Joint involvement:
  - 1 large joint: 0
  - 2–10 large joints: 1
  - 1–3 small joints: 2
  - 4–10 small joints: 3
  - >10 joints (at least 1 small joint): 5
- B. Serology:
  - −ve RF and −ve ACPA: 0
  - Low +ve rheumatoid factor or low +ve ACPA: 2
  - High +ve rheumatoid factor or high +ve ACPA: 3
- C. Acute-phase reactants:
  - Normal CRP and normal ESR 0
  - Abnormal CRP or abnormal ESR 1
- D. Duration of symptoms:
  - <6 weeks 0
  - >6 weeks 1

Common distribution of affected joints:

- Hands and feet most commonly affected (Fig. 10.5): important to ask about and examine function of hands
- Includes finger deformaties (Boutonnière, swan neck), muscle wasting (guttering) and ulnar deviation of fingers (Fig. 10.5A)
- Often symmetrical polyarthropathy:
  - Cervical spine: not common but dangerous; potential atlantoaxial subluxation resulting in spinal cord injury (a consideration with anaesthetists before extending the neck for intubation)
  - Large synovial cysts, e.g. Baker's cyst (benign swelling of bursa at the back of the knee, also called popliteal cyst)
  - Valgus (knocked knees)
  - Feet: hallux valgus/bunion (deformity of the joint at the base of the big toe), clawing of the toes and plantar callosities

Extra-articular symptoms:

- General:
  - Malaise and fatigue
- Nervous system:
  - Carpal tunnel syndrome
  - Peripheral neuropathies
  - Mononeuritis multiplex
  - Atlantoaxial subluxation: spinal cord compression
- Respiratory system:
  - Pleural effusions
  - Pulmonary fibrosis
  - Lung nodules
  - Alveolitis
- Cardiovascular system:
  - Pericarditis/serositis
  - Vasculitic rash
- Lymphoreticular system:
  - Splenomegaly
- Blood:
  - Neutropenia (Felty's)
  - Normocytic anaemia
- Eyes:
  - Sjögren syndrome (in 15%) see below.

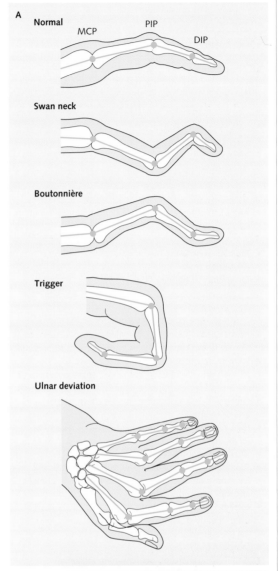

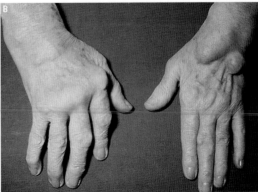

Fig. 10.5 Rheumatoid arthritis: (A) finger and hand abnormalities; (B) rheumatoid hands.

Investigations

Blood tests

- FBC: ↓ Hb, ↓ WBC, ↑ platelets
- ↑ ESR
- ↑ CRP

Antibodies:
- Rheumatoid factor (latex agglutination test)
- Anti–citrullinated peptide antibodies (anti-CCP)

Imaging

X-rays:
- Soft tissues swelling
- ↓ joint space
- Bony erosion
- Subluxation

Other imaging:
- MRI and US: show erosions earlier than plain films

Treatment

- Aim of treatment: pain control and maintain function

Conservative

- Regular exercise
- Physiotherapy
- Occupational therapy: aids.

Medical

- NSAIDs (non-steroidal anti-inflammatory drugs): treat the acute symptoms of pain, swelling and stiffness
- Intra-muscular or intra-articular steroids
- NSAIDs and steroids do not alter disease progression

Disease-modifying anti-rheumatic drugs (DMARDs):
- Given within 3–6 months: improve symptoms and outcome
- Reduce inflammation and joint erosions mostly by inhibiting inflammatory cytokines
- May take months for noticeable effect
- Require regular monitoring with blood tests
- Methotrexate and sulfasalazine are first-line choices and can be used together
- Increasingly, combinations of two DMARDs are used in early disease

Biological agents:
- Effective but expensive
- Anti-TNF: etanercept, adalimumab, infliximab
- Monoclonal antibodies, e.g. rituximab: depletes CD20+ve B-cells
- IL-1 antagonist: anakinra
- Anti-IL-6 receptor: tocilizumab
- NICE guidelines: anti-TNF only to be used after failure of two DMARDs (including methotrexate).

See table 10.3 for a summary of medications and their side effects

Table 10.3 Medications used for rheumatoid arthritis

Medication and benefits	Side effect (common but mild)	Side effect (uncommon but serious)
Methotrexate: Oral or SC Weekly Competitive dihydrofolate reductase inhibitor Given with folate	Nausea, Diarrhoea Mouth ulcers Macrocytosis with folate deficiency	Liver and lung fibrosis Myelosuppres -sion Interstitial pneumonitis Teratogenic
Sulfasalazine: Oral	Nausea Headache Rash	Liver disease Myelosuppres -sion; Oligospermia
Gold: IM injection Weekly slowly reducing to monthly injection	Mouth ulcers Rash	Proteinuria Glomerulone -phritis Widespread rash Myelosuppres -sion
Leflunomide: Oral Daily When above DMARDS have failed	Rash Oral ulcers Hypertension Teratogenic	Myelosuppres -sion Hepatoxicity
Azathioprine: Oral Often used with other DMARDs	Nausea Vomiting	Myelosuppres -sion
Hydroxychloroquine: inhibit phagocytic function No blood tests required for monitoring – useful for needle phobics	Rash	Retinopathy

Prognosis and complications

Prognosis

- 25%: long-term remission
- 50%: long-term problems
- 25%: progressive disease with severe disability and shortened life (15 years)
- 40%: stop working within 5 years of diagnosis

Poor prognostic factors:
- Female
- Joint erosions
- Nodules
- Rheumatoid factor + ve
- Increasing age
- Symmetrical pattern of arthritis
- Persistence of disease activity in first year
- Gradual onset

Complications

- Septic arthritis
- Amyloidosis

- Spinal cord compression
- Side effect of medication.

INFLAMMATORY CAUSES: SERONEGATIVE ARTHROPATHIES

PSORIATIC ARTHRITIS

Outline

- Seronegative arthritis associated with psoriasis

- Psoriasis chronic inflammatory skin condition.

Pathogenesis/aetiology

Pathology

- Synovitis and enthesitis
- Erosions start at ligament insertions

- Relates to altered inflammatory cell activation thresholds.

Who

- 10% of psoriatics

Associations:
- HLA-B27

- HLA-Cw6
- Ankylosing spondylosis more common in these patients.

A typical patient

A 30-year-old man with scaly patches over the arms, morning joint stiffness and swelling in the fingers and toes.

Clinical features

Arthritis:
- Affects small joints particularly of the hands, e.g. distal interphalangeal joints
- Also knee and wrist
- Normally asymmetrical arthritis but can be a symmetrical form that presents like rheumatoid arthritis

Skin disease:
- Symmetrical well defined red plaques with silvery scale

Nails (in 80%):
- Nail pitting
- Onycholysis: nail separation from the nail bed.

Investigations

Blood tests

- ↑ ESR and CRP

Joint aspiration

Synovial fluid:
- Inflammatory with predominantly T-cells.

Imaging

- X-rays: erosions.

Treatment

Medical

- NSAIDs/analgesics
Immunosuppressants:
- In more severe cases
- Steroid injections (IM for systemic relief or intra-articular for individual joints)

- Methotrexate
- Sulfasalazine for large joint type
- Ciclosporin
- Anti-TNF: etanercept, infliximab, adalimumab.

Prognosis and complications

Prognosis

- Better than rheumatoid arthritis.

Complications

- Arthritis mutilans (severe, rapidly erosive, deforming arthritis) in 5–15%.

ENTEROPATHIC ARTHRITIS

Outline

- Seronegative arthritis associated with inflammatory bowel disease (IBD).

Pathogenesis/aetiology

Causes

- Aetiology unknown

- Immune complexes may be relevant.

Who

- 20% of IBD patients

Associations:
- HLA-B27: 5%.

Clinical features

- Single/multiple joints (asymmetrical)
- Mostly affects knees, ankles

- Symptoms and signs of IBD.

Investigations

- Investigate as per IBD and to exclude other causes of arthritis.

Treatment

- Treat bowel disease
- NSAIDs
- Monoarthritis: steroid injections to joint

- Sulfasalazine helps both arthritis and bowel disease
- Anti-TNFα: for Crohn's.

Prognosis and complications

Prognosis

- Normally clears as IBD clears but arthritis can persist.

ANKYLOSING SPONDYLITIS

Outline

- Seronegative inflammatory arthritis affecting the spine and the sacroiliac joints
- Can lead to total fusion of the spine (ankylosis means joint stiffness)
- Extra-articular symptoms may also be present.

Pathogenesis/aetiology

Causes

- Aetiology unknown
- Autoimmune.

Pathogenesis

- Inflammation starts at sites of ligament attachment to bone (enthesitis) in the lumbar spine and sacroiliac joints
- Inflammatory changes are followed by healing with reorganisation of tissue matrix and reactive new bone formation
- Can cause bony bridges called syndesmophytes in the spine
- Upper and lower syndesmophytes slowly join, fusing the spine so that it looks like bamboo stem on X-ray
- Back pain then often stops, but the fused spine is brittle and can fracture or lead to cord compression.

Who

- Typical age: onset aged 15–30 years
- 1♀:2♂
- Men present earlier then women
- Prevalence: 0.05%

Associations:
- Psoriasis
- IBD
- Family history of any seronegative arthritis 5%
- HLA-B27 (90%).

A typical patient

A 22-year-old man with low back and buttock pain. He is stiff for two hours in the morning and cannot bend over to touch his toes.

Clinical features

Arthritis:
- Insidious onset
- Morning joint stiffness
- Lower back pain
- Loss of lumbar lordosis
- ↑ Kyphosis (curvature of the spine)
- Limited lumbar spine flexibility
- Question mark posture at final phase: kyphosis, hyperextended neck, spinocranial ankylosis (Fig. 10.6)
- Sacroiliitis causing buttock pain radiating to back of legs
- Peripheral arthritis affected (20%)

Nail changes:
- Onychylosis: nail separation from nail bed

Extra-articular symptoms:
- Malaise plus the six As:
  - **A**pical lung fibrosis (rare)
  - **A**chilles tendonitis
  - **A**nterior uveitis (30%)
  - **A**ortic regurgitation (aortitis)
  - **A**naemia
  - **A**myloidosis

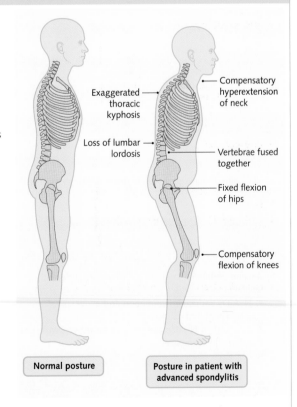

Exaggerated thoracic kyphosis

Loss of lumbar lordosis

Compensatory hyperextension of neck

Vertebrae fused together

Fixed flexion of hips

Compensatory flexion of knees

Normal posture

Posture in patient with advanced spondylitis

Fig. 10.6 Changes in posture in a patient with ankylosing spondylitis.

Investigations

- Clinical diagnosis, supported with radiology findings
- Clinical tests:
  1. Schober's test: measure of lumbar expansion. The patient touches their toes and the distance ↑ between the point 5 cm below L5 and 10 cm above L5 as they bend is measured. An increase of <5 cm suggests limited flexion
  2. Tragus to wall distance
  3. ↓ Lateral flexion: earliest loss of mobility

Blood tests

- ↑ ESR
- ↑ CRP
- HLA-B27 is very rarely used as it does not help management.

Imaging

X-ray:
- Irregular margins of sacroiliac joints
- Bone sclerosis
- 'Bamboo spine': squaring of the vertebrae and fusion (Fig. 10.7).

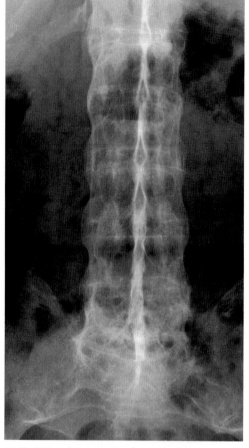

Fig. 10.7 X Ray demonstrating bamboo spine.

Treatment

The key aim of management is to maintain spinal flexibility:

Conservative

- Physiotherapy: exercise to prevent stiffening
- Sleeping with 1–2 pillows, encourage prone position (face down).

Medical

Spinal and peripheral joint disease managed differently:
- Spinal disease:
  - NSAIDs: reduce inflammation and allow spinal movement and exercise
  - Anti-TNF: if NSAIDs fail (no role for other DMARDs)
- Peripheral joint disease:
  - NSAIDs
- DMARDs: if peripheral joint disease is the dominant feature and not controlled by NSAIDs, e.g. sulfasalazine, methotrexate
- Anti-TNFα if DMARDs fail: etanercept, adalimumab, infliximab.

Surgical

- Spinal osteotomy, e.g. for kyphosis (rarely performed).

Prognosis and complications

Prognosis

- Can be progressive, remitting or recurrent
- Most lead normal lives.

Complications

- Respiratory complications due to immobility of spine and ribs
- Amyloidosis.

REACTIVE ARTHRITIS

Outline

- Arthritis triggered by reaction to:
  - GI infection
  - non-specific urethritis
- The term Reiter syndrome was formerly used to describe a type of reactive arthritis characterised by the triad of conjunctivitis, urethritis and arthritis: 'cannot see, cannot pee, cannot bend the knee'. This term has fallen from favour.

Pathogenesis/aetiology

Causes

- Often evidence of infection
- From GI cause:
  - *Salmonella*
  - *Shigella*
  - *Yersinia*
  - *Campylobacter*
- From sexually transmitted cause:
  - *Chlamydia*
  - *Ureaplasma*

Important to distinguish septic arthritis from reactive arthritis. In reactive arthritis:
1. There are no living bacteria in the joint culture
2. The joint swelling often comes after the symptoms of infection have passed.

Who

- 1♀:20♂

Associations:
- HLA-B27+ve (50%)
- Rheumatoid factor−ve.

Clinical features

Arthritis:
- Acute asymmetrical lower limb arthritis lasts days/weeks after infection
- Multiple or single joints
- Enthesitis: plantar fasciitis, Achilles tendonitis
- Knees, ankles, feet most commonly affected
- Relative sparing of wrists and hands, but get dactylitis (inflammation of the digits)
Conjunctivitis (30%):
- Iritis and anterior uveitis

Urethritis:
- Dysuria, frequency, ulceration
- Discharge
Nail changes:
- Onycholosis: nail separation from nail bed
Other symptoms:
- Hyperkeratotic skin lesions particularly on feet soles
- Mouth ulcers
- Malaise
- Fever.

Investigations

Blood tests

- ↑ ESR
- ↑ CRP

Culture and microscopy

- Joint aspirate: to exclude septic cause. Usually sterile.
- Urine
- Stool
- Throat swab
- Cervical or urethral swab.

Joint problems:
- NSAIDs
- Intra-articular steroids

Chronic disease:
- Sulfasalazine, methotrexate – both for relapsing cases
- Anti-TNFα: in severe disease

Associated disease:
- Investigate and treat any sexually treated coinfection
- Antibiotics are not effective in most cases of reactive arthritis but may help in some cases following *Chlamydia* infection

Prognosis and complications

Prognosis

- Severe symptoms can last weeks to months
- 70%: recover fully within 6 months

- 15–50%: recurrent arthritis
- 15–30%: chronic arthritis/sacroiliitis/spondylitis.

INFECTION

SEPTIC ARTHRITIS

Outline

- Joint infection
- Infection can be due to a direct injury, haematological spread or local spread from osteomyelitis

- **A medical emergency: joint can be destroyed rapidly and patient can become systemically septic.**

Pathogenesis/aetiology

Causes

Bacterial:
- *Staphylococcus aureus* (commonest cause)
- *Escherichia coli*, or Gram − ve organisms
- Gonococcus (in the sexually active, usually affects multiple joints)

- *Salmonella* (in sickle cell patients)
- TB, *Brucella* (affects the spine/sacroiliac joints).

Viral:
- EBV, HBV, mumps, varicella, coxsackie.

Pathology

- Infection leads to rapid loss of cartilage and bone and the destruction of the joint if untreated

- Granulocytes, lymphocytes and macrophages enter joint and cause inflammation with purulent exudates.

Who

Predisposing factors:
- Joint damage
- Pre-existing arthritis
- Immunosuppression
- Sickle cell

- Diabetes
- Orthopaedic procedures and prosthetic implants (need urgent removal)
- Penetrating trauma.

Clinical features

- Joint is hot, red, swollen, painful
- Loss of movement
- Sudden onset
- Systemically unwell: fever, tachycardia, hypotensive

- Usually monoarthritis, but polyarthritis in 20% (particularly in the immunosuppressed)
- Any joint can be affected: commonly hip in kids, knee in adults.

Investigations

Blood tests

- FBC: ↑ WBC
- ↑ ESR, ↑ CRP

- Culture

Aspirate joint

- Microscopy and culture with urgent Gram stain.

Imaging

- X-ray: unhelpful in the early stages, later shows bone destruction, loss of cartilage and soft tissue swelling

- US: show effusion and helps aspiration
- MRI: for deeper joints and suspected osteomyelitis

Treatment

Joint aspiration:
- Leaving pus inside a joint is harmful:
  - Remove debris
  - Pus cleared by washout
  - Open drainage or arthroscopy in severe or refractory cases only
  - Aspirate regularly

Antibiotics:
- IV antibiotics as soon as possible.
- IV flucloxallin and benzylpenicillin are a good first choice though some now advocate using a single agent
- Change regimen depending on organism seen and sensitivities
- Treatment duration: 2 weeks IV, then 4–6 weeks oral

Mobilisation:
- Avoid weight bearing initially
- Splints/plaster to protect joint and immobilise it in the acute stage
- Then early mobilisation and physiotherapy
- Analgesics.

Prognosis and complications

Prognosis

- Dependent on severity of tissue damage
- 10% mortality.

Complications

- 2° osteoarthritis
- Septicaemia
- Osteomyelitis.

OSTEOMYELITIS

Outline

- Infection of the bone
- Infection can be due to direct injury, haematological spread or local spread from septic arthritis
- Can result in ischaemic necrosis within 48 h

TB osteomyelitis:
- More destructive and resistant than other infective causes of osteomyelitis
- Haematological spread
- Often chronic, affecting only one bone (usually the long bones or spine)
- Pott's disease: TB of the spine. Collapse of vertebrae causes anterior spinal angulation.

Pathogenesis/aetiology

Causes

- *Staphylococcus aureus* (90%)
- Gram –ve bacilli and anaerobes: in diabetics
- *Salmonella*: in sickle cell patients
- *Escherichia coli, Pseudomonas, Klebsiella*: common in drug abusers.

Pathology

- Pus in the infected bone can compromise blood flow
- Reduced blood supply to the bone leads to necrosis and formation of sequestrum (dead bone)
- New bone, called involucrum forms around the necrotic area in chronic osteomyelitis.

Who

Risk factors:
- Diabetes
- Vascular insufficiency
- IVDU
- Immunosuppressed
- TB risk factors: TB osteomyelitis: in 2% of those with TB.

Clinical features

- Bone pain
- Tenderness
- Oedema
- Redness
- Warmth
- Fever, night sweats.

Investigations

Blood tests

- FBC: ↑ WBC (in 50%)
- ↑ ESR, ↑ CRP
- Cultures

Aspiration of pus and bone

- Sequestrum and involucrum seen microscopically
- TB Osteomyelitis: granulomatous inflammation with central caseous necrosis and Langhans giant cells.

Imaging

- X-rays: lytic focus surrounded by sclerotic bone
- CXR: for lung TB
- MRI: most sensitive imaging modality
- Radionuclide scanning: to highlight areas of inflammation.

Treatment

Surgical

- Surgical drainage for pressure release
- Surgical debridement
- Removal of sequestrum that can lead to further infection.

Medical

- Antibiotics with good bone penetration 2 weeks IV then 4 weeks orally: flucloxacillin and fusidic acid or clindamycin
- Analgesia for pain

TB osteomyelitis

- Quadruple antituberculous therapy
- See respiratory section
- Surgical debridement of bones and stabilisation if necessary.

Prognosis and complications

Prognosis

- 5–25%: develop chronic osteomyelitis due to delay in diagnosis, immunocompromised, extensive bone necrosis and inadequate treatment.

Complications

- Chronic osteomyelitis
- Growth retardation and deformity
- Pathological fractures
- Sepsis
- Endocarditis
- TB arthritis

AUTOIMMUNE RHEUMATIC DISEASES

SYSTEMIC LUPUS ERYTHEMATOSUS (SLE)

Outline

- Chronic, systemic, autoimmune, rheumatic disease which can affect any organ or system in the body

Discoid lupus:
- Milder variant of SLE
- Skin affected only
- Discoid erythematous plaques on the face that lead to scarring and pigmentation
- Rarely develops into SLE

Drug-induced lupus:
- Milder form of lupus often affecting skin and lungs
- Resolves with cessation of drugs:
  - Isoniazid, hydralazine, procainamide, phenytoin

Autoantibodies in SLE:
- ANA: In >95%, if −ve, SLE highly unlikely
- Anti-dsDNA and anti-ssDNA, 70–80%. Titres correlate with disease activity
- Extractable nuclear antigens:
  1. Anti-Ro: can cause neonatal heart block if present in mother
  2. Anti-La: skin disease
  3. Anti-Sm (Smith): only in lupus patients, in 15%
  4. anti-ribonucleoprotein
- Rheumatoid factor: 30%
- Anti-phospholipid antibodies
- Anti-histones: in drug-induced lupus.

Pathogenesis/aetiology

Pathogenesis

- Reduced ability to clear apoptotic cell debris from the circulation triggers stimulation and interaction of B and T cells in lymph nodes
- This results in autoantibody production which have a pathogenic effect on tissue and form immune complexes in the blood
- Complement is recruited to inflamed tissues by the immune complex deposition, resulting in depleted complement levels in the blood
- The complement deficiency leads to an immunosuppressed state

Associations, predisposing factors and triggers:
- Environmental:
  - Female hormones: pregnancy is associated with disease flare
  - UV light
  - Viral infection
- Genetics:
  - Strong family history
  - Associated with HLA-B8, HLA-DR2, HLA-DR3.

Who

- Typical age: peak age of onset 20–40 years
- 9♀:1♂

- Prevalence: 0.1%
- Commoner in Afro-Caribbeans, Asian.

A typical patient

A 26-year-old Afro-Caribbean lady with joint pain, tiredness and a rash over her cheeks has recently developed swelling of the ankles and face. She has proteinuria on dipstick testing.

Clinical features

Common but mild:
- Mild fever
- Malaise
- Fatigue
- Weight loss
- Arthralgia
- Facial malar rash: red rash over the cheeks and bridge of the nose (butterfly rash)
- Photosensitivity
- Mouth ulcers
- Raynaud's/vasculitis of fingers

Moderate severity:
- Pleurisy
- Pericarditis
- Arthritis: can lead to deformity e.g. Jaccoud's deformity (ulnar deviation of the 2nd–5th metatarsals with subluxation, not specific to SLE). Unlike in rheumatoid arthritis, arthritis is non-erosive

Severe: will need therapy with steroids and immunosuppressants:
- Renal disease:
  - Glomerulonephritis: up to 50%. Nephrotic syndrome (proteinuria, hypoalbuminaemia and oedema). If not treated successfully can lead to renal failure leading to dialysis/transplant
- Neurological disease:
  - CNS lupus (up to 60%): Anything from mild depression to psychosis and fits
- Haematological disease:
  - Anaemia
  - Thrombocytopenia
  - Neutropenia
  - Lymphopenia
- Chest/heart disease:
  - Endocarditis, myocarditis
  - Pulmonary fibrosis
  - Shrinking lung syndrome

NB: ACR criteria refers to clinical studies and is not for individual diagnosis and therefore has not been referred to here.

Investigations

Blood tests

- FBC: ↓ Hb, ↓ WBC, ↓ platelets
- U&E: monitor kidney function
- LFT: particularly albumin
- Urine protein/creatinine ratio (very important to look for nephrotic syndrome)
- Complement: ↓ C3 and C4

- ↑ ESR
- ↓/normal CRP (if ESR is raised, with a normal CRP it suggests SLE or multiple myeloma)
- Antibodies:
  - ANA and extractable nuclear antigens only at diagnosis
  - Anti-dsDNA for monitoring activity.

- CXR: for pleural effusion
- CT chest: for fibrosis
- Echo: for myocarditis, endocarditis
- Brain: MRI for cerebral lupus.

Histology:
- Skin biopsy: to diagnose lupus of skin
- Renal biopsy: classifying type of lupus nephritis (to guide treatment).

Discoid lupus:
- Topical steroids
- Monitor.

Mild cases:
- NSAIDs
- Sun block cream
- Antimalarials, e.g. hydroxychloroquine for rash, arthralgia, serositis, fatigue (side effect pigmented retinopathy and vision loss, but rare – 1 in 2000 cases)
- Flares of pain/rash: short course of oral steroids or intramuscular methylprednisolone

Severe cases:
- High-dose steroid plus immunosuppressant to induce remission then lower doses to maintain remission. Often long-term therapy required
- Immunosuppressants:
  - Methotrexate
  - Azathioprine
  - Cyclophosphamide
  - Mycophenolate
  - Rituximab
- Major side effects: immunosuppression, infertility (cyclophosphamide) bladder toxicity (cyclophosphamide) osteoporosis (steroids)

- Remitting–relapsing illness
- 90%: 10 year survival.

- Death due to infection, myocardial infarct or stroke
- Renal disease requiring dialysis and transplantation.

ANTI-PHOSPHOLIPID SYNDROME

- Persistently +ve anti-phospholipid antibodies (aPL) with either:
  - Thrombosis: arterial or venous
- Pregnancy loss: particularly second trimester
- Or both.

- Primary: patient has no other autoimmune disease
- Secondary: patient has another autoimmune rheumatic disease (usually SLE)
- Catastrophic: a rare severe form with high mortality where there are multiple infarcts in several main organs simultaneously

- aPL do not bind phospholipids directly. They bind a serum protein called beta-2-glycoprotein I, which then attaches to phospholipids on the cells membranes
- This then switches on receptors on the cell surface to alter behaviour of cells such as monocytes, endothelial cells, trophoblasts and platelets leading to clots and/or miscarriages.

- 2♀:1♂
- More common than previously thought: ~1% prevalence
- Causes up to 20% of DVTs
- Commonest cause of strokes in under 50s
- Commonest cause of recurrent miscarriage.

30-year-old lady with a history of three DVTs and two second trimester miscarriages presents to her doctor.

Clinical features

- May have no symptoms at all between events

In pregnant women:
- Miscarriage
- Pre-eclampsia
- Intra-uterine growth retardation

In the veins:
- DVT
- Livedo reticularis (net-like purplish rash on the shins from venous swelling)

In the arteries:
- Stroke
- MI
- Pulmonary embolism
- Arterial narrowing in legs
- Increasingly recognised that other symptoms occur, e.g.
  - Endocarditis
  - Migraine
  - Renal failure due to thrombosis in small renal vessels
  - Joint pain.

Investigations

- Can be measured by three tests:
  1. Anti-phospholipid/anti-cardiolipin: measures ability of antibodies in the blood to bind phospholipid. Best guide of risk of thrombosis
  2. Lupus anticoagulant: tests the ability of blood to clot in a test tube under different conditions. Clotting does not correct with the addition of normal serum. Better predictor of pregnancy problems
  3. Anti-beta-2-glycoprotein/ELISA.

Treatment

- Aim of treatment is to prevent thrombosis and pregnancy loss: so treatment continues for years in patients with thrombosis or throughout the pregnancy to avoid miscarriage
- General advice: avoid smoking, hormone replacement therapy, oral contraceptive
- aPL + ve patients with no history of DVT/pulmonary embolism:
  - No evidence to support warfarin, most are put on aspirin
- aPL + ve with one venous thrombus:
  - Warfarin aiming for INR between 2 and 3
- aPL + ve with arterial thrombosis/stroke or recurrent venous thrombosis:
  - Warfarin aiming for INR between 3 and 4
- aPL + ve and pregnant, with history of pregnancy problems:
  - Aspirin and subcutaneous heparin throughout pregnancy (warfarin is contra-indicated)
- Catastrophic anti-phospholipid syndrome:
  - Anticoagulation plus immunosuppression
  - IV immunoglobulin
  - Rituximab
  - Immunosuppression not useful in other forms.

Prognosis and complications

Prognosis

- In pregnancy. On aspirin and heparin, the live birth rate is 70%, but there is still a risk of pre-eclampsia and other complications of pregnancy.
- Risk of thrombosis remains with treatment but most do well on anticoagulation.

Complications

- Further thromboses despite anticoagulation.

SJÖGREN SYNDROME

Outline

- Chronic autoimmune condition that attacks exocrine epithelial glands, particularly the salivary and lacrimal glands
- Causes dry eyes: sicca syndrome and dry mouth: xerostomia
- Can also affect the epithelial glands of the vagina, skin, airways, joints and muscles.

Classification

- 1°: Sjögren syndrome alone
- 2°: associated with another connective tissue disorders – usually rheumatoid arthritis, SLE.

Pathogenesis/aetiology

Pathogenesis

- Lymphocytic and plasma cell infiltrate of salivary glands
Associated antibodies:
- Anti-Ro
- Anti-LA

- Rheumatoid factor
- ANAs
- High polyclonal IgG levels.

Who

- Middle aged women

Associations:
- HLA-B8
- HLA-DR3
- Other autoimmune diseases.

A typical patient

A 50-year-old lady who feels continually tired and achy, but without joint swelling. Her eyes always feel dry and gritty and her mouth is dry so that she has to carry a bottle of water at all times.

Clinical features

- Dry mouth
- Dry eyes
Systemic manifestations:
- Arthritis
- Raynaud's
- Renal involvement particularly renal tubular acidosis (20%)
- Pulmonary: fibrotic lung disease
- Parotid gland enlargement (33%)
- Vasculitis
- Purpuric lesions

- Peripheral neuropathy
- Dental care may be difficult
- Fatigue
Summary of Sjögren syndrome (**Sample**):
- **S**jögren's
- **a**rthritis
- **m**outh dry
- **p**arotid enlarged
- **l**ymphoma
- **e**yes dry.

Investigations

Conjunctival dryness:
- Schirmer's test: strip of paper inside the lower lid to measure distance of tear absorbance. <5 mm in 5 min is abnormal
- Rose Bengal staining shows corneal ulceration

Dry mouth:
- Tests of salivary flow
- Salivary gland biopsy.

Blood tests

- ↑↑ ESR (due to IgG), though CRP may be normal
Antibodies:
- Anti-Ro and anti-La antibody titres

- Rheumatoid factor +ve (often)
- ANA
- ↑ Immunoglobulins (Ig).

Treatment

Eyes:
- Hypromellose (artificial tears)
- N-acetylcysteine eye drops
- Occlusion of the punctum which drains tears
Mouth:
- Cold drinks
- Artificial saliva spray

General medical:
- Hydroxychloroquine: can help fatigue and joint pain
- Steroids: only for severe cases, e.g. neuropathy, parotid swelling.

Prognosis and complications

Prognosis

- Generally good

- Symptoms generally irritating without causing severe health problems.

Complications

- Corneal damage and blindness
- Lymphoma (6%): excess lymphocyte in salivary glands: more susceptible to mutation
- Patients with anti-Ro and or anti-La (due to SLE or Sjögren syndrome) have a 2–5% risk of delivering a baby with fetal heart block.

SCLERODERMA

Outline

- Chronic, multi-systemic, autoimmune, rheumatic disease characterised by skin sclerosis (hardening)
- Can be localised or generalised affecting the connective tissue of joints, tendons, skin, blood vessels, heart and lungs.

Classification

Localised – morphoea:
- Only affects the skin
- Includes a linear form: 'en coup de Sabre' which leaves a line down the face and/or body
- Can lead to systemic sclerosis, but rarely

Systemic sclerosis:
- Also affects internal organs:
  - Limited cutaneous ss (60%): *tight skin but only on forearms, feet and face associated with CREST syndrome*
  - Diffuse cutaneous ss (40%): *tight skin in more widespread distributions beyond the elbow. Can affect kidneys, skin, gut, heart.*

Pathogenesis/aetiology

Pathogenesis

- May be autoantibody related
- Excess collagen production
- Skin becomes oedematous and blood vessels thicken
- Fibrosis and endarteritis leads to multi-organ damage

Autoantibodies:
- Present in 80% of patients
- Classification depends on the antibody affected
- Auto-antibodies to:

- topoisomerase 1 (Scl 70): in 30% of diffuse scleroderma
- centromere antigens: associated with CREST syndrome
- RNA polymerase: in 9%
- All three antigens are important in cell division: disease affects cells dividing quickly, e.g. the skin, gut and bone marrow.

Who

- Typical age of onset: 30–40
- 15♀:1♂ in young adults
- 2♀:1♂ in elderly
- 1/10 000

Associations:
- Other autoimmune diseases
- Familial association

- Anti-Scl-70 antibodies
- HLA:
  - A1
  - B8
  - DR3
  - DR5.

A typical patient

A 33-year-old lady has always suffered from Raynaud's phenomenon in the winter. More recently she has noticed that skin over her fingers has become tight and waxy and she cannot open her mouth wide.

Clinical features

Limited cutaneous: CREST:
- **C**alcinosis (calcium deposits within the soft tissue)
- **R**aynaud's (99%) fingers go white/blue/pink in cold: commonest presenting complaint
- **E**sophageal and GI symptoms:
  - Dysphagia (due to dysmotility or stricture)
  - Gut disease
  - Watermelon stomach (dilated blood vessels of the stomach antrum resulting in watermelon–like long red lines on endoscopy)
  - Constipation/diarrhoea

- **S**clerodactyly: thickening and tightening of skin over digits
- **T**elangiectasia: localised collection of distended blood capillaries: red blanching spots.
- Must consider pulmonary hypertension which is the main serious complication in limited systemic sclerosis

Clinical features

Diffuse cutaneous:
- General: malaise, fever, weight loss, depression
- Skin changes: particularly of hands, neck and face. Tightness, hardening, shiny skin. Features: beaked nose, telengiectasia, Raynaud's develops later
- Renal: scleroderma renal crisis: hypertension, nephritic syndrome, rapid loss of renal function with rising creatinine

- Gut: oesophagitis, stricture, malabsorption, watermelon stomach, constipation, faecal incontinence.
- Lungs: pulmonary fibrosis, pulmonary hypertension (more common in limited systemic sclerosis)
- Cardiac: pericarditis, hypertension, myocarditis: heart failure, arrhythmias, MI
- Musculoskeletal: arthritis, arthralgia, tenosynovitis, myositis.

Investigations

Blood tests

- FBC: ↓ Hb
- ↑ ESR
- ↑ creatine kinase
- LFTs: monitor
- TFTs: monitor
- Autoantibodies

- Anti-topoisomerase (Scl 70)
- Anti-centromere
- Anti-RNA polymerase
- ANA
- Rheumatoid factor.

Imaging

- X-ray hands and feet: calcium deposition
- CXR
- Barium swallow or oesophageal manometry

Echo:
- CT: pulmonary fibrosis
- May need cardiac catheterisation: to diagnose pulmonary hypertension (symptoms are often mild).

Other tests

Lung function tests.

Treatment

Conservative

- Education

- Treat symptomatically

General medical

- Immunosuppressants, e.g. methotrexate
- Antifibrotic therapies, e.g. D-penicillamine, interferon
- Steroids are rarely used except where there is also pulmonary fibrosis, myositis or severe arthritis. Generally

avoided as they can increase risk of scleroderma renal crisis

Specifics

- Scleroderma renal crisis: ACE inhibitors, intravenous iloprost, ITU
- Joint pain: physiotherapy, analgesics, NSAIDs, nifedipine
- Vascular: vasodilators, remodelling potential, antioxidants
- Raynaud's: see below
- Pulmonary hypertension: prostacyclin, bosentan (anti-endothelin agent), sildenafil and sometimes prophylactic anticoagulation.

- Pulmonary fibrosis: high-dose steroids and immunosuppression with cyclophosphamide, mycophenolate or azathioprine
- Control hypertension
- Skin lubricants
- Acid reflux: prophylactic omeprazole.

Prognosis and complications

Prognosis

- Variable but normally progressive
- Better for CREST syndromes
- Very poor in pulmonary hypertension (50% of deaths)

- Death normally from lung, renal or cardiac complications:
  - 70% 10-year survival.

Complications

- Digital gangrene can occur in severe cases of Raynaud's, leading to loss of fingers or toes.

MIXED CONNECTIVE TISSUE DISEASE

Outline

- A condition with aspects of SLE, systemic sclerosis and polymyositis but not fulfilling the full diagnostic criteria for any of them

- By definition must be + ve for anti-ribonucleoprotein (anti-RNP) antibodies.

RAYNAUD'S

Outline

- Vascular disorder where the extremities change to white, blue and red, in that order, in response to cold or emotion

- Due to vasospasm of the arteries
- A phenomenon, not a disease.

Pathogenesis/aetiology

Causes

1°: Raynaud's:
- Idiopathic: exists alone. Not severe. Commoner in young women

2°: Raynaud's:
- Rheumatic disease: SLE, systemic sclerosis, rheumatoid arthritis
- Trauma

- Hypothyroidism
- Peripheral vascular disease
- Nerve compression
- Vibrating tools
- Haematological: polycythaemia rubra vera
- Drugs: β-blockers

Who

- ♀ > ♂
- Prevalence: 5%

Associations:
- Scleroderma (systemic sclerosis)

- Lupus (SLE)
- Myositis
- Sjögren syndrome
- Rheumatoid arthritis.

Clinical features

- Fingers and toes turn: white (pallor), blue (from cyanosis), then red (on reperfusion)

- Bilateral
- May be painful.

Investigations

Blood tests

- FBC, LFTs, rheumatoid factor (help to identify cause)

Autoantibodies:
- +ve ANA increases suspicion of SLE or systemic sclerosis.

Imaging

- Thermography

- Capillaroscopy of nail fold capillaries (examination of the capillaries of the nail bed under the microscope).

Treatment

Single short attacks:
- Warmth, gloves
- Heating appliances
- Stop smoking

Frequent long attacks:
- Calcium channel blockers: prevent arterioconstriction, e.g. nifedipine/diltiazem
- 5HT antagonists (vasodilate): ketanserin
- Maxepa (lowers triglycerides)

- ACE inhibitors
- Vasodilators, e.g. nitrates, prostacyclin infusion
- Fluoxetine: reduces platelet store of 5-HT
- Sympathectomy:
  - Proximal: (cervical or lumbar) if an arm or leg is most affected.
  - Digital: nerve to a single digit is severed

Severe ulcers/gangrene:
- IV Iloprost (prostacyclin), surgery, amputation.

Prognosis and complications

Prognosis

Poor indicators:
- Late onset
- Worsening symptoms
- Male
- No family history
- Abnormal capillaries
- Disease-specific ANAs.

Complications

- Digital gangrene can occur in severe cases of Raynaud's, leading to loss of fingers or toes.

MYOSITIS

Outline

- An inflammatory disorder of striated muscle.

Classification

Three major types, which are distinct diseases:
1. *Polymyositis*: occurring without rash
2. *Dermatomyositis*: muscle symptoms occur together with a characteristically distributed rash. Associated with malignancy
3. *Inclusion body myositis*: a rarer disorder occurring characteristically in older patients. The pathognomonic inclusion bodies in muscle cells are usually visible only on electron microscopy.

Pathogenesis/aetiology

Causes

- Unknown aetiology.

Pathogenesis

- Inflammation and necrosis of muscle fibres
- Myositic muscle is infiltrated with macrophages and lymphocytes
- Dermatomyositis is associated with underlying malignancy particularly in older men (10%)

Antibodies:
- ANA is usually +ve
- Myositis with anti-tRNA synthetase is called anti-synthetase syndrome. These patients frequently also have pulmonary fibrosis and arthritis.

Who

- Typical age: two peaks at 50 years and at childhood
- 2♀:1♂
- Rare.

Clinical features

Muscular symptoms:
- Muscular weakness and proximal muscle wasting of the pelvic girdle and shoulders: difficulty squatting, raising from chair and climbing stairs
- Muscle pain and tenderness (50%)

Extramuscular symptoms:
- Arthralgia and arthritis (50%)
- Dysphagia, dysphonia from oesophageal weakness
- Respiratory weakness from lung fibrosis and muscle weakness
- Raynaud's

Dermatomyositis:
- Bluish-red skin eruption of face, scalp, neck, shoulders
- Purple heliotrope periorbital rash
- Later with severe swelling of eyelids and bony prominences

- "Gottron's papules" (raised pink patches on the knuckles) (Fig. 10.8)
- Calcinosis: small hard lumps of calcium under the skin.

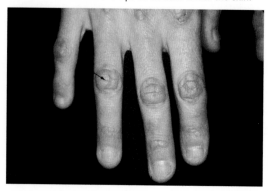

Fig. 10.8 Gottron's papules of the knuckles and fingers (arrow).

Investigations

Clinically assess muscle power

Blood tests

- ↑ ESR
- ↑ Muscle enzyme levels (creatine kinase, LDH)

- Antibodies: ANA, anti-tRNA synthetase

Physiological studies

- EMG: fibrillation potentials.

Imaging

- MRI: muscle inflammation

- Investigations for malignancy.

Other tests

- Biopsy:
  - Muscle biopsy: gold standard
  - Skin biopsy: helps in dermatomyositis.

Treatment

Conservative

- Rest

- Physiotherapy to restore muscle power.

Medical

- Prednisolone: high dose (frequently starting at 1 mg/kg daily)
- Immunosuppressives: methotrexate, azathioprine, ciclosporin if no response to steroids

- IV immunoglobulins; 3–5 day course in hospital, often repeated monthly for 3–4 months. If unresponsive to immunosuppressants
- Rituximab: particularly for anti-synthetase syndrome
- Cyclophosphamide for pulmonary fibrosis

Cases irresponsive to treatment

- Consider:
  - Is there underlying malignancy?
  - Is it inclusion body myositis: often responds poorly to treatment

- Is it anti-synthetase syndrome?
- Is it myositis? Could be muscular dystrophy: repeat biopsy.

Prognosis and complications

Prognosis

- Adults have a better prognosis than children unless malignancy is involved

- Maintain remission with low-dose steroids

Complications

- Respiratory failure due to respiratory muscle weakness.

MARFAN SYNDROME DISORDER

Outline

- An inherited disorder where a defect in the elastic fibres of collagen leads to long limbs and a tendency to heart disease.

Pathogenesis/aetiology

Causes

- Autosomal dominant inheritance

- Mutation in fibrillin-1: needed for synthesis of elastic fibres in connective tissue.

Who

- 1♀:1♂
- 0.03% of population

- Family history (75%).

Clinical features

Musculoskeletal:
- Tall
- Arachnodactyly: long slender fingers and toes
- Slender long limbs
- Scoliosis
- Pes planus
- High arched palate
- Flexibility

Cardiovascular:
- SOB
- Palpitations
- Chest pains
- Aneurysms: ascending aorta
- Aortic dissection
- Aortic valve regurgitation
- Cardiac murmurs

Pulmonary:
- Spontaneous pneumothorax
- Obstructive sleep apnoea

Occular:
- Myopia (short sighted): from partial upwards dislocation of eye lens.

Investigations

- Clinical diagnosis
- ECG
- Echo.

Treatment

Prevention of aortic dissection:
- Monitor: annual echo
- β-blockers
- Surgery if aortic diameter >5 cm suggesting an aneurysm.

Prognosis and complications

Prognosis

- Shorter life expectancy due to cardiovascular complications.

Complications

- Aortic aneurysm
- Dissection
- Mitral valve prolapse.

EHLERS–DANLOS SYNDROME

Outline

- Group of genetic disorders from a defect in collagen synthesis
- Abnormal/deficient collagen
- Affects skin, blood vessels and joints
- Six types: type III is the commonest and is a cause of hypermobility
- Type IV has the worst prognosis and commonest cause of complications.

Pathogenesis/aetiology

- Autosomal inheritance: dominant or recessive
- Gene mutations: pro-collagen.

Who

- Prevalence: 1/5000
- Rare
- Up to 10% or more of the population have some degree of hypermobility.

Clinical features

- Joints: hypermobility, unstable and flexible. Overstretched ligaments result in dislocation and subluxation
- Bones: sunken chest, scoliosis
- Skin: elastic, fragile, bruises easily, scars poorly
- Eye: near sighted
- Vascular and organs: fragility can result in the bursting of the aorta or gut wall
- General: fever, malaise, weight loss.

- Dislocation and subluxation.

Treatment

- No satisfactory treatment
- Avoid contact sports.

Prognosis and complications

Prognosis

- Type IV: shortened life span

Complications

Type IV:
- Arterial aneurysms
- Pneumothorax
- Heart valve prolapse
- Rupture of blood vessels.

METABOLIC BONE DISEASE

OSTEOPOROSIS

Outline

- A disease where the bone mineral density (BMD) is reduced, leading to brittle bones that fracture easily
- Normal bone structure with loss of bone mass rather than a defect in mineralisation/composition
- World Health Organisation defines:
  - Osteoporosis: BMD >2.5 standard deviations (sd) below peak bone mass (T-score of < -2.5)
  - Osteopenia: BMD 1–2.5 sd below peak bone mass (T score of −1 to −2.5).

Classification

- 1° *osteoporosis*: mainly affects trabecular (spongy) bone due to:
  - either: low turnover (↓ osteoblasts/postmenopausal)
  - or: high turnover (↑ osteoclasts)
- 2° *osteoporosis*: mainly affects cortical bone due to:
  - endocrine disorders
  - rheumatological disease
- malignancy
- GI causes
- anaemia
- lung disease
- Drugs: anticonvulsants, steroids, chemotherapy, heparin, alcohol
- Poor nutrition, e.g. anorexia.

Pathogenesis/aetiology

Pathogenesis

- Bone mass density peaks at 20–30 years and then declines
- Bone is continuously being formed by osteoblasts and resorbed or broken down by osteoclasts
- An imbalance of bone formation (↑ osteoclast and ↓ osteoblast activity) and remodelling results in thin, brittle bones in osteoporosis

Factors that affect bone mass density:
- Hormonal state: lack of oestrogen (oestrogen is protective), e.g. in menopause, Cushing's
- Age: osteoblasts decrease their activity in old age
- Genes: affects peak bone mass
- Exercise: ↓ activity increases risk
- Diet: calcium deficiency (often in girls)
- Osteoclast activity is stimulated by IL-I and TNF from blood monocytes and bone marrow cells.

Who

- 4♀:1♂
- 5% (50% of over 80s)
Risk factors:
- Smoking
- Family history
- Immobility
- Low peak bone mass
- Caucasians
- Early menopause
- Postmenopausal
- Drugs: steroid therapy, heparin, anti-convulsants, alcohol
Disease:
- Premature ovarian failure
- Hypogonadism in men
- Hyperparathyroidism (↑ bone resorption)
- Hyperthyroidism (↑ bone turnover)
- Addison's disease.

A 65-year-old lady has noticed increasingly stooped posture and loss of height. She suddenly develops severe back pain without significant trauma.

- Entire skeleton affected
- Asymptomatic, unless presenting with a fracture
- Fractures can occur silently leading to kyphoscoliosis and loss of height with no pain
- Fractures particularly in:
  - neck of femur: if cortical bone is affected
- distal radius: Colles fracture (posterior displacement of the wrist)
- vertebrae: if trabecular bone is affected. Particularly thoracic and lumbar vertebrae: leads to loss of height, lordosis and kyphoscoliosis. Can affect neurological structures

- PTH
- Vitamin D

Bone profile:
- ALP: normal
- Calcium: normal
- Phosphate: normal.

- X-ray
- DEXA, estimates BMD (see p. 426).

- FRAX Score: 12 point score to calculate 10 year probability of fracture. useful for deciding whether to commence 1° prevention with medication.

The aim of treatment is to prevent future fractures by reducing the rate of fall of bone density:
- Bisphosphonates, e.g. alendronate. Inhibits osteoclast activity and therefore reduces bone resorption
- Calcium/vitamin D supplements
- Calcitonin: reduces pain from acute osteoporotic fractures by reducing bone resorption
- Hormone replacement therapy in high risk women, e.g. oestrogens, given for ~10 years around menopause (side effects: cancer, VTE). In women with a uterus, progesterone is given with oestrogen to reduce risk of uterine cancer.
  Selective oestrogen receptor modulator, e.g. raloxifene, activate oestrogen receptors on bone:

- Strontium ranelate
- Recombinant PTH derivatives
- Early intervention to reduce pain and maintain mobility
Prevention:
- Exercise
- Calcium-rich diet
- No smoking
- No alcohol
- Hormone replacement therapy
- Reduce risks of falls.

- Poor if fractured neck of femur in elderly patients (50% survival at 6 months in the elderly)

- If no fracture, prognosis is good.

- Fracture

- Nerve root compression.

- Vitamin D deficiency, leading to inadequate mineralisation and the softening of bones
- Mineral content is low but bone density is normal.

- Osteomalacia: deficiency occurs after the fusion of the epiphyses (in adults)
- Rickets: deficiency before fusion of epiphyses (in children)

Pathogenesis/aetiology

Causes

- Vitamin D deficiency:
  - Poor diet
  - Malabsorption
  - Lack of sunlight: important in vitamin D synthesis in the skin
  - Renal disease
  - Liver disease

- Vitamin D resistance: congenital conditions
- Drugs: anticonvulsants induce liver enzymes breaking down 25-hydroxyvitaminD
- Phosphate deficiency.

Pathogenesis

- Vitamin D is needed for the uptake of calcium from food (see Endocrinology Chapter 9)

- Reduction leads to decalcification of bone.

Who

- Those with little exposure to sunlight, e.g. housebound, elderly.

A typical patient

A 45-year-old lady whose lifestyle and dress mean that she has very little exposure to sunlight. She has widespread bony pain.

Clinical features

Rickets:
- Valgus (knock-knees)
- Chest deformities: rachitic rosary (prominent costochondral joints with bead like appearance under the skin)
- Skull deformities
- Symptoms and signs of hypocalcaemia

Osteomalacia:
- Bone pain
- Fractures (neck of femur)
- Proximal myopathy: waddling gait, unable to rise from a chair.

Investigations

Blood tests

- ↓ 25 (OH) vitamin D

Bone profile:
- Calcium: low
- Phosphate: low
- ALP: high.

Imaging

X-ray:
- Rickets: worn metaphyseal surfaces (Fig. 10.9)
- Osteomalacia: loss of cortical bone, partial fractures at the scapula, femoral neck and pubic rami, Looser's zones (partial fracture seen as low density lines in bones on X-ray)

Bone scan:
- Increased isotope uptake.

Other tests

- Biopsy:
  - Non-mineralised bone
  - Definitive investigation

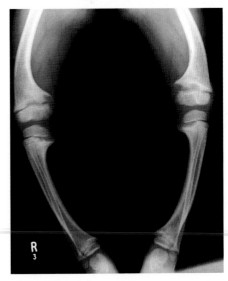

Fig. 10.9 Rickets: convexity of both legs, with fraying, splaying and cupping at the epiphysis.

Treatment

Vitamin D deficiency:
- Vitamin D tablets daily, e.g. cholecalciferol
- Intramuscular vitamin D injection
Malabsorption or vitamin D resistant:
- Calciferol tablet (much higher doses)

Renal disease:
- Alfacalcidol (vitamin D analogue)
Monitor calcium levels in all cases.

Prognosis and complications

Prognosis

- If treated with sufficient vitamin D then symptoms may improve considerably.

Complications

- Fracture.

PAGET'S DISEASE

Outline

- Chronic disease of the bones leading to enlarged and deformed bones of the skull, pelvis, backbone and long bones
- Can affect single (15%) or multiple (85%) bones
- Pagetic bone is hypervascular: can rarely result in arterio-venous shunting causing high output heart failure.

Pathogenesis/aetiology

Causes

- Aetiology unknown.

Pathogenesis

- ↑ Bone turnover: ↑ osteoclast resorption of bone with disorganised remodelling by osteoblasts
- Resultant bones are large, deformed and weak

Histology:
- Resorption pits with large multinucleate osteoclasts.

Who

- Typical age: disease of the elderly
- ♀ > ♂
- Incidence 5–11%
- N. Europeans
- Rare in black and Asian population.

A typical patient

A 70-year-old man whose hats no longer fit with some leg pain and bilateral pedal oedema. Blood tests show an isolated high ALP.

Clinical features

- May be asymptomatic or mild
- See fig. 10.10A for a summary of the systemic features of Paget's.

Musculoskeletal

- **Pain** and tenderness: commonest symptoms
Bone enlargement and deformity:
- Affected bone: skull > femur > clavicle > tibia
- Varus: bow legs, curvature of long bones
- Leontiasis ossea (lion face): bony overgrowth of facial skeleton so that it is too heavy for the neck
- Occlusion of skull foramina:
  - Headaches
  - **Deafness** from nerve compression and ossicle changes
  - Optic atrophy
  - Cord compression: paraparesis

- Platybasia = (flattening of skull base) and compression of posterior fossa structures
Fractures:
- Microfractures and fractures
- Chalk stick fractures = (fracture perpendicular to the long bone axis)
- Compression fractures of spine leading to cord injury, kyphosis

Cardiovascular complications

- **Cardiac failure**.

Investigations

Blood tests

Bone profile:
• Calcium: normal
• Phosphate: normal
• ALP: high.

Imaging

X-rays:
• Bone enlargement and deformity
• Coarse trabeculation
• Patchy osteolysis, sclerosis (Fig. 10.10B) and cortical thickening

Isotope bone scan:
• Increased uptake due to increased turnover (differential diagnosis: metastatic cancer).

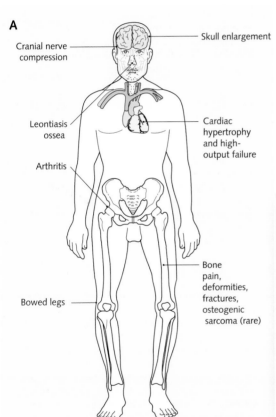

A

Cranial nerve compression

Skull enlargement

Leontiasis ossea

Cardiac hypertrophy and high-output failure

Arthritis

Bowed legs

Bone pain, deformities, fractures, osteogenic sarcoma (rare)

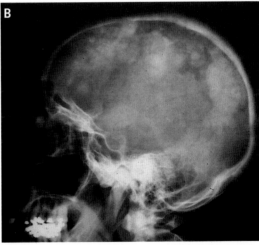

B

Fig. 10.10 (A) Systemic features of Paget's. (B) Multifocal sclerotic patches, which are cotton wool-like and characteristic of Paget's disease.

Treatment

• Often no treatment required
• Bisphosphates (alendronate) for 6 months: inhibits osteoclast activity (reducing resorption)

• Calcitonin for 3–6 months: inhibits osteoclast activity
• Analgesia
• Surgical correction of deformities.

Prognosis and complications

Complications

- 2° sarcoma in <1%
- 2° osteoarthritis
- Neurovascular complications
- Heart failure
- Renal calculi.

CRYSTAL ARTHROPATHY

GOUT

Outline

- A defect in uric acid (urate) metabolism causes it to accumulate in the blood. This can lead to deposition of urate crystals in joints, kidneys and soft tissues
- Serum urate >0.4 mmol/L

Disease progression:
- Asymptomatic hyeruricaemia
- Acute gout
- Recurrent attacks
- Chronic gout: chronic disability with joint erosion and formation of tophi (urate deposits in the soft tissue). Occurs about 10 years after initial attack

Summary: **GOUT**:
- **G**reat toe
- **O**ne joint 75%
- **U**ric acid ↑
- **T**ophi

Lesch–Nyhan syndrome:
- Hypoxanthine–guanine phosphoribosyltransferase deficiency
- Inherited defect of urate metabolism with mental retardation and self-mutilation.

Pathogenesis/aetiology

Causes

1° Gout:
- 1° uricaemia: inherited disorder

2° Gout:
- Overproduction of uric acid:
  - Psoriasis: rapid cell and purine turnover
  - Polycythaemia rubra vera
  - Leukaemia: ↑ nucleic acid turnover
  - 1° hyperparathyroidism

- Hypothyroidism
- Lesch–Nyhan syndrome
- Underexcretion of uric acid:
  - Hypertension
  - Renal disease
  - G-6-PD deficiency
  - Drugs: **alcohol**, **diuretics**, aspirin.

Pathogenesis

- Urate is a by-product of the metabolism of purines in nucleic acids
- Hyperuricaemia is due to overproduction/intake or under excretion of uric acid
- Uric acid crystals (monosodium urate) attract neutrophils which phagocytose the crystals but are unable to degrade them, resulting in inflammation:

- in joints: pannus formation (grannulation tissue in inflamed joint) can lead to fibrosis and bony ankylosis
- in soft tissue: tophi (hard crystalline deposits)
- in renal tract: urate renal calculi can cause renal failure.

Who

- Typical age: rare before puberty
- 1♀:10♂
- Prevalence 0.2% in Europe

At risk:
- Family history (30%)
- Alcoholics
- Diuretics
- Diet rich in red meat/shellfish/wine or beer.

A typical patient

An obese 50-year-old man on treatment for heart failure presents to his GP with an acute painful swelling of his big toe.

Joint problems:
- Red, painful, oedematous joints
- Can be monoarthritis or polyarticular (less common)
- Podagra: involvement of the great toe
- Other joints: midfoot, elbow, ankle, wrist or hand, fingers, knees
- Onset: sudden
- Duration: usually self-limiting, lasting a few days.
- Attacks can be separated by years

Tophi:
- Form in joints, skin, ligaments, tendons, cartilage, earlobes, kidneys, fingertips, palms, soles, olecranon, patellar bursae, eye, ear helix
- Can appear as chalky, white nodules if they break through the skin
- Can cause ulceration of overlying skin

Kidney:
- Urate stones
- Urate nephropathy: can cause renal impairment (further impairing uric acid excretion).

Blood tests

- Urate level in blood (normal urate does not exclude gout)
- U&E monitor kidney function

Joint aspiration

- Definitive test
- Polarising light microscopy to detect crystals (Fig. 10.11)
- Needle shaped
- Negatively birefringent

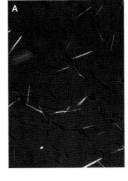

Fig. 10.11 Gout: needle-shaped, negatively birefringent urate crystals, seen under polarising light microscopy.

Imaging

X-rays:
- Early stage: soft tissue swelling
- Chronic stage: joint erosion and disruption.

Two aims of treatment:
1. Treat acute flare:

Analgesia:
- NSAIDS: Start with strongest : diclofenac, naproxen, indomethacin
- Colchicine: Inhibits leukocyte microtubular formation and migration (side effect: diarrhoea)
- Steroids: Oral or intra-articular, Use if in renal impairment (NSAIDs and colchicine are contra-indicated in renal impairment). Must exclude septic arthritis first.

2. Reduce frequency of attacks:

Conservative:
- Weight loss

Avoid:
- Purine rich food, e.g. red meat
- Diuretics
- Alcohol excess
- Aspirin (it ↑ serum urate)

Medical
- Allopurinol: xanthine oxidase inhibitor, inhibits urate production. Prevents gout long term. Not for acute cases as can precipitate an attack. Wait 3 weeks and give colchicines or NSAIDS with it. Interacts with azathioprine. (side effects: headaches, dyspepsia, diarrhoea)
- Uricosuric drugs: probenecid, sulphinpyrazone. Rarely used, contraindicated in urate nephropathy / urate renal calculi.
- Febuxostat. A new xanthine oxidase inhibitor if intolerant to allopurinol

Prognosis

- Many cases respond to change in diet and/or stopping diuretics alone
- Many more respond to allopurinol
- Severe cases with deforming arthritis are rare.

Complications

- Renal disease due to calculi.

PSEUDOGOUT

Outline

- Joint pain and gout-like symptoms from calcium pyrophosphate dihydrate crystals depositing in joints leading to arthritis
- Acute self-limiting attacks like gout but affecting different joints.

Pathogenesis/aetiology

Causes

- 1°: sporadic
- 2°: associated with:
  - diabetes mellitus
  - hyperthyroidism
  - hyperparathyroidism
- previous joint damage, e.g. surgery or illness
- haemochromatosis
- ↓ magnesium
- ochronosis.

Pathogenesis

- Calcium pyrophosphate dihydrate crystallises around joints
- Crystals build up as pseudotophi: much less common than in gout
- Chronic disease can lead to joint changes.

Who

- Typical age: >70
- ♀ > ♂
Risks:
- Dehydration
- Myxoedema
- Acromegaly
- ↓ Magnesium
- ↓ Phosphate
- Arthritis: osteoarthritis/rheumatoid arthritis.

A typical patient

A 75-year-old lady with known osteoarthritis in the left knee suddenly experiences increased pain and swelling in that knee with a warm effusion.

Clinical features

- Monoarthritis that may later become polyarthritis
- Joints affected: knees, wrists and hip. Very rarely the great toe
- Often precipitated by illness
- Check for symptoms of hypercalcaemia and hyperparathyroidism (pseudogout may be the presenting clinical feature).

Investigations

Blood tests

- ↑ WBC (not always)

Joint aspiration

- Definitive test
- Polarising light microscopy to detect crystals
- Oval or rhomboid crystals
- Positively bifringent.

Imaging

X-ray:
- Chondrocalcinosis: line of calcification deposition in intra-articular cartilage on X-ray.

Treatment

- Usually self-limiting
- Rest
- NSAIDs
- Intra-articular steroid injections
- Hydroxychloroquine: previously thought to reduce frequency of attacks, though no good evidence
- Monitor calcium and parathyroid levels and treat if necessary
- Polyarticular attacks may respond to intra-muscular steroid injection (systemic effect).

Prognosis and complications

Prognosis

- Normally self-limiting.

Complications

- 2° osteoarthritis.

MUSCULAR DISORDERS

CHRONIC WIDESPREAD PAIN/FIBROMYALGIA

Outline

- Pain in the muscle and soft tissues on both sides of the body, above and below the waist and the back lasting at least three months is called chronic widespread pain

Fibromyalgia (FM):
- A subset of this chronic widespread pain that includes all patients with chronic widespread pain who have tender spots in at least 11/18 specific sites
- Some people question the value of FM as a diagnosis since no organic abnormality in the painful tissues can be found.

Pathogenesis/aetiology

Causes

- Aetiology unknown
- Associated with (and possibly triggered by):
  - anxiety
  - depression

- chronic fatigue syndrome
- irritable bowel syndrome
- premenstrual syndrome
- hypermobility syndrome.

Pathogenesis

- Complex, involves physical and psychological components

- No organic abnormality in the painful tissues.

Who

Chronic widespread pain:
- ♀ > ♂
- Prevalence: 10%

FM:
- Prevalence: 2%.

Clinical features

- Tender trigger points (in fibromyalgia)
- Sleep disturbance
- Widespread discomfort and aches
- Fatigue
- Headache

- Numbness
- Severe cases: abnormal pain behaviour: walking, sitting or lying in abnormal posture leading to increased muscle tension and pain.

Investigations

- All investigations are normal. Performed to exclude other diagnoses.

Treatment

Aim of treatment: to improve function despite pain:
- Reassurance: explain that the pain is not causing damage to tissues and that it is OK to use the painful areas
- Exercise regime
- Pain management psychology
- Analgesics: systemic or local injections

- NSAIDs
- Antidepressants, e.g. amitriptyline at analgesic levels
- Pregabalin or gabapentin
- Acupuncture: shown to relieve symptoms (at least in the short term).

Prognosis

- The majority cannot be cured completely and people continue to live with pain.

Complications

- No complications but can result in profound loss of quality of life.

RHABDOMYOLYSIS

Outline

- Rapid breakdown of skeletal muscle leading to a build up of muscular breakdown products in the bloodstream
- Breakdown products can lead to renal damage
- Crush syndrome: traumatic rhabdomyolysis.

Pathogenesis/aetiology

Causes

- Due to injury:
  - Mechanical: crush, burns
  - Physical: fever, excess exercise, hyperthermia, infection
- Chemical: metabolic disorders, drugs, e.g. heroin, alcohol, carbon monoxide
- Inherited muscle disorder: Duchenne muscular dystrophy.

Pathogenesis

- Myoglobin, urate, creatine kinase, potassium and phosphate are released into the circulation when skeletal muscle breaks down
- Myoglobin can obstruct the kidney tubules and lead to renal failure.

Who

- $♀ < ♂$.

Clinical features

Symptoms and signs of:
- Hypovolaemia
- Hyperkalaemia
- Hypocalcaemia
- Metabolic acidosis
- Acute renal failure
- DIC.

Investigations

Blood tests

- $↓ / ↑$ potassium$^+$
- $↓ Ca^{2+}$
- $↑ ↑ ↑$ creatinine kinase (often $>1000 \times$ upper limit of normal).

Urine

- Myoglobinuria: +ve dipstick test for blood but no RBCs seen on urine microscopy

Treatment

- Mainly supportive therapy
- IV fluids
- Bicarbonates: to alkalinise the urine
- Electrolyte correction, particularly K^+
- Haemodialysis: severe cases with renal failure.

Prognosis and complications

Prognosis

- Can be fatal if patient goes into renal failure
- If survives the acute illness and renal impairment, there is a good prospect of full recovery.

VASCULITIS

GENERAL FEATURES

Outline

- Inflammation of vessel walls
- Often associated with ANCAs

p-ANCA:
- Specificity for myeloperoxidase
- Associated with microscopic polyangiitis, Churg–Strauss syndrome, Goodpasture's disease

Classical or c-ANCA:
- Specificity for serine proteinase 3
- Associated with Wegener's granulomatosus (now called granulomatosis with polyangiitis or GPA), microscopic polyangiitis, polyarteritis nodosum.

Pathogenesis/aetiology

Classification

Large vessel:
- Giant cell arteritis
- Takayasu's arteritis

Medium vessel:
- Polyarteritis nodosa
- Kawasaki disease

Small vessel ANCA +ve:
- Glomerulonephritis
- Churg–Strauss syndrome
- Wegener's ganulomatosis (GPA)

Small vessel ANCA −ve:
- Henoch–Schönlein purpura
- Goodpasture's disease
- Cryoglobulinaemia.

Who

- All are rare except giant cell arteritis

Associations:
- Rheumatoid arthritis

- Lupus (SLE)
- Polymyositis
- Allergic drug reactions.

Clinical features

Vasculitic skin lesions:
- Palpable

- Urticarial
- Non-blanching.

Investigations

Blood tests

- ↑ ESR
- ↑ CRP

- p-ANCA and c-ANCA (ANCA can be +ve in other autoimmune diseases and severe illness).

Other tests

Vessel biopsy:
- Temporal artery biopsy for giant cell arteritis, renal or lung biopsy in GPA.

Treatment

- Large vessel disease: steroids

- Medium and small vessel disease: steroids, cyclophosphamide, rituximab

Prognosis and complications

- Depend on type and system involvement.

GIANT CELL ARTERITIS (TEMPORAL ARTERITIS)

Outline

- Large vessel inflammatory granulomatous arteritis
- Affects the large arteries in the head and neck
- Associated with polymyalgia rheumatica (25%)

- Important to recognise early as can result in irreversible blindness.

Pathogenesis/aetiology

Causes

- Idiopathic vasculitis.

Pathogenesis

- Tender, thick and swollen temporal/occipital arteries
- Visual loss due to:

1. central retinal artery occlusion
2. anterior ischaemic optic neuropathy.

Who

- Typical age:>50 years
- ♀>♂.

A typical patient

A 70-year-old woman complains of pain when brushing her hair and has jaw pain on chewing food. Her blood tests showed an ESR of >100.

Clinical features

General symptoms:
- Fatigue, malaise
- Fever
- Weight loss
- Depression
- Nocturnal sweats
- Headaches

- Tenderness over temporal arteries
- Scalp tenderness: pain on combing hair, even sleeping
- Jaw claudication: jaw pain when chewing, relieved by resting
- Visual field defects
- Sudden and permanent monocular visual loss
- Polymyalgia rheumatica (see below).

Investigations

Blood tests

- Normochromic normocytic anaemia
- ↑ ESR, CRP

- ↑ ALP.

Temporal artery biopsy

- Giant cell arteritis
- Perform within 4 days of starting steroids: definitive test for diagnosis

- Normal histology does not exclude diagnosis.

Imaging

- US Doppler: halo sign (mural thickening around the flowing blood) is specific for giant cell arteritis

- PET of blood vessels.

Treatment

- Steroids even if diagnosis is only suspected: rapid relief within 24–48 h, and will prevent stroke and blindness of the other eye. Begin at 40–60 mg/day orally. Tail steroids off over months

- Calcium and vitamin D and bisphosphonates prevent osteoporosis from steroids
- If symptoms return on reducing steroids can consider a second agent, e.g. azathioprine.

Prognosis and complications

Prognosis

- After treatment, most settle after 1–2 years
- 25% need low-dose steroids for >2 years

- 85% have side effects at 10 years.

Complications

- Complications of steroids
- Monocular blindness

- Myocardial infarct.

POLYMYALGIA RHEUMATICA

Outline

- Inflammation of proximal muscles leading to pain and stiffness
- Affects muscles in shoulders, pelvic girdle, lower back, thighs, hips and neck

- Muscles are painful but not weak
- No specific findings on muscle biopsy (therefore rarely done, unlike myositis)
- Associated with giant cell arteritis.

Pathogenesis/aetiology

Pathogenesis

- Pain caused by the swelling of blood vessels in muscles

Differential diagnosis:
- Rheumatoid arthritis
- Osteoarthritis

- Polymyositis
- Malignancy
- Hypothyroidism.

Who

- Typical age: ↑ with age: 2% >60 years old
- 3♀:1♂

- Caucasian
- Northern Europe.

A typical patient

A 60-year-old woman with pain in all limbs, making it difficult to walk, climb stairs or hold up her arms.

Clinical features

Muscles:
- Symmetrical pain and stiffness in the shoulders, neck, hips, lumbar spine and limb girdles: difficulty getting out of a chair
- Worse in the morning
- Pain lasts several hours

General symptoms:
- Fatigue, malaise
- Fever
- Weight loss
- Depression
- Nocturnal sweats.

Investigations

Blood tests

- Normochromic normocytic anaemia
- ↑ ESR/CRP

- ↑ LFTs particularly ALP and GGT.

Imaging

- PET of blood vessels.

Other tests

Consider temporal artery biopsy to rule out Giant cell arteritis.

Treatment

- Steroids: start at 15–20 mg per day and reduce gradually
- The dose of steroids for polymyalgia rheumatica alone is much lower than the dose used in giant cell arteritis so it is important to distinguish whether giant cell arteritis is present
- If symptoms recur on reducing steroids, then increase dose and reduce more slowly next time
- If symptoms recur again on reducing steroids, can consider a second agent, e.g. azathioprine.

Prognosis and complications

Prognosis

- Good
- With steroids 80% of symptoms improve in days
- Treatment normally stopped after 2–4 years
- Low recurrence.

Complications

- Complications of steroids.

TAKAYASU'S ARTERITIS

Outline

- Large vessel arteritis characterised by inflammation of the aorta and major branches
- Results in thromboses, stenosis and aneurysms.

Pathogenesis/aetiology

Cause

- Aetiology unknown.

Who

- Predominantly in females aged 20–40
- Rare, except in Japan.

Clinical features

- Systemic illness: fever, weight loss
- Pain
- Tenderness: over affected arteries
- Absent or unequal peripheral pulses
- Unequal BP in the two arms
- Hypertension: due to renovascular involvement
- If aortic arch affected: upper limb and cerebral symptoms.

Investigations

Blood tests

- ↑ ESR/CRP.

Imaging

Angiography:
- Stenoses

PET scan:
- High uptake in the aortic arch and its major branches.

Treatment

Medical

- Steroids
- Immunosuppressants (azathioprine, cyclophosphamide)

Surgical

- Angioplasty or surgical bypass to improve perfusion of affected areas.

Prognosis

- 95% survival at 15 years.

Complications

- Heart failure
- Stroke.

POLYARTERITIS NODOSA

Outline

- A necrotising vasculitis of medium-sized vessels leading to thrombosis, microaneurysms, and infarction
- Patchy inflammation of artery walls
- Symptoms from ischaemic damage of affected organs.

Pathogenesis/aetiology

Cause

- Aetiology unknown
- Possible connection with HBV antibody complex deposition.

Who

- Typical age: 20–50 years
- 1♀:4♂
- Rare in UK
- Mainly middle-aged men

Associations:
- HBV surface antigen.

Clinical features

- General: fever, malaise, myalgia
- Arthritis
- Renal: hypertension, nephrotic or nephritic syndrome, renal failure
- Cardiac: myocardial infarct, pericarditis
- Asthma
- Abdominal pain
- Mononeuritis multiplex
- Vasculitic rash.

Investigations

Blood tests

- ↑ ESR/CRP
- ↑ eosinophilia
- 10% p-ANCA+ve.

Imaging

- Angiography of abdominal vessels for microaneurysms.

Other tests

- Biopsy:
  - Of affected organ.

Treatment

- Symptomatic: particularly BP control
- Steroids
- Immunosuppressive agents: cyclophosphamide, azathioprine, methotrexate
- Plasma exchange: for some severe cases (e.g. renal failure).

Prognosis and complications

Prognosis

- 40% 5-year survival

Complications

- Commonest causes of death:
  1. Renal failure
- 2. Cardiac complications.

WEGENER'S GRANULOMATOSIS (GRANULOMATOSIS WITH POLYANGIITIS)

Outline

- An autoimmune disease where there is small vessel vasculitis, particularly affecting the upper respiratory tract, lungs and kidneys
- There is multisystem granulomatous inflammation as well as arteritis.

Pathogenesis/aetiology

Causes

- Unknown aetiology
- Associated with classical c-ANCA in 90%
- c-ANCA (specific for proteinase 3).

Who

- Typical age: 40–55
- ♀=♂
- Rare: 3/100 000
- Caucasian 90%
- ANCA+ve vasculitis

Associations:
- Autoimmune disease.

Clinical features

- Upper airway disease: SOB, tracheal stenosis, rhinitis, nosebleeds, mucosal ulceration
- Pulmonary: fibrosis, cavitating nodules, haemoptysis
- Renal: necrotising glomerulonephritis leads to renal failure
- Arthritis: pain, swelling
- Eyes: scleritis, conjunctivitis
- Skin: nodules, vasculitic rash
- Ears: hearing loss
- General: weight loss, fever.

Investigations

Blood tests and sputum

- ANCA antibodies found in serum: c-ANCA (specific for proteinase 3).
- Sputum: cytology

Urine

- Proteinuria or haematuria.

Imaging

- CXR: nodular masses, pneumonic infiltrates, cavities
- CT sinuses: masses due to granulomas.

Other tests

- Biopsy:
  - Renal biopsy: necrotising glomerulonephritis
  - Sinus biopsy may show granulomas.

Treatment

- Involve the renal team.

Medical

- Aim is to:
  - achieve remission: high-dose steroid/ Immunosuppression
  - maintain remission: lower doses, may require long-term treatment
- Corticosteroids: high-dose oral or IV
- Cyclophosphamide
- Rituximab (not yet standard treatment)
- Plasma exchange can be life-saving if there is pulmonary haemorrhage or renal failure. Involves removing the disease-causing antibodies and replacing this with normal plasma by dialysis
- Co-trimoxazole in local disease.

Prognosis

- Depends on organs affected
- Better prognosis: −ve ANCA
- Untreated: mortality 80% within 1 year if extensive disease
- 5-year survival 80–90% on treatment
- Regular ANCA titre monitoring measurements – titre rises may precede disease flare.

CHURG–STRAUSS SYNDROME

Outline

- Medium and small vessel autoimmune vasculitis presenting as a triad of:
  - asthma
- systemic vasculitis
- eosinophilia.

Pathogenesis/aetiology

Causes

- Aetiology unknown. May be autoimmune or allergic response.

Pathogenesis

- Affects several systems including the lungs, skin, nerves, heart, GI system and can affect the kidneys.

Who

- Typical age: >40 years
- ♀ < ♂
- Rare.

Clinical features

- Asthma: 1st symptom to appear, sometimes many years before vasculitic symptoms
- Paranasal sinusitis
- Skin lesions: nodules, purpura
- Pulmonary symptoms: cough
- Cardiac symptoms: MI, pericarditis
- Renal symptoms: hypertension
- GI symptoms: GI bleeds
- CNS symptoms: mononeuritis multiplex.

Investigations

Blood tests

- Eosinophilia
- ANCA+ve
- Raised CRP and ESR
- U&Es to assess for renal complications.

Imaging

- CXR (if pulmonary symptoms) opacities.

Other tests

- Organ-specific tests depending on presentation, e.g. endoscopy for GI bleeds.

Treatment

- Long-term immunosuppressants:
  - prednisolone
  - azathioprine
- cyclophosphamide
- Follow-up by rheumatologists.

Prognosis and complications

Prognosis

- With treatment:
  - 1-year survival: 90%
- 5-year survival 62%.

Complications

- Depends on organs affected.

HENOCH–SCHÖNLEIN PURPURA

Outline

- A small vessel vasculitis with deposition of IgA-containing immune complexes particularly in the kidneys, skin and joints.

Pathogenesis/aetiology

Causes

- Aetiology unknown

- Often occurs following respiratory tract infection, possibly virus related.

Pathogenesis/aetiology

Pathogenesis

- Irregular granular IgA and C3 deposits in glomeruli and skin

- Similar pathogenesis to IgA nephropathy with similar renal histological findings

Who

- Typical age: <10 years old
- Commonest vasculitis in children
- ♀ > ♂

Associations:
- HLA-DR4

Clinical features

- **HENOCH S**:
  - **H**: haematuria
  - **E**: extensor distribution of purpura
  - **N**: nephritis (30–70%): proteinuria
  - **O**: onset normally preceded by viral upper respiratory tract infection

- **C**: complexes-IgA deposited/children
- **H**: has pain in joints, abdomen
- **Skin rash**: non-thrombocytopenic purpura seen mainly on the **legs and buttocks**.

Investigations

Urine

- Haematuria.

Other tests

- Biopsy:
  - Skin or renal: positive immunofluorescence for IgA or C3 deposits.

Treatment

- No treatment of proven benefit

- Normally supportive.

Prognosis and complications

Prognosis

- Usually will recover spontaneously.

Complications

- Renal disease: nephrotic syndrome and renal failure can occur (1%).

BEHÇET'S SYNDROME

Outline

- Systemic vasculitis with oral and genital ulceration and recurrent uveitis.

Pathogenesis/aetiology

Cause

- Aetiology unknown.

Who

- ♀ < ♂
- Turkey
- Iran
- Japan

- 45% develop arthritis
- Rare

Associations:
- HLA-B51.

Clinical features

- Oral ulcers, and two of:
  - genital ulcers
  - eye symptoms: uveitis
  - skin lesions: erythema nodosum (tender swellings of the shins)
  - +ve skin pathergy test

- Also:
  - arthritis: knees, ankles, wrists and elbows
  - GI: diarrhoea, colitis, abdominal pain
  - pulmonary or renal lesions
  - neurological: brainstem syndrome, meningoencephalitis, confusion.

Investigations

Pathergy test:
- Papule formation within 48 h of needle prick

- Mildly ↑ ESR/CRP in acute attacks.

Treatment

Uveitis and neurological symptoms:
- Corticosteroids
- Azathioprine
- Ciclosporin A

Erythema nodosum:
- Colchicine

Ulceration:
- Colchicine

Severe unresponsive disease:
- Thalidomide.

Prognosis and complications

Prognosis

- Mild cases may respond to colchicine alone

- Severe cases, e.g. neurological symptoms or recurrent eye problems, may need long-term steroids/immunosuppression.

PAEDIATRIC RHEUMATOLOGY

There is a big difference between the adult and child form of these diseases.

JUVENILE IDIOPATHIC ARTHRITIS

Outline

- Non-infective chronic systemic inflammatory joint disease in children

- Previously called juvenile chronic arthritis.

Classification

Oligoarthritis/pauciarticular (1–4 joints):
- Chronic synovitis
- Uveitis common
- ♀ > ♂
- Associated with ANAs
- Commonest form

Poyarthritis/polyarticular (>5 joints):
- Widespread synovitis
- No systemic features
- May show adult pattern in older children

- Uveitis can occur
- Tends to affect jaw
- Can be rheumatoid factor + ve or − ve

Systemic onset:
- Also known as adolescent onset Still's disease (to differentiate it from adult onset)
- Fever and salmon pink rash at onset, often without arthritis
- Hepatosplenomegaly, lymphadenopathy
- No antibodies recognised.

Pathogenesis/aetiology

Cause

- Aetiology unknown
- Links with:
  - genetic
  - abnormal immune response

- infection
- trauma
- emotional stress
- TNFα key molecule, overexpressed.

Who

- Typical age: rarely before 6 months
- Peaks 1–3 years and 8–12 years

- ♀ = ♂
- 1/1000.

Clinical features

General:
- Fever
- Splenomegaly
- Lasts >6 weeks

Rheumatological symptoms:
- Polyarthritis/oligoarthritis
- Synovitis
- Stiffness, pain, swelling

- Change in bone growth
- Stunted growth with deformities and retardation
- Hypoplasia of the jaw
- Rash

Eyes:
- Cataracts/uveitis (associated with oligo-disease), may be silent.

Investigations

Blood tests

- ↑ ESR/CRP

- Antibodies: ANA, rheumatoid factor.

Imaging

- Bone X-ray
- US

- MRI: to monitor disease progression.

Treatment

- By analogy with adult disease
- Multi-disciplinary team input: physiotherapy, occupation therapy, teachers, school and medical services to ensure normal life for child

Medical

- NSAIDs: ibuprofen, diclofenac
- Analgesics
- Methotrexate to suppress synovitis

Surgical

- Fusion or joint replacements.

Ophthalmology:
- For silent uveitis. All children with juvenile idiopathic arthritis should be reviewed by ophthalomologists, particularly if ANA+ve

- Anti-TNFα, e.g. etanercept
- Corticosteroids: particularly in systemic juvenile idiopathic arthritis.

Prognosis and complications

Prognosis

- 50%: long-term problems

Complications

- Infection

- 25%: arthritis as adults.

- Pericarditis.

Immunology and infectious diseases 11

Faculty Contributor: Philip Gothard

Defences against disease

External defence mechanisms

- Skin (physical barrier)
- Eyes (lysozyme, IgA)
- Gut (gastric acid, commensal organisms).

Innate mechanisms

Short lived and produced quickly, but with no memory:

- Cells:
  - Phagocytes: cells that ingest bacteria, fungi and debris and produce inflammatory molecules to assist in the immune response, e.g. neutrophils, which are mobile and travel in the blood to different sites; macrophages and monocytes, which are resident within the tissues
  - Mast cells (mobile) and basophils (resident): are important in the allergic response and release mediators such as histamine
  - Natural killer cells: kill viruses and tumour cells through cell lysis
  - Eosinophils: for protection against parasite infection
- Proteins:
  - Acute phase proteins, e.g. CRP, which is important in bacterial attack
  - Complement: a cascade of proteins synthesised in the liver for host defence; acts via two main pathways, the classical pathway, which is triggered by the antigen–antibody response; the alternative pathway, which is triggered in response to bacteria
  - Cytokines: small cell-signalling proteins involved in immune response, e.g. TNF, which is produced by macrophages against tumours; interleukins, which are produced by macrophages, neutrophils and T-cells; interferons, which are produced by T-cells (see below), natural killer cells and macrophages to enhance destruction of tumour and virally infected cells.

Adaptive mechanisms

Take longer to produce an effect but have memory and so allow a rapid response if the pathogen is encountered again. The effect is developed through the interaction of lymphocytes, B-cells and T-cells, and the production of antibodies (immunoglobulins):

- *B-cells*: produced in bone marrow and secrete antibodies, which are important in the attack of cells that are identified as dangerous, such as with a bacterial infection:
  - IgM primary response: first antibody to be produced, less specific
  - IgG secondary response: slower but more specific response than IgM; produced more rapidly after a second attack by the same antigen
- *T-cells*: produced in the thymus, and have direct roles and a role in stimulating B-cells:
  - T-helper type 1 (Th1): assist in production of cytotoxic T-cells, which kill virus-infected cells
  - T helper type 2 (Th2): activate B-cells to activate B-cells which produce antibody to immobilise bacteria
  - Cytotoxic T-cells (Tc): recognise viral antigens presented on the surface of a virally infected or otherwise damaged or dysfunctional cell by MHC molecules; the T-cell binds to the infected cell and releases cytokines, both of which lead to lysis of the damaged cell target.

Hypersensitivity reactions

These are exaggerated or inappropriate immune responses leading to tissue damage:

- They can be caused by external stimulus, e.g. pollen, persisting infections
- They can be classified into five categories (Table 11.1) (this is a common exam question).

Empirical choice of antibiotics

Although each clinical situation is different, there are some general guidelines for choosing empirical antibiotics:

- *Culture*: take plenty of blood and tissue to culture before starting treatment.

Table 11.1 The five types of hypersensitivity reactions

Type	Name	Response	Example
I	Acute allergic	Antigen induces an IgE antibody response Histamine released Reaction occurs in minutes	Hay fever Allergic reactions, e.g. to nuts
II	Antibody dependent cytotoxicity (autoimmune)	IgM, and IgG antibodies specific to cell antigen bind to cells. This leads to cell death from complement or phagocytosis	Goodpasture's disease Myasthenia gravis Haemolytic disease of the newborn
III	Immune complex mediated	Immune antigen–antibody complexes are produced and can be deposited either systematically or at the site of entry	Glomerulonephritis Vasculitis Farmer's lung disease
IV	T cell mediated Delayed	Contact with antigen leads to the activation of T cells Activates cytokines that activate macrophages Reaction peaks at 48–72 h	Granulomatous disease TB Leishmaniasis
V	Stimulatory	Antibodies against hormone receptors	Graves' disease

- *Allergy*: ask the patient for any allergies and ask exactly what happened and when; cephalosporins and carbapenems should generally not be used in patients with a clear history of severe penicillin allergy; however:
  - impurities in the early preparations of penicillin led to adverse reactions that do not occur with modern formulations
  - the benefits of using a beta-lactam may outweigh the risks in certain serious infections (e.g. pneumococcal meningitis) and so clear information on the degree of allergic reaction can help to inform this decision.
- *Appropriate antibiotics*: consult early with infectious disease physicians, microbiologists and read local hospital guidelines (Table 11.2). Table 11.3 outlines some infectious organisms and their features and table 11.4 summarises some key antibiotics, their mechanisms of action, indications and side effects.

See also system-specific infections

- Cardiology (Ch. 2): rheumatic fever, endocarditis, pericarditis
- Respiratory (Ch. 3): TB, pneumonia, empyema, lung abscess
- Gastroenterology (Ch. 4): gastroenteritis
- Hepatology (Ch. 5): viral hepatitis
- Neurology (Ch. 6): meningitis, encephalitis, brain abscess
- Renal system (Ch. 7): pyelonephritis, prostatitis
- Rheumatology (Ch. 10): septic arthritis, osteomyelitis, reactive arthritis
- Surgery (Ch. 13): cellulitis, necrotising fasciitis.

Table 11.2 Infections and appropriate antibiotic treatment

Infection	Causative organism	Treatment
Severe sepsis	Broad Gram positive and Gram negative cover	Co-amoxiclav or ceftriaxone or piperacillin/tazobactam Addition of gentamicin may help with Gram negative bacteraemia but if prolonged is associated with increased renal and ototoxicity
Risk of resistance	If recent institutional stay, recent antibiotics or previous culture data	Methicillin-resistant *Staphylococcus aureus* (MRSA): vancomycin or teicoplanin Extended spectrum beta-lactamases (ESBL): meropenem Not cephalosporins

Table 11.2 Infections and appropriate antibiotic treatment—cont'd

Infection	Causative organism	Treatment
Bacterial meningitis	*Neisseria meningitidis, Streptococcus pneumoniae, Listeria monocytogenes*	Ceftriaxone or chloramphenicol if severe penicillin allergy Add ampicillin to cover Listeria in the old, very young and pregnant
External communication	*Staphylococcus aureus* and *Pseudomonas aeruginosa*	Vancomycin and ceftazidime
Encephalitis	Usually herpes simplex virus (HSV)	Aciclovir
Brain abscess	Biopsy before treatment to identify. Look for clues of a peripheral source	Check CNS penetration of drugs: meropenem and ceftriaxone have good penetration
Pericarditis	Usually viral or TB	Microscopy and culture of pericardial fluid first
Endocarditis – native valve	50% *Streptococcus viridans* 30% *Staphylococcus aureus* 10% Enterococcus species 'HACEK' Gram negatives Culture negative – serology	Penicillin and gentamicin Flucloxacillin (vancomycin MRSA) Amoxicillin Ceftriaxone Seek advice
Endocarditis – prosthetic valve (2–3% annual risk)	First 2 months *Staphylococcus epidermidis* then usual suspects plus *Candida*	Multiple (6+) blood cultures off treatment Involve cardiothoracic surgery early
COPD	If infective: *Streptococcus pneumoniae, Haemophilus influenzae, Moraxella catarrhalis*	Amoxicillin or co-amoxiclav or doxycyline
Pneumonia	See respiratory section	
Food poisoning	*Campylobacter jejuni, Salmonella enteritidis, Shigella sonnei,* Enterohaemorrhagic *Escherichia coli*	Usually self-limiting, ciprofloxacin or azithromycin or no treatment
Cholangitis	Enteric Gram negatives	Beta-lactam and gentamicin or ciprofloxacin or Piperacillin/tazobactam
Liver abscess	Polymicrobial including anaerobes	Beta-lactam with metronidazole or piperacillin/tazobactam
	Consider amoebic liver abscess in travellers	Metronidazole then dioxanide or paramomycin
Bowel perforation	Polymicrobial including anaerobes	Beta-lactam and metronidazole or ciprofloxacin and metronidazole or piperacillin/tazobactam
Pyelonephritis	*Escherichia coli* *Klebsiella* spp.	Ciprofloxacin or co-amoxiclav Gentamicin good for bacteraemia Increasing frequency of resistant ESBL organisms particularly if recent antibiotics
Prostatitis	*Escherichia coli* *Klebsiella* spp.	Prolonged course of ciprofloxacin
Cellulitis	*Streptococcus pyogenes* *Staphylococcus aureus* (consider MRSA)	Flucloxacillin or clindamycin or beta-lactam
Necrotising fasciitis	*Streptococcus pyogenes* Polymicrobial in penetrating injuries	Surgical emergency: debridement High-dose clindamycin and penicillin and ciprofloxacin or piperacillin/tazobactam
Osteomyelitis	*Staphylococcus aureus, Mycobacterium tuberculosis, Salmonella,* others	Biopsy before antibiotics Two agents for a long time: clindamycin and ciprofloxacin is a good combination

Table 11.3 An outline of some infective organisms

Bacteria aerobes		Microorganism and outline	Disease
Cocci (spherical)	**Gram +ve** **Stain purple**	**Staphylococcus** • Seen as 'grape-like' clusters • Many species found naturally on the skin • Disease due to invasion or toxin mediated • Can produce β-lactamase that can break down β-lactam antibiotics Classification: *Coagulase +ve (causes clot formation)* • *Staphylococcus aureus*, produces extracellular toxins • May be toxin associated illness • Include MRSA subtypes *Coagulase −ve* • *Staphylococcus epidermidis*	Coagulase +ve • Skin: boils, impetigo, carbuncles, abscesses • Bone: osteomyelitis • Septic arthritis • Septicaemia *Toxin associated:* • Toxic shock syndrome • Scalded skin syndrome • Food poisoning Coagulase −ve • Wound infection • Infective endocarditis
		Streptococcus • Seen as a chain or a line as they divide along a single axis • Many species found naturally on the skin, in the respiratory tract, mouth and intestine • Can be classified according to whether they partially, completely or fail to haemolyse RBCs when plated on blood agar α haemolytic (partial haemolysis): • *Streptococcus viridans* • *Streptococcus pneumoniae* β haemolytic (complete haemolysis): Subdivided into Lancefield groups, according to the presence of antigens of the cell surface (A, B, C, F, G) • Group A: *streptococcus pyogenes*: produces toxins (streptolysin S, O, erythogenic toxin, streptokinase, hyaluronidase) • Group B *streptococcus* Non-haemolytic	**α haemolytic** *Viridans:* • Infective endocarditis • Aspiration pneumonia *Streptococcus pneumonia* • Pneumonia • Meningitis **β (complete)**, divided into: *Group A* • Pharyngitis • Impetigo • Cellulitis • Necrotising fasciitis • Scarlet fever • Sequelae: rheumatic fever, glomerulonephritis *Group B* • Neonatal sepsis • Abscesses Non-haemolytic *E. faecium:* UTI, endocarditis
		Enterococci • Occur in pairs or in chains • Gut commensals	• Urinary tract infections • Bacterial endocarditis

Bacilli (rods)	Gram −ve Stain red	**Neisseria meningitidis** • Grouped in pairs	• Meningitis • Bacteraemia • Can cause Waterhouse–Friderichsen syndrome (see Endocrinology chapter)
		Neisseria gonorrhoeae • Grouped in pairs	• Gonorrhoea (see below) • Bacteraemia
	Gram +ve	**Bacillus** • Rods	• *B. anthracis*: anthrax • *B. cereus*: food poisoning (often from rice), opportunistic infection
		Listeria monocytogenes • Common in animals, gets into the food chain • Dangerous for pregnant women as can harm the fetus	• Meningitis particularly in neonates (see Neurology chapter)
	Gram −ve	**Escherichia coli** • Intestinal commensal • *Escherichia coli* 0157 infection from eating infected meat (see Gastroenterology chapter)	• UTI (90%) See renal chapter • Neonatal meningitis • Hospital acquired pneumonia • Septicaemia • *E. coli* 01507: food poisoning, bloody diarrhoea, can lead to haemolytic uraemic syndrome
		Proteus • Intestinal commensal	• UTIs
		Salmonella	• Gastroenteritis and food poisoning (see Gastroenterology section) • Typhoid from salmonella typhi, transmitted through contaminated water (faeco–oral route) • Headache, dry cough, constipation, rising fever, relative bradycardia • Later: fever, diarrhoea, bruising, rose spots (rash) on the abdomen and thorax. In serious cases, splenomegaly, delirium and haemorrhage • Complications: osteomyelitis, meningitis, death
		Shigella • Transmitted by the faeco–oral route	• Dysentery

Continued

Table 11.3 An outline of some infective organisms—cont'd

Bacteria aerobes	Microorganism and outline	Disease
	Klebsiella • GI, urogenital and respiratory tract commensal	• UTIs • Pneumonia • Septicaemia
	Pseudomonas • Environmental organism, most live in the soil	• *P. aeruginosa*: opportunistic infection, e.g. ventilator-associated pneumonia (see Respiratory chapter), UTIs
	Haemophilus • β-lactamase-producing species • Non motile • Often found in the respiratory tract	• *H. influenzae*: meningitis, pneumonia, arthritis, osetomyelitis: affects mainly those <4 years • *H. ducreyi*: chancroid ulcer in the groin, sexually transmitted
	Legionella • Transmitted by water in aerosol form, e.g. air conditioning	• Legionnaires' disease: atypical pneumonia (see Respiratory chapter)
	Camplylobacter • Spiral, motile bacteria	• *C. jejuni*: commonest cause of food poisoning associated with chicken and pates (see Gastroenterology section). Often linked to Guillain-Barré syndrome
Anaerobes		
Cocci	**Gram +ve**	
	Anaerobic streptococci	• Abscesses
Rods	**Gram +ve**	
	Clostridium • Produce spores, exotoxins • Found in environment and GI tract • Where clostridium infection is suspected, hands should be washed well with soap and water rather than with alcoholic scrub alone as the spores are extremely resilient	• *C. perfringens*: gas gangrene, food poisoning • *C. tetani*: tetanus with contaminated wounds • *C. botulinum*: found in badly canned foods leading to severe food poisoning and botulism • *C. difficile*: pseudomembranous colitis, a normal gut commensal that causes colitis associated with antibiotic therapy particularly from clindamycin. The antibiotics kill the competing bacteria and allow the *C. difficile* to proliferate producing toxins. Can lead to toxic megacolon that can be life threatening
	Gram −ve	
	Bacteroides • β-lactamase-producing species • Normal flora of GI tract	• Abscesses

Other bacteria

Spirochaetes (Gram −ve, spiral shape important for its motility)	**Treponema** • Commensal and pathogenic	• *T. pallidum*: syphilis
	Borrelia • Commensal (oro-pharynx) and pathogenic • Transmitted by ticks and lice	• ***B. burgdorferi*: Lyme disease** transmitted by ticks • Localised rash, fever, headache, arthralgia and malaise • ~2/3 develop arthritis over months or years • May have cardiovascular and neurological symptoms • Many patients will not recall being bitten • *B. recurrentis*: relapsing fever
	Leptospira • Commensal and pathogenic • Rat acts as a reservoir	• Leptospirosis or Weil's disease: • Fever, headache, vomiting, jaundice, renal failure • Often caused by exposure to rat urine, e.g. in stagnant water
	Helicobacter pylori (see Gastroenterology chapter) • Infects the mucous lining of the stomach and duodenum • Produces urease	• Peptic ulcers • Gastritis, duodenitis • Gastric cancer
Obligate intracellular bacteria	**Chlamydia** • Not visible on Gram stain • *Chlamydia psittaci* carried by birds • Diagnosis usually serological	• *C. trachomatis*: sexually transmitted • *C. pneumoniae*: atypical pneumonia (see Respiratory chapter) • *C. psittaci*: psittacosis: atypical pneumonia (see Respiratory chapter)
	Rickettsia • Not visible on Gram stain • Transmitted by ticks, mites and lice	• Typhus: headache, rash, high fever, jaundice, delirium particularly in overcrowded areas with unsanitary conditions • Epidemics occur during times of war or famine

Continued

479

Table 11.3 An outline of some infective organisms—cont'd

Bacteria aerobes **Other organisms**	Microorganism and outline	Disease	Treatment
Fungi	• Eukaryotes, larger than bacteria • A few species are pathogenic in humans due to allergy, inflammation and tissue invasion Classification: • *Yeasts*: asexual budding: *Cryptococcus neoformans* • *Yeast-like fungi*, e.g. *Candida albicans* • *Moulds*: interlacing branching hyphae, e.g. *Aspergillus*	• *Cryptococcus neoformans*: pneumonia and meningitis particularly in immunocompromised patients. Diagnosed on Indian ink staining of CSF • *Candida albicans*: thrush, endocarditis, sepsis in the immunocompromised • *Aspergillus*: invasive infection in immunocompromised or allergic response e.g. asthma, allergic bronchopulmonary aspergillosis • *Pneumocystis*: pneumonia (AIDS defining illness)	Antifungals: • Polyene macrolides: bind to ergosterol in the fungal membrane resulting in pores in the cell wall e.g. amphotericin B, nystatin (for thrush) • Imidazoles: inhibit ergosterol synthesis e.g. clotrimazole, ketoconazole (for seborrhoeic dermatitis) • Traizoles: inhibit ergosterol synthesis e.g. fluconazole, itraconazole (both are broad spectrum but itraconazole can also be used for *Aspergillus*)
Protozoa	• Microscopic single-celled organisms Classification: • Amoebae: amoeboid movement • Flagellates: flagella (tail) present • Ciliates: cilia present for movement • Sporozoans: no appendage for locomotion	Amoebae: • *Entamoeba histolytica*: amoebic dysentery and liver abscess (see Hepatology chapter) Flagellates: • *Giardia lamblia*: giardiasis, infects the gut causing abdominal pain, explosive diarrhoea, bloating and malabsorption • *Trichomonas*: vaginitis • *Leishmania*: leishmaniasis spread by sand flies. Can be cutaneous affecting the skin, mucocutaneous (1° skin lesions spread to the mucosa) or visceral (most serious)	• *Entamoeba histolytica*: metronidazole • *Giardia*: metronidazole • *Trichomonas*: metonidazole • Malaria: see below

Helminths	• Parasitic worms Classification: • Cestodes: tape worms • Nematodes: round worms • Trematodes: flukes	• *African trypanosomes*: sleeping sickness spread by the tsetse fly. Initially causes fever, rash and headaches, then weeks or months later infection of the brain leads to convulsions, dementia, hypersomnolence and death • *American trypansomiasis*: chagras disease caused by *T. cruzi* Sporozoans: • *Plasmodium* spp: malaria	Anti-helminths • Cestodes: nicosamide, praziquantel • Nematodes: mebendazole, thiabendazole, dethycarbamazine • Trematodes: praziquantel
		Cestodes: • *Taenia solium*: eating uncooked pork containing eggs or larvae of the tapeworm causes to cysticercosis. Can affect the muscles, CNS, eyes and skin • *Taenia saginata*: from eating uncooked beef Nematodes: • *Strongyloides stercoralis*: septicaemia and meningitis • *Enterobius vernicularis*: thread worm Trematodes: • Schistosomiasis (bilharziasis): freshwater snail carriers act as vectors. The parasitic worms penetrate human skin during swimming in infected waters. Flukes invade and destroy blood vessels of the gut, bladder and liver. Causes abdominal pain, diarrhoea, hepatosplenomegaly, cirrhosis and anaemia. Infection of the bladder increases the risk of squamous cell carcinoma there (see Nephrology chapter)	

Table 11.4 Antibiotics

Group	Type	Mechanism of action	Indications	Benefits	Side effects and problems
Penicillins	• Penicillin V (oral) • Procaine (IM) • Benzylpenicillin/ penicillin G (IV)	All penicillins and their derivatives: • Inhibit bacterial cell wall synthesis by inhibition of peptidoglycan synthesis within the wall • Have a β-lactam ring as part of its structure • Are bactericidal	• Good for Gram +ve bacteria, particularly *streptococci* and *Neisseria meningitidis* • Streptococcal infection • Cellulitis • Pneumococcal pneumonia • Infective endocarditis • Syphilis • Meningitis	• Well tolerated	• Adverse reaction in 1–10%: rash and diarrhoea (common), anaphylaxis (rarer) • Destroyed by β-lacatamase that breaks down the β-lactam ring. The enzyme is produced by *S. aureus* and some anaerobes
	Flucloxacillin	• As above • β-lactamase stable	• First choice for *Staphylococcus* • Osteomyelitis • Septic arthritis • Cellulitis • Infective endocarditis		• Not effective against MRSA strains
Broad-spectrum penicillins	Amoxicillin	• As above	• For Gram +ve and some Gram –ve bacteria, e.g. pneumococcus, *Listeria*, enterococci • Good for pregnant women with UTIs		
	Co-amoxiclav (trade name: Augmentin)	• Composite of amoxicillin and clavulinic acid • Clavulinic acid is a β-lactamase inhibitor	• Sepsis • After colonic surgery • Appendicitis • Atypical pneumonia	• Anti-anaerobic activity	
Extended specificity penicillins	Piptazobactam 'Tazocin': • Piperacillin • Tazobactam	• Has β-lactamase activity • IV preparation only	• For Gram +ve and –ve, aerobic and pseudomonal infection • Good for *Pseudomonas* infection, premature babies, intensive care ventilators		

Carbapenems: • Meropenem • Ertapenem	• IV preparation only • Resistant to many β-lactamases	• Extremely good broad-spectrum activity • Good for extended spectrum beta-lactamase producing bacteria	• Given if resistant to Tazocin • Effective anti-anaerobic activity • Meropenam: good anti-pseudomonal activity	Avoid in pregnancy
Cephalosporins	• 1st generation: cefadroxil • 2nd generation: cefuroxime IV • 3rd generation: ceftazidime, cefixime, ceftriaxone	• Inhibits bacterial cell wall synthesis by inhibition of the peptidoglycan synthesis within the wall • Has a β-lactam ring as part of its structure • Has some β-lactamase activity • Bactericidal	• Cefadroxil: pregnant women with UTIs • Cefotriaxone and cefotaxime: for meningitis	• Broad spectrum • Ceftazidime is anti-pseudomonal	• Allergic reactions: 10% of those with penicillin allergies • No anaerobic effect so often used with metronidazole
Glycopeptides	• Vancomycin • Teicoplanin	• Inhibit cell wall synthesis by inhibition of peptidoglycan synthesis • Bactericidal • Not well absorbed orally	• Reserved for severe Gram +ve infections resistant to penicillins, e.g. MRSA infections and for Clostridium difficile in pseudomembranous colitis	• Very good action against Gram +ve cocci	• Nephrotoxic • Ototoxic • Rashes: red man syndrome • Increasing resistance (particularly enterococci)
Macrolides	• Erythromycin • Clarithromycin • Azithromycin	• Inhibit bacterial protein synthesis by preventing movement of the ribosome along the mRNA	• Only for Gram +ve bacteria • Good for atypical pneumonia • Erythromycin: often first-line if penicillin allergic • Azithromycin: treatment of sexually transmitted diseases	• Well tolerated	• GI upset • Jaundice • Erythromycin inhibits cytochrome P450 causing drug interactions • Avoid in pregnancy
Lincosamides	• Clindamycin	• Inhibit bacterial protein synthesis by preventing movement of the ribosome along the mRNA	• Anti-staphylococcus, streptococcus • Good bone penetration: alternative to flucloxacillin and fusidic acid	• Good anti-anaerobic activity	• High risk of pseudomembranous colitis • Avoid in pregnancy
Quinolones	• Ciprofloxacin • Levofloxacin • Moxifloxacin	• Inhibits DNA gyrase, an enzyme important for DNA replication and repair as it	• Broad-spectrum, anti-staphylococcus but not anti-streptococcus	• Good anti-pseudomonal activity	• No anaerobic effect so often used with metronidazole • GI side effects

Continued

Table 11.4 Antibiotics—cont'd

Group	Type	Mechanism of action	Indications	Benefits	Side effects and problems
		• prevents supercoiling of the DNA • Bactericidal	• Salmonella food poisoning • Children with cystic fibrosis with superimposed infection		• Tendon rupture • Avoid in pregnancy
Aminoglycosides	• Gentamicin • Netilmicin • Amikacin	• Inhibits bacterial protein synthesis by inhibiting translation • Bactericidal	• Reserved for severe Gram −ve infection • Anti-staphylococcus, not anti-streptococcus • Requires penicillin effect on cell walls before being active against streptococcus	• Good anti-pseudomonal activity	• Nephrotoxic • Ototoxic • Requires monitoring as has a narrow therapeutic index • Reduce dose with renal impairment • Avoid in pregnancy: auditory and vestibular damage
Tetracyclines	• Doxycycline • Minocycline • Tetracycline	• Inhibit bacterial protein synthesis • Affects attachment of tRNA to mRNA • Bacteriostatic	• Broad spectrum including most atypical organisms • *Chlamydia* • *Rickettsia* • *Brucella* • *Borrelia*		• Deposited in teeth causing grey staining and affect bone growth so avoid in pregnancy and children under 12 • Can exacerbate renal impairment
Dihydrofolate reductase inhibitors	• Trimethoprim • Co-trimoxazole: trimethoprim with sulfamethoxazole	• Folate is needed for DNA synthesis • Trimethoprim acts as an antifolate by inhibiting dihydrofolate reductase • Bacteriostatic	• UTIs • Respiratory tract infections • Co-trimoxazole: pneumocystis jiroveci pneumonia	• Broad spectrum • Well tolerated	• Myelosuppression • Agranulocytosis • Avoid in pregnancy
Nitromidazole	• Metronidazole	• Inhibits bacterial DNA synthesis • Bactericidal	• For anaerobic bacteria and protozoal infections	• Good for *Clostridium difficile* and anaerobic bacteria	• Headache • GI disturbance • Adverse reactions with alcohol • Avoid in pregnancy

THE SEPTIC PATIENT

Outline

- Systemic illness caused by infection
- 25% of acute medical admissions to UK hospitals are associated with infectious disease
- Severe sepsis has a high mortality

The Surviving Sepsis Campaign:
- International initiative to ↓ death from severe sepsis and septic shock
- Guidelines focus on early recognition, aggressive fluid resuscitation, use of correct empirical antibiotics and early referral to ITU
- Management of severe sepsis centres around 'bundles of care' including the resuscitation bundle which must be delivered within 6 h

- The 'sepsis six' has been developed as a simplified version of aspects of the resuscitation bundle that any health professional can deliver within 1 h. It includes:
  1. High flow O_2
  2. Blood cultures
  3. IV antibiotics
  4. IV fluid resuscitation
  5. Hb and lactate levels checked
  6. Monitor urine output hourly
- Death rates from sepsis have ↓ since the campaign was introduced.

Pathogenesis/aetiology

Causes

- Infection can be due to a large number of microorganisms in any part of the body
- The key is to identify the source of infection; until then, the surviving sepsis campaign provides a common pathway for acute management
- Construct an early differential diagnosis to focus initial investigations and empiric therapy. Remember to take a travel history

- Think about HIV infection and other causes of immunosuppression (long-term steroids, monoclonal antibody therapies, alcohol excess, renal disease, myeloma, etc.) and have a low threshold for investigating
- Common variable immunodeficiency (CVID) is a rare (1:50 000) and treatable cause of recurrent infections. Diabetes is much more common and more often missed.

Who

- Typical age: all ages at risk but extremes of life carry the highest risks due to impaired barriers and weaker immune response
- Old people may not mount a febrile response and may present late with less obvious clinical signs
- The type and degree of immunosuppression influences the likely pathogens and modifies the presentation and clinical course

- Think in broad terms of:
  - hospital acquired vs. community acquired
  - immunosuppressed vs. immunocompetent
  - acute vs. chronic
  - organ-specific vs. systemic infection.

Symptoms and signs

Systemic inflammatory response syndrome (SIRS):
- 2 or more of:
  - temperature >38 °C or <36 °C
  - heart rate >90 bpm
  - respiratory rate >20/min
  - WBC >12 or <4

Sepsis syndrome
- Systemic inflammatory response syndrome plus clinical suspicion of infection

Severe sepsis
- Sepsis and organ dysfunction; i.e. any of the following:
  - Pao_2 <8 kPa
  - Lactate >4 mmol/L
  - Oliguria (Urinary output <30 mL/h)
  - Reduced Glasgow Coma Scale

Septic shock
- Sepsis and BP <90 mmHg despite initial fluid challenge

Investigations

History:
- A detailed history including:
  - Travel times and destinations
  - Personal activities and contacts

- Previous antibiotic therapy
- Allergies

Examination:
- Keep examining the patient as their illness evolves.

- Arterial (not venous) blood lactate: useful indicator of severity
- CRP, ESR, WBC, U&Es.

- Culture ± microscopy of: blood, throat swab, sputum, urine, stool, vaginal, cervical, urethra as appropriate.

- CXR
- CT

- ECG: cardiac disease
- Echocardiogram: endocarditis

- For associated latent infections:
  - Tropical parasites in travellers
  - Transmissible viruses in IDUs
  - Genitourinary infections in the sexually active
- HIV test in those with indicator diseases or from highly endemic regions
  - TB in those from high prevalence countries.

- Take plenty of cultures at presentation, then start empiric antibiotics based on differential diagnosis
- Read the hospital guidelines for local policy. Phone the infectious diseases team to discuss the options
- Hold off broad-spectrum agents unless the patient is very sick and initial choice cannot afford to be wrong. Take plenty of cultures so that a rational decision to step down therapy can be made later
- Remove unnecessary cannulae
- Involve surgical colleagues early: excision or drainage the best approach for many localised infections
- Use imaging to guide tissue biopsy and drainage
- Stop antibiotics if the clinical picture changes and preculture if patients become unwell in hospital

Sepsis:
- Follow the guidelines for the Surviving Sepsis Campaign
- For severe sepsis follow the 'sepsis six' within the first hour.

- Most patients make a full recovery from infections
- Severe sepsis mortality rates are high (>25%) and it should be treated quickly.

- Infectious risk to others: make an early assessment; know the infection control measures to be followed.

DISORDERS ASSOCIATED WITH TRAVEL

ENTERIC FEVER

- Illness caused by *Salmonella typhi* and *Salmonella paratyphi* strains leading to systemic disease. Spread by faeco–oral route
- Also called typhoid fever
- Important cause of illness in children in the tropics; uncommon cause of progressive fever in returning travellers, particularly from South Asia
- There is syndromic overdiagnosis where there is poor access to blood and stool culture facilities
- The widely used Widal antibody test has poor specificity and is not recommended.

- Ingestion of contaminated food or water leads to a 1° gastroenteritis followed by a systemic febrile illness as the bacteria spread to the reticulo-endothelial system for phagocytosis.
- Incubation period from a few days to months; most patients develop symptoms within a few weeks of returning from travel
- Transmission persists due to asymptomatic carriage and secretion in stool and urine.

Who

- 400 cases/year are reported in the UK Health Protection Agency
- Commoner in children in endemic areas: outbreaks in areas of poor hygiene

- Carriage is associated with gallstones, bladder stones, schistosomiasis and HIV.

Symptoms and signs

Uncomplicated:
- First symptoms: prolonged fever, rigors, sweats and myalgia, in common with many systemic infections
- GI disturbance with diarrhoea or constipation and right upper quadrant pain
- Headache and dry cough
- Mild hepatosplenomegaly
- Rose spots (~0.5 cm rose-coloured macular lesions occurring in groups on the trunk or chest about 7 days after initial symptoms)

Severe (uncommon in travellers):
- Shock
- Intestinal perforation
- Lower GI bleeding
- Mycotic aneurysm (aneurysm from an infectious process): in the elderly
- Arthritis and osteomyelitis: rare confusion and reduced consciousness.

Investigations

Blood tests

- FBC: usually a normal differential white count and platelets
- LFTs: mildly raised hepatic transaminases

- CRP: mildly raised
- Normal CRP and ALT have a strong negative predictive value.

Other tests

Diagnostic:
- Blood: Gram negative rods (>80%)
- Stool cultures: positive early in infection and in asymptomatic carriage (>60%)
- Bone marrow aspirate and culture: best yield (>90%), if the clinical suspicion is high but the patient has received prior antibiotics

- Urine: *Salmonella* can occasionally be cultured
- Widal test is not useful due to poor specificity.

Treatment

Uncomplicated:
- Antibiotics:
  - Ciprofloxacin
  - Azithromycin
  - Ceftriaxone
- High levels of relative resistance to ciprofloxacin, particularly in Asia (>50%), means that it is no longer recommended as empirical therapy from this region

- Plasmid-mediated resistance often exists with amoxicillin, co-trimoxazole and chloramphenicol
Severe:
- Ceftriaxone
- Add dexamethasone if in shock
Prevention:
- Public health measures, e.g. clean water
- *Salmonella typhi* vaccine confers ~70% protection.

Prognosis and complications

Prognosis

- Can become a chronic carrier: 1%
- Untreated: mortality is about 10%

- Treated: <1% mortality.

Public health

- Notifiable disease

- Food handlers and healthcare staff should demonstrate clearance of infection with sequential stool samples before returning to work.

MALARIA

Outline

- Infection of red blood cells (RBCs) by a protozoan parasite spread by the *Anopheles* mosquito
- A leading cause of death and morbidity in the tropics, particularly in African children
- Malaria is the most important infection to consider in unwell travellers returning from the tropics

- The minimum incubation period is a week and most patients present within a month or at the latest three months after travel (but often months to years later with the benign types).

Classification

Serious:
- *Plasmodium falciparum*

Benign:
- *Plasmodium vivax*
- *Plasmodium ovale*
- *Plasmodium knowlesi*
- *Plasmodium malariae*

Plasmodium falciparum malaria is a medical emergency as patients deteriorate rapidly
If there is uncertainty about the species, treat for falciparum malaria.

Pathogenesis/aetiology

Pathogenesis

The lifecycle of malaria parasite:
- An infected female *Anopheles* mosquito bites a person and sporozoites from the saliva enter the blood and travel to the liver where they multiply and differentiate to become merozoites
- Merozoites leave the liver and invade RBC causing symptoms
- Parasites multiply 4 or 5 times in RBCs and become trophozoites and then schizonts, which are released to preinfect more RBCs
- Classically this cycle occurs every 48 h (or every 72 h for *Plasmodium malariae*) although in reality many patients have several parasites in different phases

- *Plasmodium ovale* and *Plasmodium vivax* have a latent 'hypnozoite' phase in the liver which may cause recurrences of malaria months or years after initial infection
- The key pathological process in *Plasmodium falciparum* infection is sequestration where infected RBCs adhere to the endothelial linings of small vessels causing tissue hypoperfusion and organ dysfunction
- *Plasmodium knowlesi:* has been described in patients from SE Asia, particularly Borneo. It looks like *Plasmodium malariae* on the blood film but has a replication cycle of 24 hours. It can be rapidly fatal but responds to the same treatment as other malarias.

Who

- 200 million patients infected per year world wide and >1 million deaths (mainly in African children)
- Children who grow up in high transmission (endemic) areas are likely to develop partial immunity through repeated infection or die in childhood as a consequence. This protection rapidly wanes when they leave the endemic area and upon return years later they are at similar risk to a 'naïve' traveller

- Patients from low transmission (epidemic) areas have fewer infections in childhood and are therefore more likely to experience clinical illness in adulthood.

A typical patient

A young women presents with fever that has occurred on and off over the last week with night sweats and myalgia. Careful history reveals she has recently been to see her family in Africa and did not take any malarial prophylaxis.

Symptoms and signs

Clinical features

- Almost any symptoms are compatible with malaria. The decision to test should be based on the patient's epidemiological risk
- Fever, rigors, myalgia and night sweats are common
- May also present with diarrhoea, cough or confusion and thus mimic the acute presentation of a wide range of medical emergencies
- Splenomegaly is common

Markers of severe falciparum malaria:

- Confusion/coma/seizures
- Hypoglycaemia
- Pallor from profound anaemia from damage to RBC
- Renal failure: more often due to acute tubular necrosis from dehydration and sepsis than from blackwater fever (See Complications)
- Breathlessness: due to acidosis, acute lung injury or, particularly in African children, coexistent pneumonia
- Patients may also have:
  - jaundice from haemolysis and raised bilirubin
  - disseminated intravascular coagulation
  - shock.

Investigations

Gold standard diagnosis:

- Thick blood film: most sensitive
- Thin blood film: more specific and good for determining the species and parasitaemia (the percentage of infected or parasitised RBCs on thin film)
- Parasitaemia is a good marker of severity for falciparum malaria. Severity:
  - In the UK: >2%
  - WHO guidelines for endemic regions: >5%
  - Patients may occasionally have a parasite count of >30%

- Dipstick antigen tests are increasingly used where experienced microscopists are not available (e.g. African villages or UK hospitals that seldom see malaria). They are slightly less sensitive than microscopy and cannot be used to determine the stage or parasitaemia
- Polymerase chain reaction (PCR) is used by reference laboratories to confirm infections that may have been partially treated – nucleic acid can be detected in peripheral blood 1–2 weeks after treatment

Other tests

- FBC
- Clotting
- Blood glucose
- ABG
- U&E
- Lactate
- Blood cultures
- Urinalysis
- CXR.

Treatment

- *Plasmodium falciparum* is a medical emergency
- Severe malaria should be managed in a high dependency setting.

Medical

- Most strains are sensitive to quinine so this is the drug of choice if the species is unknown or uncertain
- Quinine resistance in falciparum malaria is spreading through South-East Asia and artemisinin derivatives are the drugs of choice for patients from this region.
- All benign malarias respond to chloroquine
- *Plasmodium vivax* and *Plasmodium ovale* require an additional course of primaquine to eradicate the hypnozoite stage

Plasmodium falciparum
Severe:

- Quinine (or artesunate if available)

Uncomplicated:

- Quinine or artemisinin: artemisinin-based combination therapy (ACT); or mefloquine or malarone if not used for prophylaxis

- Patients should have daily blood films. Once the parasites have disappeared they should have a second longer acting agent such as fansidar or doxycyline to remove the low level of parasites not visible on the film
- Exchange transfusions are no longer recommended by most specialist centres

Non-falciparum:

- Chloroquine followed by primaquine

Prevention:

- Avoid bites: use repellent, wear long sleeves and socks particularly in the evenings and sleep under an insecticide-impregnated bednet

Chemoprophylaxis (98% effective) if taken properly:

- Atovaquone and proguanil (Malarone)
- Mefloquine (Lariam)
- Doxycycline.

Prognosis

- Overall mortality in UK adult travellers is 1% but this rises to 8% in the elderly
- Outcomes are worse in children in the developing world with poor access to high dependency care (>20% mortality and neurological morbidity with severe malaria)

Poor prognosis:
- Very young or elderly
- Malnourished
- Pregnant women
- Severe features:
  - Hyperparasitaemia
  - Cerebral malaria

Complications

- Blackwater fever: severe intravascular haemolysis as a complication of *Plasmodium falciparum* leading to haematuria seen as dark or black urine. May lead to kidney failure and has a high mortality

Anti-malarial side effects:
- Quinine: hypoglycaemia, tinnitus, temporary blindness
- Mefloquine: dizzy, insomnia, neuropsychiatric signs
- Doxycycline: photosensitivity, thrush, oesophagitis.

SEXUALLY TRANSMITTED DISEASES

HERPES SIMPLEX VIRUS

Outline

- A contagious virus from the human herpes family that causes cold sores and genital warts
- Two forms: HSV-1 and HSV-2

- Orogenital contact allows either virus to affect either site.

Classification

HSV-1:
- Virus enters the mouth or skin from infected saliva
- Causes cold sores
- Latent virus remains in the dorsal root trigeminal ganglion

HSV-2:
- Associated with genital, peri-genital or anal skin sites
- Usually spread by sexual contact
- Latent virus remains in the dorsal route sacral ganglia.

Pathogenesis/aetiology

Types of infection:
- Primary infection:
  - In susceptibles with no antibodies to HSV
- Recurrent infection:
  - Recurrence (reactivation) of HSV
  - Milder episodes
  - Stimuli for reactivation:
    - Stress
    - Fever
    - Exposure to ultraviolet light.

  - Tissue damage
  - Immunocompromise
Disseminated HSV:
- In immunosuppressed
- Affects organs including the liver and brain
HSV neonatal disease:
- 1 in 5000 deliveries/year
- Neonate acquires HSV in utero
- Can cause encephalitis and death.

Who

HSV-1:
- 50% of adults are HSV-1+ve
- 30% have recurrent infections
- Common in children

HSV-2:
- Sexual contact
- Causes most genital infections
- Associated with an ↑ risk of HIV infection.

Symptoms and signs

HSV-1:
Herpes gingivostomatitis:
- Primary HSV, often the first presentation
- Inflammation of the gums
- Associated with malaise, fever and lymphadenopathy
- Commonly affects children
Herpes labialis:
- HSV infects the oropharyngeal mucosa causing cold sores

- Cold sores indicate recurrent infection: pain and tingling then vesicles and crust which heals within 8–10 days
- Commonest form of HSV-1
HSV-2:
Genital herpes:
- Macules, papules and ulcers lasting 3 weeks
- Pain in the groin and thighs on recurrent infection.

Investigations

- Viruses isolated from swabs of vesicles, throat, nasopharynx, blood sample (Fig. 11.1)

HSV encephalitis:
- See Complications
- CSF (via lumbar puncture) PCR to detect HSV DNA
- CT head: to exclude other causes of presenting neurology.

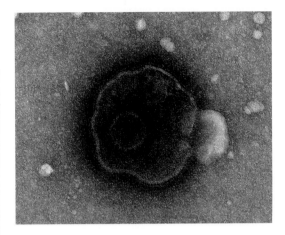

Fig. 11.1   Herpes simplex virus: 'fried egg' appearance of the herpes virus under electron microscope.

Treatment

Prevention:
- Education
- Caesarean section for expectant mothers with active infection

Treatment:
- Aciclovir: topical, oral or IV (IV for HSV encephalitis)
- Valaciclovir and famciclovir
- If HSV encephalitis is suspected, treat empirically with aciclovir.

Prognosis and complications

Prognosis

- Latency of the virus means that it remains for life

- HSV encephalitis (see below): mortality if untreated >70%.

Complications

From both HSV-1 or HSV-2:
- HSV encephalitis:
  - Encephalitis caused by HSV, often with temporal lobe symptoms
- HSV keratoconjunctivitis:
  - Unilateral or bilateral conjunctivitis

- Herpetic whitlow:
  - Painful infections of fingers
  - Common in medical and dental personnel.

SYPHILIS

Outline

- Sexually transmitted disease caused by *Treponema pallidum,* a motile spirochete
- Mimics many other diseases.
Some forms of syphilis:
- General paralysis of the insane: psychoses due to syphilis with additional features such as dementia, Argyll Robertson pupils and seizures

- Tabes dorsalis: progressive degenerative disease of the dorsal columns; symptoms include paraesthesia, ataxia, incontinence and dementia.

Pathogenesis/aetiology

Causes

Congenital:
- Vertical transmission: mother to child in utero
- Early stage: 2–6 weeks after birth
- Late stage: latent until >2 years old

Acquired:
- *Treponema pallidum* enters the host through a breach in the skin, most commonly during sex
- The initial site of infection is the site of exposure, usually the genitals, perianal area or mouth
- Also has early and late stages of presenting symptoms

Early stage:
- Primary and secondary syphilis

Early latency:
- Symptoms do not manifest until later but within 2 years. Occurs in 20%

Late stage:
- Tertiary syphilis. Very rare
- Symptoms due to gumma, which are granulomatous lesions in the liver, skin, bone (mainly skull, tibia, fibula and clavicle) and testes.

Who

- Rare in developed countries.

Symptoms and signs

Congenital syphilis:
- Early stage:
  - Stillbirth (30%)
  - Nasal discharge
  - Failure to thrive
- Late stage:
  - Teeth and bone abnormalities

Acquired syphilis:
- Primary syphilis:
  - Incubation: 10–90 days
  - Papule at site of infection
  - Ulcerates to painless solitary ulcer (chancre)
  - Regional lymphadenopathy
  - Heals within 2–3 weeks
- Secondary syphilis:
  - Systemic illness 4–10 weeks after 1° syphilis, subsides within a year

- Reddish, scaly skin rash over hands and feet that is non itchy
- Condylomata lata: warty perianal lesions
- Superficial mouth or genital ulcers (snail track)
- Sore throat
- Lymphadenopathy
- Arthralgia
- Tertiary syphilis (late stage syphilis):
  - >2 years after 1° infection
  - Almost any organ affected
  - Cardiovascular syphilis: aortic regurgitation or aneurysm, angina
  - Neurosyphilis: general paralysis of the insane, tabes dorsalis, otosyphilis
  - Bony changes, e.g. sabre tibia (convex deformity of the tibia).

Investigations

Microscopy:
- Dark ground illumination microscopy of fluid from lesions: illuminated motile spirochaetes

Serology:
- Venereal Disease Research Laboratories (VDRL) testing and rapid plasma reagin (RPR) tests. Detectable within 3–4 weeks of infection. Non-specific tests that become −ve after treatment
- *Treponema pallidum* haemagglutination assay (TPHA): confirms the RPR, remains +ve for life

Serology interpretation:
- RPR and TPHA +ve: active or treated syphilis
- RPR and TPHA −ve: no active or previous infection
- RPR −ve and TPHA +ve: treated or untreated late syphilis
- RPR +ve and TPHA −ve: false +ve RPR.

Treatment

- Antibiotics: IM benzathine penicillin for 10 days
- Alternative: doxycycline orally for 14 days

Tertiary syphilis:
- Antibiotics: IM benzathine penicillin for 4 weeks

- Alternative: doxycycline orally for 4 weeks

Follow-up:
- For 1 year after treatment
- Follow up sexual contacts.

Prognosis and complications

Prognosis

- Early syphilis: if treated, has a good prognosis

- Cardiovascular and neurological manifestations may be more permanent.

Complications

Jarisch–Herxheimer reaction:
- Malaise, fever and headache for 24 h
- Due to massive release of cytokines during antibiotic therapy in those with primary or secondary syphilis

- Treat with paracetamol/aspirin.

GONORRHOEA

Outline

- Sexually transmitted disease caused by *Neisseria gonorrhoeae*, a Gram –ve diplococcus
- Infects epithelium particularly of the:
  - urogenital tract
  - rectum
  - pharynx
  - conjunctivae
- Incubation period: 2–6 days.

Pathogenesis/aetiology

Transmission:
- Sexual intercourse

- Pregnancy: in 0.1% of pregnancies.

Who

- Typical age: adolescents and young adults
- 1♀:1.5♂
- Common

Risk factors:
- Homosexual men.

Symptoms and signs

- Asymptomatic in >50% of women, 2% of men
- Purulent discharge
- Perianal or anal discomfort
- Urethritis
- Dysuria
- Homosexual men: pruritus ani and pain

Babies:
- Preterm birth
- Neonatal conjunctivitis: ophthalmia neonatorum at 2–5 days.

Investigations

Asymptomatic:
- First catch urine for nucleic acid amplification test (NAAT)

Symptomatic:
- First catch urine

- Throat swab: culture only, no microscopy needed
- Gram stain and culture of urethral or endocervical swab
- Blood culture and synovial fluid microscopy in disseminated gonorrhoea.

Treatment

- Gonoccocal urethritis: cefixime or ceftriaxone or spectinomycin in one dose
- Neonatal conjunctivitis: erythromycin with ophthalmology review

Advice and follow-up:
- All patients should be treated for *Chlamydia* as well
- Repeat culture tests 72 h after completed treatment
- Advised to see health for partner notification and follow-up
- Partners given ceftriaxone.

Prognosis and complications

Complications

- Serious complications commoner in females
- Bacteraemia: rash and arthritis
- Acute septic arthritis
- Skin lesions

- Fitz-Hugh–Curtis syndrome (perihepatitis as a complication of pelvic inflammatory disease (PID))
- *Men*: epididymitis, prostatitis
- *Women*: salpingitis, PID
- Infertility.

CHLAMYDIA

Outline

- Sexually transmitted disease caused by *Chlamydia trachomatis*, a Gram −ve bacteria
- Incubation period: 6–14 days (longer interval than gonorrhoea)

- Also causes reactive arthritis (see Ch. 10)
Reactive arthritis:
- Conjunctivitis, urethritis, arthritis: 'Cannot see, cannot pee, cannot bend the knee'.

Pathogenesis/aetiology

Transmission:
- Sexual intercourse

- Pregnancy: in 5% of pregnancies.

Who

- Commonest sexually transmitted bacteria in the developed world

- 5–10% sexually active women infected
- Often occurs with gonorrhoea infection.

Symptoms and signs

- Asymptomatic in >50%
- Urethritis
- Discharge: not normally purulent
- Dysuria
- Women: postcoital or intermenstrual bleeding, lower abdominal pain

Babies:
- Preterm birth
- Neonatal conjunctivitis: at 7–10 days
- Pneumonia.

Investigations

- First catch urine

- Cervical or urethral swab.

Treatment

- Azithromycin single dose, od doxycycline (contraindicated in pregnancy: causes permanent tooth discoloration in fetus) for 7 days
- Erythromycin also used
- Neonatal conjunctivitis: eryrthromycin with ophthalmology review

Advice and follow-up:
- All patients should be treated for gonorrhoea as well
- Culture tests repeated 72 h after completed treatment
- Advised to see health advisers to organise partner notification and follow-up.

Prognosis and complications

Complications

- Subfertility
- Chronic pelvic pain
- Pelvic inflammatory disease (PID): 10–40%
- Adult conjunctivitis

- Reactive arthritis or Reiter syndrome: more common in men
- Epididymo-orchitis.

HUMAN IMMUNODEFICIENCY VIRUS (HIV)

Outline

- A blood-bourne virus that infects CD4+ T-cells of the immune system, leading to AIDS
- AIDS: a disease caused by the HIV virus, leading to weakening of the immune system so that the person is exposed to opportunistic infection. There are certain typical illnesses associated with AIDS that occur when the CD4 count falls low enough
- The main UK challenge is detecting cases by targeted testing.

Pathogenesis/aetiology

Pathogenesis

- HIV is a single-stranded RNA lentivirus, a subgroup of retrovirus
- Virus infects CD4+ T-cells which are important in the immune response
- HIV binds to the CD4 cell membrane via an envelope glycoprotein (gp120) and gains entry
- In the cell, viral reverse transcriptase makes a DNA copy of its RNA. Viral integrase then inserts this into the host DNA
- Once inserted, viral proteins are made constantly by the normal cell processes
- Viral proteins are cleaved by viral protease enzymes
- New viruses are assembled and released by budding from the membrane and are ready to infect new CD4+ cells
- Cell function is disrupted and eventually there is cell destruction
- Depletion of CD4+ T-helper cells makes the host susceptible to a wide array of infections

Transmission
- Sexual
- Infected blood or blood products
- Contaminated needles: IVDUs needle stick injuries
- Mother to child: parentally, perinatally, breast feeding.

Who

- ♀ > ♂
- >40 million infected worldwide (>75% in Africa)
- >70 000 infected in the UK, 30% are unaware
- First described in 1981

Risk factors:
- Concurrent STI increases susceptibility and infectiveness
- Sexual activity:
  - Unprotected sex
  - Anal sex
  - Multiple partners
  - Commercial sex work
  - Heterosexual sex is the most important mode of infection

Common presentations:
- *TB*: with any CD4 count. 23x more common in HIV
- *NHL*: with any CD4 count, associated with duration of HIV infection. 60× more common in HIV, may mimic TB so a biopsy is essential
- *PCP*: CD4 usually <200. Wide spectrum of CXR changes including pneumothoraces. Bronchoscopy yields positive results up to one week after starting treatment. Add steroids if pO$_2$ <9 kPa
- *Toxoplasmosis*: CD4 usually <200. Focal brain lesion, treat empirically and consider biopsy if alternative diagnosis suspected
- *Cryptococcal meningitis*: CD4 usually <50. Headache may be the only feature. CSF often relatively normal or lymphocytosis so need high index of suspicion for India ink or cryptococcal antigen test
- *Oesophageal candidiasis*: CD4 usually <200. Patient may present with dysphagia and no evidence of oral *Candida*.

Symptoms and signs

Stages of HIV infection

- Primary HIV infection:
  - Soon after exposure
  - Rash, fever, lymphadenopathy arthralgia, sore throat, weight loss, night sweats, fatigue, meningitis
  - Diagnosis often missed
- Seroconversion:
  - Transient, normally self-limiting illness 6–8 weeks after exposure. 'Glandular fever' type symptoms
- Asymptomatic infection:
  - May last years, some never develop AIDS
- Generalised lymphadenopathy:
  - Enlarged lymph nodes in many sites
- AIDS:
  - Proven HIV infection with an AIDS defining illness (normally with a low CD4 count)
  - Patient often has weight loss, lymphadenopathy and fever

AIDS-defining illnesses (should prompt HIV testing in a UK setting)

- Infection:
  - Recurrent bacterial infections, e.g. *Salmonella* septicaemia
  - Extrapulmonary *M. tuberculosis*
  - Histoplasmosis (fungal disease).
- Isosporiasis (parasite affecting the GI system)
- *Mycobacterium avium* complex or *Mycobacterium kansasii*
- Coccidioidomycosis
- Cryptococcosis
- Respiratory:
  - Pneumonia, recurrent: *Pneumocystis jiroveci*
  - *M. tuberculosis*
- GI:
  - CMV colitis
  - Oesophageal candidiasis
  - *Mycobacterium avium* intracellulare
  - CMV hepatitis
  - Cryptosporidiosis (protozoa causing GI disease)
- CNS:
  - Toxoplasmosis
  - Progressive multifocal leukoencephalopathy (progressive demyelination of brain white matter)
  - Cytomegalovirus (CMV) retinitis with loss of vision
  - Encephalopathy
- Reproductive:
  - Herpetic ulcers
  - Genital warts: human papillomavirus
- Malignancy:
  - Kaposi's sarcoma (tumour from human HSV8 leading to systemic disease and cutaneous lesions)
  - Lymphoma, Burkitt's or immunoblastic
  - Oral hairy leukoplakia (tumour of the mucosa presenting as a white 'hairy' patch)
  - Cervical cancer, invasive
- General:
  - Wasting syndrome.

Pretest counselling:
- Obtain informed consent
- Assure the patient of confidentiality
- Counsel regarding possible results
- Stratify risk of the patient to exposure
- Explain that the test will not detect recent infection in the last 3 months
- In patients with a known risk exposure and −ve early antibody test the antibody test should be repeated 3 months later

HIV test:
- Acute infection: p24 antigen (capsid protein of the virus) or HIV RNA
- Blood serology for anti-HIV antibodies

Monitoring HIV infection:
- Important for deciding when to start treatment and response to therapy:
  - Viral load: measure of level of viral activity. Predicts progression to AIDS, and may be undetectable (<50 copies/mL) with successful treatment
  - CD4 count: measure of degree of immunodeficiency

Further investigations:
- Screen for coexistent risks such as genitourinary infections, viral hepatitis, latent TB, cardiovascular risk factors
- Investigate for 2° infection depending on the presenting symptoms.

- Support, information and education at diagnosis

Highly active antiretroviral therapy (HAART):
- Commence when CD4 count ~350
- Initiating treatment best done by an HIV specialist
- Most patients start with two NRTIS: either a protease inhibitor or an NNRTI
- Patients must take their tablets correctly >95% of the time
- Look for genotypic drug resistance before deciding on initial therapy
- Drugs have severe side effects
  - *NRTIS*: lactic acidosis, fatty liver, loss of subcutaneous fat
  - *NNRTIS*: skin rash, hepatitis. PIs: liver toxicity, hyperglycaemia, diabetes

Nucleoside analogue reverse transcriptase inhibitors (NRTIS):
- Prevents DNA copy of viral RNA being formed

- Nucleoside analogues: zidovudine, lamivudine, didanosine, stavudine
- Nucleotide analogues: tenofovir

Non NRTIS (NNRTIS):
- Efavirenz, nevirapine

Integrase inhibitors:
- Raltegravir

Protease inhibitors:
- Prevent new virus formation
- Lopinavir, darunavir, nelfinavir, amprenavir, saquinovir, fosamprenavir, tipranvir – all boosted with ritonavir

CCR5 blockers:
- Maraviroc: blocks HIV binding receptor

Fusion inhibitors:
- Block entry of virus into the cell
- Enfuvirtide (T20)

Treatment

Prevention

- Blood screening
- Disposable equipment

- Perinatal antiretrovirals: AZT and lamivudine through pregnancy and labour (Caesarean section), then treat the neonate and avoid breast feeding.

Prognosis and complications

Prognosis

- Depends on CD4 count and viral load
- Now has an excellent prognosis and if treated with highly active antiretroviral therapy (HAART) in specialist centres the median survival is >30 years
- In the UK it is now viewed as a chronic disease, but this is not the case in the developing world

- With effective HAART, long-term prognosis is more related to cardiovascular and cancer risk than AIDS-defining infections
- Patients require aggressive control of lipids and early investigation of symptoms suggesting new malignancy.

Complications

Postexposure prophylaxis (PEP):
- Make an immediate and detailed risk assessment
- Any treatment should be started in the first hour after exposure and at the latest within 72 h

For needle stick injuries:
- Wash the wound and encourage bleeding

- Take a sample of the subject's blood and ask permission to take the donor's blood for HIV testing
- Document the injury with occupational health
- Consider accelerated HBV vaccination

For sexual risk exposures:
- Have a lower threshold for PEP if rape is suspected.

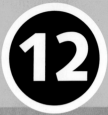
Sodium

Sodium has a number of roles in the body:

- Helps to regulate fluid balance:
  - Most sodium is extracellular and is important in determining extracellular volume control
  - Water molecules follow sodium ions by osmosis
- Plays an important role in cardiac and nervous system function.

Sodium regulation

Sodium disturbances are usually caused by water imbalances:

- Sodium regulation is largely controlled by the kidneys, and in hypovolaemia there will be increased reabsorption of sodium in the proximal and thick ascending limbs of the nephron
- There are two types of receptor involved in sodium regulation: volume receptors and osmoreceptors.

Volume receptors

Volume receptors measure and control extracellular blood volume (rather than changes in sodium concentration) but can affect sodium excretion or retention in the kidneys:

- Renal receptors:
  - Located in the afferent glomerular arteriole walls
  - Respond to low extracellular volume (or low sodium intake) to activate the renin–angiotensin system, releasing renin from the kidneys, which leads to increased BP through a number of mechanisms including increased renal sodium retention
- Extrarenal receptors:
  - High-pressure arterial baroreceptors (found in the aortic arch and internal cartotid arteries)
  - Low-pressure atrial receptors (right atrium, main thoracic veins)
  - When there is reduced extracellular blood flow, both groups initiate sympathetic activity; increasing the heart rate and causing vasoconstriction

- Low-pressure receptors also increase salt and water retention if there is reduced extracellular blood flow
- Atrial low-pressure receptors respond to high extracellular volume by releasing atrial natriuretic peptide, which increases sodium and water excretion by the kidney.

Osmoreceptors

Osmoreceptors are located in the hypothalamus and measure changes in plasma sodium concentration and osmolarity:

- In high plasma sodium concentration, they initiate thirst mechanisms and the release of ADH
- ADH is 'anti-diuretic'; that is, it reduces diuresis (production of urine) when there is too little water in the blood and, therefore, concentrates the urine
  - ADH acts at V2 receptors in the kidney to increase water absorption
  - ADH acts at V1 receptors in the arterioles causing vasoconstriction.

Potassium

Potassium also has a number of roles in the body; it is important for:

- the resting potential of cells
- the function of excitable tissues, e.g. nerves and muscle contraction (including cardiac muscle)
- fluid and electrolyte balance.

Potassium regulation

Most potassium is intracellular and so serum potassium levels will not reflect total potassium. Potassium levels are controlled by:

- the sodium–potassium ATPase (Na^+/K^+-ATPase) pump in the cell membrane, which controls the amount of potassium in cells
- pH, which has an effect on potassium in cells as potassium and hydrogen ions replace each other as they compete in exchange for sodium:

- As hydrogen ion concentration increases in acidosis, hydrogen ions move into the cell in exchange for potassium ions; this can lead to hyperkalaemia
- In alkalosis, similarly, there may be hypokalaemia
- renal excretion: mainly controlled by aldosterone (part of the renin–angiotensin system)
- extra-renal losses from the GI system.

Interpreting acidosis and alkalosis

- Can be analysed by examining pH, pCO$_2$ and bicarbonate levels (Fig. 12.1)
- The carbonic acid–bicarbonate buffering equation underlies acid–base balance
- This is also useful for interpreting ABG results.

See also

- Endocrinology (Ch. 9): calcium disorders.

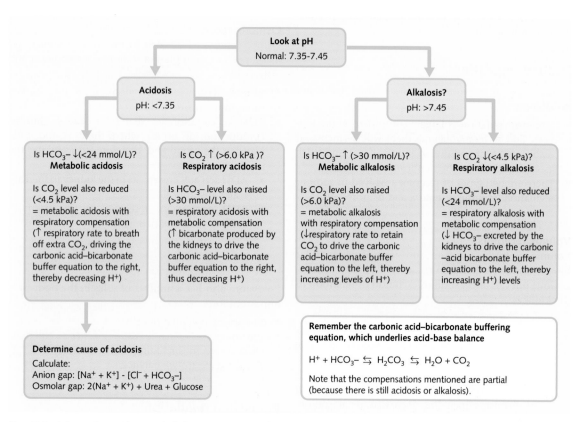

Fig. 12.1 Interpreting acidosis and alkalosis using pH and bicarbonate levels.

SODIUM DISORDERS

Normal levels: 135–145 mmol/L.

HYPERNATRAEMIA

Outline

- ↑ Serum sodium: >145 mmol/L
- Most often reflects water loss rather than sodium excess.

Pathogenesis/aetiology

Fluid loss:
- Diarrhoea
- Sweating/dehydration
- Water loss from lungs or skin

Renal loss:
- Diabetes insipidus (cranial or nephrogenic)
- Osmotic diuresis: other solutes prevent water resorption, e.g. glucose, mannitol

↓ Fluid intake:
- Mostly in the elderly, neonates and the unconscious
- Idiopathic: incorrect IV fluid replacement from too much normal saline

Endocrine changes:
- Primary aldosteronism.

Clinical features

Hypovolaemia:
- Dehydration:
  - Dry skin
  - ↓ Skin turgor
  - Postural hypotension
  - Oliguria
  - Thirst

Non-specific symptoms:
- Nausea
- Confusion
- Fever
- Fits
- Coma.

Investigations

Blood tests

- FBC: ↑ packed cell volume
- U&Es: ↑ sodium, ↑ urea (due to low concentration of water)

- ↑ Albumin
- Plasma osmolality.

Urine

- Osmolality:
  - If very low: due to diabetes insipidus
  - If very high: due to osmotic diuresis or heat stroke

- ↑ Urinary sodium.

Treatment

- Water orally
- IV dextrose 5% if oral intake not possible
- IV 0.9% saline if very severe or if there is a water deficit (and therefore sodium is not high, just concentrated)

- Correct over 48 h: rapid correction can cause cerebral oedema
- Treat underlying cause.

HYPONATRAEMIA

Outline

- ↓ Serum sodium: <135 mmol/L

- Often due to water excess.

Classification

- Hypervolaemic: due to water excess
- Hypovolaemic: due to salt loss (water follows)
- Normovolaemic: greater sodium loss than water loss
- Pseudohyponatraemia: dyslipidaemia or hyperproteinaemia results in spuriously low serum sodium concentration. Most laboratories will correct for this

- Syndrome of inappropriate ADH secretion (SIADH): ADH is secreted even when the blood is dilute and more urine should be produced. This leads to water retention and haemodilution (see Endocrinology [Ch. 9]).

Pathogenesis/aetiology

Normovolaemic:
- Glucocorticoid deficiency (cortisol will inhibit loss of sodium through the small intestine, so ↓ cortisol leads to ↑ sodium loss)
- SIADH (a diagnosis of exclusion)

Hypervolaemic (commonest cause):
- Patient is usually oedematous:
  - Renal failure, nephrotic syndrome
  - Cardiac failure
  - Cirrhosis
- Endocrine causes:
  - Addison's disease (↓ aldosterone)
  - Hypothyroidism (water retention)

Hypovolaemic:
- Dehydration
- Burns
- Diarrhoea and vomiting
- Diuretics: particularly thiazides
- Pancreatitis
- Iatrogenic
- Renal loss:
  - Salt wasting nephropathy
  - Renal tubular acidosis
  - Mineralocorticoid deficiency.

Clinical features

- Depends on cause

Hypervolaemic:
- Water moving into the brain:
  - Headache
  - Confusion
  - Convulsions
  - Coma
- Hypertension
- In some case evidence of heart failure

Hypovolaemic:
- Dehydration:
  - Dry skin
  - ↓ Skin turgor
  - Postural hypotension
  - Oliguria (↓ urine produced)
- Thirst
- Nausea
- Muscle weakness
- Anorexia.

Investigations

Blood tests

- U&Es: ↓ sodium
- Serum osmolarity: normal if pseudohyponatraemia

- Random cortisol level

Urine

Urinary sodium:
- Low sodium (<20 mmol/L):
  - If with normal kidney function consider that the patient is salt deficient from a cause other than the kidneys and they are retaining sodium

- High sodium (>20 mmol/L):
  - Consider renal failure, a salt wasting nephropathy, SIADH, diuretics, Addison's disease
  - May also be high due to bicarbonaturia in vomiting or from a metabolic acidosis.

Treatment

- Correct underlying cause

Hypervolaemic:
- Water restriction
- In emergency correct sodium levels slowly
- Diuretics to ↑ excretion of excess water
- Correct imbalance of other electrolytes

- Vaptans: new V2 receptor antagonists which promote free water loss

Hypovolaemic:
- Crystalloids or colloids to restore extracellular volume
- Correct sodium slowly to prevent central pontine myelinolysis.

POTASSIUM (K$^+$)

Normal levels of potassium: 3.5–5.0 mmol/L.

HYPERKALAEMIA

Outline

- ↑ Potassium: >5.0 mmol/L
- Requires urgent treatment
- >6.5 mmol/L is a medical emergency
- Can result in a metabolic acidosis
- Characteristic changes on ECG

Pseudohyperkalaemia:
- Measured potassium is greater than in vivo potassium due to haemolysis of RBCs in vitro releasing potassium giving a falsely high value
- High platelet counts (>1000) can interfere with laboratory tests, invalidating the result (can cause high or lower values of potassium than the true in vivo value).

Pathogenesis/aetiology

↑ Intake
- Excess potassium therapy
- Blood transfusion

↓ Renal loss:
- Renal failure (acute or chronic): very common
- Hypoaldosteronism: (aldosterone acts to ↓ potassium and ↑ sodium), Addison's disease

Release from cells:
- Diabetic ketoacidosis
- Metabolic acidosis
- Trauma: muscle injury, burns

Drugs: K-BANK (interfere with urinary excretion):
- Potassium-sparing diuretic, e.g. spironolactone
- Beta-blockers
- ACE inhibitors
- NSAIDs
- Potassium supplements.

Clinical features

- Muscle weakness, paralysis
- Kussmaul's breathing (deep, heavy breathing associated with acidosis)
- Generalised fatigue

Cardiac:
- Cardiac arrhythmias: ventricular fibrillation
- Cardiac arrest/sudden death.

Investigations

Blood tests

- U&Es

- ABG: acidosis.

ECG

- Extrasystole or bradycardia
- Tall tented T waves
- Small P wave

- Shortened P–R interval
- Wide QRS becoming sinusoidal
- Ventricular fibrillation

Treatment

If ECG changes present and potassium is >6.5 mmol/L:
- Cardioprotection (immediately):
  - Cardiac monitor
  - 10 mL of 10% calcium gluconate or calcium chloride IV over 2–3 min

To drive potassium into cells and ↓ serum potassium:
- 10 units of insulin with 50 mL 50% IV dextrose over 30 min
- Nebulised salbutamol

Other:
- Sodium bicarbonate: to correct severe acidosis
- Haemodialysis if measures fail

Subsequently:
- Monitor blood glucose hourly
- Measure potassium every 2–4 h, then daily if necessary
- Find/treat underlying cause.

HYPOKALAEMIA

Outline

- Low potassium: <3.5 mmmol/L
- If <2.5 mmol/L: urgent treatment is required

Pathogenesis/aetiology

↓ Intake:
- Dietary deficiency
- Inadequate replacement in IV fluids

↑ Renal loss:
- Diuretics: thiazides, loop diuretics
- ↓ Magnesium: magnesium needed for the cardiac Na^+/K^+-ATPase pump
- Liver failure
- Heart failure
- Renal disease

- Endocrine: hyperaldosteronism (common), corticosteroids, Cushing's, Conn's disease, congenital adrenal hyperplasia

↑ GI loss:
- Vomiting: anorexics
- Diarrhoea and laxative abuse
- Fistulae

Redistribution into cells:
- Alkalosis: excess bicarbonate, leads to potassium excretion as the two are excreted together
- Insulin.

Clinical features

In general:
- Cardiac arrhythmias
- Respiratory distress or failure
- Lethargy

Neuromuscular:
- ↓ Tendon reflexes
- Muscle weakness

- Hypotonia
- Cramps
- Tetany: spasm and twitching of muscles (particularly the face)

GI:
- Constipation
- Ileus.

Investigations

Blood tests

- U&Es: potassium, also magnesium
- TSH

- ABG.

ECG

- AF
- Small, inverted T waves
- Prominent U wave

- Prolonged PR
- ST segment depression.

Treatment

- Withdraw purgatives/laxatives
- Potassium supplements:
  - Oral: Sando-K (potassium bicarbonate and potassium chloride)
  - IV: KCl (must be given slowly). Given in diabetic ketoacidosis, severe hypoxaemia, cardiac arrhythmias

- Normalise magnesium, which can interfere with potassium levels

Overall:
- Monitor potassium and perform regular ECGs
- Treat underlying cause.

ACID–BASE INBALANCE

Figure 12.1 summarises the interpretation of blood gases.

RESPIRATORY ACIDOSIS

Outline

- Acidosis due to alveolar hypoventilation
- Failure of ventilation causes acidosis by ↑ the partial arterial pressure of CO_2 ($PaCO_2$)
- The increase in $PaCO_2$, in turn, decreases the ratio of bicarbonate to $PaCO_2$, thus decreasing pH
- Can be acute or chronic:
  - Acute respiratory acidosis:
    - $PaCO_2$ is ↑ above the upper limit of normal and the pH is low

- Chronic respiratory acidosis (with compensation):
  - $PaCO_2$ is ↑ but with a normal or near-normal pH because of 2° renal compensation:↑ bicarbonate produced by the kidneys to drive the carbonic acid bicarbonate buffer equation to the right and therefore decreasing H^+ levels as they are buffered by bicarbonate.

Pathogenesis/aetiology

Any cause of hypoventilation:
- Neuromuscular diseases:
  - Guillain–Barré syndrome
  - Myasthenia gravis
  - Muscular dystrophy
  - Motor neuron disease
  - Severe kyphoscoliosis
  - Flail chest
  - Ankylosing spondylitis

- Lung disease:
  - Chronic obstructive pulmonary disease
  - Severe restrictive lung disease
  - Obstructive sleep apnoea
- ↓ Central respiratory drive:
  - Trauma
  - Drugs (CNS depressants): opiates, barbiturates, narcotics, benzodiazepines
  - Brainstem disease
  - Encephalitis.

Clinical features

- Confusion
- Myoclonus
- Papilloedema

- Peripheral vasodilation: may ↑ ICP
- Coma
- Signs of underlying disease.

Investigations

Blood tests

- FBC: secondary polycythaemia due to chronic hypoxaemia leading to ↑ erythropoiesis. Indicated by ↑ Hb and haematocrit
- U&Es

- TSH
- ABG
- Toxicology: if suspected as a cause.

Imaging

- CXR: to identify if lung disease is the cause.

Other tests

- Lung function tests.

Treatment

- Treat cause

- Consider ventilatory support.

RESPIRATORY ALKALOSIS

Outline

- Alkalosis due to alveolar hyperventilation
- Hyperventilation leads to a ↓ $PaCO_2$
- In turn, the decrease in $PaCO_2$ increases the ratio of bicarbonate to $PaCO_2$, thus increasing pH
- This hypocapnia develops when a strong respiratory stimulus causes the lungs to remove more CO_2 than is produced metabolically in the tissues
- Can be acute or chronic:

- Acute respiratory alkalosis: $PaCO_2$ level is below the lower limit of normal and pH is high
- Chronic respiratory alkalosis (compensation): $PaCO_2$ level is below the lower limit of normal, but the pH is normal or near normal because of secondary renal compensation, where ↓ bicarbonate excreted by the kidneys drives the carbonic acid–bicarbonate buffer balance to the left, thereby ↑ H^+.

Pathogenesis/aetiology

Any cause of hyperventilation:
- Lung disease:
  - Pneumothorax or haemothorax, pneumonia, pulmonary oedema, pulmonary embolus, aspiration, restrictive and obstructive lung disease
- CNS:
  - Pain, anxiety, psychosis, stroke, meningitis, encephalitis, tumour, trauma
- Hypoxia:
  - High altitude, severe anaemia, right-to-left cardiac shunts

- Drugs:
  - Salicylates, catecholamines, nicotine, progesterone
- Endocrine:
  - Pregnancy, hyperthyroidism
- Other:
  - Sepsis, liver failure, heart failure, mechanical ventilation.

- Lightheaded
- Paraesthesia
- Numb around mouth
- Tingling in hands and feet

- Tachycardia
- Hypotension in severe cases
- Occasionally, Chvostek and Trousseau's sign present (see Hypocalcaemia in Endocrinology Ch. 9) .

Investigations

Blood tests

- U&Es: ↓ potassium
- ABG

- TSH.

Imaging

- CXR: if respiratory disease is suspected.

Other tests

- Investigations relevant to likely underlying diagnosis.

Treatment

- Usually ignored

- Treat cause.

METABOLIC ACIDOSIS

Outline

- ↓ In serum bicarbonate (HCO_3^- <22 mmol/L) due to excess H^+ (acid accumulation)
- Metabolic acidosis leads to alveolar hyperventilation to compensate for the ↑ in H^+. The ↑ respiratory rate allows the body to breath off extra CO_2, driving the carbonic acid bicarbonate buffer equation right, to ↓ H^+ levels
- The anion and osmolar gap are helpful in determining the cause of acidosis
  - The osmolar gap:
    - The difference between the laboratory measured osmolarity and the calculated osmolarity from calculated plasma solutes
    - A difference indicates that there are unmeasured osmoles in the blood such as ethanol or methanol that have been ingested
    - Calculated as: $2(Na^+ + K^+) + Urea + Glucose$
    - Causes of a high osmolar gap: ingestion of: ethanol, methanol, ethylene glycol, acetone

- The anion gap:
  - A measure of the imbalance between positive and negative ions
  - Used to determine if acidity is due to an exogenous acid (not normally present in the body, e.g. ethanol, lactic acid), or caused by build up of an endogenous acid in abnormal quantities (e.g. HCl) and so helps identify the cause
  - Calculated as: $[Na^+ + K^+] - [Cl^- + HCO_3^-]$
  - Normal anion gap acidosis (12–16 mmol/L): endogenous acid is the cause, acidity due to retention of H^+ ions or bicarbonate loss, e.g. GI or renal loss of HCO_3^-
  - High anion gap acidosis (>16 mmol/L): unmeasured exogenous acid ions such as beta-hydroxybutyrate and acetoacetate are responsible for the acidity (loss of HCO_3^- without an equal increase in Cl), e.g. lactic acidosis, ketoacidosis, salicylate toxicity, renal failure, ingestion of methanol or ethano
  - The anion gap is also useful in monitoring response to therapy.

Pathogenesis/aetiology

Increased H^+:
- Lactic acidosis: numerous causes, including circulatory failure, drugs and toxins and hereditary causes
- Ketoacidosis: diabetes, alcoholism and starvation
- Drugs (may give high osmolar gap due to ↑ in exogenous acid): salicylates, methanol, ethylene glycol, isoniazid, iron, sulphur, ammonium chloride, metformin

Failure to excrete H^+:
- Renal failure: diminished ammonia production
- Renal tubular acidosis type 1

- Hypoaldosteronism: type 4 renal tubular acidosis

Loss of bicarbonate:
- GI losses:
  - Diarrhoea
  - Pancreatic, biliary, or intestinal fistulas
  - Ureterosigmoidostomy
  - Cholestyramine
- Renal losses:
  - Type 2 (proximal) renal tubular acidosis
  - Acetazolamide therapy.

Clinical features

Cardiovascular:
- Palpitations and arrhythmias, chest pain hypotension and cardiac arrest

Respiratory:
- Hyperventilation due to respiratory compensation

Neurological:
- Headache, visual changes, fits and confusion leading to coma

GI:
- Nausea, vomiting, abdominal pain, diarrhoea

Other:
- Muscle weakness, bone pain

Special cases of metabolic acidosis:
- *Salicylate poisoning:*
  - May get tinnitus, blurred vision, and vertigo (see The acutely unwell patient, p. 14)
- *Methanol intoxication:*
  - May get visual disturbances: dimming, photophobia, scotomata and blindness.

Investigations

- ABG
- U&Es
- Lactate
- Serum osmolarity
- Glucose
- Calculate the anion and osmolar gap to help identify the cause.

Treatment

- Treat underlying cause
- In severe cases: bicarbonate replacement (give with caution as can exacerbate intracellular acidosis, contribute to volume overload, cause hypokalaemia and hypoxia).

METABOLIC ALKALOSIS

Outline

- A primary ↑ in serum bicarbonate (HCO_3^-) concentration as a consequence of a loss of H^+ from the body or a gain in HCO_3 (the kidneys usually remove excess bicarbonate)
- As a compensatory mechanism, metabolic alkalosis can lead to alveolar hypoventilation. This decreases the respiratory rate to retain CO_2, driving the carbonic acid bicarbonate buffer equation to the left thereby increasing levels of H^+.

Pathogenesis/aetiology

H^+ loss:
- Vomiting

Endocrine imbalance:
- Cushing's
- Hyperaldosteronism: volume resistant metabolic alkalosis
- Fludrocortisone

Medications:
- Ingestion of a base
- Diuretic therapy
- Glucocorticoids (has mineraolcorticoid effect in high doses)
- Antacids (e.g. magnesium hydroxide)

Clinical features

- Weakness
- Myalgia
- Polyuria
- Hypoventilation: due to inhibition of the respiratory centre
- Symptoms of hypocalcaemia may be present.

Investigations

- ABG
- U&Es (may be ↓ potassium)
- Renin and aldosterone
- Cortisol.

Treatment

- Fluid replacement: 95% of causes are volume responsive
- Replace other electrolytes, bicarbonate replaces itself
- Treat underlying cause.

Surgery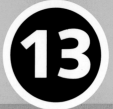

13

Faculty Contributor: Nicolas Alexander

Common surgical prefixes and suffixes

angio- vessel
chole- gall bladder/bile
colp- vagina
cyst- sac filled with fluid (also bladder)
-doch- duct
-ectomy cutting something out
enter- small bowel
fistula abnormal connection either between two organs or between an organ and the skin surface
gastr- stomach
hepat- liver
lapr- abdomen
lith- stone
mast- breast
nephr- kidney
orchid- testicle
oopher- ovaries
-pexy fixing something into place
-plasty to repair or restore
pyelo- kidney pelvis
-scopy to look inside with a camera
splen- spleen
-stomy artificial opening
thorac- chest
-tomy to cut open.

Admissions for surgery

Emergency admissions

When a patient is admitted for emergency surgery the following must be completed:

- Full history and examination
- IV access and blood tests (including a group and save)
- DVT prophylaxis:
  - Stratify risk (low/med/high)
  - Prescribe compression stockings (TEDS)
  - Prescribe suitable dose of low molecular weight heparin (LMWH)

- Ensure patient remains nil by mouth
- Prescribe:
  - adequate fluid regimen
  - antiemetics to be taken when needed
  - adequate analgesia
- Place a nasogastric tube if appropriate
- Insert catheter if appropriate
- Consent form and anaesthetic review.

Elective admissions

When a patient is admitted electively for surgery the following extra things must be completed:

- Optimise chronic conditions, e.g. diabetic control
- Consider CXR, pulmonary function tests, ECG and Echocardiogram in those with pre-existing pathology
- Anticoagulation:
  - Stop anticoagulants (e.g. aspirin, clopidogrel and warfarin) for 5 days before surgery
  - Consider switching warfarin to shorter-acting LMWH before admission because of the risk of bleeding
- Nil by mouth (food 6 h, fluid 2 h) prior to surgery.

Common medications before and after surgery

- Anxiolytics: for preoperative anxiety, e.g. benzodiazepines
- *Analgesics:* Consider the WHO analgesic ladder (originally developed for cancer patients but can be applied more generally):
  - Non-opioids: e.g. paracetamol, NSAIDs
  - Mild opioids: e.g. codeine (side effects: nausea, respiratory depression, constipation, cough suppression, sedation)
  - Strong opioids: e.g. morphine
  - Adjuvants can be added to each level as needed.
  - Postoperative patients need stronger analgesia at first, which can be stepped down
- Antiemetics
- Antibiotics to counter risk of wound infection
- IV fluids.
- Anaesthesia.

Anaesthesia

Preoperative assessments are performed to ascertain appropriate anaesthetic agent and risk; score from the American Society of Anaesthiologists Physical Status Classification System is a predictor of mortality and aids in the preoperative assessment (Table 13.1).

Table 13.1 American Society of Anaesthiologists physical status classification system

Class	Status
1	Normal healthy patient
2	Mild systemic disease
3	Severe systemic disease
4	Severe systemic disease that is a constant threat to life
5	Moribund patient not expected to live without the operation
6	Brain-dead patient whose organs are being removed for donor purposes

Local anaesthetics

- Include lidocaine, bupivicaine, benzocaine
- Prevent pain by blocking nerve conduction reversibly
- Application can be topical, by injection, nerve block, epidural
- Often injected with adrenaline to prevent spread into the systemic circulation (adrenaline is not given when anaesthetic is applied to the extremities as vasoconstriction may result in ischaemia)
- Side effects mainly result from systemic spread:
  - CNS effects: tremor, restlessness, confusion
  - Respiratory depression
  - myocardial depression.

General anaesthetics

- Multiple agents
- Application inhaled (volatile) and intravenous (e.g. propofol)
- Often anaesthesia is induced with an IV agent and maintained with volatile agents
- Side effects vary depending on agent used.

Complications after surgery

Complications should be considered in any postsurgical patient (Table 13.2).

OVERVIEW: FLUIDS AND NUTRITION

Fluid balance in the body

- Water makes up 60% of the body, divided among different compartments
- Fluid status is important when considering if a patient is dehydrated or overloaded
- In surgical patients, it is important to balance fluid input and output
- Regularly review a patient's fluid balance and adjust/stop added fluids when they start eating and drinking again
- Daily requirements:
  - Fluid: 3 L
  - Sodium: 1.5–2 mmol/kg
  - Potassium: 1 mmol/kg
- Common daily regimen (for an average 70 kg man):
  - 1 L normal saline with 20 mmol KCl
  and
  - 2 L 5% dextrose each litre with 20 mmol KCl ('One salt, two sweet').

Assessment of fluid status in a patient

- Examine the mucous membranes in the eye and under the tongue: are they moist or dry?
- Pinch the skin to see if it is dry: reduced fluid status results in decreased skin turgidity
- Assess JVP: raised in overload
- Measure BP: raised in overload
- Feel the legs and the sacrum for peripheral oedema: increased in fluid overload
- Listen to the lung bases for pulmonary oedema: increased in overload
- Measure fluid input/output (including urinary output) with fluid balance chart; urinary output should be about 30 mL/h
- Weigh the patient and compare measurements daily.

Types of intravenous fluid

- Crystalloid: electrolytes suspended in water:
  - 0.9% normal saline (isotonic)
  - 5% dextrose (hypotonic): distributes across all compartments so useful for dehydration
  - Hartman's solution (isotonic): contains physiological concentrations of electrolytes, is lactate based
- Colloid: larger molecules that remain in the intravascular compartments for longer and increase oncotic pressure (e.g. Gelofusin):

Table 13.2 Postoperative complications

Clinical features and management of postoperative complications

Complication	Time PO	Cause	Signs and symptoms	Management
Respiratory depression	<24 h	General anaesthesia (GA) or excessive analgesia	↓ RR ↓ conscious level, cyanosis	Clear airway, reverse GA or effect of analgesia
Hypovolaemia (see p. 5, chapter 1)	<24 h	Haemorrhage, inadequate fluid replacement	↓ BP, ↑ HR, ↓ urine output	IV fluids – crystalloids and packed red blood cells; return to OR if haemorrhage is active
Atelectasis	24–48 h	Poor analgesia, smoking, previous chest problems, effect of GA	↑ temp., RR ↑, ↓ O$_2$, ↓ AE bases of lungs	Analgesia, mobilization of patient; encourage deep breathing
Respiratory infection	>48 h	Poor analgesia, smoking, previous chest problems, effect of GA	↑ temp., RR ↑, ↓ O$_2$, ↓ AE and rales; ronchi, sputum production	Analgesia, mobilization of patient; nebulizers and antibiotics
Deep vein thrombosis (DVT) (see p. 581, below)	5–10 days	Operations causing immobility (e.g. pelvic orthopaedic), oral contraceptive use, malignancy	↑ temp., legs swollen, tender calf – often no physical findings except fever	Doppler ultrasound or venogram; anticoagulation if possible; if not, vena caval filter
Pulmonary embolus (PE) (see p. 107, chapter 3)	5–10 day	DVT, immobility; no signs of DVT in 50% of cases	Tachycadia, tachypnea, clear to auscultation; presents as pleuritic chest pains, multiple small PEs, or massive PE with collapse or death	ECG, V/Q scan, pulmonary angiogram anticoagulation or vena caval filter
Wound infection	5–7 days	Haematoma, contamination at operation, corticosteroid use, diabetes mellitus, malignancy, jaundice, long-duration operation	↑ temp. with red, tender, and swollen wound	Antibiotics, open wound
Urinary tract infection (see p. 304, chapter 7)	5 days	Immobility, catheterization	↑ temp., confusion in elderly, dysuria	Antibiotics
Wound dehiscence	5–10 days	Poor operative technique, wound infection, hematoma, corticosteroid use, poor nutrition, increased intra – abdominal pressure (i.e. ileus)	Red serous discharge from wound, protruding intestine	Resuscitation, return to surgery for wound closure
Paralytic ileus	>4–5 days	Normal response, but if it occurs after >4–5 days there may be intra-abdominal pathology or ↓ K$^+$, narcotics	↑ NG aspirate, abdominal distention, obstipation	Resuscitation, NG aspiration, correct electrolytes, rule out intra-abdominal pathology
Anastomotic dehiscence	5–10 days	Poor operative technique, infection, vascular insufficiency	↓ BP, ↑ temp., ↑ HR, peritonitis	Resuscitation, laparotomy, antibiotics, lavage
Pseudomembranous colitis		Following antibiotic use, due to clostridium difficile toxin	Diarrhoea, dehydration, abdominal pain	Resuscitation, oral metronidazole or vancomycin

- Risk of anaphylaxis as colloids are made from biological products
- Good where a rapid increase in BP is needed, e.g. in the acutely unwell patient whose BP has suddenly fallen to systolic BP <80 mmHg.

Additional requirements

Extra fluids are needed in certain patients where there are:

- third space losses: after surgery or in disease such as pancreatitis, the endothelium can leak and fluid can accumulate within the bowel
- insensible losses: increase with fever
- haemorrhage.

Cautions

Care should be taken in prescribing fluids for certain patients:

- In heart and liver failure: avoid sodium as it promotes water retention
- In renal failure: avoid adding potassium as kidneys control potassium homeostasis and there is a risk of hyperkalaemia
- In the elderly: be cautious with adding fluids because of the risk of developing heart failure.

Nutritional support

Possible feeding routes

- Enteral feeding: via the GI tract, options include:
  - nasogastric tube
  - nasojejunal tube (tube placed via a nostril into jejunum)
  - percutaneous endoscopic gastrectomy (PEG): feeding tube directly through skin into stomach
  - percutaneous endoscopic jejunostomy (PEJ): feeding tube through skin into the jejunum
- Parenteral nutrition (i.e. IV):
  - long-term support requires a central line with nutrition supplied IV
  - indicated if enteral nutrition is inadequate
  - complications include line sepsis and thrombosis.

Cautions

Any patient being fed after a prolonged period of inadequate nutrition is at risk of refeeding syndrome:

- commencing adequate nutrition can result in abnormal electrolytes
- therefore monitor electrolytes (particularly phosphate).

Stomas

A stoma is an opening between a body viscus and an external surface. The term is often used to describe the

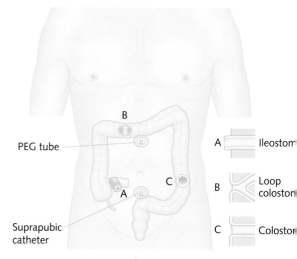

Fig. 13.1 Abdominal stoma, their locations and forms.

surgical procedure where part of the gut is removed (e.g. in cancer) and the remaining segment is brought out to the surface of the abdomen and the waste/gut contents collects in an artificial stoma bag:

- Surgical stomas from the gut can be permanent or temporary.
- Types of stoma (Fig. 13.1):
  - Ileostomy: ileum opens directly to the abdominal wall, end or loop
  - Colostomy: colon opens directly to the abdominal wall, end or loop
  - Ureterostomy: ureters open out directly to the abdominal wall bypassing the bladder and urethra.

Useful dermatological terminology

Bulla: raised lesion with fluid >0.5 cm
Vesicle: raised lesion with fluid <0.5 cm
Papule: circumscribed, raised lesion <1 cm
Plaque: a raised flat top lesion >1 cm
Nodule: circumscribed, raised lesion, like a papule but >1 cm
Crust: dried serum or exudate on the skin
Erosion: superficial loss of epidermis, heals without scarring
Erythema: red skin, blanches with pressure
Excoriation: partial or complete loss of epidermis from scratching
Lichenification: thickening of the skin and skin markings usually from constant rubbing
Macule: area of change in skin colour without elevation

Purpura: non-blanching purple or red skin
Ecchymosis: large area of purpura (a bruise)
Pustule: pus-filled lesion
Telangiectasia: abnormal visible dilatation of the blood vessels
Ulcer: lesion of the skin with full epidermal and some dermal loss.

Lesions associated with systemic disease

- Erythema nodosum:
  - Nodular, painful, blue/red lesions on the anterior surface of the shins
  - Associated with IBD, sarcoidosis, drugs (e.g. dapsone), Behçet's disease, streptococcal infection, viral infections
- Erythema multiforme:
  - Symmetrically distributed circular, target lesions with central blistering mostly found over the limbs
  - Associated with drug reactions, infection and collagen disease.

Systemic disease associated with skin lesions

- Diabetes mellitus:
  - Granuloma annulare: chronic benign condition where there is a ring of papules
  - Acanthosis nigricans: pigmented roughened areas of thickened skin found in the axilla, neck or groin
  - Necrobiosis lipoidica diabeticorum: shiny, yellow area on the shins
- Liver disease:
  - Spider naevi: spider-shaped telangiectasia in the distribution of the superior vena cava
  - Leuconychia: whitened nails due to ↓ albumin
- Sarcoid:
  - Lupus pernio: purple firm swelling of the skin often on the face
  - Erythema nodosum (see above)
- Rheumatic fever:
  - Erythema marginatum: pink rings found over the trunk which appear and disappear
- Inflammatory bowel disease:
  - Erythema nodosum
  - Pyoderma gangrenosum: ulcers with a bluish-tinged edge found over the back, abdomen and thighs
- Cancer:
  - Dermatomyositis: inflammation of striated muscle occurring together with a characteristically distributed rash
  - Acanthosis nigricans (particularly gastric cancer) (see above).

Types of lump or lesion

Lymph nodes: may become enlarged
- primary lymph node disorders: lymphoma
- secondary: to infection or malignancy
- Abscess:
  - Collection of pus (dead neutrophils) in a cavity owing to infection
  - Signs of infection: surrounding erythema, warmth, pain and swelling
  - Treatment by surgical incision and drainage, antibiotics.
- Campbell de Morgan spots/cherry angiomas:
  - Angioma formed by clusters of tiny capillaries at the skin surface
  - Appear as small non-blanching bright red or purple spots on the skin surface; occur in old age
  - No other significance
- Cyst: epithelium-lined, fluid-filled sac:
  - Dermoid cyst: teratoma containing developmentally mature tissue; can contain skin with hair follicles, sweat glands, pockets of sebum, blood, fat, bone, nails, teeth, eyes, cartilage or thyroid tissue
  - Ganglion cyst: originates from the synovial lining of a joint or tendon sheath and contain gelatinous material; can be anywhere in the body
  - Sebaceous cysts: from obstruction of the sebaceous glands in the skin; have a central black spot (punctum) and contain 'cheesy material'; remove under local anaesthesia
- Dupuytren's contracture:
  - Associated with alcoholic liver disease, diabetes mellitus, occupation (manual labour, vibration)
  - Thickening of palmar or plantar fascia
- Keloid scar
  - Difficult to treat, can attempt excision or steroids
  - Hypertrophy of collagen at the edge of a previous scar

Skin tumours: benign

- Lipoma:
  - Benign fatty lumps of adipose tissue
  - Smooth, soft swellings with imprecise margins
- Moles:
  - Benign pigmented naevi
  - 3% have two or more at birth
  - Monitor for malignant change
- Neurofibromas:
  - Associated with von Recklinghausen's neurofibromatosis (Fig. 13.2).
  - Tumours of nerves
- Papillomas:
  - Common benign epidermal tumour from skin overgrowth
  - Common in the elderly
  - Includes infective warts, basal cell warts, keratin horns, pedunculated papillomas

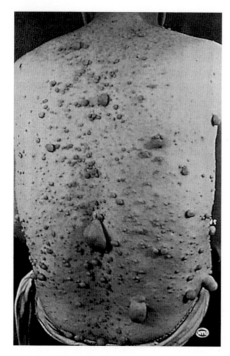

Fig. 13.2 Neurofibromatosis.

- Seborrhoeic keratosis (senile wart):
  - Appear as light–dark brown 'stuck on' patches, usually over the trunk and sun-exposed areas
  - Benign hyperplasia of the basal epithelial layer
  - No treatment needed.

Skin tumours: malignant

See malignant melanoma, basal cell carcinoma, squamous cell carcinoma, from p. 586.

Neck lumps

- Posterior:
  - Pharyngeal pouches: outpouching of the pharynx (see p. 534)
  - Cystic hygroma/lymphangioma: a congenital lymphovascular malformation usually presents in infancy

- Anterior:
  - Thyroglossal cyst: midline swelling anywhere along the migration path of the thyroid (from the posterior of the tongue to near the hyoid bone); the cyst will move when the patient protrudes their tongue as the cyst is embryologically derived from the foramen caecum of the tongue
  - Carotid body tumour: slow-growing tumour originating from the cells of the carotid body at the carotid bifurcation
  - Branchial cyst: congenital abnormality, remnant of the 2nd pharyngeal cleft that appears in young adult life
  - Parotid lumps: parotid salivary gland can become swollen in mumps, Sjögren's disease, chronic liver disease, local infection, parotid duct calculus, tumours.

Breast lumps

Benign breast neoplasms:

- Fibroadenoma:
  - 20% of breast masses
  - Discrete, smooth, well-defined mobile lumps
  - May be multiple and painful
  - Commonly found in those aged 15–25 years
  - Excision only if large, painful, growing or patient is over 40 years of age
- Phylloides tumour:
  - Similar to fibroademona but occurs in older women
  - Has malignant potential.

Malignant breast disease:

- See p. 515.

See also

- Cardiology (Ch. 2): coarctation of the aorta
- Endocrinology (Ch. 9): thyroid lumps
- Common presenting complaints (Ch. 14): abdominal pain, abdominal masses.

DISORDERS OF THE BREAST

MALIGNANT BREAST CANCER

Outline

Cancer of the breast:
- Carcinoma of the breast:
  - 20% of all cancers in women:
    - In situ:
      - Has not invaded the basement membrane
      - Ductal carcinoma in situ (20%): 50% progress to invasive ductal carcinoma. Commonest form
      - Lobar carcinoma in situ: rare, often multifocal. May not be visible on mammography
    - Invasive:
      - Ductal (75%): commonest invasive carcinoma
      - Lobular (10%): may not be visible on mammography
      - Tubular

- Medullary: begins in the milk ducts
- Papillary
- Mucinous: mucus produced by the cells
- Other cancers of the breast:
  - Paget's disease: intraductal carcinoma of the nipple (2% of breast cancers). Spreads from the epithelium of main collecting duct to the skin of the nipple. Presents as unilateral red, eczematous lesion of the nipple and areola. Usually unilateral red, oozing, crusting and unhealing sore
  - Sarcoma: very rare, tumour of spindle cells. Can arise from phylloides tumour
  - Lymphoma.

Pathogenesis/aetiology

Metastases:
- Spread to bone, liver, lungs:
  - Locally
  - Lymphatics: to axilla:
    - Level 1 – nodes inferior to pectoralis minor
    - Level 2 – nodes behind pectoralis minor
    - Level 3 – above the supraclavicular fossa, internal mammary chain
  - Haematological: particularly to bones and liver
Hormone receptors:
- Oestrogen receptor (ER) and progesterone receptor (PR) status. Important for prognosis and targeted therapy
- 60% of postmenopausal breast cancers are ER and PR+ve. Better prognosis
- Human epidermal growth factor receptor 2 (HER2) is a surface protein involved in cell development. If activated, it accelerates tumour formation. 20–30% of breast cancers over express HER2. Associated with a worse prognosis.

Grading and staging:
- Grade:
  - 1: differentiated
  - 2: moderately differentiated
  - 3: undifferentiated
- TNM staging (tumour, nodes, metastases):
  - Tis: ductal carcinoma in situ
  - T_1: <2 cm
  - T_2: 2–5
  - T_3: >5
  - T_4: fixed, skin changes
  - No: no nodes metastases
  - N1: ipsilateral nodes
  - N2: metastases to internal mammary nodes
  - M0: no distant metastases
  - M1: distant metastases

Who

- Typical age: ↑ with age, rare under 30
- 10% of UK females
- ♂: account for 1/300 cases
- Commonest cause of cancer deaths in women 15–54:
Risk factors:
- Family history:
  - 4–10% are inherited
  - Autosomal dominant genes (5% of cases):
    - BRCA1 on chromosome 17 (80% risk)
    - BRCA2 on chromosome 13
- Previous history:
  - Previous benign breast disease
  - Cancer in other breast
  - Radiation exposure

- Uninterrupted oestrogen exposure increases risk:
  - Contraceptive pill
  - Hormone replacement therapy
  - Early menarche or late menopause
  - Late 1st pregnancy
  - Few pregnancies
  - Obesity: ↑ oestrogen levels
  - Alcohol: ↑ oestrone and estradiol
- Other:
  - High alcohol or fat intake
  - Afro-Caribbean
  - Geographical factors
- Protective factors:
  - Breast feeding for >3 months
  - Exercise: probably due to affect of delaying menarche and reducing cycles.

Clinical features

- Palpable lump
- Pain 10%
- Weight loss, anorexia

Inspection:
- Skin:
  - Tethering
  - Erythema
  - Ulceration
  - Satellite nodules
  - Dimpling (peau d'orange, skin of an orange): from direct spread to the lymphatics causing blockage and causing oedema of skin between pits

- Nipple
  - Destruction/ulceration
  - Unilateral inversion or in drawing/retraction
  - Distortion, erythema, Paget's, discharge (blood)

Palpation:
- Texture: hard irregular lumps
- Mobility: fixed to skin/muscle
- Breast lump or thickening
- Swelling or lump in axilla

Location of breast cancer:
- Most cancers occur in the upper outer quadrant.

Investigations

Triple screening

1. History and examination
2. Imaging:
   - Mammography (above 35 years) and US (below 35)
   - Mammography not useful in those below 35 as breast tissue is too dense
   - Cancer changes on mammography include: spiculated lesions, masses and microcalcifications (Fig. 13.3)
3. Fine needle aspiration cytology or core biopsy

For grading and staging

- Blood tests: FBC, U&Es, LFTs

Imaging

- CXR
- Bone scan
- Abdominal US
- CT: brain/thorax
- MRI
- Biopsy: of the lump and sentinal node biopsy where dye is injected into the area around the cancer and the first node that the cancer is likely to spread to is identified and excised.

Prevention

- Breast screening: two view mammography every 3 years for women aged 50–70 years

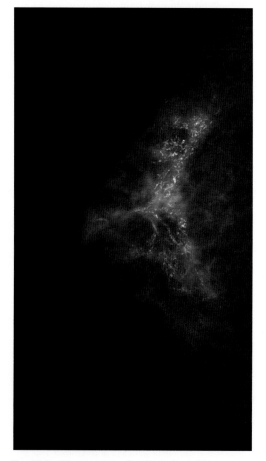

Fig. 13.3 Mammogram showing a branching calcification consistent with carcinoma.

Treatment

T_1, T_2:
- Wide local excision: removal of lump combined with:
  - sentinel node biopsy: (biopsy of the first nodes reached by the tumour) if the lymph node is clear, axillary clearance can be avoided
  - axillary lymph node sampling: removal of lower axillary nodes, which if affected are cleared
  - axillary clearance: removing axillary nodes below axillary vein
  - radiotherapy
- Simple mastectomy: >3.5 cm lump or nipple involved. Need for radiotherapy driven by grade of disease as well as spread to nodes
- Mastectomy and wide local excision have similar survival rates
- All surgery requires chemotherapy and/or hormone therapy
- Reconstructive surgery: at initial mastectomy or at a later date

T_3, T_4:
- Chemotherapy, radiotherapy
- Salvage mastectomy

Paget's disease:
- Mastectomy

M1 (distant metastases):
- Palliation
- Bone disease: bisphosphonates, analgesia, radiotherapy

- Hormonal therapy
- Chemotherapy
- Aspiration of pleural effusions
- Dexamethasone and radiotherapy for cerebral metastases

Endocrine therapy:
- Aim to reduce oestrogen
- Aromatase inhibitors (anti-oestrogen), e.g. arimidex effective in 75% of postmenopausal women who have only peripheral oestrogen
- Tamoxifen: ER blocker if ER+ve (side effects: Endometrial cancer risk, menopausal symptoms, stroke, hot flushes, pulmonary embolism), 5% of ER−ve women respond
- Oophorectomy: removal of ovaries and therefore ovarian oestrogen in premenopausal women
- Molecular therapy: herceptin (Trastuzumab): monoclonal antibody to target HER2

Cytotoxic chemotherapy:
- Reduce recurrence/death by 20%
- For recurrent disease, large tumours, premenopausal women
- Anthracycline, taxane
- 5-Fluorouracil, epirubicin, cyclophosphamide (FEC; side effects are nausea, exhaustion, vomiting, hair loss, suppressed bone marrow, infertility).

Prognosis and complications

Prognosis

- Metastatic disease: life expectancy is 2–3 years
- Mastectectomy: 50% recurrence locally from 1° tumour

- Poor prognostic factors:
  - Skin ulceration
  - Palpable enlarged liver

Complications

From radiotherapy:
- Arm oedema
- Brachial plexopathy
- ↓ arm mobility
- Soft tissue necrosis
- Rib fractures
- Radiation pneumonitis

- Radiation-related heart disease
- Carcinogenesis

From axillary treatment:
- Nerve injury
- Wound complications
- Reduction in shoulder movement
- Lymphoedema: postoperatively 10%.

UROLOGICAL DISORDERS

EPIDIDYMAL CYST

Outline

- A fluid-filled cyst of the head of the epididymis (Fig. 13.4)
- Distended with milky fluid
- Can be single or multiple
- Spermatocele: cyst filled with sperm, more opalescent and milky than a pure epidydimal cyst

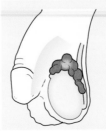

Fig. 13.4 Epididymal cyst: small firm mass that is cystic and within the epididymis (separate from the testes).

Pathogenesis/aetiology

Causes

- Unclear cause
- From the collecting tubules of the epididymis
- Possibly due to obstruction which may arise due to trauma.

Who

- Typical age: develops in adulthood
- Commonest cystic condition encountered in scrotum.

A typical patient

A man presents after noticing a painless swelling on self examination.

Clinical features

- Painless cystic mass at head of epididymis
- Can get above the lump and it separates from the testes
- May be multiple cysts
- Asymptomatic but larger cysts can be uncomfortable.

Investigations

Clinical examination

- Transilluminates
- Lump is separate from the testes.

Imaging

- US.

Other tests

- Aspiration: to distinguish an epididymal cyst from a spermatocele.

Treatment

Conservative

- If asymptomatic or small.

Surgical

- Spermatocelectomy: if discomfort or pain (pain may persist though).

Prognosis and complications

Prognosis

- Benign condition.

Complications

- Risk of damage to the epididymis.

HYDROCELE

Outline

- Hydrocele: an accumulation of serous fluid in a bodily cavity
- Hydrocele testis: serous fluid around the testicle between the tunica vaginalis and tunica albuginea (Fig. 13.5).

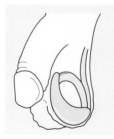

Fig. 13.5 Hydocele: fluid in the tunica vaginalis that surrounds the testicle; a cystic mass that transilluminates.

Pathogenesis/aetiology

Causes

1°:
- Children: the processus vaginalis (part of the peritoneal sac) can descend with the testes and if connected to the abdomen, can fill with peritoneal fluid. Note the difference between a hydrocele and hernia; if fluid comes down it is a hydocele, if bowel, it is a hernia, they have the same cause (a patent processus vaginalis)
- Adults: the tunica vaginalis produces excessive fluid

2°:
- Infection: orchitis
- Malignancy: testicular tumours can present with a hydrocele
- Trauma.

Who

- Typical age: common in those >40

- Commonest cause of scrotal swellings.

A typical patient

A man notices a painless swelling in the testis which changes in size.

Clinical features

- Develop slowly
- Large and tense
- Usually lies in front of the testes and contains straw-coloured fluid
- On palpation it is possible to feel above the swelling

- Lump cannot be separated from the testes
- Transilluminates
- Can appear blue in a tense hydrocele.

Investigations

- Clinical examination.

Imaging

- US: important to distinguish between hydrocele and tumour.

Treatment

- Small: no treatment
- Larger: US to exclude tumour prior to surgical treatment
- Infants: no repair as 95% will resolve spontaneously by age of 2. Ligation of the patent processus vaginalis is cosmetic

- Do not aspirate unless excluded tumour; otherwise, risk of spread to external inguinal nodes.

Surgical

- Lord's repair: drain fluid and evert tunica vaginalis
- Jaboulay's repair: invert the sac around the spermatic cord

- Emergency surgical exploration if associated with swollen and acutely tender testis as can be due to acute torsion of the testis.

Prognosis and complications

Prognosis

- Primary hydrocele is a benign condition, but secondary hydrocele outcome depends on cause.

VARICOCELE

Outline

- An abnormal enlargement of the veins (pampiniform plexus) in the scrotum draining the testicles (Fig. 13.6)
- Usually left sided.

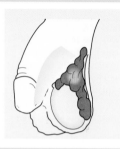

Fig. 13.6 Varicocele: dilated tortuous veins in the pampiniform plexus.

Pathogenesis/aetiology

Causes

- Defective valves
- Compression of the vein by a nearby structure; may be a presentation of renal carcinoma.

Who

A typical patient

A man presents with swollen testis and complaining of a dragging sensation in his scrotum. On palpation the testis feels like 'a bag of worms'

Clinical features

- Testicular pain
- Heavy feeling
- Shrinking of testes
- Large veins
- Blood vessels: feels like 'a bag of worms'
- Does not transilluminate
- Can feel above the lump and is separate from the testes
- Reduced fertility.

Investigations

Imaging

- US scan.

Treatment

- Scrotal support
- Surgical ligation of testicular vein
- Percutaneous embolisation.

Prognosis and complications

Prognosis

- Successful treatment may reduce the risk of infertility.

Complications

- Infertility: a common reason for seeking help.

EPIDIDYMO-ORCHITIS

Outline

- Inflammation of the testis and epididymis due to infection (Fig. 13.7).

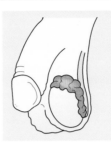

Fig. 13.7   Epididymitis: a non-cystic, very painful mass

Pathogenesis/aetiology

Causes

- Young: viral e.g. mumps
- Older: bacterial e.g. *Escherichia coli* UTI, *Chlamydia trachomatis*, *Neisseria gonorrhoeae*, TB >.

Who

A typical patient

A man presents with acute scrotal pain and pain on passing urine.

Clinical features

- Acute and severe testicular pain
- Pain may be referred to right iliac fossa
- Tender, erythematous and warm testes
- Urethral discharge
- Lower urinary tract symptoms
- Fever
- Epididymis separate from testicle
- Elevation of the testes by hand relieves pain (pain persists if due to testicular torsion).

Investigations

Urine

- microscopy and culture

Imaging

- US (in children) due to association with vesicoureteric reflux disease and abnormalities of ureteric insertion.

Other tests

- Sexual screen

Treatment

Antibiotic therapy

Prognosis and complications

Prognosis

- Resolution with antibiotic therapy
- Recurrence suggests underlying anatomical anomaly.

Complications

- Infertility.

BALANITIS

Outline

- Inflammation of the foreskin and glans.

Pathogenesis/aetiology

Causes

- Infection from *Staphylococcus, Streptococcus*

Risk factors:
- Young boys with phimosis (see below)
- Diabetes mellitus.

Who

A typical patient

A man presents with dysuria and on examination the doctor is unable to retract his foreskin.

Clinical features

- Can present with retention due to pain and swelling.

Investigations

- Clinical examination.

Treatment

- Antibiotics
- Circumcision.

Prognosis and complications

Complication

Recurrent balanitis can lead to scarring and the need for circumcision.

PHIMOSIS

Outline

- Narrowing of the opening of the foreskin
- Inability to retract the foreskin.

Pathogenesis/aetiology

Causes

- 2° to infection and scarring
- Physiological in infants
- Preputial adhesions holding the foreskin to the penis.

Who

A typical patient

A patient complains that he cannot retract his foreskin.

Clinical features

- Painful intercourse
- Bleeding of the foreskin
- Recurrent infection.

Investigations

- Clinical examination.

Treatment

- Treat any infection
- Trial of steroid cream can treat preputial adhesions
- Circumcision.

Prognosis

- Most resolve with conservative treatment.

PARAPHIMOSIS

Outline

- Swelling of the glans from tight foreskin being retracted and not replaced
- Prevents venous return leading to oedema and ischaemia of the glans.

Pathogenesis/aetiology

Causes

- Can occur after catheterisation, an erection, masturbation.

Who

A typical patient

A man who has had a catheter inserted notices a tender glans.

Clinical features

- Tender swollen glans with tight foreskin
- Bleeding.

Investigations

- Clinical examination.

Treatment

- Manually reduce oedema with compression and squeeze foreskin and glans
- Surgical: dorsal slit may be needed.

Prognosis and complications

Prognosis

- Good outcome if treated early.

Complications

- Obstructed venous return causes oedema and swelling.

HYPOSPADIAS

Outline

- Abnormal position of urethral opening in development failure.

Pathogenesis/aetiology

- Urethra can open anywhere on the ventral surface of the penis.

Who

A typical patient

A paediatric doctor notices a 'hooded' foreskin at postnatal check and that the urethral opening is not in the anatomical position.

Clinical features

- Typically 'hooded' foreskin or absent foreskin
- Abnormal opening of urethra.

Investigations

- Clinical examination.

Treatment

- Paediatric surgery
- Should not have cultural circumcision as the foreskin is used in reconstruction.

Prognosis and complications

Prognosis

- Good outcome with surgical correction.

Complications

- Fistula after repair.

UNDESCENDED TESTIS (CRYPTORCHIDISM)

Outline

- Testes do not descend properly during their embryological development.

Pathogenesis/aetiology

- Unilateral pathology is more common than bilateral
- Bilateral undescended testes are associated with endocrine abnormalities.

Pathogenesis

- Testes normally develop on the posterior abdominal wall and descend at 28–34 weeks
- If they fail to descend, they can lie anywhere between the abdomen and the groin
- 80% of undescended testes are palpable in the inguinal canal.

Who

- Incidence: 3% at birth, 1% at one year
- Commoner in premature babies.

A typical patient

On routine postnatal check the paediatrician notices that the testis is not in the scrotum.

Clinical features

- Impalpable testes

Investigations

Clinical examination

- Testes not palpable within the scrotal sac
- May be palpable at the scrotal ring or inguinal canal.

Imaging

- US
- MRI.

Other tests

- Laparoscopy

Treatment

Orchidopexy:
- Surgical fixation of the undescended testis into place
- Ideally by the age of 2
- Aim is to bring the testis to an examinable position and to prevent torsion or trauma

- Testes are fixed in the scrotum in a subdartos pouch

Age-specific considerations:
- Monitor if <1 year old at diagnosis.

Prognosis and complications

Prognosis

- If diagnosed before age 1, testes may still spontaneously descend.

Complications

- Infertility
- Increased risk of testicular malignancy
- Torsion
- Trauma.

TESTICULAR TORSION

Outline

- Twisting of the testis in the tunica vaginalis
- Urological emergency as the blood supply to the testis is compromised and can infarct within hours
- Usually unilateral.

Pathogenesis/aetiology

Causes

- Testis at risk of twisting as it hangs relatively freely from its mesentery
- Normally history of trauma or exertion

Differential diagnosis:
- Torsion of the hydatid of Morgagni: embryological remnant of the testes
- Epidydimo-orchitis.

Who

- Typical age: peak incidence at 12–25 years, often around puberty.

A typical patient

A teenage boy has sudden-onset acute scrotal pain.

Clinical features

- Sudden-onset testicular pain
- Severe pain: in scrotum and lower abdomen
- Hot, swollen testis
- Tender vas deferens
- Erythema of scrotal skin due to ischaemia and oedema
- Testis lies abnormally: horizontally or retracted
- Nausea and vomiting
- Associated hydrocele
- History: mumps, trauma, sore throat, dysuria.

Investigations

- **Surgical emergency, do not delay for unnecessary tests.**
  - Surgical exploration

Blood tests

- FBC, U&Es

Urine

- Urine dipstick: exclude infection

- Analgesia
- Urgent surgery: if in any doubt to prevent ischaemia
- If viable: bilateral fixation (orchidopexy)

- If not viable: orchidectomy, with fixation of the other testicle.

Prognosis and complications

Prognosis

- Good outcome with early intervention.

Complications

- Loss of testis
- Testicular atrophy

- Infertility due to anti-sperm antibodies.

TESTICULAR TUMOURS

Outline

- Cancer of the testis (Fig. 13.8)
- Bilateral in 5%
Types:
- *Seminomas* (40%): a germ cell tumour, commoner in those aged 30–65 years. Aggressive. Can excrete human chorionic gonadotrophin (hCG)
- *Teratomas* (10%): commoner in younger men aged 20–30 years
- *Mixed* (40%)
- *Leydig or Sertoli tumours*: rare
- *Lymphomas*: older men

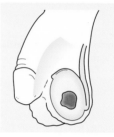

Fig. 13.8 Testicular tumour: a solid mass that is part of the testicle.

Pathogenesis/aetiology

Staging:
- I: confined to testes
- II: lymph nodes below diaphragm

- III: above diaphragm
- IV: extralymphatic spread.

Who

- Commonest malignancy in males aged 15–44
- <2% of male malignancy
- Prevalence: 0.007%

Risk factors:
- Undescended testes (10%)
- Infertility

A typical patient

A 25-year-old man presents with a testicular lump that he noticed on self examination.

Clinical features

- Painless testicular mass
- Able to palpate above the mass
- Does not transilluminate

- Leydig or Sertoli tumours can produce oestrogens and androgens leading to feminisation and virilisation, e.g. gynaecomastia.

Investigations

Serum tumour markers

In seminomas:
- Placental alkaline phosphotase

In teratomas:
- Beta-hCG: can detect easily on urine dipstick
- α-fetoprotein.

Imaging

- US

- CXR, CT: for metastases.

Other tests

- Excision biopsy.

Treatment

- Monitor with tumour markers

- Sperm banking if fertility is an issue.

Surgical

- Orchidectomy if confined to testis: occlude spermatic cord to decrease risk of spread

- Further treatment depends on grade and stage

Radiotherapy

- Seminomas are radiosensitive

- Teratomas are less sensitive

Chemotherapy

- For widespread tumours

- Teratomas with metastases: bleomycin, etoposide, cisplatin.

Prognosis and complications

Prognosis

- Stage I: 96–100% 5 year survival
- Stage IV: 55–75% 5 year survival

- Recurrence likely at 18–24 months so monitoring is important.

Complications

- Infertility
- Metastases to:
  - lymph nodes: to para-aortic lymph nodes as testes descend along the para-aortic path

- lungs
- liver
- (not bone).

CANCER OF THE PENIS

Outline

- Cancer of the penis.

Pathogenesis/aetiology

Pathogenesis

- Squamous cell carcinoma

- Spreads locally to inguinal nodes.

Who

- Typical age: in elderly
- Rare, particularly in circumcised men

- Occurs more often in humid, hot countries.

Clinical features

- Bloody discharge
- Ulcer

- Painful lesions
- Lymphadenopathy.

Investigations

- Biopsy

- CT.

Treatment

- Radiotherapy for small lesions.

Surgical

- Amputate if urethra involved
- Partially amputate if >2 cm penis unaffected

- Circumcision if early detection.

Prognosis and complications

Prognosis

- Carcinoma in situ 5-year survival: 90%
- Local lymph node involvement 5 year survival: 60%

- Distal spread 5 year survival: 20%.

Complications

- Ulceration

- Distal metastases.

HERNIAS

GENERAL FEATURES

Outline

- Protrusion of an organ or tissue through the walls of its cavity into an abnormal position
- Consists of the sac, its contents and the hernial orifice

Abdominal hernias:

- Hiatus hernia: see 'Disorders of the oesophagus' below
- Epigastric/ventral: through the linea alba that runs down the midline of the abdomen
- Umbilical
- Paraumbilical
- Spigelian: (lateral ventral hernia) through the spigelian fascia (between rectus abdominis medially, and semilunar line laterally), often develop at or below the linea arcuata. Due to lack of posterior rectus sheath
- Maydl's: herniating double loop of bowel, strangulated part can reside as single loop inside bowel cavity
- Littre's: hernial sac with Meckel's diverticulum
- Obturator: through obturator foramen, above the pubic rings
- Femoral
- Inguinal
- Gluteal
- Lumbar: through lumbar triangles
- Amyand hernia: contains appendix.

Pathogenesis/aetiology

Causes

Congenital:
- These do not regress spontaneously
- Infantile inguinal/umbilical

Acquired:
- Weakness of an opening and straining from:
  - Chronic cough
  - Chronic constipation
  - Severe muscular effort
  - Obesity
  - Ascites
  - Previous surgery
  - Iatrogenic
  - Infective
  - Traumatic
  - Neoplastic

Definitions:
- *Incisional hernia*: arising though a weakness created from a previously made incision
- *Reducible*: hernia can be returned to former position
- *Irreducible*: cannot be reduced to former position
- *Incarceration*: hernial contents are fixed inside due to adhesions. This is a surgical emergency.
- *Obstructed*: bowel contents within the hernia are obstructed
- *Strangulated*: the orifice of the hernia restricts the blood supply and ischaemia occurs. This is a surgical emergency.
- *Sliding hernia*: the organ is part of the hernial sac
- *Richter's*: only part of bowel wall is herniated so hernia can be strangulated without obstruction. Common in femoral hernias.

Who

- Depends on the hernia.

Clinical features

- A lump: typically on straining, coughing, standing or lifting. May disappear on lying down or when pressed on by patient
- Pain
- Cannot get above a hernia
- Can occur in several locations (Fig. 13.9)

Abdominal hernias – typically:
- Reducible
- Audible bowel sounds over the hernia
- Cough impulse: expansile but not if incarcerated or strangulated
- Strangulation: constant pain with tachycardia. Overlying skin is red and oedematous, with an irreducible mass. Symptoms of obstruction.

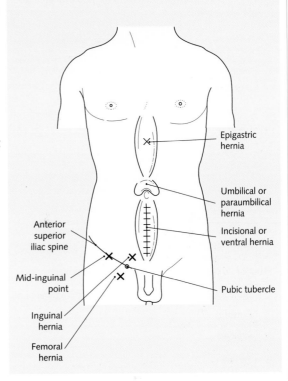

Fig. 13.9 Location of hernias.

Labels: Epigastric hernia; Umbilical or paraumbilical hernia; Incisional or ventral hernia; Pubic tubercle; Anterior superior iliac spine; Mid-inguinal point; Inguinal hernia; Femoral hernia

Investigations

- Clinical examination of a hernia:
  - Stand up
  - Expose umbilicus to mid-thigh
- Cough
- Identify location and direction of bulge movement.

Treatment

- Surgery with sutures or mesh repair. Mesh reduces risk of recurrence
- Elective surgery for reducible hernias
- Emergency surgery for strangulated or incarcerated hernias.

Prognosis and complications

Complications

- Obstruction
- Strangulation
- Richter's hernia: often gets reduced, and then perforates, causing peritonitis.

FEMORAL HERNIA

Outline

- Bowel protrudes through the femoral canal (Fig. 13.10)
- Normally the canal contains only fat and lymph
- Mass is found below and lateral to the pubic tubercle and extends upwards.

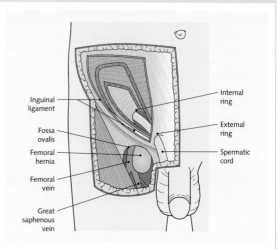

Fig. 13.10   Femoral hernia.

Pathogenesis/aetiology

Table 13.3 compares femoral and inguinal hernias.

Table 13.3   Comparison of femoral and inguinal hernias

Femoral	Inguinal
Smaller	Larger
♀ > ♂	♀ < ♂
Mass below and lateral to pubic tubercle. Protrudes medial to the epigastric vessels	Mass above and lateral to pubic tubercle (but can be medial)
Strangulation more likely	Strangulation less likely
15%	60% indirect 25% direct

Who

- ♀ > ♂.

A typical patient

An elderly female has a tender groin swelling.

Clinical features

- Mass in upper medial thigh pointing down leg
- Neck of the hernia felt inferior and lateral to pubic tubercle

- Often irreducible
- Likely to strangulate: tender, colicky abdominal pain.

Investigations

- Clinical examination of a hernia as above.

- All should be repaired quickly due to risk of strangulation
- Surgery: suture inguinal ligament to pectineal ligament.

Prognosis

- Poor recognition leads to damage of hernia contents.

Complications

- Strangulation: more likely than for inguinal hernias as the lacunar ligament which forms the medial border is sharp-edged.

INGUINAL HERNIA

Outline

- Protrusions of bowel through the inguinal canal.
  - May be direct or indirect (Fig. 13.11).

Classification

Indirect hernia 80%:
- Passes through the deep and superficial inguinal rings
- May be congenital from patent processus vaginalis or acquired from weakness through the deep ring
- Bowel travels along the inguinal canal with spermatic cord and often extends to scrotum

Direct hernias 20%:
- Enter directly through the superficial ring
- Acquired from a weakness in the transversalis facia in Hasselbach's triangle
- Triangle boundaries: inguinal ligament, inferior epigastric vessels and the lateral border of rectus abdominus

Structures

- *Deep ring:* at the midpoint of the inguinal ligament
- *Superficial ring:* a split in the external oblique aponurosis
- *Processus vaginalis:* projection of peritoneum from when testes develop as they descend from abdomen to the scrotum forming the inguinal canal
- *Midpoint of the inguinal ligament:* midpoint between the anterior superior iliac spine and the pubic tubercle. Surface marking of the deep inguinal ring
- *Mid-inguinal point:* midpoint between the anterior superior iliac spine and pubic symphysis. Surface marking of femoral artery

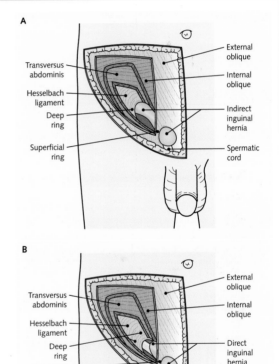

Fig. 13.11   Inguinal hernia: (A) indirect; (B) direct.

Pathogenesis/aetiology

Table 13.4 summarises the differences between direct and indirect hernias:

Table 13.4 Differences between direct and indirect hernias

Indirect	Direct
Through superficial and deep rings	Through deep ring
Congenital or acquired	Acquired
Children and adults	Adults
Will not reduce at once	Reduces spontaneously on lying
High risk of strangulation	Rarely strangulates

Who

- ♀ < ♂
- 7% of population

- Prevalence: more common than femoral hernias.

A typical patient

A male presents with a painful lump in his groin.

Clinical features

- Groin lump
- Bulge in the inguinal region

- Unable to get above the lump
- Protrudes with coughing.

Investigations

- Clinical examination of a hernia as above
To differentiate between types of inguinal hernias (often requested in OSCEs but realistically not accurate nor does it alter management):
- Reduce the hernia while patient is supine

- Apply pressure with thumb over the deep ring (at the midpoint of the inguinal ligament)
- Ask the patient to stand and cough
- If hernia is restrained it is indirect, if it is not restrained it is direct.

Treatment

Surgical

- In all children and infants: complete herniotomy as quickly as possible to prevent incarceration

- Herniotomy: operative ligation of hernia sac at deep ring.

Prognosis and complications

Prognosis

- Good outcome with surgical repair.

Complications

- Recurrence

- Incarceration.

PARAUMBILICAL/UMBILICAL HERNIA

Outline

- Bowel herniates through a weakness in the umbilicus (true hernia) or area just next to it (paraumbilical hernia).

Pathogenesis/aetiology

Paraumbilical hernias:
- Acquired
- Occurs in adults
- Bowel protrudes through a canal bordered by the umbilical fascia posteriorly, linea alba anteriorly and rectus sheath laterally

True umbilical hernia:
- Congenital defect
- 3% of births
- Due to failure of closure of the umbilical ring through which the umbilical vessels pass
- Recurrence in adults, e.g. in pregnancy or ascites.

Who

Risk factors:
- Obesity

- Ascites.

Clinical features

- Paraumbilical hernias: able to see the umbilicus as a semicircle

- Umbilical hernias: mass bulges directly from the umbilicus.

Investigations

- Evident on clinical examination.

Treatment

Paraumbilical hernia:
- Surgery: repair of the rectus sheath with sutures or mesh

True umbilical hernia:
- Surgery rarely required in children as most resolve by age 3

- Reserve surgery for those persisting after age 5 and a defect >1 cm
- Can consider surgery in preschoolers for cosmetic reasons

Prognosis and complications

Prognosis

- Good outcome.

Complications

- Incarceration rare

- Ulceration if hernia is very large.

DISORDERS OF THE GI TRACT

DISORDERS OF THE OESOPHAGUS

OESOPHAGEAL PERFORATION

Outline

- Perforation of the oesophagus.

Pathogenesis/aetiology

Causes

- Iatrogenic: commonest cause, e.g. from endoscopy
- Ingesting sharp foreign body or corrosive agent

- Boerhaave syndrome from forceful/prolonged vomiting.

A typical patient

- A patient who has just had a routine OGD suddenly collapses.
- A rugby playing medical student who has drunk excessive alcohol comes to A&E with severe chest pain.

Clinical features

- Sudden severe pain in the chest, back and neck
- Fever
- Hypotension
- Surgical emphysema in left supraclavicular fossa.

Investigations

Imaging

- Erect CXR: air in mediastinum
- Contrast swallow (with water-soluble contrast agent)
- Endoscopy
- CT.

Treatment

- Nil by mouth
- IV antibiotics
- IV fluid
- Chest drain for infected pleural space
- Surgical repair if necessary
- Find and treat cause

If Iatrogenic perforation:
- Nasogastric tube
- proton pump inhibitor
- antibiotics.

Prognosis and complications

Prognosis

- High mortality rate.

Complications

- Mediastinitis
- Empyema.

PHARYNGEAL POUCH

Outline

- Outpouching of pharynx
- Usually above the upper sphincter of the oesophagus; between the upper border of cricopharyngeus muscle
- and lower border of inferior constrictor muscle of the pharynx
- Corresponds with a potential weak area called Killian's dehiscence.

Pathogenesis/aetiology

Causes

- Peristalsis against resistance from uncoordinated muscular spasms
- Food can collect in the pouch and expand, causing dysphagia.

Who

A typical patient

A patient presents to his GP complaining of bad breath.

Clinical features

- Asymptomatic
- Food regurgitation from the diverticulum
- Dysphagia
- Gurgling sounds
- Halitosis (bad breath)
- Neck lump: usually to left side of neck.

Investigations

- Barium swallow.

Treatment

Surgical

- Excision of pouch by open surgery
- Endoscopic stapling between pouch and oesophagus which opens the pouch and allows it to drain freely.

Prognosis and complications

Prognosis

- Surgery is curative.

Complications

- Perforation during endoscopy if scope enters diverticulum rather than the oesophagus.

HIATUS HERNIA

Outline

- Herniation of the stomach or gastro-oesophageal junction through the diaphragmatic hiatus into the thoracic cavity

Classification (Fig. 13.12)

- *Sliding hiatus*: 80%. Gastro-oesophageal junction is pulled through the diaphragmatic hiatus into the thorax
- *Rolling/para-oesophageal*: 15%. Stomach rolls up through the hiatus beside the oesophagus. The junction remains in the same place within the abdomen
- *Mixed*: 5%.

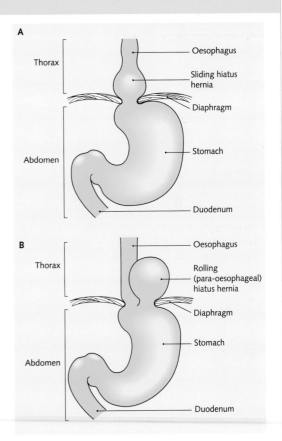

Fig. 13.12 Types of hiatus hernia. Sliding (A) and Rolling (B).

Pathogenesis/aetiology

Causes

- Increased abdominal pressure
- Low-fibre diets

- Laxity of the diaphragmatic hiatus
- Peri-oesophageal attachments.

Who

- Typical age: incidence: ↑ after 50 years
- ♀ > ♂

Risk factors:
- Obese.

A typical patient

An obese patient presents with symptoms of GORD.

Clinical features

- Asymptomatic unless associated reflux
- Reflux oesophagitis in 50%

- Retrosternal burning pain.

Investigations

- Barium swallow

- CXR: may show air fluid level or stomach in chest.

Treatment

Conservative

- Lose weight
- Stop smoking

- Smaller meals earlier in the evening.

Medical

- Antacids
- Proton pump inhibitors, e.g. omeprazole

- H$_2$ receptor antagonists, e.g. ranitidine
- Alginate preparations.

Surgical

- If medication fails
- Nissen fundoplication (open or laparascopically): mobilise fundus of stomach and wrap around lower

  oesophageal sphincter, which causes a high-pressure area to prevent reflux.

Prognosis and complications

Prognosis

- Benign course

Complications

- Reflux oesophagitis, which can then result in:
  - Oesophagitis
  - Oesophageal stricture and dysphagia
  - Ulceration
  - Anaemia

- Mucosal erosions
- Bleeding: haematemesis/melaena
- Aspiration pneumonia
- Asthma due to aspiration of acid.

DISORDERS OF THE STOMACH

PYLORIC STENOSIS

Outline

- Narrowing of the pyloric sphincter of the stomach leading to severe vomiting.

Pathogenesis/aetiology

Pathogenesis

- Stenosis is at the entrance of the small intestines from the stomach

In babies:
- Due to hypertrophy of smooth muscle of the pylorus

In adults:
- May be due to scarring from a previous ulcer, malignancy or external compression.

Who

- Typical age: 2–6 week old babies, but can also occur in adults
- 1♀:5♂
- Incidence: 1 in 300–400 children

Associations:
- First-born males
- Caucasians
- Strong family history.

A typical patient

A patient with known gastric cancer presents with vomiting 1-2 hours after eating.

Clinical features

- Weight loss: from obstruction
- Dehydration

Investigations

Clinical examination

- Succession splash: sound made by shaking free fluid and air or gas in a hollow organ or cavity.

Blood tests

- Electrolyte disturbance
- Hypochloraemic, hypokalaemic, metabolic alkalosis.

Imaging

- Barium studies
- Endoscopy

Treatment

- Fluid resuscitation
- Correct dehydration and biochemical abnormalities with fluids
- In babies: surgical Ramstedt pylorotomy to divide muscle fibres of pylorus
- In adults: establish feeding route (e.g. naso-jejunal feeding tube to bypass the obstruction) and treat obstruction e.g. NSAIDs if due to peptic ulcer disease, surgery if an operable malignancy, stent if inoperable malignancy.

Prognosis and complications

Prognosis

- Surgery is curative in babies.

Complications

- Metabolic alkalosis.

PERFORATED PEPTIC ULCER

Outline

- Rupture of a peptic ulcer leading to acute peritonitis
- (See Peptic ulcer disease in Gastroenterology chapter)
- Commonest site is the first part of the duodenum
- **A surgical emergency.**

Pathogenesis/aetiology

- Anterior ulcers: tend to perforate
- Posterior ulcers: tend to haemorrhage.

Pathogenesis

- 30% of perforated gastric ulcers are malignant
- 90% of perforated ulcers are associated with *H. pylori*.

Who

- Rare with *H. pylori* treatment.

Clinical features

Symptoms

- Sudden severe pain: begins in epigastrium, becomes generalised
- Vomiting.

Signs

- Peritonism
- Patient lies still
- Rigid abdomen
- Rebound tenderness
- Percussion tenderness
- Absent bowel sounds.

Investigations

- Clinical diagnosis.

Blood tests

- FBC
- U&Es
- Clotting
- Amylase: slightly ↑.

Imaging

- Erect CXR: air under diaphragm in 70% (Fig. 13.13).
- CT

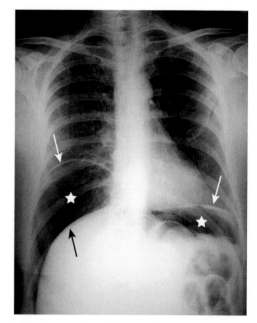

Fig. 13.13 Perforated gastric ulcer; a large amount of free air (white stars) seen underneath the diaphragm (white arrows) on erect CXR. The top of the liver (black arrow) is made visible by the air above it.

Treatment

- Resuscitation

Conservative

- Fluids and antibiotics if surgery cannot be performed.

Surgical

- Laparotomy
- Duodenal: washout and patch

Medical

- Long-term acid suppression with anti-*H. pylori* treatment.

- Nil by mouth, nasogastric tube

- Gastric: excise ulcer and repair defect: biopsy for malignancy

Prognosis and complications

Complications

- Peritonitis

- GI bleeding due to erosion into gastric (or rarely pancreatic) vessels.

DISORDERS OF THE BOWEL

SMALL BOWEL OBSTRUCTION

Outline

- Obstruction of the small bowel
- Severe tenderness implies ischaemia of the bowel
Distinguishing small bowel from large bowel:
- *Small bowel*: have valvulae conniventes (membranous folds of the small intestine) that cross the lumen completely and are seen to cross the entire width on X-ray, appearing as a 'laddering' effect (Fig. 13.14)
- *Large bowel*: have haustra that only partly cross the lumen width and appear as interrupted lines on X-ray.

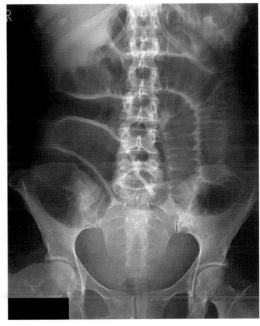

Fig. 13.14   AXR showing dilated small bowel loops in obstruction.

Pathogenesis/aetiology

Causes

Within the lumen:
- Large polyps
- Intussusception
- Gallstone
- Faeces/food bolus
- Swallowed foreign body

Within the bowel wall:
- Benign stricture
- Malignancy
- Infarction

- Crohn's disease
- Ileus: ↓ bowel motility and peristalsis causing functional obstruction

Outside the bowel:
- Adhesions: commonest cause, particularly postoperatively
- Strangulated hernia: 2nd commonest cause
- Volvulus (see below)
- Intussusception.

Who

A typical patient

A patient complains of colicky abdominal pain with bile-stained vomiting and abdominal distension.

Clinical features

Symptoms

- Early: vomiting
- Late: constipation, may not be complete

- Severe pain: intermittent colicky spasms in the central abdomen. Pain higher in abdomen than in large bowel obstruction.

Signs

- Abdominal distension (less than in large bowel obstruction)

- Increased bowel sounds: tinkling

Ileus (reduced bowel motility)

- No pain, bowel sounds are absent

Strangulation

- Patient more ill than expected. Sharper pain, focal tenderness. Peritonism is the key sign with fever and tachycardia. Requires urgent surgery.

Investigations

Clinical examination

- Rectal examination

- Hernia examination.

Blood tests

- FBC
- U&Es

- Lactate: ↑ in ischaemia
- ↑ Amylase.

Imaging

- Plain AXR: bowel distension and air-fluid levels, central gas shadows and no gas in large bowel (Fig. 13.14).

Treatment

- Fluid resuscitation
- 'Drip and suck':
  - Drip: IV fluid
  - Suck: nasogastric tube to remove bowel secretions and allow the gut to rest
- Determine cause
- Small bowel obstruction can be treated conservatively in adults

Specifics:
- Emergency surgery: if ischaemic bowel or incarcerated hernia
- Hernia: herniotomy and manually release obstruction.
- *Adhesions*: likely if previous surgery and no evidence of ischaemia. Treat conservatively. If no improvement, laparotomy and adhesiolysis (division of adhesions)
- *Ileus and incomplete obstruction*: can be managed conservatively.

Prognosis and complications

Prognosis

- Spontaneous resolution in a proportion without intervention.

Complications

- Strangulation: mesentery twists and can lead to gut ischaemia.

LARGE BOWEL OBSTRUCTION

Outline

- Obstruction of the large bowel
- Severe tenderness implies ischaemia of the bowel

- In 20% of patients the large bowel cannot decompress into the small bowel due to the competency of the ileocaecal valve. This can lead to perforation.

Pathogenesis/aetiology

Causes

Within the lumen:
- Polypoid tumour
- Intussusception

Within the bowel wall:
- Colon cancer
- Diverticulitis
- Benign strictures
- Infarction

- Constipation/impacted faeces
- Crohn's disease

Outside bowel:
- Volvulus (twisting of bowel around its mesenteric attachment, see below)
- Adhesions
- Strangulated hernia
- Intussusception.

Who

A typical patient

An elderly patient presenting with abdominal distension and absolute constipation.

Clinical features

Symptoms

- Earlier: complete constipation
- Late: vomiting

- Pain: colicky spasms, severe and more constant than in small bowel obstruction.

Signs

- Abdominal distension: from obstructed bowel loops becoming distended with fluid and flatus

- Anaemia.

Investigations

Blood tests

- FBC
- U&Es

Imaging

- AXR: gas shown proximal to the blockage. Colonic dilatation with a cut-off (Fig. 13.15)
- Sigmoidoscopy
- Barium enema to confirm level of obstruction.
- CT

- Lactate: ↑ in ischaemia
- ↑ Amylase.

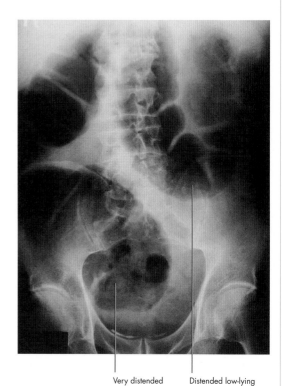

Very distended caecum

Distended low-lying transverse colon

Fig. 13.15 AXR showing distended caecum in large bowel obstruction.

Treatment

- Fluid resuscitation
- 'Drip and suck':
  - Drip: IV fluid

- Suck: nasogastric tube to remove bowel secretions and to allow the gut to rest
- Determine cause.

Surgical

- **Emergency surgery**: if ischaemic bowel
- Stenting: endoscopically or by radiological guidance
- Laparotomy: if the caecum is wide or evidence of peritonitis

- Less urgent bowel obstruction can be treated with water-soluble enemas.

Prognosis and complications

Prognosis

- Depends on cause.

Complications

- Perforation: normally occurs in the caecum as it is the thinnest region.

MESENTERIC ISCHAEMIA: ACUTE

Outline

- Acute restriction in blood supply to the gut
- Can affect any bowel segment: normally affects the small bowel.

Pathogenesis/aetiology

Causes

Those with risk factors for vascular disease:
- Arterial:
  - Thrombotic 35%
  - Embolic 35%
- Venous thrombosis

- Vasculitis
- Trauma
- Radiotherapy
- Strangulated bowel.

Who

A typical patient

A vasculopath presenting with severe central abdominal pain.

Clinical features

- AF with abdominal pain
- Acute severe abdominal pain: constant, central or around RIF
- Redcurrant jelly stool
- Abdominal tenderness

- Peritonitis
- Rapid hypovolaemia
- Shock with minimal abdominal signs.

Investigations

Blood tests

- ↑ Hb (due to plasma loss)
- ↑ WBC

- ↑ Amylase
- Persistent metabolic acidosis.

Imaging

- AXR: gasless abdomen
- Arteriography

- Angiography
- CT or MRI.

Treatment

- Fluid resuscitation
- Antibiotics: gentamicin, metronidazole

- Heparin
- Surgery.

Prognosis and complications

Prognosis

- Poor for arterial thrombosis and non-occlusive disease

- Better for venous and embolic ischaemia

Complications

- Septic peritonitis

- Progression to multi-organ dysfunction mediated by bacterial translocation across the dying gut wall.

MESENTERIC ISCHAEMIA: CHRONIC

Outline

- Chronic restriction in blood supply to the gut
- Less urgent.

Pathogenesis/aetiology

Causes

- Combination of reduced blood flow with atherosclerotic vessels
- Affects small or large bowel.

Who

- ♀ > ♂

A typical patient

An elderly female has a tender groin swelling.

Clinical features

Small bowel:
- Severe abdominal pain: colicky and after eating
- Rectal bleeding
- ↓ Weight and malabsorption

Large bowel:
- Lower left-side abdominal pain
- Diarrhoea
- Pyrexia
- Tachycardia
- Rectal bleeding
- Leucoytosis.

Investigations

- Angioplasty
- Barium enema
- MRI angiography.

Treatment

Conservative

- Fluid replacement
- Antibiotics

Surgical

- Resection with stoma formation for gangrene.

Intervention

- Percutaneous transluminal angioplasty
- Endovascular stent insertion.

Prognosis and complications

Prognosis

- Discrete lesion: symptoms can improve with intervention

Complications

- Gangrenous ischaemic colitis
- Acute ischaemia causing peritonitis and hypovolaemic shock.

VOLVULUS

Outline

- Twisting of bowel around its mesenteric attachment
- Can produce rapid obstruction by strangulation.

Pathogenesis/aetiology

- Normally occurs in the sigmoid
- Can also occur in the caecum and small intestine.

Who

- Typical age: the elderly

Risk factors:
- Constipation.

A typical patient

As with bowel obstruction.

Clinical features

- Constipation
- Colicky pain

- Abdominal distension.

Investigations

- AXR: characteristic coffee bean shape (Fig. 13.16).

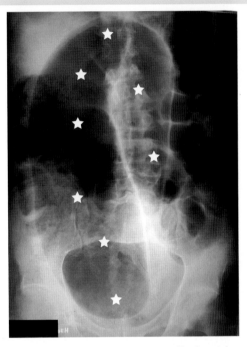

Fig. 13.16 AXR showing characteristic 'coffee bean' shape of grossly dilated sigmoid colon in sigmoid volvulus (starred).

Treatment

- Decompression of the volvulus: leads to excess defecation of faeces. With:
  - A flatus tube or

- Sigmoidoscopy
- Colectomy if recurrent.

Prognosis and complications

Prognosis

- Good with early intervention.

Complications

- Perforation.

DIVERTICULAR DISEASE

Outline

- Diverticulum: outpouching of gut wall
- Diverticulosis: diverticula are present
- Diverticular disease: condition where there are symptomatic diverticula in the colon associated with pain and disturbed bowel habit
- Diverticulitis: inflamed diverticula
- In diverticulitis, pain is due to inflammation of the diverticula; in diverticular disease, pain is due to muscular spasm of the bowel wall.

Features:
- Commonest in sigmoid colon: causes 95% of complications
- Rarely symptomatic if in small intestine
- Never in rectum
- A benign condition: not premalignant.

Pathogenesis/aetiology

Causes

- Unknown
- Congenital

- Acquired: more common
- High fibre diet reduces likelihood of disease.

Pathogenesis

- Diverticula protrude through weakened areas in the muscular intestinal wall near blood vessels

- Low fibre diet may cause ↑ pressure in the colon from more vigorous and longer contractions causing mucosal herniation at sites of weakness
- Pain is due to spasm of the bowel muscle.

Who

- Typical age: mainly in the elderly. >60% of those over 80 years

- Predominately a Western disease.

Clinical features

- Usually asymptomatic
- Constipation and/or diarrhoea
- Abdominal pain in left iliac fossa
- Bloating
- Disturbed bowel habit
- Severe bleeding
- Nausea
- Flatulence
- Weight loss (may be severe)
- Pneumaturia (gas/air in urine) from a colovesicular fistula
- Massive painless haemorrhage: arterial bleed

Diverticulitis:
- As above plus
  - Pyrexia
  - ↑ WBC
  - ↑ CRP and ESR
  - Tender abdomen
- Peritonism
Perforated diverticulitis:
- More sudden onset of pain, signs and symptoms suggestive of acute diverticulitis
- Ileus
- Generalised signs of peritonitis
- Shock
- Erect CXR: free gas under the diaphragm.

- Rectal examination.

Imaging

- Sigmoidoscopy
- Colonoscopy
- Barium enema (Fig. 13.17)
- CT more useful than US.

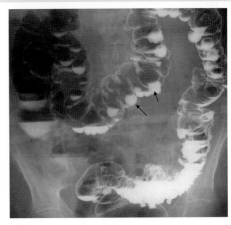

Fig. 13.17 Barium enema showing smooth outpouchings (arrowed) in diverticular disease.

Treatment

Conservative

- High fibre diet
- Mebeverine and peppermint oil
- Mild attacks can be managed at home with bowel rest, intake of only fluids and antibiotics (co-amoxiclav or metronidazole)

- If oral fluids cannot be tolerated or uncontrollable pain, admit: nil by mouth, IV fluids and antibiotics.

Surgical

- Required in 20% of severe cases.

Prognosis and complications

Complications

- Obstruction: inflammatory mass from fibrosis and stricture formation
- Perforation: 40% mortality
- Infection
- Fistulae: colovesicular most common

- Haemorrhage
- Abscess: often in the liver or bowel wall
- Cystitis: if fistulated into the bladder wall
- No predisposition to carcinoma of colon
- Incidental findings can be treated conservatively.

COLONIC POLYPS

Outline

- A polyp is an elevation of tissue projecting from a mucous membrane
- Colonic polyps project into the colonic lumen

- May be multiple
- Malignant potential

Adenomatous polyps

- 70–80% of polyps
- Benign tumours of neoplastic epithelium
- Sporadic or familial

Types:
1. Tubular adenoma (75%):
   - Multiple in 25% cases
   - Most are <2 cm diameter
   - Malignant risk is <5% but they account for most colorectal carcinomas

2. Villous adenoma (10%):
   - Large, occur in recto-sigmoid colon
   - Fibrovascular stalks, covered by neoplastic epithelium
   - 40% contain invasive carcinoma
3. Mixed (15%)

Hamartomatous polyps

- Benign tumours
  - *Type 1: juvenile polyps:*
    - Low malignant potential
    - Dominantly inherited
    - In children and teens

- *Type 2: Peutz–Jeghers syndrome:*
  - Rare, autosomal dominant
  - Hamartomatous polyps throughout tract
  - Pigmentation of skin around lips, gums, palms and soles
  - Malignant potential <3%.

Causes

- No definite cause
- Genetic associations (see below)

Other polyps:
- Familial adenomatous polyposis (FAP):
  - Autosomal dominant
  - Mutation in *APC* (adenomatous polyposis coli gene) on long arm of chromosome 5
  - Hundreds of adenomatous polyps throughout the gut at an early age
  - Commonly present in teens
  - Leads to colon cancer unless large bowel is removed
  - Many also have congenital hypertrophy of the retinal pigment epithelium (CHRPE)

- Gardner syndrome:
  - Autosomal dominant
  - Multiple colonic adenomas with bony osteomas and epidermoid cysts
  - Variant of FAP
  - Mutation in *APC*
- Inflammatory polyps:
  - In inflammatory bowel conditions, e.g. pseudopolyps in ulcerative colitis
- Metaplastic (or hyperplastic) polyps:
  - Normally small, multiple, slightly raised
  - Not malignant
  - No treatment needed.

Who

- Adenomatous polyps in 10% of population
- Most colonic carcinomas originate from polyps.

Clinical features

- Usually asymptomatic: most found incidentally. Can cause:
  - obstruction
  - anaemia

- diarrhoea in villous adenoma
- bleeding: frank or microscopic
- tenesmus (sensation of incomplete emptying).

Investigations

Stool:
- Faecal occult blood as part of national Bowel Cancer Screening Programme.

Imaging

- Barium enema

- Colonoscopy with biopsy and polypectomy.

Genetic studies

- If familial syndrome suspected.

Treatment

- Endoscopic polypectomy (removal of polyp)
- Surgical polypectomy: for some large right-sided polyps
- Screening: for at-risk patients

Familial adenomatous polyposis:
- Counsel carriers
- Prophylactic colectomy
- After colectomy they remain at risk of small bowel cancer (commonest cause of death is duodenal adenocarcinoma).

Prognosis and complications

Prognosis

- After removal of adenomatous polyps, 50% recur.

Complications

- Malignancy: 5% of polyps removed are found to have invasive carcinoma

- Intussusception: particularly in infants as polyp can act as apex
- May prolapse through the anus.

APPENDICITIS

Outline

- Inflammation of the appendix
- Obstruction of the appendix with infection superimposed

- Inflammation progresses to surrounding tissues and peritoneum
- Felt in right iliac fossa (RIF)
- **Commonest surgical emergency.**

Pathogenesis/aetiology

Pathogenesis

- The appendix becomes obstructed from a faecolith (faeces inside) or hypertrophy of lymphoid tissue following infection or in rare cases carcinoma
- The obstructed mucosa ulcerates and bacteria multiply
- The blood supply to the appendix is via an end-artery and when it is blocked, gangrene develops

- An acutely inflamed appendix may:
  - resolve
  - become gangrenous and perforate
  - become surrounded by loops of bowel to wall off the infection, causing a mass to develop.

Who

- Typical age: any age, commonest in children and young adults
- 6% lifetime incidence

- Commonest surgical presentation needing an operation
- 1/1000 pregnancies (not commoner but more fatalities and perforations).

A typical patient

A 25-year-old student presents with a one-day history of fever with severe pain that began centrally and then moved to the RIF. He has guarding in the RIF and rebound tenderness.

Clinical features

Pain:
- Begins as central periumbilical pain: in the early stages inflammation is confined to the appendix wall, affecting only the visceral wall, which leads to poorly localised pain
- Pain migrates to the RIF: as inflammation spreads, it affects the parietal peritoneum, which is more clearly localised

- Somatic pain settles at McBurney's point (2/3 of way along umbilicus to anterior superior iliac spine)
- Worse on movement or coughing; patients tend to lie still.

Symptoms

- Patient unwell
- Vomiting

- Anorexia
- Constipation ± diarrhoea.

Signs

- Guarding in RIF
- Rebound/percussion tenderness

- Rovsing's sign: pain more in RIF than the left iliac fossa when the left iliac fossa is pressed
- Fever.

Investigations

Clinical examination

- Rovsing's sign
- Temperature

- Rule out ectopic pregnancy in females of reproductive age.

Blood tests

- ↑ WBC

- ↑ ESR and CRP.

Imaging

- US: useful to rule out other pathology

Alvarados scoring system

- **MANTRELS**:
  - **M**igratory pain (1)
  - **A**norexia (1)
  - **N**ausea (1)
  - **T**enderness (2)
  - **R**ebound tenderness (1)
  - **E**levated temperature (1)

- **L**eucocytosis (2)
- **S**hift of WBC to left i.e. increase in percentage of neutrophils
- Score <5 unlikely
- Score 5–6 doubtful
- Score >6 likely.

Treatment

- Prompt appendectomy
- Incision in RIF over McBurney's point

Appendiceal mass:
- IV fluids
- Antibiotics: metronidazole and cefuroxime.

Prognosis and complications

Prognosis

- Good with early intervention
- Late intervention particularly in children associated with a high mortality

- Preschool appendicitis present late and have worse outcomes.

Complications

- Wound infection
- Abscess (pelvic)
- Perforation
- Ileus (paralytic)

- Faecal fistula
- Hernia (right inguinal)
- Obstruction due to adhesions.

MECKEL'S DIVERTICULUM

Outline

- A congenital diverticulum protruding into the ileum
- Remnant of vitello intestinal duct which connects the midgut to the yolk sac in the embryo

- Usually disappears during embryological development
- Can become inflamed, mimicking appendicitis.

Pathogenesis/aetiology

- '2222':
  - 2% of population
  - 2 foot proximal to iliocaecal valve

- ~2 inch long
- If symptomatic, normally before the age of 2.

Who

- Most frequent malformation of the GI tract

- Commonest cause of massive lower GI bleeding in children.

Clinical features

- Asymptomatic
- Similar presentation to appendicitis if inflamed

- Rectal bleeding: if it contains an ectopic gastric mucosa
- Volvulus or intussusception.

Investigations

- Laparotomy

- Technetium scan: for bleeding.

Treatment

- Surgical excision.

Prognosis and complications

Prognosis

- Resection is curative.

Complications

- Volvulus: if it is tethered to the abdominal wall
- Intussusception: by forming the apex

- Obstruction of the intestine
- Haemorrhage.

INTUSSUSCEPTION

Outline

- One segment of bowel telescopes into an adjacent part of bowel (Fig. 13.18)
- Commonly proximal to the ileocaceal valve
- Can result in obstruction
- Occurs in children
- Life threatening.

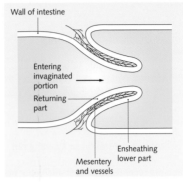

Fig. 13.18 Intussusception.

Pathogenesis/aetiology

Causes

- Mesenteric lymph node hypertrophy following viral illness acts as the lead point in the majority

- May be driven by a factor acting as the apex or lead point of the intussusception, e.g.:
  - Meckel's diverticulum
  - polyp
  - tumour (more in adults).

Who

- Typical age: mostly children under 1 year.

Clinical features

Symptoms

- As for small bowel obstruction

Signs

- Redcurrant jelly stool: blood and mucus (late sign)

- Obstruction and shock develop over 24–48 h.

Investigations

- US

- CT

Treatment

- Surgical reduction or resection and primary anastomosis.

Prognosis and complications

Prognosis

- Good outcome, even if resection required.

Complications

- Strangulation and infarction: inner layer of intestine has its blood supply cut in intussusception, increasing the risk of gangrene.

DISORDERS OF THE RECTUM AND ANUS

HAEMORRHOIDS (PILES)

Outline

- Enlargement of the spongy vasculature around the anus, usually following constipation
- Can become bulky/loose, protrude to become piles
- Normally occur where superior rectal vessels enter the muscle; at the 3, 7, 11 o'clock positions (Fig. 13.19).

Classification

- 1st degree: remain in rectum
- 2nd degree: prolapse on defecation or straining but return spontaneously
- 3rd degree: prolapse on defecation or straining but need digital reduction
- 4th degree: remain permanently prolapsed.

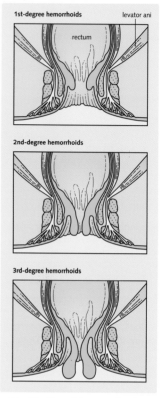

Fig. 13.19 Classification of haemorrhoids.

Pathogenesis/aetiology

Pathogenesis

- Anus lined by spongy vasculature tissue, anal cushions, which are important for anal closure
- Cushions are covered in a layer of mucosa containing branches of superior rectal artery and superior rectal vein
- Vessels loosen due to:
  - constipation with straining
  - congestion from pregnancy, tumour, portal hypertension
  - gravity.

Who

- Typical age: middle age
- Prevalence: 50% of the population.

A typical patient

A 55-year-old man presents after noticing fresh blood on his stool and toilet paper. He has not had any pain during defecation.

- Bright red rectal bleeding, often coating stools or dripping after defecation
- Associated with constipation
- Mucous discharge

- Pruritus ani
- Severe anaemia
- Painless as no sensory fibres
- Asymptomatic.

- Abdominal examination
- Rectal examination

- Proctoscopy
- Rigid sigmoidoscopy.

1st and 2nd degree haemorrhoids

- Conservative
  - ↑ fibre and fluid intake, avoid straining on defecation, analgesia, ice, bed rest
- Medical:
  - Laxatives, topical Anusol

- Interventions:
  - Rubber band ligation
  - Sclerotherapy: injection of phenol with almond oil to shrink smaller haemorrhoids, can be repeated
  - Cryotherapy
  - Infra-red coagulation of the vessels.

3rd/4th degree haemorrhoids

- Surgical: haemorrhoidectomy, day case removal of haemorrhoid tissue.

Treatment of complications

- Bed rest, analgesia, laxatives, antibiotics and surgery.

Prognosis

- Conservative measures often adequate.

Complications

Early:
- Pain
- Urinary retention
- Haemorrhage
- Constipation
- Infection

Late:
- Strictures
- Thrombosis
- Ulceration
- Faecal incontinence
- Strangulated piles: prolapsed piles can be strangulated by anal sphincters and ulcerate or infarct.

ANAL FISSURE

- Break in the skin lining the anal canal
- Midline split, normally at 6 o'clock position but can be at 12 o'clock

- Acute or chronic
- May be a symptom of an underlying disease
- Pain exacerbated by anal sphincter spasm.

Causes

- Constipation or diarrhoea
- Trauma
- Crohn's disease

- Syphilis
- Herpes.

- ♀ > ♂.

Clinical features

- Acute throbbing pain after and during defecation
- Rectal bleeding
- Sentinel pile: small skin tag at the base of the anal fissure.

Investigations

- Examination: fissure may be visible
- Rectal examination (may be too painful)
- Sigmoidoscopy.

Treatment

Conservative

- High fibre diet
- Avoid straining.

Medical

- Ointments to relax the sphincter muscle: glyceryl trinitrate paste, local anaesthetic, Botox injection
- Laxatives.

Surgical

- Usually for chronic cases
- Lateral sphincterotomy: partial division of the external anal sphincter to relax the sphincters, ↓ pressure and

promote healing. Gold standard. Complications include incontinence in <2%.

Prognosis and complications

Prognosis

- Conservative measures often effective.

Complications

- Recurrence of fistula.

ANAL FISTULA

Outline

- A fistula is an abnormal connection between two epithelial surfaces

Fistula in ano:

- Opening between anal canal and skin surface
- Fistula can be high or low (origin of fistula track; Fig. 13.20):
  - High fistulae cross the sphincter muscles
  - Low fistulae do not cross the sphincter muscles (95%)

Parks' classification:

- Intersphincteric ~70%
- Transsphincteric ~25%
- Suprasphincteric ~5%
- Extrasphincteric ~1%.

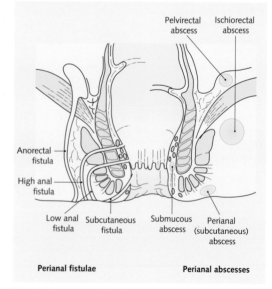

Fig. 13.20   Perianal fistulae and abscesses.

Pathogenesis/aetiology

Pathogenesis

- Often complication of a perianal abscess

- External opening is too small for proper drainage and spontaneous resolution.

Causes

- Abscess
- Rectal inflammatory disease: Crohn's disease
- Direct infiltration: carcinoma

- Radiotherapy
- TB
- Diverticular disease.

Who

- Any time in adult life.

Clinical features

- Purulent discharge from fistula opening
- Pain: if filled with pus
- Pruritus ani: if discharge makes perianal skin wet
- Symptoms may be episodic

Goodsall's rule (Fig. 13.21):
- Describes path of fistula between openings
- Fistulae anterior to the anus open to the anus in straight line
- Fistulae posterior to the anus have a curving track and open in the midline posteriorly
- Important to help locate the trajectory and internal opening of the fistula during surgery.

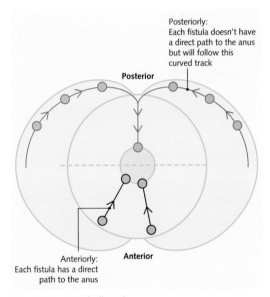

Posteriorly:
Each fistula doesn't have a direct path to the anus but will follow this curved track

Posterior

Anteriorly:
Each fistula has a direct path to the anus

Anterior

Fig. 13.21 Goodsall's rule.

Investigations

- Examination under anaesthesia
- Fistulogram: dye injected into distal orifice to identify the opening

- Endoanal US
- MRI.

Treatment

Low fistulae:
- Cut fistula open by inserting a metal probe into the fistula and making an incision through the tissue and onto the probe
- Packed afterwards to ensure healing

High fistulae:
- Not treated as above as danger of anal sphincter damage

- Seton (a silk suture) is passed through the fistula track and tied on the outside to form a loop. The suture is gradually tightened so that it slowly cuts through the sphincter to the surface, with fistural healing by scar tissue formation
- Deep fistulae may require a colostomy to permit adequate healing of the fistula
- If secondary to Crohn's disease, treat conservatively.

Prognosis and complications

Prognosis

- Low fistulae: good outcome
- High fistulae: risk of sphincter damage.

Complications

- Recurrence
- Sphincter damage.

PERIANAL ABSCESSES

Outline

- An abscess: a localised collection of pus that has accumulated in a cavity (see Fig. 13.20)
- Risk of necrotising infection.

Classification

- Perianal abscess: 60%
- Ischioanal abscess: 20%
- Intersphincteric abscess: 5%
- Supralevator abscess: 4%.

Pathogenesis/aetiology

Causes

- Simple skin infection
- Anal gland infection
- Supralevator abscess:
  - Crohn's disease
  - Diverticulitis.

Who

Risk factors:
- Crohn's disease
- Diabetes mellitus
- Carcinoma.

Clinical features

- Perianal abscess: perianal discomfort, worse when sitting
- Ischioanal abscess: fever, chills, not visible on examination
- Intersphincteric: rectal pain
- Discharge.

Investigations

- Rectal examination
- Swab for microscopy and culture
- If abscess contains bowel flora, suspect fistula

Treatment

- Incision and drainage under general anaesthesia, then packed and left to heal
- Antibiotics.

Prognosis and complications

Prognosis

- Curative incision unless underlying fissure.

Complications

- Fistula formation in 30%.

PILONIDAL SINUS

Outline

- Track from skin surface between the buttocks, often containing hairs
- Asymptomatic until sinus becomes infected and presents as an abscess.

Pathogenesis/aetiology

At risk:
- Excessive body hair

- Prolonged sitting.

Who

- Typical age: teenagers, young adults
- 1♀:4♂.

A typical patient

A hirsute teenage girl presenting with recurrent natal cleft infections.

Clinical features

- Infections
- Discharge

- Abscess.

Investigations

- Clinical examination.

Treatment

Conservative

- Anal hygiene
- Shave hair.

Medical

- Antibiotics.

Surgical

- Incision and drainage for abscess with packing
- Second procedure at a later date to excise the tract.

Prognosis and complications

Prognosis

- Good outcome with adequate surgical clearance.

Complications

- Recurrence.

RECTAL PROLAPSE

Outline

- The walls of the rectum protrude through the anus and become visible outside the body
- Due to excessive straining and a lax sphincter.

Classification

- *Complete prolapse*: entire rectum protrudes
- *Partial prolapse*: only the rectal mucosa prolapses

- *Internal intussusception*: the rectum collapses but does not exit the anus.

Pathogenesis/aetiology

Causes

- Chronic constipation
- Multiparity in women: damages the pudendal nerves, resulting in sphincter weakness
- Weakness of the pelvic floor
- Sigmoid redundancy: following prolonged dilatation of the sigmoid colon
- Lax anal sphincter.

Who

- Typical age: occurs at the extremes of life
- 5♀:1♂.

Clinical features

- Rectal bleeding: mucosal ulceration from stool trauma
- Mucosal discharge
- Incontinence
- Tenesmus: feeling of incomplete defecation
- Discomfort
- May present as a semi-emergency if it becomes oedematous and ulcerated.

Investigations

- Clinical diagnosis
- Sigmoidoscopy: to investigate for ulcers
- Endoscopic US: to determine presence of muscle damage.

Treatment

- May resolve spontaneously, particularly in children
- High fibre diet
- Reduce strain on defecation

Partial prolapse:
- Phenol injection: reduces scarring
- Rubber band ligation

- Delorme's procedure: local excision of redundant rectal mucosa, very good for elderly

Complete prolapse:
- Rectopexy: fixation of the rectum to the abdomen
- Delorme's procedure if patient is not fit for surgery.

Prognosis and complications

Prognosis

- Most resolve without complex surgery.

Complications

- Incontinence (75%)
- Recurrence.

DISORDERS OF THE PANCREAS

PANCREATITIS: ACUTE

Outline

- Inflammation of the pancreas by autodigestion
- Leads to further inflammation with oedema, fat necrosis, vascular destruction and haemorrhage.

Classification

Acute, mild:
- Mostly self-limiting with minimal organ dysfunction

Acute severe, 20%:
- Necrosis and widespread haemorrhage from destruction of blood vessels
- Potentially fatal from multi-organ failure

Pseudocyst:
- Walled off collection of pancreatic secretions, drained from damaged ducts. Fibrotic tissue surrounds secretions forming a fluid-filled pseudocyst
- Found within or next to the pancreas
- Suspect in any patient with persisting or recurring symptoms after acute pancreatitis
- Complications include haemorrhage or rupture.

Pathogenesis/aetiology

Causes

- **GET SMASHED:**
  - **G**allstones: commonest (50%)
  - **E**thanol: (20%)
  - **T**rauma
  - **S**teroids
  - **M**umps
  - **A**utoimmune
- **S**corpion venom
- **H**yperlipidaemia/hyperparathyroidism/ hypercalcaemia
- **E**RCP: iatrogenic
- **D**rugs: e.g. azathioprine
- 20% are idiopathic.

Pathogenesis

- Inflammation damages pancreatic cells, releasing digestive enzymes
- Auto-digestion of the pancreas and further inflammation result in a destructive cycle
- Auto-digestion of blood vessels can result in haemorrhage: seen in the flanks (Grey Turner's sign) and bruising at the umbilicus (Cullen's sign)
- Extracellular fluid becomes trapped in the peritoneum and gut (3rd space losses)
- Inflammation finally leads to necrosis, infection and multi-organ failure, which carries a high mortality.

Who

- Incidence: 5–10/100 000 per year in the West.

A typical patient

A 60-year-old publican presents to A&E with severe upper abdominal pain that came on suddenly and radiates to the back with vomiting. You notice that he is jaundiced.

Clinical features

Symptoms

- Sudden upper abdominal pain radiating to the back
- Relieved on sitting forward
- Nausea and vomiting.

Signs

- Epigastric tenderness (soft abdomen with normal bowel sounds)
- Jaundice: if biliary tree obstructed
- Cullen's sign: periumbilical bruising and discoloration
- Grey Turner's sign: flank bruising and discoloration
- Fever
- Tachycardia

If severe necrotising pancreatitis:
- Shock: pale and sweaty (from retroperitoneal fluid loss)
- Tachypnoea: may indicate metabolic acidosis or ARDS
- Absent bowel signs: ileus
- Rigid abdomen

Scores to predict clinical outcome:
- Ranson's, Glasgow, APACHE II, SAP (simplified acute physiology)

Glasgow criteria: **PANCREAS**
- **P**aO$_2$ <8.0 kPa
- **A**ge >55 years
- **N**eutrophils >15 $\times$ 10^9/L
- **C**alcium <2 mmol/L
- **R**enal function urea >16 mmol/L
- **E**nzymes: LDH >600 i U/L
- **A**lbumin <32 g/L
- **S**ugar: blood glucose >10 mmol/L
- Severe pancreatitis defined as $\geq$3 criteria detected within 48 h (refer to ICU).

Investigations

Blood tests

- ↑ Pancreatic enzymes
- ↑↑ Amylase: >1000 U/L (biliary cause leads to higher amylase than alcoholic cause). Note that amylase may be raised (but not this high) for any cause of acute abdomen
- ↑ Serum lipase: more specific than amylase, but less readily available

- Biochemistry: ↓ albumin, ↓ calcium, ↑ urea
- ↑ Glucose
- LFTs: ↑ AST in acute pancreatitis suggests gallstone aetiology
- FBC: ↑ WBC
- ↑ CRP.

Imaging

- CXR: air under diaphragm if bowel perforation
- CT scan: better visualisation of the pancreas than with US and can identify pseudocysts

- US: to detect biliary cause such as gallstones.

Treatment

Treatment depends on severity of inflammation, and needs to be regularly reassessed:
- Mild:
  - Supportive
- Severe:
  - Resuscitate
  - Intensive care if Glasgow criteria severity score is >3
- Support:
  - O$_2$
  - Nil by mouth: insert nasojejunal tube for feeding beyond pancreas. Should be initiated early, particularly in ICU to avoid pancreatic stimulation and complications from bowel flora:

- IV fluid resuscitation: often excessive 3rd space losses
- Analgesia: opiates
- Antiemetics
- Insulin: to control hyperglycaemia
- Antibiotics: not in early stage as inflammation not infection causes peritonitis. Given 5–7 days later for infection
- Proton pump inhibitor: to reduce gastric acid secretion
- Hourly monitoring.

Surgical

- ERCP and gallstone removal
- Elective laparotomy: for pancreatic abscess, necrosis

- Elective endoscopic US-guided drainage of pseudocysts (see below).

Prognosis and complications

Prognosis

- Mild cases: low mortality, normally recover within 7 days
- General mortality: 5–10%

- Poor prognostic indicators: renal failure, ARDS
- Infected necrosis is commonest cause of death

Complications

Local:
- Phlegmon: non-suppurative inflamed mass
- Pancreatic abscess
- Pseudocysts
- Duodenal obstruction
- Thrombosis: in splenic/gastric arteries causing bowel necrosis
- Splenic artery pseudoaneurysm
- Fistulae

Systemic:
- ARDS
- Sepsis and shock: 5% within 1 week of presentation
- Multi-organ dysfunction syndrome
- Secondary diabetes
- Malabsorption due to lack of enzymes for food breakdown
- Hypocalcaemia
- Death.

PANCREATITIS: CHRONIC

Outline

- Sustained, irreversible inflammatory disease of the pancreas
- Duct plugging by abnormal secretions or repeated inflammation promotes gland distortion, increasing the likelihood of further pancreatitis
- Initially the pancreas is enlarged; it then shrinks and hardens due to fibrosis and calcification.

Pathogenesis/aetiology

Causes

- Alcohol
- Obstruction of pancreatic duct
- Hyperparathyroidism
- Hypercalcaemia
- Hyperlipidaemia
- Biliary disease
- Cystic fibrosis
- Genetic: rare autosomal dominant hereditary pancreatitis
- 40% unknown.

Who

- Typical age: presents in 5th decade
- 0.01% of Western population

Clinical features

- Epigastric pain radiating to the back, relieved on sitting forward
- Jaundice
- Bloating
- Symptoms of malabsorption, e.g. steatorrhoea: from ↓ lipase, ↓ weight/anorexia.

Investigations

Stool:
- ↓ faecal elastase.

Imaging

- AXR: calcification of pancreas
- US
- CT.

Treatment

Conservative

- Alcohol cessation
- Low fat diet.

Medical

- H_2 receptor blocker, e.g. ranitidine, or proton pump inhibitor, e.g. omeprazole
- Pancreatic supplements with meals, e.g. Creon
- Analgesia, lipase, fat-soluble vitamins (vitamins A, D, E and K).

Surgical

- For unresolving pain
- Pancreaticojejunostomy: draining the pancreatic duct to the jejunum
- Coeliac plexus block for pain
- ERCP if gallstone aetiology.

Prognosis and complications

Complications

- 70% have local complications:
  - Pseudocysts: common
  - Biliary obstruction
  - Ascites
- Gastric varices
- Type 1 diabetes
- Pancreatic carcinoma
- Aneurysm.

MALIGNANCY OF THE GASTROINTESTINAL TRACT

OESOPHAGEAL CANCER

Outline

- Cancer of the oesophagus
Benign tumours:
- Leiomyomas
- Lipomas
- Haemangiomas
- Benign polyps
Malignant tumours:
- Squamous cell carcinoma:
  - 90% of oesophageal malignancies worldwide

- Presents in the 5th decade
- Commoner in males
- Associated with achalasia, Plummer–Vinson syndrome, diet
- Most affects the lower oesophagus
- Adenocarcinoma:
  - Mostly associated with Barrett's oesophagus
  - Most in distal oesophagus.

Pathogenesis/aetiology

Risk factors:
- **BAD SPACeS:**
  - **B**arrett's
  - **A**lcohol
  - **D**iet: smoked and pickled food, ↓ fruit and vegetables intake, salted food

- **S**moking
- **P**lummer–Vinson syndrome
- **A**chalasia
- **C**oeliac disease
- **S**tricture.

Who

- Typical age: middle-aged and elderly populations
- 1♀:3♂
- 5% of all cancers
- 8th commonest cancer in the UK

- Incidence of adenocarcinoma is rising in the West
- High incidence in China and Japan
Associations:
- Human papilloma virus (squamous cell carcinomas).

A typical patient

A 65-year-old man presents with 2 months progressive dysphagia and weight loss.

Clinical features

Symptoms

- Progressive dysphagia: initially solids, then liquids
- Odynophagia: pain on swallowing
- Significant weight loss
- Haematemesis

- Hoarseness
- Vomiting
- Cough.

Signs

- Anaemia
- Anorexia
- Lymphadenopathy

- Hepatomegaly
- Ascites.

Investigations

Blood tests

- FBC: ↓ Hb

- LFTs: deranged with liver metastases

Endoscopy

- OGD with biopsy

Imaging

- Barium swallow: if patient cannot tolerate endoscopy or stricture is high: will need endoscopy with biopsy if abnormal
- Staging:
  - CT

- Endoscopic US
- MRI
- PET
- Bronchoscopy: if suspect bronchial involvement.

Treatment

No metastasis (33%)/no locally advanced disease

Surgical:
- Surgical resection, operative mortality: 5–10%
- Access depends on site of tumour. Can be transthoracic resection or trans-hiatal oesophagectomy: allows removal of the oesophagus through an abdominal and neck incision with less complications than transthoracic resection

Chemotherapy and radiotherapy:
- Pre- and postoperative

Metastasis (66%)/locally advanced disease

- Mostly treated palliatively
- Chemotherapy
- Radiotherapy: good for squamous cell carcinoma. Can be external or intraluminal (brachytherapy)

- Dilation of strictures with stenting
- Laser photocoagulation of the tumour

Prognosis and complications

Prognosis

- Poor survival rates
- Mostly present late, when tumour is large enough to cause dysphagia

- 10% 5-year survival overall
- After successful resection: prognosis 50%.

Complications

- Complications of metastases
- Obstruction
- Perforation

- Aspiration pneumonia: obstruction can lead to overflow of oesophageal contents
- Fistulae between trachea and oesophagus
- Malnutrition.

GASTRIC CARCINOMA

Outline

- Cancer of stomach.

Classification

- 90% adenocarcinomas
- 4% lymphomas
- 3% carcinoids
- 2% sarcomas

Histological subtypes: Lauren classification of adenocarcinomas:
- Intestinal type: glandular adenocarcinoma: well-circumscribed glandular formation that is mucin secreting
- Diffuse types: poorly localised. Infiltrates the whole stomach wall causing it to become fibrosed and rigid described as **linitis plastica: (leather bottle)**. It spreads locally to invade adjacent structures. It has a worse prognosis than the intestinal type.

Pathogenesis/aetiology

Risks:
- *H. pylori*
- Dietary nitrates: smoked or pickled food, ↓ fruit and vegetables intake
- Smoking: ↑ 1.5–3 × risk
- Chronic gastritis: ↑ 2–4 × risk
- Alcohol

- Blood group A
- Ulcers: chronic change
- Gastric polyps
- Previous gastric surgery
- Familial: abnormalities of E cadherin-cellular adhesion molecule (a tumour suppressor)
- Vitamin C is protective.

Pathogenesis

- Early cancer consists of a nodule or ulceration confined to the mucosa and submucosa that invades the muscularis propria

Areas affected:
- Pylorus/antrum 50%
- Cardia 25%
- Body 25%
- Lesser curve of stomach.

Who

- Typical age: ↑ with age
- ♀ < ♂
- 6th commonest cancer
- 2.5% of cancer deaths
- Incidence is declining
- Incidence higher in Japan and China.

A typical patient

A 50-year-old man presents with weight loss and haematemesis.

Clinical features

Symptoms

- Nausea
- Anorexia
- Weight loss
- Bowel change
- Haemorrhage/upper GI bleeding (rarer)
- Vomiting with outflow obstruction if tumour is near pylorus
- Abdominal pain
- Dyspepsia
- Dysphagia: difficulty swallowing, if there is gastro-oesophageal obstruction.

Signs

- Palpable epigastric mass in 50%
- Virchow's node (in 30%): cancer spreads to left supraclavicular lymph node. This is Troisier's sign
- Succussion splash: splashing sound on auscultation caused by residual gastric fluid due to an obstruction in the antrum of the stomach
- Associated skin manifestations: acanthosis nigricans (pigmented warty skin found in body folds, e.g. neck, axilla or groin)
- Abdominal swelling from abdominal mass, or if metastases; ascites or hepatomegaly.

Investigations

Blood tests

- FBC: ↓ Hb
- LFTs: deranged with liver metastases.

Endoscopy

- Gastroscopy with biopsy.

Imaging

- Barium meal

Staging:
- CT
- Endoscopic US
- MRI
- PET.

Treatment

Non-metastatic/no locally advanced disease

Surgical:
- If operable, remove cancer
- If confined to the stomach: gastric resection and radical resection of lymph nodes
- If early detection: endoscopic mucosal resection
- Tumours in distal 2/3: partial gastrectomy with Roux en Y anastomosis to prevent bile reflux
- Upper stomach carcinoma: total gastrectomy

Chemotherapy and radiotherapy:
- As adjuvant treatment

Metastatic/locally advanced disease

- Mainly palliative
- Proton pump inhibitors: to reduce bleeding from ulcerating tumours
- Argon plasma coagulation: an endoscopic procedure where a high current is delivered through a jet of argon gas to control bleeding
- Haemostasis for polypoid gastric tumours
- Laser therapy: for tumour debulking or haemorrhage
- Analgesia
- Antiemetics
- Chemotherapy: mostly palliative, increases survival
- Radiation; not valuable

Surgery:
- Palliative to relieve outlet obstruction, e.g. endoscopic stents for restrictions or bypass procedures.

Prognosis and complications

Prognosis

- Presents late, poor prognosis
- 5 year survival overall: 20%

- Influenced by depth of invasion.

Complications

- Metastases

- Krukenberg's tumours are secondary tumours in the ovaries whose primary site is the breast or GI tract.

SMALL BOWEL TUMOURS

Outline

Classification

Malignant:
- Adenocarcinoma (50%): mostly from pre-existing adenomatous polyps
- Carcinoid tumour (10%): low-grade malignancy

- Leiomyosarcomas
- Sarcomas: GI stromal tumours (GISTs)
- Lymphomas.

Pathogenesis/aetiology

Risks:
- Adenocarcinoma: ↑ incidence in Crohn's disease and coeliac disease.

Who

- Rare

- <5% of GI tumours.

Clinical features

Present late with intestinal obstruction or anaemia:
Benign:
- Incidental findings
- Bleeding
- Intussusception

Malignant:
- Abdominal pain
- Diarrhoea
- Anaemia
- Weight loss.

Investigations

Blood tests

- FBC: ↓ Hb, ↓ MCV

Imaging

- CT: abdomen
- Barium follow through

- Capsule endoscopy
- MRI: small bowel.

Treatment

- Surgical resection

- Chemotherapy (radiotherapy of little value).

Prognosis and complications

Prognosis

- Dependent on tumour.

COLORECTAL CARCINOMA

Outline

- Cancer of the large bowel
- 90% occur sporadically, 10% are linked to hereditary cause
- Mostly adenocarcinomas
- Most occur with ulcers

Sites of tumours

- 65% rectosigmoid
- 5% descending colon
- 10% transverse colon
- 15% ascending colon
- Right sided tumours have worse prognosis as they present later.

Classification: Dukes

- A: confined to bowel wall
- B: through bowel, no metastasis
- C: regional lymph nodes affected:
  - C1: highest node not involved
  - C2: highest node involved
- D: distant metastases

NICE guidelines for urgent referral for suspected bowel cancer:
- >40 years: rectal bleeding with a change of bowel habit for >6 weeks
- >60 years: rectal bleeding OR a change in bowel habit for >6 weeks
- Any man or non-menstruating woman with unexplained iron-deficiency anaemia.

Pathogenesis/aetiology

Risk factors:
- Polyps (see Gastroenterology chapter)
- IBD
- Previous cancer, particularly of bowel
- Diet: ↓ fibre and vegetables, ↑ animal fat and bile salts. Poor diet may ↑ transit time and exposure to swallowed carcinogens
- Genetics: inherited or acquired mutations, e.g. *KRAS*, *APC* (adenomatous polyposis coli gene) on chromosome 5, p53

Linked to family history:
- Positive family history ↑ risk 2–3 ×
- Familial adenomatous polyposis: polyps that lead to colon cancer (see Gastroenterology, chapter 4)
- Hereditary non-polyposis colorectal cancer: ↑ risk of developing tumours when young
  - Mostly right-sided tumours
  - Also ↑ incidence of other malignancies
  - Autosomal dominant, with incomplete penetrance
  - Gene found on chromosome 2, also linked with *APC* (adenomatous polyposis coli gene).

Who

- Typical age: >70 years
- 1♀:1♂
- 2nd commonest cancer in UK
- Lifetime incidence: 1 in 27
- Higher incidence in developed countries
- Rarer in Africa and Asia.

A typical patient

An elderly patient presents with altered bowel habit and weight loss.

Clinical features

- Presentation depends on site

Right side of colon:
- Diarrhoea
- RIF mass
- Anaemia
- Weight loss
- Abdominal pain

Left side of colon:
- Constipation
- Bleeding
- Mucus
- Tenesmus

- Rectal mass
- Abdominal pain

Rectum:
- Tenesmus: sensation of incomplete emptying
- Proctalgia fugax: episodic severe rectal pain, may be caused by spasms of rectum

General:
- Rectal bleeding: dark/bright red, usually mixed with stool
- Weight loss
- Can be asymptomatic
- 30% present as emergencies.

Signs

- Iron deficiency
- Abdominal mass
- Hepatomegaly: due to metastases.

Investigations

Blood tests

- FBC: ↓ Hb
- U&Es, LFTs (for metastases)
- Carcinoembryonic antigen (CEA): to monitor disease activity

Genetic screening

- Familial adenomatous polyposis.

Imaging

- Colonoscopy with biopsy. Investigation of choice
- Barium enema: 'apple core' constriction (Fig. 13.22)
- CT: also important for staging
- MRI/endorectal US: gold standard imaging.

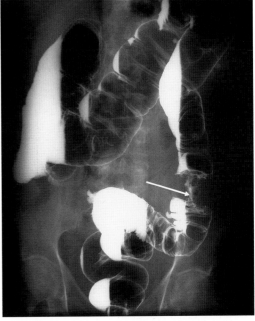

Fig. 13.22 Barium enema showing the typical apple core appearance (arrowed) of colon cancer.

Treatment

Treat according to Dukes' classification:
- Dukes' A: no chemotherapy
- Dukes' B: adjuvant chemotherapy
- Dukes' C: tumour controlled by chemotherapy – postoperative chemotherapy is effective:
  - First line: 5-FU and folinic acid
  - Second line: irinotecan/oxaliplatin
- Dukes' D: resect liver metastases, improves overall survival

Surgical procedures:
- Caecum and right colon affected: right hemicolectomy
- Transverse segment affected: extended right hemicolectomy
- Descending colon affected: left hemicoloectomy
- Sigmoid colon affected: sigmoid colectomy

- Rectum affected: anterior resection
- Low in rectum affected: abdomino-perineal resection with permanent colostomy

Radiotherapy:
- Preoperatively

Chemotherapy:
- Reduce Dukes' mortality, also palliative

Screening:
- Colonoscopy: good for those at high risk
- Faecal occult blood: tests for small amounts of blood in the faeces. In England, those aged 60–75 are routinely offered screening every two years. National flexible sigmoidoscopy screening for left sided polyps and cancers is due to commence 2014/5.

Prognosis and complications

Prognosis

- Generally not metastasised at presentation
- Dukes' classification 5-year survival rate:
  - A: 85%
  - B: 67%
  - C: 37%
  - D: <10%, with liver resection of metastases, 60% 3 year survival
- Overall survival <40% at 5 years.

Complications

- Metastases (commonly to the liver).

ANAL CANCER

Outline

- Cancer of the anus
- Mainly carcinoma originating in squamous mucosa of anal canal.

Pathogenesis/aetiology

Risks:
- Syphilis and warts: related to human papilloma virus infection
- Bowen's disease: squamous carcinoma in situ.

Who

- Typical age: mainly in the elderly
- 5♀:♂
- Uncommon.

A typical patient

An elderly patient presents with painful rectal bleeding.

Clinical features

- Rectal bleeding
- Perianal pain
- Change in bowel habit
- Local pruritus
- Rectal mass
- Stricture
- Inguinal lymphadenopathy.

Investigations

- Clinical examination
- Biopsy.

Treatment

- Radiotherapy
- Chemotherapy.

Surgical

- Local excision for carcinoma in situ.

Prognosis and complications

Prognosis

- Good if treated early.

Complications

- Local invasion
- Incontinence.

CARCINOID TUMOURS

Outline

- Neuroendocrine amine precursor uptake and decarboxylation system (APUD) tumours
- Arise from endochromaffin (neural crest) cells
- Form diverse group of tumours that can arise anywhere in the gut but also elsewhere: ileum, rectum, ovary, testis, lungs
- May be secretory, e.g. 5HT, somatostatin, vasoactive intestinal peptide, gastrin, insulin, bradykinin, tachykinin, substance P, glucagons, ACTH, PTH, thyroid hormones
- Malignant potential dependent on origin.

Pathogenesis/aetiology

Pathogenesis

- Mostly slow growing
- 10%: part of MEN1 (see specific section) syndrome
- 10%: occur with other neuroendocrine tumours

Carcinoid syndrome:
- Symptoms occur when hormones from carcinoid tumours are released into the general circulation
- Occurs in 5% of cases

- Isolated GI carcinoid tumours do not produce the syndrome as endocrine products undergo first-pass metabolism as they drain via the liver
- However, once the tumour has metastasised to the liver, tumour products can drain into the systemic circulation, leading to carcinoid syndrome
- Carcinoid lung tumours can cause carcinoid syndrome without metastasising as they drain directly to the systemic circulation.

Who

- Typical age: <40 years
- 1♀:1♂

- Rare.

Clinical features

- Many are asymptomatic

Early:
- Diarrhoea
- Haemorrhage
- Depends on site
- GI tumours: abdominal pain, diarrhoea. May be appendicitis, obstruction, intussusception
- Lung tumour: wheeze, SOB

Carcinoid syndrome:
- Flushing
- Wheezing
- Right-sided cardiac lesions 50%
- Skin rash
- Bronchospasm
- Regurgitation
- Intestinal colic
- Diarrhoea
- Borborygmi: abdominal gurgle from movement of gas and fluid within the intestine.

Investigations

- Urinary 5-hydroxyindoleacetic acid (5-HIAA; derivative of serotonin): for diagnosis and monitoring
- Tumour marker: chromogranin A
- CXR, bronchoscopy for lung carcinoid

- US or CT for metastases
- Octreotide scan: radioactively labelled octreotide is injected into the blood, attaching to tumour cells with receptors for somatostatin so that they can be identified.

Treatment

Tumour therapy:
- Curative resection: if isolated primary
- Surgical debulking
- Embolisation of hepatic metastases
- Radiofrequency ablation
- Radiolabelled octreotide

Carcinoid syndrome:
- Octreotide (somatostatin analogue): blocks release of tumour mediators, counters peripheral effects. Prevents massive carcinoid crisis
- Loperamide for diarrhoea
- Interferon-α: a good adjuvant for octreotide.

Prognosis and complications

Prognosis

- Most survive 5–10 years from diagnosis

- Median survival if metastases at presentation: 38 months.

Complications

- Metastasis: common, in 80% of large tumours

- Carcinoid crisis: if tumour outgrows its blood supply. Life-threatening condition with vasodilation, hypertension, tachycardia bronchoconstriction, hyperglycaemia.

ENDOCRINE TUMOURS OF THE PANCREAS

Outline

- Multiple hormones can be produced; normally one hormone predominates
- Much rarer than exocrine pancreatic tumours.

Classification

- *Insulinoma*: from islet cells, causes hypoglycaemia. Majority are benign
- *Glucagonoma*: from alpha cells of the pancreas leading to ↑ glucagon and blood glucose
- *Somatostatinoma*: from delta cells of the pancreas leading to ↑ somatostatin
- *VIPoma*: produces vasoactive intestinal peptide, which stimulates water and electrolyte secretion from the gut
- *Gastrinoma*: see below.

Pathogenesis/aetiology

- An endocrine gland is a ductless gland manufacturing hormones directly into the blood.

Causes

- Can occur alone or as part of MEN (see Ch. 9).

Who

- Typical age: ↑ with age
- Rare
- Associations:
  - MEN1 patients: 80% have a pancreatic tumour.

Clinical features

Insulinoma:
- Weight gain, hypoglycaemic episodes

Gastrinoma:
- Peptic ulcer disease symptoms, diarrhoea from excess acid

Glucagonoma:
- Diabetes mellitus, weight loss, stomatitis, weakness, migratory erythematous rash

Somatostatinoma:
- Triad of:
  - diabetes
  - steatorrhoea
  - gallstones

VIPoma:
- Diarrhoea and dehydration.

Investigations

- ↑ Plasma gastrin levels
- ↑ Insulin
- Low blood sugar levels
- Serum hormone levels by radioimmunoassay
- IV injection of labelled octreotide: increased uptake in tumour.

Imaging

- CT with contrast (pancreas protocol) is the investigation of choice for staging
- US
- MRI
- Duodenoscopy
- ERCP.

Treatment

- Resection not usually possible
- Usually palliative
- Octreotide for VIPomas
- Chemotherapy and radiotherapy not of value.

Surgical

- Bypass with a stent: to relieve jaundice if obstructed common bile duct
- Most insulinomas are cured with surgical resection

Prognosis and complications

Prognosis

- About 90% of insulinomas are benign
- Glucagonoma, somatostatinoma and gastrinoma likely to be metastatic at presentation with poor prognosis. Most die within a year.

Prognosis and complications

Complications

- Obstruction: biliary and pancreatic
- GI bleeds
- Hypoglycaemic coma

- Dehydration
- Arrhythmias
- Malnutrition.

GASTRINOMA: ZOLLINGER–ELLISON SYNDROME

Outline

- Gastrin-secreting tumour of the G cells
- Originates mainly in the pancreas (though can also occur in the stomach, duodenum and ovaries)

- Gastrin leads to increased gastric acid secretion by the stomach
- Often difficult to detect as small in size.

Pathogenesis/aetiology

- ~50% malignant

- Can be part of MEN1 syndrome (see Endocrinology section).

Pathogenesis

- Gastrin is a hormone normally produced by the G cells of the stomach, duodenum and pancreas
- It stimulates the parietal cells in the stomach to secrete gastric acid

- Hypersecretion of gastrin from any location causes ↑ gastric acid leading to GI ulcers and malabsorption.

Who

- Typical age: 30–50
- ♀ < ♂

- Rare.

Clinical features

- Peptic ulceration
- Diarrhoea

- Abdominal pain from excess acid
- Symptoms and signs of malabsorption.

Investigations

- ↑ Plasma gastrin levels aid diagnosis but there are other causes of hypergastrinaemia.

Imaging

- CT scan
- MRI

- Angiography
- Intraoperative US in pancreas.

Treatment

Medical

- Treat ulcers

- Proton pump inhibitors.

Surgical

- For tumour and ulcers.

Prognosis and complications

Prognosis

- Depends on size of tumour and whether it has spread.

VASCULAR DISEASE

LYMPHOEDEMA

Outline

- Abnormal collection of lymph fluid in the tissues, leading to swelling
- Legs most commonly affected.

Pathogenesis/aetiology

Causes

1°:
- Congenital:
  - *Milroy's disease*: congenital lack of lymphatics, presents at birth
  - *Yellow nail syndrome*: lyphoedema, pleural effusions, thick opaque nails, bronchiectasis
- Praecox: adolescence
- Tarda: 30–40 year olds

2°:
- Due to blockage of lymphatics:
  - Fibrosis
  - Previous surgery
  - Radiotherapy
  - Infection (e.g. filariasis)
  - Trauma
  - Tumour.

Who

A typical patient

A woman presents with a swollen arm following treatment for breast cancer.

Clinical features

- Peripheral oedema worse on standing
- Initially pitting, over time there is an inflammatory response in the skin leading to thickening and non-pitting oedema
- Unilateral or bilateral
- Skin changes: hyperkeratosis, infection.

Investigations

- Doppler US
- CT or MRI
- Lymphangiography.

Treatment

- Treat underlying cause

Conservative

- Leg elevation, particularly at night
- Compression stockings
- Physiotherapy
- Treat secondary skin changes
- Weight loss.

Medical

- Antibiotics if infective cause.

Surgical

- Debulking operation but only for severe lymphoedema.

Prognosis and complications

Prognosis

- Some resolution from conservative treatment
- Best managed by specialist service.

Complications

- Pain
- Ulceration.

ARTERIAL DISEASE

ACUTELY ISCHAEMIC LIMBS

Outline

- Inadequate flow of blood to upper or lower limbs, due to a sudden change in blood flow
- Tissues cannot adapt to sudden reduction in O_2
- Lower limb more commonly affected
- **Emergency: 4–6 h to save limb.**

Pathogenesis/aetiology

Causes

Emboli and thrombosis are the commonest causes:
- Embolus: commonly from the heart (e.g. in AF) or an aneurysm

- Thrombosis in pre-existing atheroma
- Trauma
- Graft occlusion after vascular surgery.

Who

- Patient often has a past history of vascular disease (cardiac, claudication).

A typical patient

A vasculopath presents with limb pain at rest of sudden onset.

Clinical features

- **6 Ps:**
  - **P**ale
  - **P**ulseless
  - **P**ain
  - **P**erishing with cold
  - **P**aralysed
  - **P**araesthethic

NB: Final two indicate severe ischaemia and danger of limb loss
- Sudden onset
- Progresses to gangrene
- Ischaemic rest pain: a symptom of critical ischaemia.

Investigations

- Identify cause.
- Clinical examination: peripheral pulses, AF, mitral stenosis, aneurysms

- Arteriogram.

Treatment

Treat quickly to save the limb:
- Embolic cause:
  - Local thrombolysis, e.g. tissue plasminogen activator (tPA)
  - Surgical embolectomy: Fogarty catheter where a tube is passed past the clot, a balloon at the end is inflated and then pulled back, pulling the clot away with it:

- Postoperatively:
  - Find source of embolus
- Thrombotic cause:
  - Arteriogram
  - Bypass surgery
  - After flow is restored: fasciotomy (division of deep fascia of the calf to prevent damage if muscles swell):
- Postoperative:
  - Anticoagulants: heparin.

Prognosis and complications

Prognosis

- Mortality 22%

- Amputation 16%.

Complications

- Postoperative reperfusion injury and acute renal failure

- Compartment syndrome: muscle swelling from ischaemia in a closed compartment.

CHRONIC ISCHAEMIC DISEASE

Outline

- Inadequate flow of blood normally to the lower limbs, due to a chronic change in blood flow
- Tissues adapt to ↓ O_2 supply by forming collateral vessels.

Pathogenesis/aetiology

Causes

- Always atherosclerosis
Predisposing factors:
- History of other ischaemic problems
- Atherosclerosis
- Diabetes mellitus
- Hyperlipidemia
- Family history
- Smoking.

Who

Associations:
- Young heavy smokers: Buerger's disease (vascular disease of medium-sized blood vessels).

A typical patient

A vasculopath presents with intermittent pain on walking.

Clinical features

Stages of ischaemia:
1. *Intermittent claudication:*
   - Leg cramps (calves/feet) during exercise, relieved by rest
   - Measured by claudication distance (distance before symptoms produced)
   - Blockage of the femoropopliteal segment: causes calf pain
   - Blockage of the iliac artery: causes buttock pain and impotence (Leriche syndrome)
2. *Rest pain:*
   - Ischaemia of muscles and soft tissue at rest.
   - Usually at night: patient may hang leg over bed to ↑ blood supply

- Pain mainly over metatarsal head (area of least blood supply)
- Ischaemia is critical and viability of leg is at risk
3. *Gangrene*
   - Tissue is black
Symptoms and signs:
- Absent pulses
- Cool, white legs
- Punched out ulcers
- Postural or dependent colour change
- Skin changes
- Hair loss and brittle nails on affected digits
- Prolonged capillary refill.

Investigations

Bedside tests:
- Capillary refill >5 s
- Buerger's test: raise legs while lying flat to see if and when they go pale. Normally pink even at 90°. Severe ischaemia if positive test at <20 °
- Ankle brachial pressure index (ABPI): use a cuff and US Doppler probe for the measurements, then divide the higher of the systolic pressures of the ankles (dorsalis

pedis or posterior tibialis) for each leg by the higher of either brachial BPs:
- Normal radio: >1
- Claudication: 0.6–0.9
- Rest pain: 0.3–0.6
- Caution in diabetics with hardened uncompressible calcified atherosclerosis giving false negative results.

Blood tests

- FBC
- U&Es
- Lipids
- Platelets
- Clotting profile.

Imaging

- Contrast arteriography
- Colour duplex imaging allows visualisation of blood flow.

Treatment

Intervene if:
- disabling claudication/rest pain
- critical limb ischaemia

Conservative treatment:
- Stop smoking
- Exercise
- Lose weight
- Antiplatelets: aspirin
- Lipid-lowering drugs: statins
- Diabetic control
- Monitor: can do so over many years

Critical ischaemia:
- ABPI 0.5–0.7: refer to outpatient specialist
- 0.3–0.5: urgent referral
- <0.3: urgent referral to vascular emergency on call team

Interventions:
- Percutaneous angioplasty: widening of the obstructed blood vessel normally via access through the brachial or femoral vein. Useful for short stenoses in big arteries
- Bypass graft surgery:
  - Aortic or iliac artery occlusion: aorta bifemoral bypass graft
  - Distal occlusion: femoral-popliteal bypass graft often using the long saphenous vein
- Sympathectomy: chemically or surgically to relieve pain if revascularisation is impossible
- Amputation: relieve pain and reduce likelihood of death.

Prognosis and complications

Prognosis

- The more distal the occlusion, the lower the likelihood of successful bypass
- Femoral distal bypass: 50% remain patent after 1 year.

Complications

- Progression to critical ischaemia
- Aneurysmal dilatation
- Other vascular problems, e.g. coronary or carotid artery disease
- Infection of ischaemic tissue, particularly in diabetics.

ANEURYSM

Outline

- Abnormal dilatation of the arterial wall or chamber of the heart
- Normally due to a weakened arterial wall

Classification (Fig. 13.23)

- True aneurysm: arterial dilatation. Can be:
  - fusiform: spindle shaped, tapered at both ends
  - saccular: sac or berry shaped
- False aneurysm: leak in an artery causes a collection of blood to pool around the vessel. The blood is confined by surrounding tissue and continues to communicate with that inside the vessel.

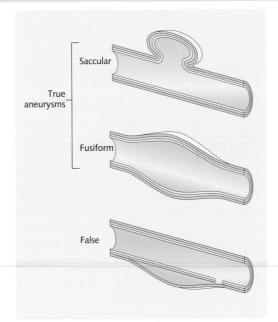

Fig. 13.23 Different types of aneurysm.

Pathogenesis/aetiology

Causes

- Atherosclerosis: dilatation and thinning of the wall
- After trauma
- Congenital, e.g. berry aneurysms
- Infective or inflammatory: tertiary syphilis leads to thoracic aneurysms, TB, *Staphylococcus*, pneumococci, *Salmonella*

- Connective tissue disease: rheumatoid arthritis, ankylosing spondylitis, Marfan syndrome, Ehlers–Danlos
- Vasculitis: polyarteritis nodosa, Kawasaki syndrome, giant cell arteritis.

Who

- Typical age: rare before age 50
- ♀ < ♂

Risk factors:
- Diabetes
- Smoking
- Hypertension
- Hyperlipidaemia.

Clinical features

- Prominent expansile mass on palpation
Sites:
- Aortic:
  - Ascending
  - Abdominal 95%
  - Supra-renal aorta
  - Iliac

- Non-aortic:
  - Subclavian
  - Splenic
  - Hepatic
  - **Femoral 20%**
  - **Popliteal 70%:** 50% have a coexisting aortic aneurysm. Less common than abdominal aneurysm
  - Berry aneurysm: arteries in circle of Willis in the brain.

Investigations

Imaging

- US

- CT.

Treatment

- Repair or replacement of the damaged vessel

- False aneurysms: direct thrombin injection.

Prognosis and complications

Complications

- Rupture and haemorrhage: risk depends on size and rate of increase
- Pressure on adjacent structures: ureter, vertebral and renal vessels, thoracic compression of airways (persistent cough, aortic root dilatation)

- Infection
- Thrombosis or embolisation.

ABDOMINAL AORTIC ANEURYSM

Outline

- Abnormal dilatation of the wall of the aorta in the region of the abdomen.

Classification

- Infrarenal: 90%

- Suprarenal: 10% (higher mortality during surgery).

Pathogenesis/aetiology

Causes

- See above.

Pathogenesis

- Normally fusiform aneurysm.

Who

- 1♀:3♂
- Prevalence: 5% of >50 years

- One of the commonest causes of sudden death.

A typical patient

A vasculopath is found to have a pulsatile mass on routine abdominal examination.

Clinical features

Unruptured:
- Often asymptomatic
- Abdominal or back pain
- Abdominal expansile, pulsating mass
- Upper GI haemorrhage from fistulation in the bowel

Ruptured abdominal aortic aneurysm:
- Abdominal pain radiating to the back or groin
- Dilated abdomen
- Signs of shock: pallor, tachycardia, collapse.

Investigations

- Don't waste time

- Aim to: confirm diagnosis, determine extent, identify location and determine if leaking or bleeding.

Imaging

- **US**: best, cheap and can estimate aneurysm size
- CT/MRI: can be helpful in stable patient with uncertain diagnosis

- X-ray: calcification on plain X-ray.

Treatment

Unruptured:
- <5.5 cm: examination and US every 6 months
- >5.5 cm or rapidly expanding: consider surgery as risk of rupture
- Surgery: replacement of the aneurysm with a synthetic graft either with an endoluminal approach (via the femoral artery) known as endovascular aneurysm repair or open surgery
- Suprarenal aneurysms require re-implantation of the renal vessels and other affected arteries to the aorta

Ruptured abdominal aortic aneurysm:
- Emergency:
  - ABC approach: O_2, fluids, blood
  - Vascular surgeon needed
  - Clamp aorta above and below leak. Open aneurysm and insert a graft
  - Prophylactic antibiotics: cefuroxime, metronidazole
  - Postoperative: ICU, ventilation, dialysis.

Prognosis and complications

Prognosis

- Mortality:
  - Unruptured and treated: 5%
  - Unruptured: 10%

- Ruptured and treated: 50%
- Ruptured untreated: 100%

Complications

- As above
- In addition:
  - Renal failure
  - Fistulae
  - Acute ileus

- Surgical complications (5%), e.g. spinal/mesenteric ischaemia
- Late surgical complications: graft infection, aorto-enteric fistula, development of a false aneurysm.

DISSECTING AORTIC ANEURYSM

Outline

- Blood separates the layers of the aortic wall so that there are two longitudinal lumens instead of one
- **An emergency as the vessel can rupture and due to further complications**

- If the dissection progresses proximally (i.e. back towards the heart) it can cause acute MI, if it dissects distally (i.e. towards the renal arteries) it can lead to organ hypoperfusion by occluding vessels branching off from the aorta.

Classification

- *Type A* (70%): involves the ascending aorta, proximal to the left subclavian artery origin and may involve descending aorta

- *Type B* (30%): not involving the ascending aorta, distal to the origin of the left subclavian artery.

Pathogenesis/aetiology

Aortic dissection risk factors:
- Anything that weakens the arterial wall:

- **ABC**:
  - **A**therosclerosis/**A**geing/**A**ortic aneurysm
  - ↑ **BP**/**B**aby (pregnancy)
  - **C**onnective tissue disorders (Marfan syndrome, Ehlers–Danlos syndrome).

Pathogenesis

- An intimal tear allows blood to enter the second layer, the media causing the layers of the arterial wall to separate and leading to a blood-filled 'false' channel
- The false channel can obstruct vessels originating in the path of the dissection

- It can rupture and if the dissection affects the attachments of the aortic valve, can cause aortic incompetence and MI as the coronary arteries originate from the aortic root above the aortic valve
- The commonest site for the dissection is the thoracic aorta.

Who

- Typical age: peak incidence 40–60 years

- $♀ < ♂$.

A typical patient

A vasculopath presents with a tearing interscapular pain.

Clinical features

- Sudden tearing chest pain that radiates to the back, chest, neck or abdomen
- Can mimic a myocardial infarct
- Peripheral pulses may be absent

- BP and pulse may be different on each arm: radio-radial delay if the vascular supply of one arm is affected more than the other
- Neurological symptoms due to involvement of spinal arteries
- Shock: if rupture occurs.

Investigations

Imaging

- ECG
- CXR: wide mediastinum

- CT/MRI
- Transoesophageal echocardiogram.

Treatment

- **Emergency**
- Resuscitate

Type A:
- **Emergency**
- Manage surgically
- Aortic root replacement

Type B:
- Usually managed medically
- Antihypertensives: beta-blockers
- Managed surgically under certain conditions such as organ or limb ischaemia.

Prognosis

- Acute operative mortality <25%.

Complications

- Myocardial infarct
- Hemiplegia (if carotid is affected)
- Renal ischaemia and acute renal failure if renal arteries are occluded
- Acute lower limb ischaemia.

CAROTID ARTERY DISEASE

Outline

- Disease of the carotid arteries mostly from atheroscleosis
- Normally at sites of division into internal and external carotid arteries
- Can lead to stroke or TIA as the internal carotid artery supplies the brain.

Pathogenesis/aetiology

Causes

- Primarily atherosclerosis
- Associated with smoking and hypertension.

Who

- Typical age: >65 years
- ♀<♂.

A typical patient

A vasculopath presents with a stroke.

Clinical features

- TIA
- Stroke
- Asymptomatic bruit of carotid artery.

Investigations

Imaging

- Duplex carotid US scanning: detect stenosis
- Angiography
- CT or MRI.

Treatment

Conservative and medical

- ↓ smoking and fat, ↑ exercise
- Control hypertension
- Antiplatelet therapy
- Statins.

Surgical

- If symptomatic and stenosis is >70%, perform a carotid endarterectomy: the stenosed carotid artery is opened, obstructing material removed and the artery repaired.

Prognosis and complications

Prognosis

- Narrowing of the external carotid artery is not problematic due to multiple collaterals.

Complications

- Carotid endarterectomy leads to stroke in 10%.

VENOUS DISEASE

VARICOSE VEINS

Outline

- Tortuous, lengthened, dilated superficial veins with incompetent valves
- Mostly refers to veins of the legs, but can occur anywhere, e.g. anus, oesophagus, abdominal wall

Sites of incompetent valves:
- *Saphenofemoral junction*: commonest site
- *Saphenopopliteal junction* in popliteal fossa behind knee
- *Perforating veins*: can be the mid-thigh or medial calf perforators.

Pathogenesis/aetiology

Pathogenesis

- The leg comprises a deep and superficial system of veins (Fig. 13.24):
  - *Superficial*: great and small saphenous veins, perforator veins
  - *Deep*: popliteal, femoral, tibial veins
- Normally blood flows from the superficial to the deep veins directly and via perforating veins
- The deep venous circulation is at a higher pressure than the superficial venous system but valves prevent back-flow. The two main valves are the saphenofemoral and the saphenopopliteal valves
- Varicose veins occur if:
  - the valves are incompetent
  - the perforating veins are incompetent
  - in post-thrombotic syndrome: thrombosis prevents blood flow and causes pooling
- These mechanisms allow blood to reflux and pool in the superficial veins which have thinner walls than the deep veins.

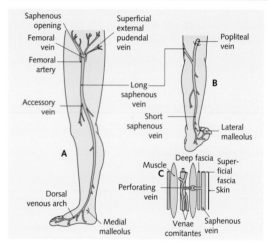

Fig. 13.24 Veins of the legs: (A) long saphenous; (B) short saphenous; (C) perforators.

Causes

- 1°:
  - Unknown: commonest cause
  - Congenital valve absence: rare
- 2°:
  - Obstruction to venous flow:
    - Abdominal mass
  - Ascites
  - Pelvic tumour
  - Pregnancy: impaired venous return and progesterone-induced venous dilatation
- Valve destruction:
  - e.g. DVT.

Who

- ♀ > ♂
- 10–20% of the population
Risk factors:
- Use of oral contraceptive pill
- Obesity
- Family history
- Standing for long periods of time: certain occupations.

Clinical features

- Often asymptomatic
Varicose veins symptoms:
- **AEIOU**:
  - **A**ching: dull ache, cramping and restlessness
  - **E**czema
  - **I**tching
  - **O**edema (pitting)
  - **U**lceration: from poor circulation
  - **U**gly: veins are visibly larger
- Lipodermatosclerosis: skin hardness due to chronic inflammation
Ask:
- What worries patient? Cosmetic issues or pain?
- Pain: aching worse after standing? Associated swelling of ankles?
- Family history of varicose veins?
- History of DVT/pulmonary embolism?.
- Number of pregnancies?

Investigations

Clinical examination

- Inspect
- A cough impulse at the saphenofemoral junction suggests valve incompetence
- Tap test:
  - Calf veins are tapped: if there is an incompetent valve the thrill is transmitted to saphenous vein in the thigh (interrupted if competent valves present)
- Trendelenburg's test:
  - Locates presence and site of incompetent valves
  - The patient lies down and the affected leg is elevated to drain the superficial veins

- A tourniquet is placed around the leg and the patient then stands
- If the defective valve is above the tourniquet, the veins below will not fill until the tourniquet is released
- If the defective valve is below the tourniquet level, the veins will fill on standing
- The test can be repeated distally to assess the level of the incompetent valve but is unreliable below the knee

Imaging

- Doppler US probe:
  - Listen for flow in incompetent valves

- Duplex scanning:
  - Duplex marking of perforators
- Venography.

Treatment

Conservative:
- Education
- Avoid prolonged standing
- Support stockings
- Lose weight
- Exercise

Surgical

For valve or perforator incompetency:
- High ligation (tying off) at the saphenofemoral junction and partial stripping of the vein to remove it
- Followed by multiple avulsions for tributaries to prevent pooling of blood further down the leg
- Postoperatively legs bandaged tightly and elevated for 24 h

Injection sclerotherapy:
- Mainly done for minor pathology or slight changes identified postsurgery
- Sclerosant injected at multiple sites causing a chemical thrombophlebitis to occlude the vein
- Vein is compressed for a few weeks to avoid thrombosis.

- Better than sclerotherapy long term
- Not for surgery if the cause of the varicose veins are 2° to malignancy
For post-thrombotic syndrome:
- Treat as for DVT with venous drainage and elastic stockings.

Prognosis and complications

Prognosis

- Early intervention helps prevent ulceration and dermatofibrosis.

Complications

- Oedema
- Thrombosis
- Stasis
- Dermatitis
- Ulceration
- Pain
- Bleeding

- Infection
- Thrombophlebitis
Postoperative complications:
- Wound sepsis
- Nerve damage
- Haematoma
- DVT.

DEEP VEIN THROMBOSIS (DVT)

Outline

- Obstruction of a deep vein by a thrombus (blood clot)
- Can dislodge and impact in a pulmonary vein causing a pulmonary embolism
- Post-thrombotic syndrome is another serious complication
- Most common in the lower limb

Lower limb DVTs:
- Proximal veins (above knee): high risk of embolism
- Veins below the knee: less likely to embolise, but clots can move into the proximal veins
Upper limb DVTs:
- ↑ incidence due to Hickman lines.

Pathogenesis/aetiology

Causes

- Virchow's triad of factors:
  1. ↓ *Flow rate*: immobility, varicose veins
  2. *Vessel wall damage*: trauma
  3. *Abnormal blood consistency*: hypercoagulability, e.g. malignancy, thrombophilia, nephrotic syndrome

Differential diagnoses:
- Cellulitis
- Haematoma
- Lymphoedema.

Who

- Common
- Incidence: 0.05–0.12%
- 25–50% of surgical patients

Risk factors:
- Age
- Obesity

- Immobility
- Malignancy
- Surgical patients
- Past history of DVT or pulmonary embolism
- Pregnancy
- Oral contraceptive pill.

A typical patient

A young woman who is taking the oral contraceptive pill presents with calf pain following a long-haul flight.

Clinical features

- Asymptomatic (65% of calf vein thromboses)
- Unilateral (unless multiple DVTs)
- Pain
- Swelling
- Hot
- Erythema
- Venous dilatation
- Tenderness
- Mild fever
- Unilateral pitting oedema
- Impaired skin circulation, venous gangrene

Wells' criteria:
- Used to predict likelihood of a DVT: consider imaging if score is >2:
  - Active cancer (1)
  - Calf swelling (1)
  - Whole leg is swollen (1)
  - Pitting oedema (1)
  - Collateral (non-varicose) superficial veins (1)
  - Pain localised along deep venous system (1)
  - Paralysis, paresis, or recent cast immobilisation of lower extremities (1)
  - Bedridden >3 days, or major surgery in last 4 weeks (1)
  - Alternative diagnosis is as likely (minus 2).

Investigations

Blood tests

- FBC, U&Es, LFTs, clotting

D dimer:
- A fibrin degradation product. Always ↑ in a DVT, but not specific

Imaging

Doppler US:
- Non-invasive
- Visualises thromboses (particularly proximal DVTs)
- Investigation of choice

Contrast venography:
- Contrast injected and X-rays taken
- Gold standard
- Invasive
- Rarely done.

Other tests

Thrombophilia tests: only if history is suggestive of a coagulopathy

Treatment

Suspected DVT

- Mostly treated as outpatients, certain criteria for treating as an inpatient
NICE guidance (May 2011)
- Mechanical interventions:
  - Graduated elastic stockings for post thrombotic syndrome
  - Inferior vena cava filler if contraindication for medical coagulation
- Pharmacological interventions:
  - LMWH: continued until warfarin treatment is begun and the therapeutic target INR is attained. Unless due to malignancy when LMWH is continued instead of warfarin

- Vitamin K antagonist e.g. Warfarin: Target INR 2–3 (with regular monitoring). Anticoagulated for 3–6 months if there is a definite trigger that has been eliminated and this is the 1st event. Ongoing treatment if there are persistent multiple risk factors or this is the second episode
- Factor Xa inhibitors, e.g. fondaparinux, rivaroxaban.
Thrombolysis
- For certain criteria in DVT and PE

Primary prevention

- Prophylaxis for surgery: mobilise early postoperatively, antiembolism compression stockings, LMWH, intermittent pneumatic compression devices

(devices applying intermittent pressure usually to legs to ↓ clot risk).

Prognosis and complications

Prognosis

- Significant mortality.

Complications

- Pulmonary embolism: >90% of acute pulmonary embolisms are from proximal DVTs
- Paradoxical embolism: rare, due to an ASD allowing the clot to cross into the left sided circulation causing systemic infarcts, e.g. stroke
- Recurrence of thrombosis

- Phlegmasia cerulea dolens: severe, acute, massive obstruction of a major limb vein and its tributaries. Leads to sudden swelling, oedema, and gangrene. Rare, but risk of pulmonary embolism
- Post-thrombotic syndrome (1/3 patients at 5 years): pain, swelling and leg ulcers.

OBSTRUCTED SUPERIOR VENA CAVA

Outline

- Obstruction of the superior vena cava (the vessel carrying blood from the body back to the heart)

- Usually leads to distension of veins in the upper part of the body.

Pathogenesis/aetiology

Causes

- Malignancy including lymphomas are commonest cause.

Who

A typical patient

An elderly patient with diagnosis of lymphoma presents with dilated neck veins.

Clinical features

- Plethoric (red) face
- Headaches
- Swelling of upper body, arms and neck
- Chemosis: conjunctival swelling

- Dizziness
- Distended jugular veins
- Dilated superficial veins on chest.

Investigations

- History often suggests cause.

- Radiotherapy: for malignant cause
- Stenting.

- Depends on response of malignancy to treatment.

SKIN DISEASE

ULCER (LEG OR OTHER)

An abnormal breach in an epithelial surface.
Classification of ulcers by edge (Fig. 13.25):

- **S PURE**:
  - **S**loping edge (e.g. venous stasis ulcer)

- **P**unched out (e.g. trophic, arterial)
- **U**ndermined (e.g. pressure, TB)
- **R**olled (e.g. basal cell carcinoma)
- **E**verted (e.g. squamous cell carcinoma).

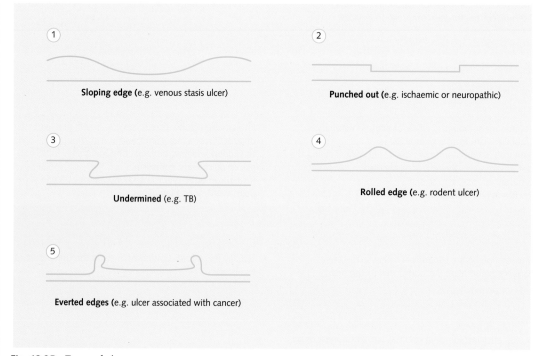

Sloping edge (e.g. venous stasis ulcer**)**

Punched out (e.g. ischaemic or neuropathic**)**

Undermined (e.g. TB**)**

Rolled edge (e.g. rodent ulcer**)**

Everted edges (e.g. ulcer associated with cancer**)**

Fig. 13.25 Types of ulcer.

- *Venous* (80%): increased pressure in the superficial system damages venous valves, e.g. varicose veins or DVTs
- *Arterial* (2%): vasculitis, peripheral vascular disease. Associated with gangrene of the toes in 10%
- *Mixed*: arterial and venous (15%)

- *Neuropathic*: chronic alcohol excess, peripheral neuropathy, diabetes, tabes dorsalis
- *Neoplastic*: squamous cell carcinoma, basal cell carcinoma
- *Infection*: syphilis
- *Trauma*
- *Drugs*.

Who

- Prevalence: 2% in the developed world

Risk factors:

- Trauma
- Diabetes mellitus
- Peripheral vascular disease
- IBD (pyoderma gangrenosum)
- Steroid use
- Varicose veins.

Clinical features

- Location can help identify cause (Fig. 13.26)
- Venous leg ulcers:
  - Affects the lower leg, particularly over the medial malleolus, along the greater saphenous vein
  - Evidence of pigmentation and lipodermatosclerosis
  - Painless
- Arterial leg ulcers:
  - Affects the anterior aspect of the shin or the dorsum of the foot
  - Associated signs of peripheral ischaemia, e.g. gangrene
  - Pain
- Pressure sores and neuropathic ulcers:
  - Affects bony prominences such as the heel and plantar aspect of the first metatarsal head
  - Painless, reduced sensation
  - Foot is warm with good blood supply.

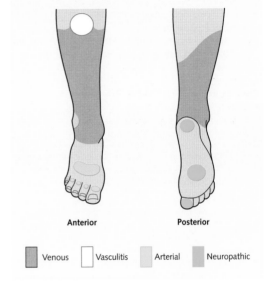

Anterior   Posterior

Venous   Vasculitis   Arterial   Neuropathic

Fig. 13.26   Location of leg ulcers according to cause.

Investigations

- Determine cause

Clinical examination

- Site, shape, skin changes, arterial examination.

Blood tests

- FBC
- ESR, for vasculitis
- VDRL (Venereal Disease Research Laboratory) test, for syphilis.

Microbiology

- Culture swab, for infection.

Imaging

US:

- *Arterial*: duplex Doppler to determine if cause is arterial or venous, ankle brachial pressure index: see ischaemic disease above.
- *Venous*: duplex Doppler, venogram.

Other tests

Biopsy:
- If malignancy is suspected.

Treatment

- Treat cause

Conservative

- Usually reviewed in primary care:
  - Prevention is key
  - ↓ Risk factors, e.g. smoking

- Skin care: clean, protect from injury
- Avoid standing still/crossed legs
- Refer to ulcer clinic/community nurse

Medical and bandaging

- Dress ulcer: moist environment over ulcer to promote epithelial regrowth
- Pressure bandaging: only if ankle brachial pressure index is >0.8 (not if history of peripheral vascular disease)

- Elevation
- Topical agents; silver sulfadiazine, gentamicin
- If dirty: antiseptic, deslough dressing
- Hospital admission if necessary.

Surgical

- Large ulcer: consider skin graft

- Treatment of varicose veins.

Prognosis and complications

Prognosis

- Early intervention by specialist service optimises outcome.

Complications

- Eczema of leg

- Cellulitis.

MALIGNANT MELANOMA

Outline

- Malignant tumour of the melanocytes, the pigment cells of the basal layer of the skin that produce melanin

- Most serious form of skin cancer, can kill, metastasises early.

Classification

1. *Lentigo maligna melanoma*: a melanoma in situ. A patch of brown pigmented skin which can develop into a papule, signalling invasive tumour. Usually on the face, progresses slowly
2. *Acral lentiginous*: like lentigo maligna but affects the palm, sole, or under the nail and normally presents late

3. *Superficial spreading (80%)*: flat tumour with variable pigmentation that grows slowly, better prognosis, commonest form of melanoma
4. *Nodular malignant melanoma*: most aggressive form, rapidly growing pigmented nodule.

Pathogenesis/aetiology

Causes

- Excessive UV exposure
- May be genetic element: ↑ risk with a family history and tumour suppressor gene is frequently mutated or deleted in melanoma cell lines

Staging systems:
Breslow thickness:
- Measure of local invasion by depth in millimetres, important for prognosis
Clark's staging:
- Another measure of local invasion by a scale of 1–5 from 'confined to the epidermis (in situ)' to 'penetration of the subcutaneous tissue.

Who

- Typical age: more common in the elderly
- ♀1: ♂1.3
- Incidence increasing most likely due to sun exposure

Risk factors:
- Sun exposure
- Fair or red haired people
- Positive family history
- Atypical mole syndrome: can lead to malignant melanoma.

A typical patient

A changing mole is noted on self-examination.

Clinical features

- Mostly found on the skin
- Suspect changing moles particularly if irregular edge and variation in pigmentation
- Melanomas are assessed according to the ABCDE or Glasgow 7 checklist: presence of features on these lists makes melanoma more likely.

Glasgow 7 checklist; refer if >3 points:
- Major (2 points per feature):
  1. Change in size
  2. Change in shape: irregular border
  3. Change in colour: irregular pigmentation
- Minor (1 point per feature):
  4. Diameter >7 mm
  5. Inflammation
  6. Oozing/bleeding
  7. Itch/odd sensation.

ABCDE (Fig. 13.27):
- A: asymmetry of mole
- B: border irregularity
- C: colour variegation: irregular pigmentation
- D: diameter >6 mm
- E: evolving: consider any changes in size, shape, colour.

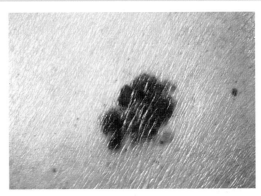

Fig. 13.27 Malignant melanoma.

Investigations

- Histological analysis:
  - Clark's level: depth of invasion
- Breslow thickness: thickness of tumour
- Sentinel node biopsy to predict prognosis.

Treatment

Prevention:
- UV avoidance and burning
- Sun protection
- Self-examination for suspicious lesions

Treat (based on Glasgow 7 point checklist):
- One major: excise urgently
- Any minor: add to suspicion
- Excise and ensure borders of tissue are clear.

Prognosis and complications

Prognosis

- Mortality: 1.9/100 000/year in UK
- Tumours <1 mm thick 5-year survival: 90%
- Tumours >3.5 mm: 5-year survival rate is <35%.

Complications

- Metastases: common
- Can occur in the retina leading to excision of the eye (consider this if a patient presents with a glass eye and hepatomegaly in examinations).

BASAL CELL CARCINOMA

Outline

- Cancer of the basal cells of the skin, the deepest of the five layers of the epidermis
- Commonest skin cancer
- Also called a rodent ulcer.

Pathogenesis/aetiology

Causes

- UV light/sun exposure
- Carcinogenic chemical.

Pathogenesis

- Grows slowly
- Highly invasive but rarely metastasises
- Causes local destruction, e.g. to bone.

Who

- Typical age: commoner in the elderly
- ♀ < ♂
- Commonest malignant skin tumour

Risk factors:
- Positive family history
- Fair skinned
- ↑ Sun exposure.

Clinical features

- Pearly pink nodule with rolled edge and central scab which may ulcerate (Fig. 13.28)
- Overlying telangiectasia
- Areas of pigmentation
- Usually on exposed skin areas: 90% found on the face (e.g. side of nose, eyelids).

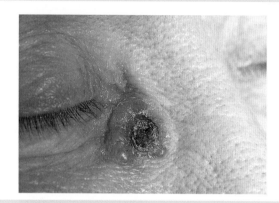

Fig. 13.28 Basal cell carcinoma with pearly nodule and crust.

Investigations

- Clinical examination

- Biopsy.

Treatment

- Excise
- Cryotherapy (freezing) with curettage (removing around the area with a knife) for non-critical sites or in the elderly
- Radiotherapy if large/unable to excise

- Photodynamic therapy (light applied to the basal cell carcinoma that has been made sensitive to light using a photosensitiser). Leads to tissue destruction.

Prognosis and complications

Prognosis

- Good
- Metastases are rare

- 5% recur at 5 years.

Complications

- Locally destructive.

SQUAMOUS CELL CARCINOMA

Outline

- Cancer of the squamous cell layer of the skin
- More aggressive than basal cell carcinoma
- May arise in pre-existing solar keratoses or Bowen's disease

Bowen's disease:
- Squamous cell carcinoma in situ.

Pathogenesis/aetiology

Causes

Often seen on damaged skin:
- UV light/sun exposure
- Smoking
- Infection: human papilloma virus subtypes

- Immunosuppression
- Chronic inflammation, e.g. venous leg ulcers; if this is the cause it is called a Marjolin's ulcer.

- Less common than basal cell carcinoma.

A typical patient

An elderly patient presents with a facial lesion on sun-exposed skin.

Clinical features

- Firm, irregular, crusted nodules that can ulcerate (Fig. 13.29)
- Everted, hard edges
- Lesions often kerototic (excessive growth of horny tissue of the skin)
- Rapid growth
- Usually on sun-exposed sites.

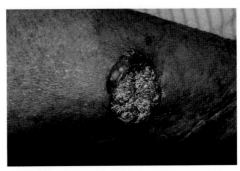

Fig. 13.29   Squamous cell carcinoma.

Investigations

Clinical examination

- Examine regional lymph nodes.

Other tests

- Biopsy.

Treatment

- Excise
- Radiotherapy
- Avoid curettage.

Prognosis and complications

Prognosis

- Metastases are rare, but can metastasise, particularly to regional lymph nodes
- Invasive.

CELLULITIS

Outline

- Infection of the subcutaneous tissue with inflammation, pain and erythema.

Pathogenesis/aetiology

Causes

- Commonly *Streptococcus pyogenes* or *Staphylococcus aureus*
- More likely where there is a break in the skin for the bacteria to enter or the host is immunocompromised.

Who

Risk factors:
- Diabetic patients
- Vascular disease
- Leg ulcers
- Lymphoedema
- Obesity
- IVDU.

- Local pain, tenderness, swelling, erythema
- May be pus or discharge
- Often affects the legs
- Systemically unwell: fever, malaise.

- Clinical examination
- Swab if appropriate.

- CRP, FBC.

Check local guidelines:
- Mild (oral):
  - Treated as outpatients
  - Penicillin V and flucloxacillin or co-amoxiclav or erythromycin (if penicillin allergic)

- Severe (IV):
  - IV benzylpenicillin and IV flucloxacillin (for *Staphylococcus*)
  - IV fluid
  - Analgesia.

- Good if treated early.

- Infection of deeper structures, e.g. bone.

NECROTISING FASCIITIS

- Rapidly spreading infection of the subcutaneous tissue leading to destruction of the muscle, fat and tissue
- Life-threatening illness
- Most serious form of streptococcal infection.

- Bacterial infection of layer of fascia beneath the skin by group A beta-haemolytic streptococcus
- More likely where there is a break in the skin for the bacteria to enter
- Toxin production causes shock and organ failure.

- Rare

Risk factors:
- Elderly and postoperation
- History of minor trauma.

- Begins as mild cellulitis that progresses
- Pain with erythema
- May develop blistering, purple skin discoloration and necrosis

- Systemic features: fever, drowsiness, diarrhoea, vomiting shock.

Blood tests

- FBC
- U&Es

- Blood and tissue cultures.

Imaging

- CT/MRI.

Other tests

- Tissue biopsy.

Treatment

- Immediate surgical debridement
- ICU

- High-dose broad-spectrum antibiotics: IV benzylpenicillin: IV clindamycin (turns off toxin production by the organism).

Prognosis and complications

Prognosis

- High mortality.

Complications

- Limb loss
- Renal failure

- Septic shock.

GANGRENE

Outline

- Death of tissue from a poor blood supply:
  - Wet gangrene: tissue death and infection
  - Dry gangrene: no infection

- Gas gangrene: death and decay of tissue infected by the bacteria *Clostridium perfringens*. Bacterial toxins cause connective tissue decay with gas generation.

Pathogenesis/aetiology

- More common in the extremities or areas under pressure.

Causes

- Poor circulation: peripheral vascular disease, diabetes
- Trauma

- Infection.

Who

- Rare.

Clinical features

- Brown or black tissue
- Loss of sensation

- May have pain in the area adjacent to the gangrene
- Strong odour and discharge if infected.

Investigations

Infection screen

- Blood cultures.

Treatment

- Debridement
- Amputation
- Antibiotics

Gas gangrene:
- Remove dead tissue
- Antibiotics

Prognosis and complications

Prognosis

- Early intervention allows salvage of affected tissue.

Complications

- Amputation
- Death.

TAKING A HISTORY

How to take a basic history

- Introduce yourself
- Ask the patient for their name, age and occupation

Presenting complaint

- 'What has brought you in today?'

History of presenting complaint

- When the main problem started?
- How it has been since then?
- Any associated problems?

If the patient describes any pain obtain a precise description of the pain by going through the SOCRATES questions:

- **S**ite of pain?
- **O**nset: precipitators, sudden or insidious progression
- **C**haracter
- **R**adiation: does the pain radiate to any other site?
- **A**ssociated symptoms
- **T**iming of the pain: when did it start? Does it recur?
- **E**xacerbating or relieving factors
- **S**everity:
  - How does the problem affect the patient's daily lifestyle
  - Address the risk factors for the top differential diagnoses.

Past medical history

- Do you have any medical conditions?
- Is there anything that you see the doctor regularly for?
- Are you under any consultants and if so, where?
- Have you ever suffered from one of the following? (use MJTHREADS):
  - **M**yocardial infarction
  - **J**aundice
  - **T**B
  - **H**ypertension
  - **R**heumatic fever
  - **E**pilepsy
  - **A**sthma
  - **D**iabetes
  - **S**troke.

Surgical history

Have you ever had any operations?

Drug history

- What medicines are you currently taking?
- Do you buy any medicines in the chemist/health store?
- Do you have any allergies, in general or to any medications?

Family history

- Is there anything that runs in the family?
- Think of risk factors associated with the differential diagnoses and ask specifically for these.

Social history

- Where do you live?
- Who with?
- Are you able to manage all the normal activities of daily living (ADLs)?
- Do you get any help at home?
- How much exercise do you do and how easy is it for you to get around?
- Smoking history
- Alcohol and recreational drug history
- Have you been travelling recently?
- Do you have any pets?

Systems review

Run through the various symptoms of each system to see if anything has not been considered (Table 14.1).

Concluding remarks

- ICE, ask—What are your:
  - **i**deas
  - **c**oncerns
  - **e**xpectations of your symptoms?
- Repeat back to the patient the key things discussed:
  - Have I missed anything out?
  - Would you like to add anything?
  - Do you have any questions?
- Thank the patient for their time.

Table 14.1 Symptoms grouped by system

Cardiovascular	Respiratory	Gastrointestinal	Genitourinary	Nervous system	General
Chest pain?	SOB?	Abdominal pain?	Change in frequency?	Headaches?	Weight loss?
Palpitations?	Cough? Is it productive?	Nausea and vomiting?	Nocturia?	Dizziness?	Fatigue?
SOB?	Haempotysis?	Bowel changes?	Incontinence?	Loss of consciousness?	Appetite?
Syncope?	Wheeze?	Dyspepsia?	Poor stream?	Changes in hearing?	Rashes?
Ankle swelling?	Breathlessness?	Dysphagia?	Hesitancy?	Changes in sight?	
Intermittent claudication?	Chest pain?	Melaena or haematemesis?	Dysuria?		

The surgical sieve

The surgical sieve (TIN CAN MED DIP) is used to narrow down the possible causes of any disorder:

- Trauma
- Inflammation (physical/chemical/infective)
- Neoplastic (benign, malignant, 1°/2°)
- Circulation/vasculitic
- Autoimmune
- Nutritional
- Metabolic
- Endocrine
- Drugs
- Degeneration
- Iatrogenic/idiopathic
- Psychosomatic.

Remember: common things are common.

CARDIOVASCULAR

CHEST PAIN

Description

- Very common presenting complaint
- Must be taken seriously as could represent a number of emergency conditions which must be ruled out in any patient presenting with chest plain

Pleuritic pain:
- Pain due to inflammation of the pleura
- Characterised by pain that is worse on inspiration that causes the patient to catch their breath

- Occurs in **PPPPP**:
  - **P**ulmonary embolism
  - **P**neumonia
  - **P**neumothorax
  - **P**leural effusion
  - **P**ericarditis.

Causes

Four key emergencies to exclude in those with chest pain:
1. *Myocardial infarction (MI)*: dull, tight ache, with heaviness, like 'an elephant standing on one's chest', radiating to the left arm, neck or jaw, more severe at rest:
   - Only on exertion: consider stable angina
   - At rest with increasing frequency: consider unstable angina
   - With vomiting, sweating, often lasting >30 min: consider probable myocardial infarction (MI)
2. *Aortic dissection*: severe tearing chest pain radiating to the back
3. *Pulmonary embolism (PE)*: pleuritic chest pain with breathlessness and tachycardia, may be associated with leg swelling (DVT). May be no signs on ECG or CXR
4. *Pneumothorax*: breathlessness, sudden onset, may be history of trauma, or asthma/COPD

Cardiovascular causes:
- Angina; dull, crushing pain, relieved by rest and glyceryl trinitrate (GTN). Radiates to jaw/neck/arms
- Pericarditis: central sharp pain, worse with movement, relieved on sitting forward

Respiratory causes:
- Pleural effusion: stony dullness on chest percussion
- Empyema
- Pneumonia: fever, cough

Gastrointestinal causes:
- Reflux oesophagitis: burning pain worse when lying flat and relieved by antacids
- Oesophageal spasm/rupture
- Peptic ulcer

Musculoskeletal causes:
- Muscular skeletal pain is usually sharp, well localised with tender area on palpation:
  - Costochondritis (=inflammation of the costosternal or costochondral joints. A benign condition)
  - Bony metastases
  - Rib fractures
  - Herpes zoster

Psychogenic causes:
- Depression
- Anxiety.

What to ask for and associated symptoms

Ask the patient:
- Use **SOCRATES**:
  - **S**ite of pain?
  - **O**nset: precipitators, sudden or insidious progression?
  - **C**haracter: sharp or dull?
  - **R**adiation: does the pain radiate to any other site?
  - **A**ssociated symptoms?:
    - Cough: pneumonia
    - Dyspnoea: PE, pneumothorax
    - Calf swelling: PE
    - Fever: pneumonia
    - Palpitation
    - Nausea and vomiting: MI
    - Sweating
  - **T**iming?
  - **E**xacerbating or relieving factors?:
    - Relieved sitting forward: pericarditis

- Relieved by:
  - ○ glyceryl trinitrate: angina (early relief), oesophageal spasm (late relief)
  - ○ antacids: reflux oesophagitis
  - Worse on deep inspiration and causes catching of breath: pleuritic pain
- **S**everity?
- Have they had any recent long travel or surgery or swelling in their legs: PE
- Do they have any cardiac risk factors?:
  - Hypertension
  - Ischaemic heart disease
  - Family history (under age 55)
  - Hyperlipidaemia
  - Diabetes mellitus
  - Smoking history
  - In young people with chest pain ask about cocaine use, which can induce MI.

Clinical examination

- Pain replicated by pressing on the chest: costochondritis
- Blood pressure different in each arm with tearing pain radiating to the back: consider aortic dissection
- ↓ Air entry on one side on auscultation: pneumothorax.

Blood tests

- FBC, CRP: Look for any signs of infection
- Serum cardiac markers: useful for cardiac causes
- Arterial blood gases: useful for PE, serious pneumonia
- D-dimers: useful to exclude PE, non-specific if the test is positive.

ECG

- S1, Q3, T3 pattern, tachycardia or right heart strain pattern: PE
- ST segment changes in:
  - MI: ST elevation or depression
  - pericarditis: saddle shaped ST segments
  - myocarditis: non-specific
- New-onset left bundle branch block: MI
- Perform serial ECGs to monitor for dynamic changes, especially if suspecting ischaemia.

Imaging

- CXR: very useful for pneumonia, pneumothorax, effusion, aortic dissection (widened mediastinum)
- Echocardiogram: useful for pericardial effusion
- CT if aortic dissection is suspected
- CT pulmonary angiogram (CTPA): for suspected PE.

- Analgesia
- Rule out emergencies: ABC if necessary
- Treat specific cause.

PALPITATIONS

- Abnormal heartbeats, described by the patient as an unusual awareness of their heart beat
- Noticed as rapid/forceful/irregular/missing beats
- May be harmless but can be life-threatening
- Can compromise blood supply to the brain leading to syncope or sudden death.

Tachycardias (fast beats):
- Pathological causes:
  - Atrial fibrillation: commonest occurrence
  - Atrial flutter
  - Pathological arrhythmias
  - Thyrotoxicosis
  - Anaemia
- Physiological causes:
  - Exercise
  - Fever
  - Pregnancy
- Anxiety
- Response to drugs: caffeine, nicotine, alcohol, cocaine, amphetamine, ecstasy

Bradycardias (slow beats):
- Athletes
- Ischaemia
- Hypothyroidism
- Hypopituitarism
- Hypothermia
- Response to drugs: beta-blockers, digoxin.

See also Bradycardias and tachycardias on p. 15.

Ask the patient:
- To tap out rate and rhythm with their finger
- Ask them to describe the heartbeat:
  - Rapid or slow?
  - Regular or irregular?
  - Forceful?
- Missed beats?
- Continuous or occasional?
- Precipitating and relieving factors?
- How long has it been going on?
- How long do the palpitations last?
- Previous heart conditions?

What to ask for and associated symptoms

- Risk factors for heart disease?
- Family history of sudden cardiac death, e.g. in hypertrophic obstructive cardiomyopathy?
- History of thyroid disease?
- Drug history including illicit drugs?
- Alcohol intake?
- Caffeine intake?

- Associated symptoms?:
  - Dizziness
  - Syncope
  - Chest pain
  - Breathlessness
  - Anxiety.

Investigations

Clinical examination

- Cardiac examination.

Blood tests

- FBC
- U&Es
- TFTs (thyrotoxicosis or hypothyroidism)

- Glucose
- lipids
- Drug concentrations.

Cardiac examinations

- ECG, possibly 24 h ECG or longer, or exercise stress test

- Echocardiogram: especially if abnormal ECG.

Management

- Treat underlying cause
- Anti-arrhythmic medication if indicated

- Consider electrophysiology and ablation.

RESPIRATORY

SHORTNESS OF BREATH (SOB)

Description

- Feeling of breathlessness, also called dyspnoea
The Medical Research Council's dyspnoea scale:
1. Breathlessness only on strenuous exercise
2. Short of breath hurrying up a slight hill
3. Has to stop for breath when walking
4. Stops for breath after 100 m
5. Too breathless to leave the house
Orthopnoea:
- Breathlessness on lying flat
- From the redistribution of blood to ↑ venous return to the heart when lying down. The extra load on the heart leads to pulmonary congestion

- Often due to heart failure but can be other causes such as chronic respiratory disease
- If a patient describes orthopnoea, ask how many pillows are used at night: the more they use, the worse the condition
Paroxysmal nocturnal dyspnoea (PND):
- Breathlessness, anxiety and a feeling of 'struggling to breath' waking the patient at night, usually after a few hours of sleep
- Caused by similar features to orthopnoea or Cheyne–Stokes breathing in sleep. Suggests cardiac cause.

Causes

Respiratory:
- Sudden:
  - Airway obstruction: foreign body
  - Aspiration
  - Pulmonary embolus (PE)
  - Pneumothorax: unilateral pain
- Acute:
  - Acute asthma: wheeze
  - Pneumonia: cough, fever, malaise
  - Exacerbation of a chronic condition
- Chronic:
  - Asthma
  - Fibrosing lung disease (sarcoid, ankylosing spondylitis, cryptogenic fibrosing alveolitis)

- Chronic obstructive pulmonary disease (COPD)
- Lung cancer: haemoptysis, weight loss
- Tuberculosis
- Pleural effusion
- Allergic bronchopulmonary aspergillosis (ABPA)
Cardiac:
- Heart failure/pulmonary oedema
- Angina
- Aortic/mitral stenosis
- Arrhythmias
Musculoskeletal:
- Neuromuscular disease
- Chest wall deformities, e.g. kyphosis

Causes

Systemic:
- Sudden
  - Anaphylaxis
  - Hyperventilation
  - Anxiety.

- Acute-chronic
  - Thyrotoxicosis
  - Metabolic acidosis
  - Fever
  - Neurological disease
  - Anaemia
  - Obesity.

What to ask for and associated symptoms

Ask the patient:
- Onset: sudden or gradual
- How long has it been going on: minutes, hours or months?
- Exercise tolerance? Does it affect daily activity?
- History of respiratory or cardiac disease?
- Atopy: asthma, eczema, allergies?
- Pets?
- History of smoking?
- Occupational history: check for exposure to dust?
- How many pillows are used at night to prevent breathlessness: orthopnoea?
- Does breathlessness wake the patient at night: PND?

Associated symptoms?:
- Cough: is it productive? (see below)
- Wheeze: suggestive of COPD or asthma
- Stridor: suggests upper airway obstruction
- Dizziness: hypertrophic obstructive cardiomyopathy, ventricular tachycardia, aortic stenosis
- Haemoptysis
- Chest pain
- Fever
- Ankle swelling or oedema: heart failure
- Palpitations: arrhythmias
- Sweating, vomiting?: myocardial infarction.

Investigations

Clinical examination

- Respiratory examination: look for cyanosis, clubbing, auscultate the chest

- Cardiac examination.

Blood tests

- FBC, U&Es
- ABG

- Immunological tests where appropriate (*Aspergillus* precipitins; $\alpha 1$ anti-trypsin, etc.).

Imaging

- CXR, CT, CTPA (if suspecting pulmonary embolism).

Other tests

Lung function tests:
- Spirometry
- Peak expiratory flow
- Bronchoscopy if suspect aspiration or foreign body

Cardiac tests:
- ECG
- Echocardiogram
Microbiology:
- Sputum and blood

Management

- ABC if acutely unwell
- Oxygen

- Treat underlying cause.

COUGH

Description

- Explosive expiration caused by irritation in the respiratory tract
- Prevents aspiration

- Can be:
  - Acute: <3 weeks
  - Chronic: >8 weeks
  - No cause found in 15% of cases of chronic cough.

Causes

Acute cough:
- Acute infection: often viral
- Post nasal drip
- Pressure on the trachea: e.g. from goitre, tumour
- Inhaled foreign body

Chronic cough:
- Productive:
  - *Purulent, yellow or green* (suggests infective cause)
    - Pneumonia (acute presentation)
    - Bronchiectasis: often large quantities of sputum
  - Blood stained:
    - Pulmonary oedema: pink frothy
    - Tuberculosis (TB)
    - Pulmonary embolus (PE)
    - Lung cancer
    - Bronchiectasis

- Clear, mucoid/black specks suggesting tar staining
  - Chronic obstructive pulmonary disease (COPD)
- Non-productive:
  - Respiratory causes:
    - Lower tract: asthma, pulmonary fibrosis, sarcoidosis, Wegener's granulomatosis, Goodpasture's disease, polyarteritis nodosa
  - Gastrointestinal causes:
    - Gastro-oesophageal reflux disease (GORD)
  - Cardiovascular:
    - Left ventricular failure
  - Other:
    - Drugs: ACE inhibitors, irritants
    - Smoking.

What to ask for and associated symptoms

Ask the patient:
- How long have they had the cough?
- Onset acute or gradual?
- Productive or non-productive?
- If productive, any colour change?
- Does anything make the cough worse? Asthma may be worse at night
- Does anything make the cough better?
- Smoking history?
- Drug history?

- Occupation? Certain occupations may lead to dust exposure

Associated symptoms?:
- Haemoptysis
- Wheeze: asthma, COPD
- Shortness of breath
- Weight loss: cancer, TB
- Pleuritic chest pain: PE
- Trauma.

Investigations

Acute cough:
- None usually needed for acute cough with no significant associated symptoms

Chronic cough:
- For chronic cough, consider the following investigations:

Blood tests

- FBC, U&Es, CRP and ESR: rule out infection, malignancy, vasculitis

- Autoantibodies, e.g. anti-glomerular basement membrane antibodies if suspecting Goodpasture's disease.

Imaging

- CXR
- Echocardiogram
- CT if suggested by other imaging

- Fibre-optic bronchoscopy ± bronchoalveolar lavage.

Other tests

- Peak flow for asthma
- Sputum culture: useful for infection, e.g. TB
- Spirometry

- CT pulmonary angiogram (CTPA): pulmonary embolism
- Oesophageal pH studies: for gastro-oesophageal reflux

Management

- Treat cause.

HAEMPOTYSIS

Description

- Coughing up blood
- May originate from:
  - upper respiratory tract: nose, mouth, nasopharynx
  - lower respiratory tract
  - upper GI tract: stomach (often brown or black).

In 50% no cause found.

Causes

Respiratory causes:
- Infection: TB, COPD exacerbation, lung abscess, bronchiectasis, pneumonia
- Lung cancer
- Pulmonary oedema
- Pulmonary embolism (PE)
- Foreign body
- Airway trauma: may be iatrogenic, e.g. from bronchoscopy

Cardiovascular causes:
- Mitral stenosis: rare
- Left ventricular failure: rare
- Pulmonary hypertension
- Iatrogenic: Swan-Ganz catheter insertion

Other causes:
- Coagulation disorders
- Trauma
- Arterio-venous malformation
- Wegener's granulomatosus
- Goodpasture's syndrome.

What to ask for and associated symptoms

Ask the patient:
- Volume of blood coughed up?
- Colour?
- Any associated sputum: what volume or colour?
- Any other sites of bleeding: suggestive of 'other causes', e.g. coagulation disorders, Wegener's or Goodpasture's
- Any history of smoking?: lung cancer
- History of trauma/childhood infections?
- Occupation?: some occupations linked to lung cancer
- TB exposure?

- Past medical history?: coagulation disorders
- Associated renal disease?: Wegener's or Goodpasture's

Associated symptoms?:
- Cough
- Chest pain
- Breathlessness
- Fever, night sweats, ↓ appetite with weight loss: suggestive of cancer or TB
- Nose bleeds: Wegener's.

Investigations

Blood tests

- FBC, U&Es, CRP and ESR
- Clotting screen
- Autoantibodies if appropriate, e.g. ANA, rheumatoid factor, ANCA (Wegener's granulomatosis),

Anti-glomerular basement membrane antibodies (Goodpasture's disease).

Imaging

- CXR: infection, malignancy, pulmonary oedema
- Echocardiogram

- Fibre-optic bronchoscopy
- CT.

Other tests

- Mantoux test/IGRA: tests for TB
- ECG: Cardiac causes

- CTPA: For suspected PE

Management

- Treat cause.

CYANOSIS

Description

- Abnormal blue discoloration of the skin from ↑ quantities of deoxyhaemoglobin

Classification

- *Central*: cyanosis centrally due to right-to-left shunt or inadequate oxygenation of the blood

- *Peripheral*: cyanosis in the peripheries from poor peripheral circulation; may be physiological (cold) or pathological (e.g. heart failure).

Causes

Central:
- ↓ Oxygen saturations: severe respiratory disease, PE, cyanotic congenital heart disease
- Abnormal haemoglobin

Peripheral:
- Central causes
- Raynaud's phenomenon
- Acrocyanosis (cyanosis of the extremities)
- Vascular occlusion.

What to ask for and associated symptoms

- Centrally: blue tinge of the lips and underneath the tongue.

- Peripherally: blue discoloration of the hands

Investigations

Central:
- ABG
- Investigations guided by clinical history and examination

Peripheral:
- Need to exclude vascular occlusion.

Management

- Treat cause.

GASTROENTEROLOGY AND HEPATOLOGY

DYSPHAGIA

Description

- Dysphagia: difficulty in swallowing
- Aphagia: unable to swallow

- Odynophagia: pain on swallowing
- Most disorders of the oesophagus include dysphagia.

Causes

Intraluminal

- Oesophageal infection or inflammation

- Obstruction: tumour, foreign body.

Extraluminal–extramural

- Malignancy
- Pharyngeal pouch
- Hiatus hernia

- Goitre
- Vascular structures, e.g. aortic aneurysm.

Extraluminal–intramural

- Strictures, benign, malignant
- Achalasia: aperistalsis of the muscular wall of the oesophagus
- Oesophageal spasm

- Plummer–Vinson syndrome: middle-aged women with iron deficiency anaemia
- Presbyoesophagus: dysmotility associated with age.

Systemic

- Scleroderma: failure of peristalsis
Neurological:
- Myasthenia gravis

- Parkinson's disease
- Bulbar and pseudobulbar palsy
- Motor neuron disease.

What to ask for and associated symptoms

Ask the patient:
- How long has it been going on?
- What is difficult to swallow?:
  - Solids: mechanical obstruction
  - Liquids: functional, motility dysfunction
- Where does food get stuck?
- Is food regurgitated immediately?

- Progressively worsening: malignancy
- Episodic or continuous?
- Family history?
Associated symptoms?:
- Weight loss: malignancy
- Pain: malignancy, oesophagitis, oesophageal spasm.

Investigations

Blood tests

- FBC
- U&Es: to assess for dehydration.

Endoscopy

- 1st line. Visual assessment and therapeutic intervention

Imaging

- Barium swallow: good for motility disorders, pharyngeal pouch, achalasia
- CT: for staging extent of malignant disease.

Other tests

- Oesophageal pH studies: for gastro-oesophageal reflux disease
- Manometry: to assess lower oesophageal sphincter and peristalsis function. Important in achalasia
- Biopsy.

Management

- Treat cause.

NAUSEA AND VOMITING

Description

- Vomiting: ejection of the gastric contents through the mouth
- Nausea: the sensation of feeling about to vomit
- Vomiting is often due to a vagal reflex involving the chemoreceptor trigger zones or direct stimulation of the vomiting centre (central vomiting).

Causes

Gastrointestinal causes:
- Intestinal obstruction
- Paralytic ileus
- Inflammation or infection: appendicitis, cholecystitis, pancreatitis, gastroenteritis

Metabolic causes:
- Uraemia
- ↑ Calcium
- ↓ Sodium
- Diabetic ketoacidosis
- Addison's disease
- Do not forget pregnancy in women of fertile ages

Nervous system causes:
- Meningitis
- Migraine
- ↑ Intracranial pressure
- Brainstem lesions

- Head injury
- Autonomic neuropathy
- Motion sickness
- Meniere's disease: disorder of the inner ear affecting hearing and balance and leading to a triad of tinnitus, deafness and vertigo

Cardiac causes:
- Myocardial infarct

Drugs:
- Commonly:
  - Antibiotics
  - Cytotoxics
  - Digoxin
  - Opiates
  - Chemotherapy drugs
  - Alcohol.

What to ask for and associated symptoms

Ask the patient:
- How long has it been going on for?
- Any precipitants?
- Any relationship to meals?
- Amount of vomit?
- Content of the vomit: liquid, bile, blood, coffee grounds
- Past medical and family history, e.g. inflammatory bowel disease?
- Possibility of pregnancy?
- Any recent history of new medications?

- Any recent travel?

Associated symptoms?:
- Related to the gastrointestinal system:
  - Abdominal pain
  - Change in bowel habit: diarrhoea
  - Haematemesis.
- Related to the nervous system:
  - Headaches
  - Fever
  - Vertigo.

Investigations

Clinical examination

- Abdominal examination
- Look for signs of dehydration

- Examination of the nervous system if applicable.

Blood tests

- FBC, U&Es, LFTs, ESR, CRP

- Blood glucose: diabetic ketoacidosis.

Imaging

- CXR: erect if suspect bowel perforation
- Abdominal X-ray
- Abdominal US

- Abdominal CT
- Cranial CT if suggestion of ↑ intracranial pressure.

Management

- Treat cause
- Fluids if signs of dehydration
Antiemetics: **DASH**:
- **D₂ receptor antagonist:**
  - For neoplastic disease, radiation sickness, drug-induced vomiting:
    - Metoclopramide: good for migraine
    - Domperidone: does not cross the blood–brain barrier so has fewer central side effects
    - Haloperidol
    - Prochlorperazine: vertigo, labyrinth disorders
  - Side effects: extrapyramidal

- **A**nticholinergics:
  - Act on the vomiting centre. For palliative care, motion sickness, e.g. hyoscine bromide
  - Side effects: drowsy, blurred vision, dry mouth, difficulty micturating
- **S**erotonin antagonists:
  - Good for side effects of chemo- or radiotherapy, e.g. ondansetron
    - Side effects: constipation, rash, flushing, headache
- **H₁** antagonists:
  - Good for any cause of nausea: vertigo, motion sickness, Meniere's disease, e.g. cyclizine, cinnarizine
  - Side effects: drowsiness, dry mouth, blurred vision.

CONSTIPATION

Description

- Infrequent (bowels opening <3x per week) or difficult passage of hard stool with straining
- The reduction in frequency compared with normal is important

- Any change in bowel habit: consider cancer especially in the middle-aged–elderly
NICE guidelines for urgent referral for suspected bowel cancer:
- >40 years: rectal bleeding with a change of bowel habit for >6 weeks
- >60 years: rectal bleeding OR a change in bowel habit for > 6 weeks.

Causes

Gastrointestinal causes:
- Simple constipation: no cause
- ↓ Dietary fibre
- Painful anal conditions, e.g. anal fissure
- Medical disorders:
  - Diverticular disease
  - Inflammatory bowel disease (IBD)
  - Irritable bowel syndrome (IBS)
  - Coeliac disease
- Surgical:
  - Malignancy (local)
  - Appendicitis
  - Ischaemic bowel
  - Intestinal obstruction

Systemic causes:
- Immobility
- Dehydration
- ↑ Calcium
- ↑ Potassium
- Neurological: Parkinson's disease
- Depression
- Malignancy
- Pregnancy
- Endocrine: hypothyroidism, diabetes, hyperparathyroidism
- Drugs: (**A COIL**) **a**nticholinergic drugs, **c**alcium channel blockers (verapamil), **o**piates, **i**ron, **l**ithium.

What to ask for and associated symptoms

Ask the patient:
- What is your normal bowel habit?
- Duration of symptoms?
- Frequency of defecation?
- Does it occur with liquid stool: overflow diarrhoea
- Appetite/diet fibre intake?
- Drug history (including 'over-the-counter' medication)?

- Foreign travel?

Associated symptoms?:
- Weight loss?: malignancy
- Fever
- Pain
- Diarrhoea: IBD, IBS, diverticular disease.

Investigations

Clinical examination

- Examination per rectum (PR).

Blood tests

- FBC: anaemia, iron deficiency

- U&Es (especially Ca), LFTs, TFTs (hypothyroidism)

Other tests

- Faecal occult blood (FOB): detects small quantities of blood in the faeces.

- Colonoscopy with biopsy: especially if ruling out malignancy

Imaging

- Abdominal X-ray
- Abdominal US

- Abdominal CT.

Management

- Treat cause

Conservative

- ↑ Fibre and fluid

- ↑ Exercise

Medical

- Laxatives **BOSS:**
  - **B**ulking agents:
    - ↑ Faecal mass, e.g. methylcellulose, bran
  - **O**smotic agents:
    - Draw water into large bowel, e.g. lactulose, Movicol, magnesium salts

- **S**timulants:
  - ↑ Intestinal secretions and motility, e.g. senna, bisacodyl
- **S**ofteners:
  - Soften the stools, making it easier to pass, e.g. docusate sodium (oral), arachis oil (PR).

DIARRHOEA

Description

- ↑ Frequency or amount of loose stool
- Any change in bowel habit: consider cancer especially in the middle-aged–elderly (see NICE guidelines above)

Steatorrhoea:
- Passage of pale bulky stools containing fat
- >6 g of fat in 24 h.

Causes

Gastrointestinal causes:
- Infective
- Malignancy
- Malabsorption
- Inflammatory bowel disease (IBD)
- Irritable bowel syndrome (IBS)
- Diverticular disease

Systemic causes:
- Endocrine: hyperthyroidism, Addison's, diabetes
- Anxiety
- Bacterial overgrowth: in the elderly or with proton pump inhibitor therapy
- Bile salt malabsorption
- Drugs:
  - Laxatives, antibiotics, SSRI antidepressants, metformin, orlistat.

What to ask for and associated symptoms

Ask the patient:
- What is your normal bowel habit?
- Duration of symptoms?
- Frequency of defecation?
- Colour: black (melaena)?
- Blood?: infection (*Shigella, Salmonella, Campylobacter, Escherichia coli*), IBD, malignancy
- Mucus?: IBS, polyps, malignancy
- Floating stool?: malabsorption
- Smell?: malabsorption, infection, melaena
- Normal appetite and diet?

- With constipation?: think overflow
- Drug history (including 'over-the-counter' medicines)?
- Family history of bowel problems?: IBD, malignancy
- Foreign travel?
- Contacts with others with diarrhoea?

Associated symptoms?:
- Weight loss: malignancy, malabsorption
- Fever
- Pain
- Vomiting.

Investigations

Clinical examination

- Examination per rectum (PR).

Blood tests

- FBC: anaemia, iron deficiency

- U&Es, LFTs, TFTs (hyperthyroidism), CRP.

Other tests

Colonoscopy with biopsy
Stool samples:
- Microbiology:
  - Ova, cysts and parasites
  - Bacterial culture
  - Viral culture and PCR: norovirus, enterovirus
  - *C. difficile* toxin

- Faecal occult blood (FOB) (see above)
- Faecal elastase.

Imaging

- AXR
- Abdominal US

- Abdominal CT.

Management

- Treat cause
- Rehydration
- Absorptive agent: Kaolin

- Reduce GI motility
- Opiates: codeine, loperamide.

DYSPEPSIA

Description

- Indigestion, recurrent epigastric discomfort
- A non-specific group of symptoms relating to the upper GI tract including pain, nausea, vomiting, bloating, fullness, heartburn, anorexia, early satiety

Rome criteria: For use with functional dyspepsia:
- Epigastric pain
- >12 weeks/year
- Associated with nausea, epigastric bloating.

Causes

Local causes:
- Gastro-oesophageal reflux disease (GORD)
- Peptic ulcer disease
- Infection: *Helicobacter pylori*
- Inflammation
- Malignancy: oesophageal or gastric
- Hiatus hernia
- Zollinger–Ellison syndrome: rare
- Food intolerance

Systemic causes:
- Infection
- Alcohol

- Smoking
- Systemic sclerosis
- Drugs:
  - NSAIDs
  - Steroids
  - Calcium channel blockers
  - Bisphosphonates
  - Nitrates
  - Theophyllines
  - Anti-muscarinics
  - Anticoagulants.

Ask the patient:
- Smoking history?
- Alcohol intake?
- Drug history?: recent aspirin or NSAID use, anticoagulants, steroids

Associated symptoms?:
- Weight loss
- Chest pain
- Heart burn
- Cough
- Hiccups
- Fullness and bloating
- Nausea and vomiting
- Anorexia
- Pain or discomfort related to hunger, specific foods, time of the day

Red flags (alarm symptoms):
- If present, suggests an ↑ risk of malignancy.
  - Vomiting
  - Unintentional weight loss
  - GI bleeding
  - Dysphagia/odynophagia
  - Anaemia
  - Epigastric mass
  - Haematemesis/melaena
  - Jaundice
  - Previous gastric ulcer/gastric surgery
  - Age >55 years.

Investigations

Clinical examination

- Abdominal examination: feel for abdominal mass

- Troisier's sign: lymphadenopathy in left supraclavicular fossa (Virchow's node) in gastric cancer

Blood tests

- FBC: anaemia and signs of bleeding

Other tests

Microbiology:
- *H. pylori* testing

ECG:
- To rule out atypical presentation of chest pain and MI
Endoscopy

Imaging

- Barium meal
- Manometry

- 24 h oesophageal pH studies
- Abdominal US.

Management

Conservative

- Weight reduction
- Smoking cessation
- Alcohol cessation

- ↓ Chocolate/caffeine
- Stop NSAID use
- Elevate head of bed

Medical

- *Helicobacter pylori* eradication therapy if it is the causative agent
1. Acid suppression:
   - Proton pump inhibitor (PPI): lansoprazole, omeprazole
   - H$_2$ receptor antagonists: ranitidine

2. Antacids (neutralise acid): aluminium and magnesium hydroxide
3. Mucosal protection:
   - Prostaglandin analogue: misoprostol
   - Alginate: Gaviscon
   - Chelates: sucralfate.

GASTROINTESTINAL BLEEDING

Description

- Bleeding from the gastrointestinal tract
- **May be a medical emergency**

Classification:
- *Upper GI bleed*: bleed from the mouth to the 2nd part of the duodenum
- *Lower GI bleed*: bleed from the 2nd part of the duodenum to the rectum

Prognosis:
- Mortality 5–10%

Complications:
- Poor prognosis if:
  - Old age
  - Shock
  - Continued bleeding
  - Hb <8 g/dL
  - Comorbidity
  - Requires >5 units of blood transfused.

Causes

Oesophageal causes:
- Oesophagitis
- Oesophageal cancer
- Mallory–Weiss tear: 10% of upper GI bleeds
- Oesophageal varices: 10–20% of upper GI bleeds

Gastric causes:
- Gastric ulcer: 50% of major upper GI bleeds
- Gastritis: 20% of upper GI bleeds
- Gastric cancer: 5% of upper GI bleeds

Small bowel and colonic causes:
- Malignancy
- Diverticulitis.
- Ulcerative colitis (UC)
- Crohn's disease
- Gastroenteritis
- Ischaemic colitis
- Duodenal ulcer
- Polyps
- Angiodysplasia: rare

Rectal causes:
- Malignancy

Anal causes:
- Haemorrhoids
- Anal fissure
- Anal fistula

General causes:
- Infectious diarrhoea
- Drugs:
  - Antiplatelet agents: aspirin, clopidogrel, dipyridamole
  - Warfarin
  - Newer anticoagulants e.g. dabigatran
  - Steroids
  - NSAIDs
  - Alcohol

What to ask for and associated symptoms

Ask the patient:
- Where is the blood coming from and what colour is it?:
  - *Haematemesis*: vomiting blood. Either bright red (fresh blood) or 'coffee ground like' if altered by gastric acid. Indicates an upper GI bleed
  - *Melaena*: black, sticky, smelly, tar-like stool. Caused by haemoglobin that has been altered by digestion and oxidation as it passes through the gut, therefore usually caused by an upper GI bleed
  - *Haematochezia*: fresh blood per rectum. Likely to be caused by a lower GI bleed or from blood that has passed rapidly from the upper GI tract
- Is the blood mixed in with the stool or coating it?

- How much blood is there?
- Are you taking any new medication?
- Any history of binge drinking?: Mallory–Weiss tear
- History of liver disease?: oesophageal varices

Associated symptoms and signs?:
- Acute haemorrhage: hypotension and collapse
- Weight loss: cancer
- Ascites and signs of chronic liver disease: oesophageal varices
- ↑ Prothrombin time
- Epigastric pain
- Chest pain
- Signs and symptoms of anaemia

Investigations

Clinical examination

- Pulse and BP: look for postural drop

- Examination per rectum (PR).

Blood tests

- FBC: ↓ Hb
- U&Es: ↑ urea with normal creatinine due to high protein (from blood) absorbed in the gut
- LFTs: to assess for liver disease

- Amylase
- Clotting screen
- Group and save: if transfusion is necessary
- ABG.

Urine

- Monitor urine output.

Imaging

- Erect CXR: gas under diaphragm indicates bowel perforation

- Barium enema
- Angiography: lower GI bleeding.

Other tests

The Rockall score (see Table 14.2):
- Endoscopy once haemodynamically stable: for diagnosis and intervention: injection, thermal coagulation, laser, glue, endoclips. Emergency endoscopy in acute bleed.

- Used to determine prognosis in acute GI bleeds and risk of rebleed. A score of >8 indicates a high risk of death

Table 14.2 The Rockall score

Variable	Score 0	Score 1	Score 2	Score 3
Age (years)	<60	60–79	>80	
Shock (systolic BP)	No shock	Systolic BP >100, pulse >100	Systolic BP<100	
Comorbidity	No major comorbidity		Heart failure, IHD, other major comorbidity	Renal failure, liver failure, metastatic cancer
Diagnosis	Mallory–Weiss tear only	All other diagnoses	Upper GI malignancy	
Evidence of recent bleeding on endoscopy	None		Blood in upper GI tract, adherent clot, visible vessel	

Acute GI bleed:
- ABC approach
- Oxygen: high flow
- IV access
- IV fluid resuscitation and consider blood transfusion
- Correct clotting abnormalities
- Urgent endoscopy (once stable):
  - Identify site
  - Stop bleeding with adrenaline, sclerotherapy, variceal bands
  - Treatment specific for ulcers and varices (see Chapters 4 and 5)
- If risk of rebleeding: IV protein pump inhibitor infusion following therapy

Interventional radiology:
- To identify and embolise the vessel
Surgical:
- **Urgent surgical intervention if:** failure to stop bleeding
Medical:
- Antibiotics if septic
- Postoperatively *Helicobacter pylori* eradication if relevant, long-term medication for acid suppression
Smaller bleed:
- May resolve spontaneously
- Lifestyle advice:
  - Alcohol cessation
  - Avoid NSAIDs.

ABDOMINAL PAIN

- Pain in the abdomen
- Can be direct or referred
Types of pain:
- Colic:
  - Pain due to the obstruction of a hollow viscus surrounded by smooth muscle
  - The smooth muscle contracts in peristaltic waves to overcome the obstruction and these contractions cause pain
  - Patients typically curl their legs up and move around to↓ the pain
  - Biliary colic does not come in waves but is continuous.
- The acute abdomen:
  - Sudden, severe abdominal pain
  - Often a medical/surgical emergency
  - May present with peritonitis

- Peritonitis:
  - Inflammation of the peritoneum (abdominal cavity lining)
  - **A surgical emergency**
  - Pain is worse with movement
  - Typical presentation:
    - Lying still to try to ↓ the pain
    - Board-like rigidity of the abdomen
    - Guarding: reflex contraction of the abdominal wall
    - Absence of bowel signs
    - Shock: pale, sweaty, with sunken eyes, weak pulse and shallow breath
  - The peritoneum is innervated by somatic nerves so the pain is localised to the inflammatory site
  - Causes include bowel perforation.

Causes

General:
- Inflammation
- Colic

The acute abdomen:
- Ruptured organ
- Appendicitis
- Peritonitis
- Acute pancreatitis
- Mesenteric ischaemia
- Diabetic ketoacidosis.
- Acute pyelonephritis
- Spontaneous bacterial peritonitis (SBP)
- Ectopic pregnancy

Gastroenterological:
- Gastro-oesophageal reflux disease (GORD)
- Dyspepsia
- Peptic ulcer disease
- Gastroenteritis
- Diverticulitis
- Adhesions
- Malignancy: oesophagus, stomach, colon
- Appendicitis
- Mesenteric adenitis: inflammation of the mesenteric lymph nodes
- Meckel's diverticulitis
- Intestinal obstruction
- Strangulated hernia

Hepatobilary:
- Pancreatitis
- Cholecystitis
- Cholangitis: infection in the biliary tract
- Gallstones causing biliary colic, cholangitis or cholecystitis
- Biliary colic
- Hepatitis
- Malignancy: biliary tree

Pancreatic:
- Pancreatitis
- Pancreatic cancer

Vascular:
- Ruptured abdominal aortic aneurysm (AAA)
- Mesenteric embolus or thrombosis
- Ischemic colitis

Urological:
- Renal colic
- Urinary tract infection (UTI)
- Testicular torsion
- Urinary retention

Gynaecological:
- Ectopic pregnancy
- Ovarian cyst
- Pelvic inflammatory disease.

What to ask for and associated symptoms

Ask the patient:
- Obtain a precise description of the pain using 'SOCRATES':
  - **S**ite of pain
  - **O**nset: precipitators, sudden or insidious progression
  - **C**haracter
  - **R**adiation: does the pain radiate to any other site
  - **A**ssociated symptoms?:
    - Vomiting
    - Haematemesis
    - Change in bowel habit
    - Rectal bleeding
    - Dysuria with urinary frequency: UTI
    - Vaginal discharge: pelvic inflammatory disease
    - Fever
  - **T**iming
  - **E**xacerbating or relieving factors
  - **S**everity
- Past medical/family history?
- Menstrual history?

Investigations

Blood tests

- FBC, U&Es, LFTs, CRP
- Amylase: pancreatitis
- Blood glucose: diabetic ketoacidosis
- ABG.

Urine

- Urinalysis: UTI, diabetic ketoacidosis, ectopic pregnancy.

Imaging

- Erect CXR: gas under the diaphragm suggests a perforated organ
- AXR
- US
- CT

Other tests

- Endoscopy
- Laparoscopy.

Management

Treat cause
- The acute abdomen:
  - Resuscitate if necessary
  - Oxygen
- IV fluid resuscitation
- Urgent surgery if:
  - **ruptured organ**
  - **peritonitis**.

ABDOMINAL MASSES

Description

Best classified by position:
- Right upper quartile:
  - Liver mass/abscess
  - Enlarged kidney: tumour or polycystic disease
- Left upper quartile:
  - Splenomegaly (see below)
  - Colonic cancer
  - Pancreatic cancer
  - Pancreatic cysts/ pseudocyst
  - Diverticulitis
  - Enlarged kidney: tumour or polycystic disease
- Right lower quartile:
  - Appendicitis
  - Cancer of the large intestine
  - Caecal carcinoma
  - Ovarian cyst
  - Ectopic pregnancy
  - Lymphadenopathy
  - Crohn's disease
- Left lower quartile:
  - Diverticulitis
  - Sigmoid carcinoma
  - Ovarian cyst
  - Ectopic pregnancy
  - Splenomegaly
  - Lymphadenopathy.

Causes

Other causes:
- General:
  - Crohn's disease
  - Carcinoma: stomach or bowel
  - Tuberculous mass
  - Enlarged kidney or renal transplant
  - Undescended testicular tumour
  - Mucocele
  - Faeces
  - Intussusception
- Arising from pelvis:
  - Fibroids, uterine mass, bladder
- Umbilical:
  - Appendix mass or abscess
  - Umbilical or periumbilical hernia
  - Sister Mary Joseph's nodule: nodule protruding from umbilicus, a sign of metastasis of a cancer of the abdomen
  - Aortic aneurysm
  - Pancreatic pseudocyst.

What to ask for and associated symptoms

Ask the patient:
- How was it noticed?
- How long has it been there?
- Has it changed in size or shape?
- Any associated pain?
- Any change in menstrual cycle?
- Any other masses?

Associated symptoms?:
- Vomiting
- Change in bowel habit
- Change in micturition
- Rectal bleeding
- Weight loss and lethargy: malignancy
- Pain.

Investigations

Clinical examination

- Lymphadenopathy: supraclavicular, axillary and inguinal nodes.

Blood tests

- FBC, U&Es, LFTs, CRP
- Amylase: pancreatitis
- Blood glucose
- ABG.

Urine tests

- Urinalysis.

Imaging

- AXR: erect and supine
- US
- CT

Special tests

- Endoscopy
- Laparoscopy
- Laparotomy.

Management

- Depends on cause.

PRURITUS ANI

Description

- Itching of the anus
- Particularly if moist or soiled.

Causes

Local causes:
- Idiopathic (50%)
- Anal fissure
- Anal fistula
- Haemorrhoids
- Crohn's disease
- Neoplasia

- Faecal soiling: poor hygiene, diarrhoea, incontinence
- Anal discharge leading to moisture in the region: skin tags, polyps
- Infection: threadworms, *Candida*

Systemic causes:
- Anxiety
- Skin disease: psoriasis, eczema, *Candida*.

What to ask for and associated symptoms

Ask the patient:
- Is pruritus localised or general?
- Any skin conditions?
- Any change in bowel motions?
- Faecal soiling?
- Recent antibiotic therapy: causing *Candida*

- Any mood changes?

Associated symptoms?:
- Skin disease
- Skin tags
- Anal discharge
- Depression or anxiety.

Investigations

Clinical examination

- Examine the anus and rectum for skin tags, haemorrhoids, skin disease, discharge and soiling.

Blood tests

- FBC, U&Es, LFTs, ESR and CRP.

Other tests

- Urine analysis
- Stool culture

- Sellotape swab: for threadworms
- Biopsy: anal carcinoma.

Management

- Anal hygiene
- Anaesthetic cream

- Treat cause.

HEPATOMEGALY

Description

- Enlarged liver: mild, moderate or massive
- Liver edge may be smooth (hepatitis, congestive heart failure) or irregular (malignancy)

- May be tender if inflamed
- May be pulsatile in tricuspid regurgitation.

See Hepatology chapter 5.

Causes

- Commonly: malignancy, alcoholic liver disease, congestive cardiac failure

Infective causes:
- Hepatitis
- Epstein–Barr virus

Malignancy:
- Hepatocellular carcinoma (HCC)
- Myelofibrosis
- Myeloproliferative disorders
- Leukaemia
- Metastasis

Liver disease:
- Cirrhosis (in early phase)
- Fatty liver disease

Biliary tract disease:
- Primary biliary cirrhosis,
- Primary sclerosing cholangitis
- Extrahepatic obstruction

Metabolic disease:
- Wilson's disease
- Glycogen storage disease
- Haematochromatosis

Haematological:
- Sickle cell disease
- Thalassaemia

Cardiac:
- Congestive heart failure
- Constrictive pericarditis.

Ask the patient
- Travel history?
- Sexual history: hepatitis?

Associated symptoms and signs?:
- Weight loss: malignancy

- Splenomegaly (see Hepatosplenomegaly below)
- Fever: infective causes
- Jaundice: hepatitis, biliary tract obstruction, cholangitis
- Stigmata of chronic liver disease: spider naevi, gynaecomastia, ascites.

Blood tests

- FBC, U&Es, LFTs, ESR and CRP
- Clotting profile
- Blood culture
- Antibody screen: for autoimmune hepatitis, primary biliary cirrhosis and primary sclerosing cholangitis

- Hepatitis serology
- Alpha feto-protein: ↑ in HCC
- Iron studies: haemochromatosis.

Imaging

- US

- CT

Other tests

- ERCP and MRCP: ductal abnormalities
- Bone marrow aspiration: haematological malignancies

- Liver biopsy.

- Treat cause.

SPLENOMEGALY

Description

- Enlarged spleen
- Normally located under the 9th, 10th and 11th ribs on the left side in Traube's space
- Palpable when about 3 times its original size
- Splenomegaly can be classified into massive, moderate and mild

Causes of massive splenomegaly:
- Gaucher's disease (lysosomal storage disease)
- Malaria
- Myelofibrosis
- Visceral leishmaniasis (kala-azar)
- Chronic myeloid lymphoma (CML)
- Polycythaemia rubra vera
- Thalassaemia.

Causes

Infective causes:
- Bacterial: tuberculosis, typhoid, syphilis
- Viral: Epstein–Barr virus (EBV), cytomegalovirus (CMV), hepatitis
- Protozoal: malaria

Inflammation:
- SLE, rheumatoid arthritis, amyloid, sarcoid

Haematological:
- Leukaemia, lymphoma, myelofibrosis, polycythaemia rubra vera, thalassaemia, sickle cell disease, hereditary spherocytosis, pernicious or iron deficiency anaemia

Hepatic:
- Portal hypertension

Metabolic disease:
- Gaucher's disease

Neoplastic:
- Primary tumours
- Metastases.

Ask the patient:
- Foreign travel?
- Family history?

Associated symptoms?:
- Fever: infective and inflammatory causes, malignancy
- Anaemia: neoplastic or haematological disease

- Lymphadenopathy: glandular fever (EBV), haematological malignancies
- Weight loss: malignancy
- Night sweats: lymphoma, TB
- Hepatomegaly (see Hepatosplenomegaly below)
- Arthritis: inflammatory causes.

Clinical examination

- Distinguish mass as a spleen rather than a kidney (see Enlarged kidney below).

Blood tests

- FBC, U&Es, LFTs
- ESR
- Calcium
- Serum angiotensin converting enzyme (ACE): sarcoid
- Blood film: malaria

- Culture: infection
- Antibody screen: SLE, RA
- Monospot test: EBV
- Viral serology.

Imaging

- CXR: bilateral hilar lymphadenopathy suggests lymphoma, sarcoid or TB

- US
- CT.

Other tests

Bone marrow aspirate:
- Haematological malignancies.

Management

- Depends on cause.

HEPATOSPLENOMEGALY

Description

- Enlarged liver and spleen.

Causes

Infective causes:
- Epstein–Barr virus (EBV)
- Cytomegalovirus (CMV)
- Hepatitis
Inflammation:
- Amyloid

Haematological:
- Leukaemia
- Lymphoma
- Myelofibrosis
- Thalassaemia
- Sickle cell disease
Chronic liver disease:
- Causing portal hypertension.

What to ask for and associated symptoms

Associated symptoms?:
- Fever

- Anaemia: blood disease.

Investigations

As above.

Management

- Depends on cause.

HYPOSPLENISM/ASPLENISM

Description

- Hyposplenism: small spleen

- Asplenism: no spleen.

Causes

Asplenism:
- Splenectomy: due to:
  - trauma
  - hypersplenism

Hyposplenism:
- Sickle cell: from splenic infarction
- Coeliac disease.

Ask the patient:
- Previous operations/splenectomy?

Associated signs and symptoms?:
- Anaemia
- Hepatomegaly.

Investigations

Clinical examination

- Scar if spleen has been removed.

Blood tests

- FBC, U&Es, LFTs
- Clotting profile
- Blood film: Howell–Jolly bodies: DNA fragments seen in RBC in hyposplenism (see p. 613).

- Cultures
- Immunoglobulin screen.

Imaging

- AXR
- Abdominal US

- Abdominal CT.

Other tests

- Bone marrow aspirate.

Management

- Depends on cause
- Particularly vulnerable to encapsulated microorganisms

- Need:
  - vaccinations for pneumococcus, meningococcus, *Haemophilus influenzae b*
  - antibiotic cover for life: penicillin V.

NEUROLOGICAL

HEADACHE

Description

Primary:
- Headache is the primary symptom, no underlying structural lesion, e.g. tension headaches or migraine

Secondary:
- Headache is the symptom of the primary cause, e.g. brain tumour.

Causes

Acute single episode:
- Sinusitis: tender face, post nasal drip
- Infection: meningitis/encephalitis. Signs of meningism include: irritability, neck stiffness, photophobia, positive Kernig's sign (knee extension is painful/worsens headache)
- Head injury
- Acute closure glaucoma

Sudden onset:
- Subarachnoid haemorrhage (SAH): may cause signs of meningism from meningeal irritation
- Subdural haematoma

Acute recurrent attacks:
- Migraine: auras, vomiting, sensitivity to light
- Cluster headaches: recurring, severe unilateral eye pain, often recurring at the same time of day. Associated with autonomic symptoms: runny and blocked nose, lacrimation

- Glaucoma: red eyes, haloes, fixed dilated oval pupil, low visual acuity, worse in the early evening
- Analgesic-dependent headache: overuse of mild opiates. Stop analgesic and give amitriptyline

Progressive: investigate all headaches of this nature:
- ↑ Intracranial pressure (ICP): worse in the morning, may wake patient at night associated with vomiting, dizziness and visual disturbance
- Giant cell arteritis: jaw claudication, tender scalp in the elderly, unilateral headache. Threat to vision if untreated

Chronic headache:
- Tension headache: tight 'vice-like band around the head', low mood, stress, commoner towards the end of the day
- Chronically ↑ intracranial pressure (ICP)
- Drugs: substance withdrawal, glyceryl trinitrate, nifedipine, dipyridamole.

What to ask for and associated symptoms

Ask the patient:
- Obtain a precise description of the pain using 'SOCRATES':
  - **S**ite of pain
  - **O**nset: precipitators, sudden or insidious progression
  - **C**haracter
  - **R**adiation: does the pain radiate to any other site
  - **A**ssociated symptoms?
    - Loss of consciousness: SAH, ↑ ICP
    - Localising signs
    - Papilloedema: tumour, benign intracranial hypertension, malignant hypertension
  - Neck stiffness: meningism
  - Visual disturbances: migraine, glaucoma
  - Drowsiness
  - Vomiting
  - Fever and rash: meningitis
  - **T**iming
  - **E**xacerbating or relieving factors
  - **S**everity
- Any family history
- Pregnancy (pre-eclampsia).

Investigations

Clinical examination

- Fundoscopy: look for evidence of glaucoma, papilloedema (=swelling of the optic disc due to raised intracranial pressure)
- Tenderness of superficial temporal artery with jaw tenderness: giant cell arteritis
- Neurological examination.

Blood tests

- FBC, U&Es, CRP
- ESR: high in temporal arteritis, infection, malignancy
- Culture.

Imaging

If diagnosis unclear:
- CT or MRI head: space occupying lesions.

Other tests

- Intraocular pressure measurements: glaucoma
- Lumbar puncture for CSF analysis and an opening pressure: useful for meningitis, subarachnoid haemorrhage (xanthochromia) and benign/idiopathic intracranial hypertension (opening pressure is diagnostic and therapeutic). Contraindicated if ↑ ICP
- Temporal artery biopsy: giant cell arteritis
- Angiography: for vascular malformations.

Management

- Treat cause
- Cluster headache: high flow O_2 and sumatriptan. Prophylaxis, steroids, verapamil
- Tension headache: relaxation, amitriptyline, analgesics
- Migraine: early antiemetic and paracetamol, progressing to triptans
- SAH: after angiography, endovascular coiling of aneurysm or clipping
- Giant cell arteritis: steroids immediately.

CONFUSION

Description

- Disordered and disorientated thinking
- May be chronic (e.g. dementia) or acute (delirium)
- May be permanent (e.g. dementia) or temporary due to a reversible cause (e.g. vitamin B_{12} deficiency)
- Common in the elderly

Delirium:
- Confusion with an impairment in consciousness
- Often associated with infection

Dementia:
- Progressive disturbance of multiple higher cortical functions including memory, orientation and language without loss of consciousness
- A symptom, not a diagnosis.

Causes

Causes **DDELIRIUMM**:

- **D**rugs or withdrawal: analgesia, antiemetics, steroids. Consider alcohol withdrawal if occurring a few days after hospital admission
- **D**ementia: see Neurology section
- **E**lectrolyte imbalance: ↑calcium, urea, ↓ sodium
- **L**ow oxygen: cardiac failure, respiratory problems
- **I**nfection
- **R**educed organ function: renal, liver or respiratory failure
- **I**ntracranial pathology: stroke, epilepsy, tumour
- **U**rinary retention
- **M**etabolic causes: hyperglycaemia, hypoglycaemia, thyroid disorders, thiamine and B_{12} deficiency
- **M**alignancy: leads to confusion due to hyperviscosity, medications, ↑ calcium, mass effect in the brain, organ failure

Additional causes of confusion:

- Psychiatric causes
- Up to 30% of surgery complicated by delirium.

What to ask for and associated symptoms

Ask the patient (or their relatives):

- How long has it been going on for?
- Any impaired consciousness?
- Any precipitating factors?
- Recent head injury?
- Past medical history?
- Drug use (including alcohol)?

Associated symptoms?:

- Weakness: stroke
- Sensory deficit: thiamine deficiency, B_{12} deficiency
- Dysuria: UTI
- Fever: infection
- Weight loss: malignancy

Risk factor assessment (from NICE guidelines on delirium):

- On presentation to hospital a person is at risk of delirium if they are:
  - >65 years
  - Have dementia or cognitive impairment
  - Current hip fracture
  - Severe illness.

Investigations

Clinical examination

- Glasgow coma scale (GCS) score: check for any impairment in consciousness
- Neurological examination
- Oxygen saturations.

Blood tests

- FBC, U&Es, LFTs, TFTs and CRP
- ABG
- Toxicology screen
- Blood glucose: hyper- or hypoglycaemia.

Urine

- Dipstick: UTI
- Microscopy and culture

Imaging

- CT of head if intracranial pathology is suspected

Other tests

Sputum:

- Microscopy and culture
- EEG.

Management

- Depends on cause
- Correct reversible causes
- Small doses of sedative drugs: haloperidol, lorazepam
- Prognosis is worse if it occurs with pre-existing dementia.

Prevention

NICE have guidance on preventing delirium in hospital, including:

- ↓ distress
- Calm environment, especially at night
- Prevention of dehydration or constipation by ensuring good fluid status
- Good lighting and signage (clocks or calendars)
- Encouraging mobilisation or exercise
- Good nutrition
- Review multiple medications.

VERTIGO AND DIZZINESS

Description

Vertigo:
- Illusion of movement
- Usually the illusion of rotational movement ('the room is spinning'), worse with movement
- Often with vomiting, sweating or pallor
- Due to pathology of the inner ear labyrinth or the 8th cranial nerve and its connections
- Distinct symptom from dizziness

Dizziness:
- An imprecise term to describe the feeling of spatial disorientation and instability
- The term is often used by patients to describe their perception of vertigo, light-headedness, faintness, syncope or disequilibrium.

Causes

Vertigo:
- Disorders of the ear labyrinth:
  - Labyrinthitis
  - Otitis media
  - Meniere's disease: vertigo, hearing loss, tinnitus
  - Benign paroxysmal positional vertigo (BPPV): crystals in the inner ear are dislodged and move to the semicircular canal leading to positional vertigo
  - Otic barotraumas: damage to the ear due to differences in pressure in the middle and outer ear. Caused by diving or flying
- 8th cranial nerve:
  - Acoustic neuroma: tumour of the 8th cranial nerve leading to loss of consciousness, seizures, facial weakness, dysphagia, diplopia
  - Ototoxic drugs, e.g. aminoglycosides (gentamicin)
  - Infection: herpes zoster virus (Ramsey Hunt syndrome)
- Brainstem disease:
  - Stroke
  - Migraine
  - Tumour
  - Infection: encephalitis
  - Multiple sclerosis
- Dizziness:
  - Anaemia
  - Hypoglycaemia
  - Anxiety
  - Hypoventilation
  - Postural hypotension
  - Pyrexia.

What to ask for and associated symptoms

Ask the patient:
- How long has it been going on for?
- Sudden or gradual onset?
- Constant or recurrent attacks?
- Drug history?: aminoglycosides
- Any relation to head movement?: BPPV
- Recent ear surgery?
- Recent diving or flying?

Associated symptoms?:
- Nausea
- Vomiting
- Sweating
- Ear symptoms: discharge, pain, tinnitus, deafness
- Neurological symptoms: facial weakness, dysarthria, dysphagia, seizures, loss of consciousness
- Aura: suggests a peripheral lesion.

Investigations

Clinical examination

- Lying and standing blood pressure: postural hypotension
- Hearing assessment: Rinne's and Weber's tests, audiometry
- Hallpike manoeuvre: to assess labyrinth pathway and BPPV. The patient quickly lies down with the head tilted to one side; in BPPV there is nystagmus after a brief latent period
- Caloric tests: cold then warm water in the auditory canal normally causes contralateral and then ipsilateral nystagmus. Reflex is lost with 8th cranial nerve pathology.

Blood tests

- FBC, ESR.

Imaging

- CT or MRI of the head.

Other tests

- ECG: arrhythmias.

Management

- Depends on cause

BPPV:
- The Epley manoeuvre: movement of the head repositions the ear crystals from the semicircular canal so that they do not cause symptoms.

LOSS OF VISION

Description

- Loss of vision unilateral or bilateral.

Causes

Sudden visual loss:
- Stroke: homonymous hemianopia
- Papilloedema
- Giant cell arteritis: pain, jaw claudication, scalp tenderness
- Amaurosis fugax: painless fleeting loss of vision to one eye like a 'curtain drawn' across the visual field
- Central retinal vein or artery occlusion
- Optic neuritis
- Retinal detachment: symptoms include sudden ↑ of floaters and flashes of light. It is an emergency and requires urgent ophthalmology referral

- Tumour, e.g. pituitary tumour (bitemporal hemianopia)
- Drugs: quinine, methanol
Gradual visual loss:
- Diabetic retinopathy
- Glaucoma: peripheral field loss
- Cataract
- Age-related macular degeneration: central field loss
Visual disturbance:
- Migraine
- Retinal detachment
- Vitreous haemorrhage

What to ask for and associated symptoms

Ask the patient:
- Did it occur suddenly or gradually?
- Any precipitating symptoms or factors?
- Any pain?
- Past medical history?: cardiovascular risk factors
- Drug history?

Associated symptoms?:
- Red eye
- Pain
- Floaters: small deposits in the vitreous humour that appear like black spots moving across the visual field
- Scalp tenderness and jaw claudication: giant cell arteritis.

Investigations

Clinical examination

- Eye examination including fundoscopy.

Blood tests

- ESR

- Blood glucose.

Imaging

- CT or MRI.

Other tests

- Intraocular pressure measurements

- Temporal artery biopsy.

Management

- Ophthalmology referral

- If high index of suspicion for giant cell arteritis, start steroids immediately.

BLACKOUTS

Description

- Transient loss of consciousness
- Causes include: neurological, cardiovascular or endocrinological causes

Syncope:
- Faint from an interruption in cerebral perfusion

- Recovery is spontaneous normally without long lasting effects
- Vasovagal syncope is the commonest cause (simple fainting).

Causes

Neurological:
- Migraine: aura
- Seizure: associated with tongue biting, urinary and faecal incontinence
- TIA (rare presentation)
- Subarachnoid haemorrhage: rare presentation
- Intracranial mass lesion

Cardiovascular:
- Vasovagal syncope: pallor, feel hot, dizzy and sick just before passing out. Can be caused by fear, emotion, prolonged standing

- Arrhythmias: sick sinus syndrome, tachycardias
- Postural hypotension: lying/standing BP difference >20 mmHg. Caused by hypovolaemia, autonomic neuropathy and drugs

Endocrinological:
- Hypoglycaema

Others:
- Hypoxia
- Drugs: antihypertensives, diuretics, opiates.

What to ask for and associated symptoms

Ask the patient or witness:
- Presyncope:
  - Warning signs?
  - Aura?
  - Recent head movement: consider vertebrobasilar insufficiency
- Attack:
  - Were there any witnesses?
  - Circumstances of event?
  - Loss of consciousness?
  - Injured by fall?
  - Incontinence or tongue biting: epilepsy.

Ask the patient:
- Postsyncope
  - What do they remember? What is the first thing recalled on coming round: fits tend to be confused
  - Speed of recovery
  - Muscle pain afterwards?: suggest tonic/clonic seizure
- General questions:
  - Any previous episodes?
  - Cardiac risk factors?
  - History of head trauma?

Associated symptoms?:
- Nausea, weakness, change in vision: vasovagal syncope
- Palpitations.

Investigations

Clinical examination

- Lying and standing blood pressure: postural hypotension

- Cardiovascular and neurological examination.

Blood tests

- FBC, U&ES, LFTs, TFTs
- Blood glucose: hypoglycaemia

- Toxicology screen
- ABG.

Urine

- Urinalysis: ketones in diabetic ketoacidosis.

Imaging

- CXR: pulmonary oedema, infection
- Echocardiogram: in adults, especially if they have an abnormal ECG

- CTPA: for suspected pulmonary embolism
- MRI of the head: to exclude structural lesions in seizures.

Other tests

- ECG: especially in young people, may need 24 h or longer recording

- EEG: little use in the elderly

Management

- Treat cause

Vasovagal:
- Reassurance
- Food and fluid intake
- Improve sympathetic nervous system and prevent pooling: calf/hand pumping
- Sympathomimetics.

COMA

Description

- Unarousable unconsciousness
- Equates to a GCS <8

Due to impaired function of either or both of:
- Reticular activating system (RAS): responsible for arousal and located within the brainstem
- Both cerebral hemispheres

Brainstem reflexes:
- The brainstem connects the brain to the spinal cord
- Brainstem death occurs when the brainstem no longer functions. Certification needs to be made by two senior doctors independently
- The function of the brainstem is assessed by the brainstem reflexes, including:
  - Gag reflex
  - Pupillary light reflex
  - Corneal reflex
  - Vestibulo-ocular reflex.

Causes

Neurological causes:
- Stroke
- Epilepsy
- Tumour
- Infection: meningitis, encephalitis
- Trauma

Metabolic causes:
- Glucose: ↑ or ↓
- Diabetic coma
- Hypoxia
- Hypovolaemia
- Uraemia
- Hypothermia
- Hepatic encephalopathy
- Hypothyroidism

Organ failure:
- Cardiac failure
- Respiratory failure
- Renal failure
- Liver failure

Trauma:
- Head injury, vascular event

Drugs:
- Opiates
- Sedatives
- Alcohol

Toxins:
- Carbon monoxide.

What to ask for and associated symptoms

Ask relatives and witnesses:
- Determine history surrounding event including symptoms beforehand
- Past medical history: including diabetes, epilepsy, cardiovascular risk factors, drug abuse
- Drug or alcohol abuse

Associated symptoms?:
- Fever
- Prior headache: trauma, subarachnoid haemorrhage, tumour
- Injuries: trauma.

Investigations

Clinical examination

- Glasgow Coma Scale (GCS) score (see Chapter 1)
- Neurological examination
- Eyes:
  - Pinpoint pupils: opiate overdose
  - Small pupils: brainstem lesions
  - Dilated pupils: amphetamines, hypoglycaemia, brainstem death, cocaine

- Fundoscopy: to look for ↑ intracranial pressure
- Vestibulo-ocular reflex (by the doll's head manoeuvre in comatose patients): if pupils are fixed on the same point in space when the head is moved quickly then the brainstem from 3rd to 7th nucleus is intact

Blood tests

- FBC, U&Es, LFTs, TFTs, CRP
- Glucose
- Toxicology screen

- ABG
- Cultures.

Investigations continued

Urine

- Urinalysis: ketones in diabetic ketoacidosis
- Toxicology screen
- Microscopy and culture.

Imaging

- CXR: pulmonary oedema, infection
- CT or MRI of the head
- Echocardiogram: cardiac causes

Other tests

- ECG
- EEG: for epilepsy or encephalopathy.
- Lumbar puncture: contraindicated in comatose patients without imaging first.

Management

- Resuscitation
- ABC approach (see Chapter 1).

GAIT DISORDERS

Description

- Disorders in walking
- Can be from a structural or neurological cause.

Causes

Summary of types of gait and their causes (see Table 14.3).

Table 14.3 Types of gait and their causes

Type of gait	Gait description	Cause
Neurological causes		
Cerebellar ataxia	Unsteady; wide based gait: feet wide apart	Cerebellar pathology
Sensory ataxia	Stomping Romberg's test +ve	Dorsal column pathology (sensory perception)
Apraxic gait	Like 'walking on ice', hesitant steps Difficulty initiating walking	Frontal lobe disease
Myopathic gait	Waddling gait due to proximal leg weakness	Duchenne's dystrophy
Spastic gait	Scissor gait Thighs strongly adducted so legs cross as the patient walks	Spastic paraparesis or bilateral hemiparesis, cerebral palsy
Unilateral Foot drop	High step Weakness of tibial and peroneal muscles	Peroneal nerve palsy
Parkinsonian gait	Festinant gait (small, shuffling, accelerating steps, as if trying to catch up with one's self) Slow starting, stopping and turning	Parkinson's disease
Hemiparetic (one sided weakness) gait	Fixed extension of a lower limb causing the leg to swing round when walking May also have ipsilateral fixed flexion of the upper limb	After stroke Cerebral palsy
Structural causes		
Antalgic gait:	Limping from walking whilst in pain	Pain
Trendelenburg gait	Waddling with pelvis tilted to the normal side, and the trunk tilted to the weak side to compensate for this Trendelenberg test +ve	Weak hip abductors or pain

Ask the patient:
- Change in gait?
- How long has it been going on for?
- Any precipitating event?
- Head or limb trauma?
- Worse in the dark: sensory ataxia (due to loss of visual cues)

Associated symptoms?:
- Pain
- Any sensory loss: sensory ataxia.

Clinical examination

- Full motor and sensory neurological examination
- Assessment of walk (see Figure 14.1).

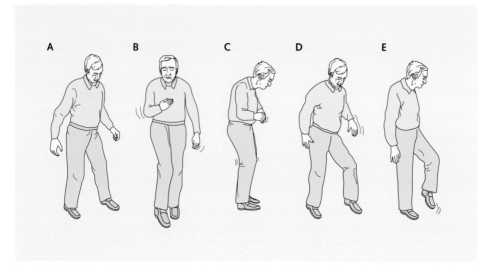

Fig. 14.1 Disorders of gait. (A) Cerebellar ataxia, (B) hemiparetic, (C) parkinsonian, (D) sensory ataxia, and (E) unilateral footdrop.

Romberg's test:
- A test of proprioception. The patient stands with feet together and eyes closed. A positive result is any falling or swaying and suggests any ataxia is sensory in nature, e.g. due to peripheral neuropathies or conditions affecting the dorsal columns of the spinal cord.

Trendelenburg test:
- The patient stands on one leg at a time. The pelvis should not tilt; if it does tilt, the side that tilts is normal ('the sound side sags'). A positive test suggests pain in the hip or weak abductor muscles.

Imaging

- X-ray: hip, knees, spine
- CT or MRI of the head: if central nervous system cause suspected.

Other tests

- EMG and nerve conduction studies: for myopathic gait, foot drop or sensory ataxia.

- Depends on cause.

RENAL DISORDERS

ENLARGED KIDNEY

Description

- Enlargement of the kidney

For the differences between an enlarged spleen and enlarged left kidney, see Clinical examination pages, the Gastrointestinal system p. 650.

Causes

Unilateral enlarged kidney:
- Solitary cyst or tumour
- Infection: TB, abscess
- Hydronephrosis: build up of urine in the renal pelvis and calyces causing distension normally due to obstruction of urine outflow

Bilateral:
- Polycystic kidney disease
- Hydronephrosis.

What to ask for and associated symptoms

Ask the patient:
- Change in urinary frequency?: hydronephrosis
- History of TB?
- Family history?: adult polycystic kidney disease

Associated symptoms?:
- Haematuria
- Dysuria
- Loin pain
- Anaemia
- Weight loss: malignancy.

Investigations

Clinical examination

- Abdominal examination

- Blood pressure.

Blood and urine tests

- FBC, U&Es, CRP, ESR

Urinalysis.

Imaging

- CXR
- X-ray of kidneys, ureters, bladder (KUB)
- US KUB

- IV urogram (IVU)
- MRI.

Other tests

- Renal biopsy.

Management

- Depends on cause.

Description

- Blood in the urine
- >2 red blood cells (RBCs) per high power field
- Dipstick-positive haematuria must be sent for microscopy to determine presence of RBCs
- Suggests renal tract disease
- 35% with frank haematuria have urological malignancy

- Haematuria characterises nephritic from nephrotic syndrome, see nephrotic syndrome, in chapter 7

Causes of urine discoloration:
- These can be confused with haematuria: eating beetroot, haemoglobinuria, myglobinuria, porphyria, drugs, e.g. rifampicin (orange urine), nitrofurantoin (orange/brown urine)

Causes

BURPS:
- **B**ladder:
  - Calculi
  - Tumour
  - Trauma
  - Infection
  - Cystitis
- **U**rethra and ureters:
  - Calculi
  - Tumour
  - Trauma
- **R**enal:
  - Nephritic disease
  - Tumour
  - Trauma

- Infection
- Cystic disease
- Interstitial nephritis
- **P**rostate:
  - Carcinoma
  - Prostatitis
  - TB
- **S**ystemic causes:
  - Bleeding disorders
  - Leukaemia
  - Anticoagulants
  - Haemoglobinopathies
  - Sickle cell disease
  - Endocarditis
  - Drugs: NSAIDs, antibiotics in high dose.

What to ask for and associated symptoms

Ask the patient:
- Systemically well or unwell?
- Clarify origin of the blood (urethra, rectum or vagina)?
- Is the urine blood stained from the start, middle, end or throughout the urine stream?
- Is it definitely blood?: rule out false positives
- If there any pain? Is it loin pain or pain on passing urine?: distinguishes between aetiologies
- History of trauma?
- Medical history?: diabetes, kidney stones, infection including TB, high blood pressure
- Drug history? NSAIDs, anticoagulants

Associated symptoms?:
- Weight loss: malignancy
- Infection: dysuria, frequency
- Pain: painless haematuria is more sinister.

Painful haematuria	Painless haematuria
UTI	Cancer of urinary tract
Kidney stones	Infection
	Nephritic syndrome

Investigations

Blood tests

- FBC, U&Es, CRP

- Clotting screen: for bleeding disorders.

Urine

- Dipstick
- Microscopy and culture

- Early morning samples: for TB.

Imaging

- X-ray of kidneys, ureters, bladder (KUB)
- IV urogram

- US or CT: for soft tissue

Other tests

- Cytoscopy: bladder lesions
- Angiography: exclude arterio-venous (AV) malformations.

- Renal biopsy: if cause remains unexplained.

Management

- Treat cause

- Refer to a urologist.

PROTEINURIA

Description

- Protein in the urine
- May be due to a renal or non-renal cause; significant proteinuria is usually from a renal cause
- Occurs in nephrotic syndrome and glomerular disease

Protein levels:
- Normal: 40–80 mg/day

- Proteinuria: >150 mg/day
- Glomerular disease: >2 g/day
- Nephrotic syndrome >3.5 g/day
- Microalbuminuria: ↑albumin found in the urine in the range of 30–300 mg/day. It is one of the earliest evidence of diabetic glomerular disease.

Causes

TO BUG:
- **T**ubular:
  - Acute tubular necrosis (ATN)
  - Renal transplant
  - Chronic nephritis
  - Heavy metal poisoning
- **O**verflow:
  - Myeloma: Bence Jones protein
  - Acute pancreatitis: amylase

- **B**enign:
  - Pregnancy
  - Exercise
  - Acute illness: infection
  - Recent intercourse (men)
- **U**rinary tract infection (UTI)
- **G**lomerular:
  - Glomerulonephritis: see Chapter 7, causes include lupus and diabetes.

What to ask for and associated symptoms

Ask the patient:
- Systemically well or unwell?
- Appearance of urine?
- Volume of urine?
- Other urinary symptoms?
- Pain?

- Medical history?: recent urine infection

Associated symptoms?:
- Nephrotic syndrome: oedema
- Nephritic syndrome: haematuria, hypertension, oedema, oliguria and symptoms of uraemia.

Investigations

Blood tests

- FBC, U&Es, CRP

- Glucose: diabetes mellitus.

Urine

- Urinary Bence Jones proteins (myeloma)
- Microscopy, especially for casts
- Culture

To measure proteinuria:
- Dipstick gives rapid, crude measure
- Protein: creatinine ratio from spot urine
- 24 h urine collection.

Imaging

- X-ray of kidneys, ureters, bladder (KUB)
- IV urogram
- Renal US.

Management

- Treat cause.

POLYURIA

Description

- Increased urine output
- >3.5 L/24 h

Pathogenesis:
- Antidiuretic hormone (ADH) is a hormone produced in the brain that ↑ the amount of water reabsorbed in the distal convoluted tubules and collecting tubules of the kidney
- The greater the amount of ADH produced, the more water is reabsorbed and less urine is produced.

Causes

Too much fluid intake:
- Polydipsia: drinking a lot

Diuresis:
- Hyperglycaemia.
- Hypercalcaemia
- Hyperurea
- Drugs: diuretics, mannitol

Diabetes:
- Diabetes insipidus: cranial or nephrogenic (see endocrinology section)
- Diabetes mellitus: causes osmotic diuresis

Renal failure:
- Acute or chronic.

What to ask for and associated symptoms

Ask the patient
- Duration of polyuria?
- True polyuria or ↑ frequency: infection
- Drug history?: diuretics, renal disease
- Family history?: diabetes, renal disease

Associated symptoms?:
- Polydipsia
- Thirst
- Weight loss: diabetes, malignancy (hypercalcaemia).

Investigations

Water homeostasis:
- Weigh patient
- Strict fluid balance monitoring

Blood tests

- FBC, U&Es (calcium, daily sodium), calcium, glucose, LFTs, osmolarity.

Urine

- Dipstick: glucose
- Microscopy and culture

- Osmolarity
- 24 h urine collection: to quantify amount

Imaging

- CT or MRI of head

Other tests

- Renal biopsy.

Endocrine tests:
- Water deprivation test with desmopressin (ADH analogue): test confirms DI and can distinguish between cranial/nephrotic cause (see Chapter 9).

Management

- Treat cause.

OLIGURIA

Description

- Reduced urine output: <300 ml/24 h

Anuria:
- No urine produced
- Likely indicates obstruction of bladder outflow or of both the ureters.

Causes

Prerenal causes

- Dehydration
- Hypotension

- Hypovolaemia
- Cardiac failure.

Renal causes

- Acute renal failure
- Acute glomerulonephritis

- Acute interstitial nephrosis
- Acute tubular nephrosis.

Postrenal causes

- Obstruction of ureters or bladder outflow: stones, tumours, blocked catheter.

Ask the patient:
- Duration of oliguria?
- If catheterised, is it blocked?
- Past medical history? stones, renal disease

Associated symptoms?:
- Thirst.

Investigations

- Assess fluid status
- Blood pressure.

Blood tests

- FBC, U&Es, calcium, bicarbonate, phosphate, magnesium, urate, glucose.

Urine

- Mid stream urine microscopy
- 24 h urine collection

- Sodium and osmolarity.

Imaging

- Renal tract US: for obstruction

- Dimercaptosuccinic acid (DMSA) scan: radionuclide scan to test renal function, including scarring and damage, which is often used for children who have had a UTI.

Other tests

- Cystoscopy: for obstruction

Management

- Treat cause.

GENERAL PRESENTING COMPLAINTS

FEVER

Description

- Temperature >37.5°C
- Pyrexia of unknown origin (PUO): persistent unexplained fever for >3 weeks
- In 25% of cases the cause is never discovered

Febrile neutropenia:
- Fever in a neutropenic patient
- Neutrophils: $<1 \times 10^9$
- Complication of chemotherapy.
See also The septic patient in Chapter 11.

Causes

Infective causes: 25%:
- Bacterial: tuberculosis (TB), abscess, subacute bacterial endocarditis, typhoid
- Viral: HIV, cytomegalovirus (CMV), Epstein–Barr virus (EBV), influenza, dengue fever
- Fungal: *Candida*, aspergillosis
- Protozoal: malaria, toxoplasmosis
Malignancy: 20%:
- Lymphoma
- Leukaemia

Connective tissue disease: 20%:
- Lupus (SLE)
- Rheumatoid arthritis
- Temporal arteritis
Others:
- Disease of the CNS leading to poor thermoregulation
- Myocardial infarction
- Sarcoid
- Crohn's disease.

What to ask for and associated symptoms

Ask the patient:
- Foreign travel
- Contact with other people with fever
- Contact with animals
- Sexual history
- Bites
- Immunisation history
- Drug history

Associated signs and symptoms?:
- Weight loss
- Rash
- Diarrhoea
- Sweating
- Pruritus
- Lumps
- Lymphadenopathy: lymphoma.

Investigations

See investigations for 'The Septic patient, Chapter 11'.

Management

- Depends on cause
- Supportive
- Paracetamol
- Fluids
- Antibiotics if relevant, especially in febrile neutropenia.

WEIGHT LOSS

Description

- Due to ↓ energy intake or ↑ energy output
- Important to exclude malignancy.

Causes

With normal appetite:
- Malabsorption
- Endocrine: hyperthyroidism, diabetes

With anorexia:
- *Psychological*: anorexia nervosa, bulimia, depression, schizophrenia, neglect
- *Malignancy*: produces high metabolic rate or leads to anorexia

- *Endocrine*: phaeochromocytoma, hypopituitarism, diabetes, adrenal insufficiency
- *Infection*: HIV, TB, helminth infection
- *Chronic inflammation*: connective tissue disease
- *GI*: dysphagia, peptic ulcer disease, inflammatory bowel disease (IBD)
- *Neurological*: motor neuron disease, myopathies, dementia
- *Organ failure*: cardiac, renal or respiratory.

What to ask for and associated symptoms

Ask the patient:
- What is your normal diet and appetite?
- Normal levels of physical activity?
- Perception of body image?: eating disorders
- Change in bowel habit? GI causes
- Stool changes?: floating, smelly stool: steatorrhoea in malabsorption
- Difficulty swallowing?: dysphagia

- Past medical or family history?
- Drug and alcohol history?

Associated symptoms?:
- Fevers
- Sweats
- Malaise: feeling generally unwell
- Rash.

Investigations

Blood tests

- FBC, U&Es, LFTs, TFTs, calcium (malignancy), glucose, CRP
- Cultures.

Urine

- Dipstick
- Urinary 24 h collection for catecholamines (phaeochromocytoma).

Imaging

- CXR: TB, malignancy
- AXR.

Other tests

- Endoscopy
- HIV antibodies
- Short Synacthen test: Addison's disease (see Chapter 9).

Management

- Depends on cause.

WEIGHT GAIN

Description

- Increase in weight.

Causes

↑ In fluid:
- Oedema
- Renal or cardiac failure
- Lymphatic obstruction

↑ In fat:
- Endocrine causes: hypothyroidism, Cushing's disease, polycystic ovary syndrome

- Overeating

↑ In muscle:
- ↑ Androgenic steroids
- Growth hormone: acromegaly

Other:
- Pregnancy
- Drugs: corticosteroids, antipsychotics, antidepressants.

What to ask for and associated symptoms

Ask the patient:
- What is your normal diet and appetite?
- Normal levels of physical activity?
- Perception of body image: eating disorders?
- Drug history?
- Possibility of pregnancy?

Associated symptoms?:
- Hair growth, acne: Cushing's disease or syndrome
- Lethargy, goitre, dry skin: hypothyroidism
- Irregular periods: polycystic ovary disease.

Investigations

Blood tests

- FBC, LFTs
- U&Es: ↓ potassium in Cushing's disease

- TFTs: hypothyroidism
- Glucose.

Hormone tests

- Random cortisol level
- Low-dose dexamethasone test: Cushing's disease (see Chapter 9)

- FSH/LH: polycystic ovary disease.

Imaging

- CT or MRI: hypothalamic disorders

- Abdominal US: polycystic ovary disease.

Management

- Depends on cause.

OEDEMA

Description

- The accumulation of fluid in the tissues
- May be localised or general

- Due to ↑ hydrostatic pressure (pressure driving fluid out of the capillaries) or ↓ oncotic pressure (form of osmotic pressure driving fluid into the capillaries).

Pitting oedema

- When finger pressure is applied for a few seconds to the area of swelling, indentation occurs

- More common than non-pitting.

Non-pitting oedema

- No indentation occurs when applying pressure
- Due to protein in the interstitial fluids that are not properly drained and which retain the water

- Causes include lymphoedema.

Causes

Increased hydrostatic pressure:
- Heart failure
- Drugs: vasodilators, e.g. nifedipine/amlodipine

Decreased oncotic pressure:
- Renal failure: due to low albumin which is a significant part of oncotic pressure. Part of nephrotic or nephritic syndrome
- Liver failure: low albumin
- Malabsorption
- Lymphadenopathy

Local causes of oedema: **VITAL**:
- **V**enous: deep vein thrombosis (DVT), varicose veins, venous insufficiency
- **I**nfection
- **T**rauma
- **A**llergy
- **L**ymphoedema: impaired lymphatic drainage often secondary to breast cancer.

What to ask for and associated symptoms

Ask the patient:
- How long has it been going on?
- Local or generalised oedema?
- Any precipitating factors?: e.g. infection or trauma
- Past medical history? Previous cardiac or renal impairment?
- Drug history?: vasodilators, calcium antagonists

Associated symptoms?:
- Erythema: infection
- Weight loss: malignancy
- Nephritic syndrome: haematuria, hypertension, oliguria
- Nephrotic syndrome: frothy urine (from proteinuria).

Investigations

- Blood pressure.

Blood tests

- FBC, U&Es, LFTs, CRP

- Albumin: ↓ in nephrotic syndrome, systemic or chronic illness, postoperatively.

Urine

- Evidence of proteinuria (see above).

Imaging

- Doppler of deep veins or venography: DVT

- Lymphangiography: lymphoedema.

Management

- Depends on cause.

LYMPHADENOPATHY

Description

- Enlarged lymph nodes

- Can be localised or general.

Causes

Malignancy:
- Normally enlarge slowly and is painless:
  - Leukaemia
  - Lymphoma
  - Myeloproliferative disease
  - Metastases

Infective causes:
- Normally enlarge quickly:

- Bacterial: TB, syphilis
- Viral: HIV, cytomegalovirus (CMV), Epstein–Barr virus (EBV)
- Protozoal: toxoplasmosis

Other causes:
- Sarcoid
- Rheumatoid arthritis (RA)
- Amyloidosis.

What to ask for and associated symptoms

Ask the patient:
- Time course of lymph gland enlargement?
- Are they painful?: associated with infection

Associated symptoms?:
- Splenomegaly
- Fever

- Pain with alcohol: haematological malignancy
- Symptoms from local structures: mass, pain, erythema
- Night sweats, weight loss: lymphoma, TB
- Rash: lupus, sarcoid
- Joint pain: lupus, RA
- Weight loss: malignancy.

Investigations

Blood tests

- FBC, U&Es, LFTs, ESR
- Clotting profile
- Culture
- Antibody screen: lupus, rheumatoid arthritis

- Monospot test: for EBV
- Viral serology.

Imaging

- CXR: bilateral hilar lymphadenopathy: lymphoma, sarcoid and TB

- US
- CT.

Other tests

- Fine needle aspiration of the lymph node
- Excision biopsy

- Bone marrow aspirate: haematological malignancies.

Management

- Depends on cause.

PRURITUS

Description

- Itching
- Can be local or generalised in cause

- Local causes include dermatological disease and scabies.

Causes

Generalised causes: **BLINKED**:
- **B**lood disease, e.g. iron deficiency, polycythaemia
- **L**iver disease: due to bile salt deposition within the skin
- **I**nfection, immunological disease
- **N**eoplasm

- **K**idney disease: chronic due to uraemia
- **E**ndocrine: hyper- or hypothyroidism, diabetes mellitus, Hodgkin's disease
- **D**ermatological disease, **D**rugs: oral contraceptive, opiates, alcohol.

What to ask for and associated symptoms

Ask the patient:
- How long has it been going on?
- Location of pruritus?
- Exacerbating and relieving factors?
- Drug history?
- Systemically well or unwell?

Associated symptoms?:
- Rash
- Jaundice
- Anaemia
- Lethargy
- Weight loss
- Lymphadenopathy.

Clinical examination

- Examine **all** the skin.

Blood tests

- FBC, U&Es, TFTs, LFTs, ESR, glucose.

Urine

- Dipstick: renal disease.

Other tests

- Lymph node biopsy: lymphoma.

Management

- Depends on cause.

FATIGUE

Description

- Tiredness for a long period of time
- Often presents to GP as 'tired all the time'
- Can be caused by chronic illness.

Causes

Endocrine:
- Diabetes mellitus
- Addison's disease
- Hyperthyroidism, hypothyroidism

Social:
- Overwork
- Reduced sleep

Haematological:
- Anaemia

Chronic disease:
- Malignancy
- Renal disease
- Cardiac failure

Drugs:
- Tricyclic antidepressants

Psychological/neurological:
- Depression
- Myalgic encephalomyelitis (ME) or chronic fatigue syndrome.

What to ask for and associated symptoms

Ask the patient:
- How long has it been going on?
- How are they generally?

Associated symptoms?:
- Pallor: anaemia
- Weight loss.

Investigations

Blood tests

- FBC: anaemia
- ESR: infection
- U&Es: renal disease

- TFT: hypothyroidism
- Glucose: diabetes.

Management

- Depends on cause

- If no cause found: consider chronic fatigue syndrome, suggest lifestyle changes and follow-up for development of further symptoms.

BACK PAIN

Description

- Common

- Normally transient (<6 weeks) and does not need investigation or bed rest.

Red flag signs: need further investigation

- <20 or >55 years
- Wakes patient at night
- T1–L2 region
- Recent or acute onset
- History of malignancy or signs suggestive of systemic cancer such as weight loss

- Immunosuppression
- Pain ↑ or unrelieved by rest
- Recent infection anywhere
- Prolonged use of steroids
- Disturbance of bladder or bowel.

Causes

Congential causes:
- Ankylosing spondylitis: pain early in the morning
- Scoliosis: lateral curvature of the spine
- Spondylolisthesis: displacement of a vertebral body.

Malignancy:
- Primary tumour
- Metastases
- Myeloma

Spinal problems:
- Prolapsed disc: worse when coughing
- Fractures

Bone disease:
- Degenerative joint disease

- Rheumatoid arthritis
- Paget's

Metabolic:
- Osteoporosis (causing fractures)
- Osteomalacia
- Cushing's disease.

Infective:
- Osteomyelitis
- Pott's disease: tuberculosis of the spine

Other:
- Pregnancy
- Trauma: of muscle, bone or ligaments
- Psychosomatic: depression and anxiety worsens.

What to ask for and associated symptoms

Ask the patient:
- When did it start and how has it progressed?
- Motor or sensory symptoms?
- Bladder or bowel affected?
- Pain worse on movement or rest?

Associated symptoms?:
- Weight loss: malignancy
- 15–30 years:
  - Prolapsed disc
  - Trauma
  - Fractures
  - Ankylosing spondylitis
  - Pregnancy

- 30–50 years:
  - Degenerative joint disease
  - Prolapsed disc
  - Malignancy
- >50 years:
  - Osteoarthritis
  - Osteoporosis
  - Paget's: chronic disease of the bones leading to enlarged and deformed bones of the skull, pelvis, backbone and long bones
  - Malignancy
  - Myeloma.

Investigations

Clinical examination

- Back and musculature
- Neurological examination

- Breast examination to rule out breast cancer leading to back pain.

Blood tests

- FBC, U&Es, LFTs, ESR and CRP

- Prostate specific antigen (PSA): prostate cancer, often metastasises to the bones.

Urine

- Bence Jones protein: myeloma.

Imaging

- Spinal X-ray
- MRI: for cord compression, myelopathy (pathology of spinal cord), cysts, haemorrhages

- Technetium scan: hot spots for inflammation or malignancy
- Bone scan.

Management

- Treat underlying cause
- Analgesia
- Physiotherapy.

FALLS IN THE ELDERLY

Description

- Falls are more common in the elderly
- Due to a wide range of causes related to physiological effects of ageing with additional pathology.

Causes

Neurological causes:
- Cognitive impairment
- Loss of vision: cataract
- Impaired autonomic function
- Impaired balance and increased sway
- Peripheral neuropathy
- Previous stroke disease or dementia

Cardiovascular:
- Postural hypotension

- Arrhythmias and conduction defects

Muscular:
- Muscle weakness

Infection
- Anywhere

Other:
- Polypharmacy: >4 drugs
- Hypoglycaemia.

What to ask for and associated symptoms

Ask the patient or witnesses:
- Previous history of falls?
- Loss of consciousness?
- Do they recall any preceding dizziness, confusion, headache or leg weakness?
- Relation to postural change?
- First thing they remember coming round: fits tend to be confused?

- Speed of recovery?
- Was there any injury as a result of the fall?
- Drug history: polypharmacy, postural hypotension
- Medical history? Cardiac risk factors

Associated symptoms?:
- Weakness
- Change in vision
- Confusion.

Investigations

Clinical examination

- Lying and standing blood pressure: postural hypertension
- Cardiovascular and neurological examination.

Blood tests

- FBC, U&Es, LFTs and TFTs
- Blood glucose: hypoglycaemia
- Cultures.

Urine

- Microscopy and culture.

Imaging

- CXR: for infection
- MRI: if seizure is suspected to rule out structural lesions.

Other tests

Cardiac investigations:
- ECG

Management

- Majority of falls are due to postural instability
- Evidence based single intervention: exercise programmes
- Multifactorial interventions proven effective include:
  - Hazard modification
  - Review of medication
  - Exercise.

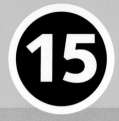
CARDIAC EXAMINATION

Introduction: WIPER

Wash hands
Introduce yourself
Permission: ask permission to examine
Expose patient correctly
Reposition: sit patient up at 45°.

Examination

- General inspection; is the patient well or unwell?
- Look at each of the areas outlined below.

Hands

- Peripheral cyanosis: blue discoloration of the extremities:
  - Causes: peripheral vasoconstriction, cold, hypoxia, Raynaud's phenomenon (see p. 447)
- Capillary refill: to assess adequacy of perfusion
  - Normal time is <2 s
- Clubbing of the nail (convex shape): loss of the nail angle:
  - Cardiac causes: cyanotic heart disease, infective endocarditis and atrial myxoma
  - Other examinations list other causes
- Koilonychia: spooning of the nails (concave shape):
  - Seen in iron deficiency
- Osler's nodes: painful papular red lesions on the finger pulps:
  - Deposition of immune complexes, most commonly in infective endocarditis
- Janeway lesions: painless macular lesions on the palmar aspect of the hand:
  - Deposition of immune complexes, most commonly in infective endocarditis
- Splinter haemorrhages: dark vertical lines under the nails:
  - Associated with infective endocarditis and trauma
- Arachnodactyly: long slender (spider-like) fingers:
  - Feature of Marfan's disease, of which aortic regurgitation is a complication.

Arm and neck

- Pulses: radial, brachial, carotid pulses looking for rate, rhythm, volume and particular characteristics
- BP: consider in both arms (to look for radio-radial delay) and lying and standing BP for postural hypotension.

Pulse characters and their associations

- Collapsing pulse: any condition which causes a hyperdynamic circulation with increased stroke volume and decreased peripheral vascular resistance, e.g. pregnancy, anaemia, high-output cardiac failure, thyrotoxicosis, aortic regurgitation, CO_2 retention
- Slow rising/low volume pulse: cardiogenic shock and aortic stenosis
- Jerky pulse: hypertrophic obstructive cardiomyopathy
- Pulse pressure: difference between systolic and diastolic pressures:
  - Narrow pulse pressure: aortic stenosis
  - Wide pulse pressure: aortic regurgitation
- Pulsus paradoxus (exaggeration of the normal fall in BP on inspiration): right heart strain owing to obstruction such as tamponade and pulmonary embolus
- Pulsus alternans (alternating weak then strong pulse): left ventricular impairment
- Biphasic pulse (double peak to the pulse): aortic stenosis with regurgitation, hypertrophic obstructive cardiomyopathy
- Radio-radial delay: dissecting aortic aneurysm, subclavian stenosis
- Radio-femoral delay: dissecting aortic aneurysm, coarctation of the aorta
- Postural hypotension: lying/standing BP difference >20 mmHg; wait 2 min after the change in position to look for a postural drop; caused by hypovolaemia, autonomic neuropathy (diabetes mellitus and Parkinson's disease), drugs.

Face

- Eyes:
  - Conjunctival pallor in anaemia
  - Xanthalasma (periorbital fat deposits) in hypercholesterolaemia
  - Corneal arcus (white arc around the cornea) in hypercholesterolaemia

- Mouth:
  - Central cyanosis (blue discoloration under the tongue)
  - Dentition, poor hygiene a risk factor for bacteraemia in infective endocarditis
- Neck:
  - JVP: a measure of central venous pressure, with a biphasic wave form (Fig. 15.1) measured at the internal jugular, between the heads of sternocleidomastoid, over the muscle (normally <4 cm above the right atrium); Table 15.1 outlines the clinical significance of JVP signs.

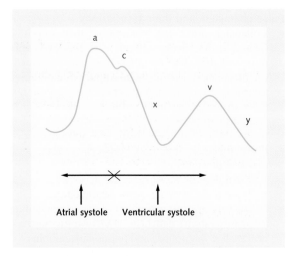

Fig. 15.1 The JVP waveform. A wave, atrial systole; C wave, tricuspid valve closure; V wave, atrium fills against a closed tricuspid valve; X descent, ventricular systole; Y descent, tricuspid valve opens.

Table 15.1 Clinical significance of JVP signs

JVP sign	Associated condition
Raised JVP	Fluid overload Right heart failure SVC obstruction
No visible JVP	Haemorrhage Dehydration
Large A wave	Pulmonary hypertension Pulmonary stenosis Very large/cannon wave: heart block, ventricular tachycardia
No A wave	Atrial fibrillation
Large V wave	Tricuspid regurgitation
Rapid Y descent	Constrictive pericarditis

Chest

Inspect
- Scars: sternotomy, mitral valvotomy, thoracotomy, vein harvesting scars in the legs and arterial harvesting in the arms
- Implantable devices, e.g. pacemaker.

Palpate
- Apex beat (the most forceful downward and outward (inferolateral) point): determine character and displacement:
  - Hyperdynamic and displaced in valvular regurgitation
  - Sustained and undisplaced in aortic stenosis
  - Tapping and undisplaced in mitral stenosis
  - Jerky apex in hypertrophic obstructive cardiomyopathy
- Right ventricular or parasternal heave: increased right ventricular volume, e.g. pulmonary hypertension
- Thrills: palpable murmurs over the precordium caused by turbulent flow.

Auscultate
Main questions to ask while listening to the heart
Timing sounds with carotid pulse:
- Can I hear heart sounds 1 + 2?
- Are they normal, soft or loud?
- Are there any additional sounds such as an S3, S4, systolic or diastolic murmurs?
- If so, what is the nature of an additional sound (see below): Do murmurs radiate? Do they increase or decrease while breathing in and out.

Main areas to auscultate
Four areas (Fig. 15.2; remember by 'A Place To Meet'):

Aortic valve
Pulmonary valve
Tricuspid
Mitral valve.

- Ask the patient to lean onto their left side and then while holding their breath in expiration, listen over the apex with the bell for the mid-diastolic rumbling murmur of mitral stenosis.
- Then sit the patient forward and while holding their breath in expiration, listen at the lower left sternal edge with the diaphragm for the early diastolic murmur of aortic regurgitation.

Heart sounds
S1: closure of mitral valve on the left (and tricuspid valve on the right)
S2: closure of aortic valve on the left (and pulmonary valve on the right)

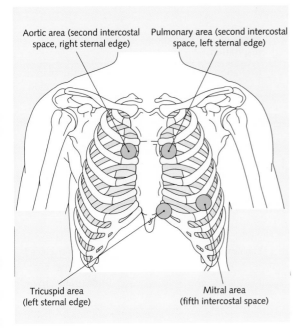

Aortic area (second intercostal space, right sternal edge)

Pulmonary area (second intercostal space, left sternal edge)

Tricuspid area (left sternal edge)

Mitral area (fifth intercostal space)

Fig 15.2 Four main areas for auscultation.

S3: rapid ventricular filling:
- Benign in the young or athletes
- Pathogenic S3 is higher pitched and occurs with poor left ventricular function, constrictive pericarditis or restrictive pericarditis (sounds like Ken-Tuc-Kee)

S4: atrial constriction from blood against a stiff ventricle:
- Always pathogenic, e.g. in aortic stenosis (sounds like Ten-E-See).

Types of cardiac murmur
Summarised in Table 15.2. Note, the heart rate increases on inspiration and decreases on expiration.
- RILE RULE:
  - Right-sided murmurs are louder on inspiration
  - Left-sided murmurs louder on expiration.

To complete the cardiovascular examination

- Feel for peripheral and sacral oedema
- Examine peripheral pulses and feel for abdominal aortic aneurysm
- Listen for carotid bruits
- Auscultate the back of the chest: for evidence of left ventricular dysfunction (pulmonary oedema)
- View a 12 lead ECG.

RESPIRATORY EXAMINATION

Introduction: WIPER

Wash hands
Introduce yourself
Permission: ask permission to examine
Expose patient correctly, from waist upwards
Reposition: sit patient up at 45°.

Examination

General inspection; is the patient well or unwell?

Hands

- Peripheral cyanosis: blue discoloration of the peripheral extremities
- Clubbing of the nails (convex shape): loss of the nail angle:
  - Respiratory causes: fibrosing alveolitis, lung abscess, bronchiectasis, bronchial carcinoma
  - See other examinations for other causes
- Tar staining: evidence of smoking
- CO_2 retention flap: indicates CO_2 retention
- Anaemia: skin fold pallor.

Arm and neck

- Radial pulse
- JVP (Fig. 15.1): elevated in cor pulmonale
- Trachea: feel for displacement, left/right shift
- Cricosternal distance: distance between sternum and cricoid should be three fingers; is reduced in patients with severe airflow limitation, e.g. COPD, hyperinflated chest
- Cervical lymphadenopathy (Fig. 15.4).

Eyes

- Conjunctival pallor: anaemia
- Ptosis: Horner's syndrome associated with a Pancoast's tumour and lung cancer

Mouth

- Central cyanosis.

Chest

- Respiratory rate: normally 12–15 breaths/min
- Asymmetry of chest expansion
- Tracheal tug, intercostal and subcostal recession: from increased effort in breathing
- Scars: thoracotomy, sternotomy.

Table 15.2 Visual representation of heart sounds

Murmur	Valve lesion	Patient position	Phase of respiration	Radiation	Other features
Mid-diastolic, low and rumbling, listen with bell of stethoscope, loud S_1, OS	Mitral stenosis OS S_1 A_2 P_2 S_1 S_2	Lying on left side	Expiration	None	Tapping non-displaced apex; often associated with atrial fibrillation; pulmonary hypertension may occur with loud P_2 and TR
Pansystolic, listen with diaphragm of stethoscope, soft S_1	Mitral regurgitation S_1 A_2 P_2 S_1 S_2	On back at $45°$	Expiration	To axilla	Thrusting, displaced apex, may be associated with atrial fibrillation
Ejection systolic murmur, listen with diaphragm, may get reversal of S_2 due to prolonged LV emptying	Aortic stenosis S_1 A_2 P_2 S_1 S_2	On back at $45°$	Expiration	To carotid arteries	Heaving, non-displaced apex; slow-rising, low-volume pulse
Soft, blowing early diastolic murmur, heard in tricuspid area, soft S_2, may hear Austin Flint murmur, listen with diaphragm	Aortic regurgitation S_1 A_2 P_2 S_1 S_2	Sitting forward	Expiration	None	Thrusting, displaced apex; waterhammer (collapsing) pulse, wide pulse pressure, Duroziez sign, Quincke sign, pistol shot femorals, de Musset sign

The second heart sound (S_2) has two components: A_2 (aortic value closure) and P_2 (pulmonary valve closure). LV, left ventricle; OS, opening snap; S1, first heart sound; TR, tricuspid regurgitation.

Signs of hypoxia

- Cyanosis
- Confusion
- Visual hallucinations

Signs of CO_2 retention

- Bounding pulse
- Drowsy
- Tremor
- Flap
- Headache
- Papilloedema.

Palpation, percussion and auscultation

After detailed inspection, palpate, percuss and auscultate first the front of the chest of the patient, then ask them to lean forward and inspect, palpate, percuss and auscultate the lung areas on their back.

Palpate

- Ask if there is any pain
- *Apex beat*: check for displacement; should be 5th intercostal space, mid-clavicular line
- *Expansion*: assess for equal air entry and degree of expansion
- *Tactile vocal fremitus (TVF)*: ask the patient to say '99' and feel for vibration with the edge of the hand at each lung lobe.

Percussion

At each lung lobe listen for dullness. Percuss the clavicles.

Auscultate

Ensure each lung lobe is auscultated. Do not forget the axillae:

- *Vocal resonance*: ask patient to say '99' and listen for vibration at each lung lobe. Can do either TVF or vocal resonance (not necessary to do both).

Consolidation increases vibration on TVF, and the sound is transmitted more clearly; in pleural effusion there are fewer vibrations felt on TVF and poorer transmission of sound.

- Sounds on auscultation:
  - *Vesicular breathing*: normal sounds of breathing, inspiratory sound is longer than expiratory; ensure when listening that air entry is equal and good on both sides
  - *Bronchial breathing*: inspiratory and expiratory phase are the same length; heard in consolidation, localised fibrosis
  - *Stridor*: harsh inspiratory sound caused by upper airway obstruction
  - *Wheeze*: musical sound heard in the expiratory phase caused by air passing through a narrowed airway in lower airway obstruction; heard in asthma, COPD
  - *Crackles or crepitations*: caused by opening of closed bronchioles in inspiration, with coarse crackles from proximal areas (e.g. bronchiectasis), fine crackles from distal airways (e.g. pulmonary oedema or fibrosis)
  - *Whispering pectoriloquy*: whispered high-pitch sounds heard over consolidation
  - *Pleural rub*: localised creak or groan from inflammation or roughness of the pleural surfaces rubbing together; sounds like treading on fresh snow
  - *Cheyne–Stokes respiration*: cyclical variation in respiration rate, where breathing becomes slower, may stop for a few seconds then speeds up to a peak and then slows again; occurs in heart failure, sleep at altitude and when the sensitivity of the respiration centres in the brain become impaired in coma states.

Figure 15.3 summarises the findings on respiratory examination and interpretation

To complete the respiratory examination

SOAP:
Sputum sample,
O_2 saturation,
Ankle and sacral oedema,
peak flow.
   Also:

- CXR if indicated
- Check for lymphadenopathy (Fig. 15.4).

GI SYSTEM EXAMINATION

Introduction: WIPER

Wash hands
Introduce yourself
Permission: ask permission to examine
Expose patient correctly: from 'nipples to knees'
Reposition: lie patient flat.

Fig. 15.3 Findings on respiratory examination and interpretation

	Consolidation	Pneumothorax	Pleural effusion	Lobar collapse	Pleural thickening
Chest radiograph	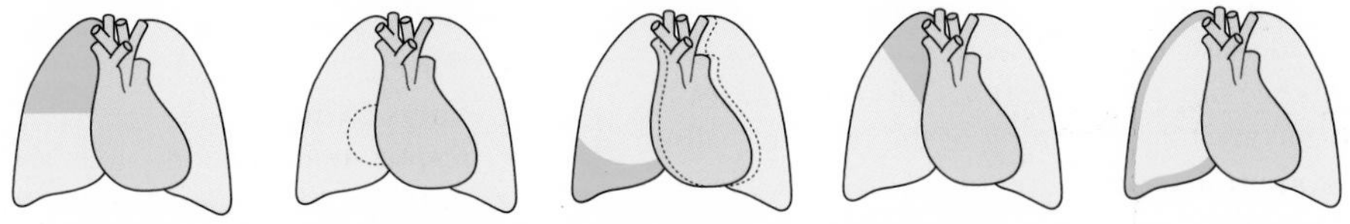				
Mediastinal shift and trachea	None	None (simple), away (tension)	None or away	Towards the affected side	None
Chest wall excursion	Normal or decreased on the affected side	Normal or decreased on the affected side	Decreased on the affected side	Decreased	Decreased
Percussion note	Dull	Resonant	Stony dull	Dull	Dull
Breath sounds	Increased (bronchial)	Decreased	Decreased	Decreased	Decreased
Added sounds	Crackles	Click (occasional)	Rub (occasional)	None	None
Tactile vocal fremitus or vocal resonance	Increased	Decreased	Decreased	Decreased	Decreased

Fig 15.3 Findings on respiratory examination and interpretation.

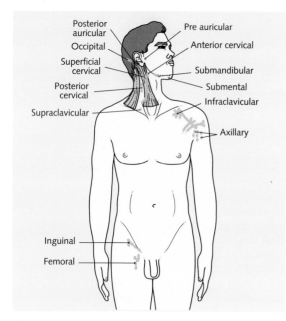

Fig 15.4 Examination of lymph nodes.

Examination

General inspection

Is the patient well or unwell?

Hands

- Palmar erythema: redness of the palms, causes include pregnancy and liver cirrhosis
- Clubbing of the nail (convex shape): loss of the nail angle:
  - Gastroenterological causes: inflammatory bowel disease, coeliac disease, liver cirrhosis
  - See other examinations for other causes
- Leuconychia: whitening of the nails in ↓ albumin
- Koilonychia: spooning of the nails in ↓ iron
- Dupuytren's contracture: fixed flexion of the hand bringing the fingers towards the palm:
  - Causes include alcohol abuse, cirrhosis, diabetes, idiopathic
- Tremor: in alcohol withdrawal
- Liver flap (asterixis): myoclonic jerk on cocking the wrists back with hands outstretched:
  - Causes include hepatic encephalopathy and CO_2 retention.

Arm

Radial pulse.

Neck

- JVP (Fig. 15.1) with patient lying at 45°: liver failure
- Virchow's node: enlarged left supraclavicular lymph node associated with metastatic gastric cancer.

Eyes

- Pallor of mucosa: anaemia
- Jaundice: of the sclera
- Xanthelasma: from hypercholesterolaemia, e.g. in primary biliary cirrhosis
- Keiser–Fleischer rings: seen on slit-lamp examination in Wilson's disease

Mouth

- Glossitis: inflammation of the tongue in vitamin B_{12} deficiency
- Dry tongue: dehydration
- Ulcers: Crohn's disease
- Angular stomatitis: cracking lips, inflammation at edges of mouth caused by iron or vitamin B_{12} deficiency

Chest

- Spider naevi: small dilated vessels on the skin in the distribution of the superior vena cava, seen in chronic liver disease
- Gynaecomastia: breast tissue in males caused by ↑ oestrogen levels (e.g. in cirrhosis), drugs (steroid, omeprazole, digoxin, spironolactone, oestrogen, cannabis), persistent pubertal gynaecomastia, primary hypogonadism, Klinefelter's syndrome, testicular tumours, hyperthyroidism.

Abdomen

- Distension from 5Fs: fluid, foetus, faeces, fat, flatus (wind)
- Caput medusae: dilated abdominal veins from portal hypertension
- Body hair distribution: ↓ with low testosterone levels
- Scars (Fig. 15.5).

Palpation and percussion

Light palpation

- Palpate the nine areas of the abdomen (see Fig. 15.6)
- Watch the patient's face for anxiety or distress, palpating the tender region last
- Assess for tenderness, guarding, rebound tenderness (pain worse when releasing palpating hand).

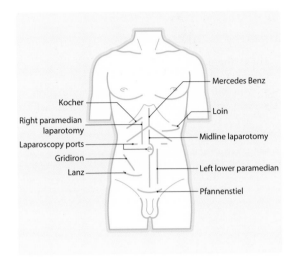

Fig. 15.5 Scars of the abdomen to look out for in GI examination.

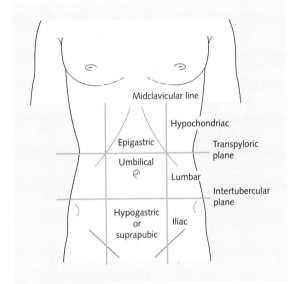

Fig. 15.6 The nine areas of the abdomen.

Deep palpation

- Feel the nine segments more deeply
- Assess for masses
- Feel for an abdominal aortic aneurysm (a pulsatile and expansile mass)

Palpate and percuss

- Liver, spleen and kidneys
- Distinguishing a kidney from the spleen (Table 15.3).

Table 15.3   Distinguishing a kidney from the spleen

Kidney	Spleen
Ballotable	Non ballotable
Moves downwards late in inspiration	Moves downwards medially towards the umbilicus early in inspiration
No notch	Notch present
Can palpate above it	Cannot palpate above
Resonant on percussion	Dull on percussion

Percussion

Percuss for:

- shifting dullness seen with ascitic fluid
- the bladder (dull to percussion).

Auscultation

- Bowel sounds: may be over- or underactive
- Renal bruits: auscultate over both the renal arteries (2.5 cm up and 2.5 cm lateral from the umbilicus).

To complete the abdominal examination

- Obtain stool sample for analysis
- Check the hernial orifices: umbilical/femoral/inguinal
- Ask the patient to cough and look for any abdominal hernias
- Rectal examination
- Urine dipstick.

PERIPHERAL SENSORY NEUROLOGICAL EXAMINATION

Introduction: WIPER

Wash hands
Introduce yourself
Permission: ask permission to examine
Expose patient correctly: depending on if it is an upper or lower limb examination
Reposition.

Examination

- General inspection; is the patient well or unwell?
- Look for **DWARFS**: **d**eformities, **w**asting, **a**symmetry, **r**ashes, **f**asciculations, **s**cars.

Light touch (dorsal column)

- Use a cotton wool swab on each upper or lower limb dermatome (Fig. 15.7).

Pain (spinothalamic tract)

- Use a neurological pin on each dermatome.

Temperature (spinothalamic tract)

- Use a cold tuning fork on each dermatome.

Proprioception (dorsal column)

- Ask the patient to close their eyes. Hold their big toe or thumb at the sides of the nail between two fingers. Then move the most distal joint using your other hand. Move the toe in stages up or down. Ask them at any point if you have moved their toe up or down.

Vibration (dorsal column)

- Ask the patient to close their eyes. Vibrate a 128 or 256 Hz tuning fork on their most distal bony prominence on the big toe or thumb. Ask them to tell you when you stop the fork vibrating. Move up the bony prominences until they detect vibration.

To complete the peripheral sensory examination

- Thank the patient for their time
- Complete the examination by saying:
  - you will do a full neurological examination
  - you will complete some imaging, e.g. MRI, or nerve study tests.

PERIPHERAL MOTOR NEUROLOGICAL EXAMINATION

Introduction: WIPER

Wash hands
Introduce yourself
Permission: ask permission to examine
Expose patient correctly: depending on if it is an upper or lower limb examination
Reposition.

Examination

General inspection

- Is the patient well or unwell?
- Look for **DWARFS**: **d**eformities, **w**asting (LMN disease), **a**symmetry, **r**ashes, **f**asciculations (LMN disease), **s**cars.

Tone

- Look for rigidity and spasticity (hypertonia)
- Clasp knife (on performing a quick stretch, patient resists movement and then sudden release, a measure of spasticity): UMN lesion
- Lead pipe (resistance through a range of movements): extrapyramidal lesion (Parkinson's)
- Cogwheel rigidity (tremor with lead pipe): Parkinson's disease
- Hypotonia: LMN lesions
- Lower limb:
  - Ask the patient to relax their leg and roll their leg on the bed
- Upper limb:
  - Ask the patient to relax their hand
  - Hold the patients hand in yours and, using the other hand to steady their elbow
  - Move the hand around in different directions to assess tone.

Power

Tables 15.4 and 15.5 summarises the assessment of movements in the lower and upper limbs and the

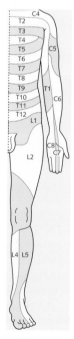

Fig. 15.7 Dermatomes of the lower and upper limbs.

Table 15.4 Assessment of movements in the lower limbs

Movement	Instruction	Muscle/myotome
Hip flexion	Lift your leg straight off the bed, keep it up	Iliopsoas/L1, L2
Hip extension	Straighten your knee and don't let me bend your leg	Quadriceps/L3, L4
Hip adduction	Keep your knees together and don't let me pull them apart	Hip adductors/L2, L3
Knee flexion	Bend your knee and keep it bent	Hamstrings/L5, S1
Ankle dorsiflexion	Pull your foot up toward your nose, don't let me push it down	Tibialis anterior and long extensors/L4, L5
Plantiflexion (toward the floor)	Point your foot down to the bed, keep it there	Gastrocnemius/S1
Knee extension	Press your legs flat against the bed and don't let me pull them up	Gluteal muscles/L5, S1

Table 15.5 Assessment of movements in the upper limbs

Movement	Instruction	Muscle/myotome
Shoulder abduction	Bend your elbow and hold your arms up and out to the side. Don't let me push them down	Deltoid/C5
Elbow flexion	Bend your elbow and don't let me straighten it	Biceps/C5, C6
Wrist extension	Cock your hands up like this and don't let me stop you	Wrist extensors/C7
Finger extension	Straighten your fingers out and don't let me push them down	Finger extensors/C8
Grip	Grip my fingers	Finger flexors/C8, T1
Thumb abduction	[with palms flat] Point your thumb to the ceiling and don't let me push it down	Abductor policis brevis/C8, T1, median nerve
Index finger abduction	Spread your fingers wide and don't let me push them together	Abductors (dorsal interossei)/T1, ulnar nerve

myotomes responsible. Assess power by testing each of the movements described in the tables and compare power between each limb.

Power of each movement is graded on the Medical Research Council scale 0–5:

0: no movement
1: minor movement
2: movement but not against gravity
3: movement against gravity, not against gravity
4: weaker than full strength
5: full power.

Reflexes

Test reflexes using a tendon hammer.

If no reflex is elicited ask the patient to clench their teeth for reinforcement.

- Grade reflexes as:
  - −: absent
  - +: normal
  - ++: brisk/exaggerated (UMN disease)
- Lower limb:
  - Knee jerk: L3–L4 (mediated by nerve roots L3 and L4)
  - Ankle jerk: S1
  - Test the Babinski reflex by using an orange stick: running it along the lateral side from the back of the foot and then across the top towards the big toe; normally toes curl down, upwards response in newborns and in UMN lesions
- Upper limb:
  - Biceps: C5–Cc6
  - Supinator: C6
  - Triceps: C7.

Coordination/cerebellar signs

Lower limb
- Ask the patient to lift their leg up straight and then place their heel on their other knee and run it down towards their toes and then to lift it off the toes back to the knee and repeat this action making circular movements
- Repeat with the other leg.

Upper limb
- Ask the patient to place one finger on their nose. Place a finger in front of them and ask them to move their finger back and for between their nose and your finger as fast and accurately as they can. Repeat this with the other hand:
  - Assess for past pointing, which occurs in cerebellar damage
- Dysdiadochokinesis: the patient places the palm of their hand on top of their other hand; they then turn the top hand over so the back of their hand now rests on the hand below. Get them to repeat this movement quickly several times. Ask them to repeat this with the other hand.

Gait
- Test gait by asking the patient to walk to the other side of the room and walk back, making sure they are stable enough to be safe.

To complete the peripheral motor examination

- Thank the patient for their time
- Complete the examination by saying:
  - you will do a full neurological examination
  - you will complete some imaging, e.g. MRI, or nerve study tests.

Patterns of altered movement and sensation

Neurological signs are dependent on location of the lesion. Figure 15.8 summarises the patterns of altered movement and sensation.

It is always useful to consider if a change in the motor system is caused by LMN or UMN damage and where the damage originates.

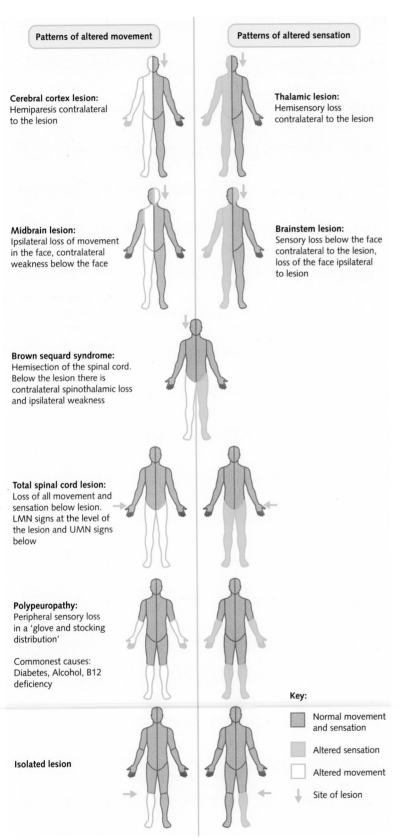

Patterns of altered movement

Patterns of altered sensation

Cerebral cortex lesion:
Hemiparesis contralateral
to the lesion

Thalamic lesion:
Hemisensory loss
contralateral to the lesion

Midbrain lesion:
Ipsilateral loss of movement
in the face, contralateral
weakness below the face

Brainstem lesion:
Sensory loss below the face
contralateral to the lesion,
loss of the face ipsilateral
to lesion

Brown sequard syndrome:
Hemisection of the spinal cord.
Below the lesion there is
contralateral spinothalamic loss
and ipsilateral weakness

Total spinal cord lesion:
Loss of all movement and
sensation below lesion.
LMN signs at the level of
the lesion and UMN signs
below

Polypeuropathy:
Peripheral sensory loss
in a 'glove and stocking
distribution'

Commonest causes:
Diabetes, Alcohol, B12
deficiency

Isolated lesion

Key:

▨ Normal movement
and sensation

▨ Altered sensation

☐ Altered movement

↓ Site of lesion

Fig. 15.8 Patterns of altered
movement and sensation.

Index